Nurse Practitioner
Manual of Clinical Skills

Sue Cross BSc(Hons) PGCE RN NPDip International Liaison for RCN NPA

Sue Cross trained as an SRN at the Royal Masonic Hospital in London. She left nursing for some time to raise a family and then returned to school nursing in 1987. She later worked in a small rural practice in Bedfordshire as a practice nurse and during this time, in 1991, successfully completed the first Nurse Practitioner course at the Royal College of Nursing in London.

Along with Myfanwy Rimmer, Sue was a founder member of the RCN Nurse Practitioner Committee and later became Chair of the Association. Her major interest was to develop relations with other nurse practitioners around the world and she has worked closely with the American Academy of Nurse Practitioners to achieve this goal. For this work she has been awarded a fellowship with the American Academy.

She was employed from 1991 by the National Asthma and Respiratory Training Centre in Warwick as Director of Training and in 2001 moved to Liverpool to work for the Respiratory Education Resource Centres as International Project Manager, developing respiratory training for health professionals abroad.

Myfanwy Rimmer

BSc(Hons) Health Studies NPDip QN RGN

Myfanway Rimmer trained as a nurse in Manchester, undergoing a combined paediatric and general course at Booth Hall Children's Hospital and North Manchester General. She moved to Berkshire in 1969 and worked at the Royal Berkshire Hospital, then spent twenty six years in Primary care working as a District Nurse, Practice Nurse. For the next ten years she worked alongside five GPs as a Nurse Practitioner.

She completed her Nurse Practitioner diploma and BSc degree at the Royal College of Nursing I.A.N.E. Myfanwy became an active member of the Nurse Practitioner Committee in the early years of its existence. Locally she has been very involved in teaching, course developments and Practice Nurse development. She was board nurse member for Wokingham PCG 1999–2001.

Myfanwy is currently working as a nurse practitioner at the Slough Walk-in Centre, a nurse-led government sponsored project offering instant access to health care for the citizens of Slough and the surrounding area, and part time with a small two-doctor practice in Finchampstead, Berkshire.

For Baillière Tindall:

Senior Commissioning Editor: Ninette Premdas
Project Development Manager: Karen Gilmour
Project Manager: Gail Murray
Designer: George Ajayi

www.harcourt-international.com

Bringing you products from all Harcourt Health Sciences companies including Baillière Tindall, Churchill Livingstone, Mosby and W.B. Saunders

▶ **Browse** for latest information in books, journals and electronic products

▶ **Search** for information on over 20 000 published titles with full product information including tables of contents and sample chapters

▶ **Keep up to date** with our extensive publishing programme in your field by registering with **eAlert** or requesting postal updates

▶ **Secure online ordering** with prompt delivery, as well as full contact details to order by phone, fax or post

▶ **News** of special features and promotions

If you are based in the following countries, please visit the country-specific site to receive full details of product availability and local ordering information

USA: www.harcourthealth.com

Canada: www.harcourtcanada.com

Australia: www.harcourt.com.au

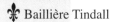 Baillière Tindall   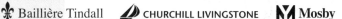 CHURCHILL LIVINGSTONE   Mosby   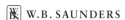 W.B. SAUNDERS

Nurse Practitioner Manual of Clinical Skills

Edited by

Sue Cross BSc(Hons) PGCE RN NPDip International Liaison for RCN NPA

and

Myfanwy Rimmer BSc(Hons)Health Studies NPDip QN RGN

Foreword by

Barbara Stilwell FRCN
Scientist, Department of Organization of Health Services Delivery (OSD), Evidence for Information and Policy (EIP), World Health Organization, Geneva, Switzerland

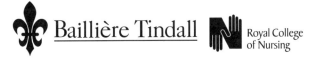

EDINBURGH • LONDON • NEW YORK • PHILADELPHIA • ST LOUIS • SYDNEY • TORONTO • 2002

BAILLIÈRE TINDALL

An imprint of Harcourt Publishers Limited

© Harcourt Publishers Limited 2002

♣ is a registered trademark of Harcourt Publishers Limited

First published 2002

ISBN 0 7020 2518 6

British Library Cataloguing in Publication Data
A catalogue record for this book is available from the British Library

Library of Congress Cataloging in Publication Data
A catalog record for this book is available from the Library of Congress

Note
Medical knowledge is constantly changing. As new information becomes available, changes in treatment, procedures, equipment and the use of drugs become necessary. The editors, contributors and the publishers have taken care to ensure that the information given in this text is accurate and up to date. However, readers are strongly advised to confirm that the information, especially with regard to drug usage, complies with the latest legislation and standards of practice.

The
publisher's
policy is to use
**paper manufactured
from sustainable forests**

Printed in China

CONTENTS

Contributors		ix
Foreword		xi
Chapter 1	How to Use this Book *Sue Cross and Myfanwy Rimmer*	1
Chapter 2	Health Promotion *Rosie Walsh*	3
Chapter 3	Blood Disorders *Frances Simpson*	16
Chapter 4	Dermatology *Jill Peters*	33
Chapter 5	The Eye and External Adenexa *Anna Hunter*	65
Chapter 6	Head and Neck *Wendy Johnson*	77
Chapter 7	Respiratory System *Linda Pearce*	94
Chapter 8	The Cardiovascular System *Morag White*	116
Chapter 9	The Gastrointestinal System *Jane Bayliss*	137
Chapter 10	Endocrine Disorders *Rosie Walsh*	158
Chapter 11	Nervous System *Daphne Miller*	173
Chapter 12	Musculoskeletal Disorders *Nicola Nurse*	200
Chapter 13	Genito Urinary Conditions *Claire Pratt*	222
Chapter 14	Contraception, Sexuality and the Menopause	
	Part 1 Contraception and Sexuality *Sue Reed*	243
	Part 2 Menopause *Myfanwy Rimmer*	258
Chapter 15	The Gynaecological System *Mary Rawlinson*	267
Chapter 16	Mental Health and the Nurse Practitioner in Primary Health Care *Ruth Davies and Deborah Humble*	282
Chapter 17	Care of the Child *Katie Barnes and Debra Sharu*	295
Chapter 18	Care of the Older Adult *Soline Jerram and Sylvia Newson*	318
Index		333

A colour plate section appears between pages 64 and 65.

CONTRIBUTORS

Katie Barnes   RGN RSCN BSc(Hons) MSc MPH CPNP
Katie Barnes is a Certified Paediatric Nurse Practitioner
(CPNP) who immigrated from the USA in 1997. Originally a
Bostonian, she received her undergraduate nurse training
from Northeastern University in 1986 and subsequently
moved to New York City, where she completed her Master of
Science degree in Pediatric Primary Care at Columbia
University in 1989. After achieving her National Board
Certification as a PNP, she was named as a Fellow in the
National Association of Pediatric Nurse Practitioners. In New
York, she worked with disenfranchised children on mobile
medical units within the homeless and foster care systems.
This was followed by a PNP position in paediatric
haematology at Columbia-Presbyterian Medical Center until
she travelled to the jungles of Guatemala, where she worked
for 12 months with Mayan children in rural villages. She
returned from Central America to conduct community-based
research for the Columbia University School of Public Health,
where she also completed a Master of Public Health in 1996.
She currently lives in Suffolk, where she continues her
practice as a paediatric nurse practitioner and works as a
lecturer in Child Health at Suffolk College, Ipswich.

Jane Bayliss BSc(Hons) RGN RM RHV NPDip PGCHE
Jane Bayliss was one of the first nurse practitioners to qualify
from the Royal College of Nursing in 1992. Jane worked in
primary care as a nurse practitioner for five years before
becoming a freelance consultant and part-time lecturer at the
University of Central England (UCE) in Birmingham. Since
1999, Jane has worked as a full time senior lecturer leading
the Practice Nurse degree programme and the Nurse
Prescribing roll-out programme at UCE. She has recently
taken up the post as Training Manager with North Walsall
Primary Care Group to lead a new and innovative multi-
agency learning programme. This programme provides
protected time for general practitioners, practice nurses and
other primary health care staff to learn together to implement
the National Service Framework guidelines.

Ruth Davies   BSc(Jt Hons) MSc RMN RGN RNT Dip Couns
Ruth Davies was involved with the RCN Nurse Practitioner
programme since its inception, firstly as specialist lecturer in
communication and latterly as programme director. Her major
clinical interests are mental health, communication and
counselling in health care settings.

Deborah Humble   BSc(Hons) NPDip RGN
Deborah Humble currently works as a nurse practitioner in a
south-west London, nurse-led NHS walk-in centre. She
previously spent six years working in general practice, where
she developed a special interest in mental health.

Anna Hunter   BSc(Hons) NPDip RGN OND
Anna Hunter is currently a nurse practitioner at the Kent
County Ophthalmic and Aural Hospital in Maidstone, and a
Nurse Fellow at Canterbury, Christchurch University College,
where she teaches physical examination and health
assessment on the degree programme for Advanced Clinical
Nursing Practice.

Soline Jerram   BSc(Hons) Nurse Practitioner RGN EN(M)
Soline Jerram is currently Lead Nurse Practitioner for
primary care services to nursing and residential home
residents in Bognor Regis. Her role involves clinical
assessment, screening and review of acute and chronic
conditions, and general support of the care providers in the
private sector. In collaboration with local general
practitioners, the service is aimed at providing proactive,
health educational care for older adults living in community
homes. Over the past two years Soline has been directing a
research project looking at the cost effectiveness of nurse
practitioner services to older adults, and received the Nurse
2000 Nursing Older Adults award for her work in this area.

Wendy Johnson   BSc(Hons) RN DipN(Lond) NPDip
Wendy Johnson is currently Nurse Consultant in Primary
Care, Tooting NHS Walk-in Centre. She has a background in
general practice, where she has extensive experience in a
variety of practice settings. As one of the first nurse
practitioners to qualify in the UK, she pioneered and
promoted the role. Wendy has a particular interest in
education, and works as a freelance lecturer, teaching a
variety of primary care professionals. She co-founded
Practitioners' Associates Ltd, an organisation dedicated to
providing continuing education for advanced practice health
professionals. Her work has been published widely in a
variety of nursing journals.

Daphne Miller   PGCUT BSc(Hons) NPDip SRN
Daphne Miller is currently a lecturer in nursing at the
University of Ulster, Northern Ireland, where she is Pathway
Co-ordinator for the Postgraduate Diploma/Master of Science
in Advanced Nursing, Nurse Practitioner Pathway, and
Module Option Leader of the BSc(Hons) Community Nursing
General Practice Nurse option. Daphne also works part-time
as a nurse practitioner in a general practice surgery in
Belfast.

Sylvia Newson   BSc(Hons) NPDip RGN DN Cert CPT NP
Sylvia Newson trained as a district nurse in Portsmouth and
later moved to Seaford, where she undertook her Community
Practice Teacher training and her Nurse Practitioner
Diploma. There is a large elderly population within
Eastbourne and surrounding areas and, having spent many
years working as both a district nurse and more recently as
nurse practitioner, Sylvia has become extremely skilled in
working with this patient group. She is currently employed as
a Senior Practitioner, District Nursing with Eastbourne and
County NHS Trust. Her role involves providing clinical
supervision for district and practice nurses, implementing
evidence-based practice and facilitating practice development.

Nicola Nurse   BSc(Hons) RGN ENB 199, 998, A33
A career specialising in accident and emergency nursing has
led Nicola Nurse into the field of autonomous practice. After
completing her nurse practitioner degree at the Royal College
of Nursing Institute, she has continued to pursue a particular
interest in the assessment, management and provision of
excellent care for patients with musculoskeletal injuries by

the emergency nurse practitioner, and the provision of education and support for nurses preparing for autonomous practice in this field. Nicola is employed currently as a lecturer practitioner at the Florence Nightingale School of Nursing and Midwifery, King's College London, where she is the course leader for courses to prepare experienced nurses for autonomous practice. She spends clinical time at the Minor Injuries Unit, Guy's Hospital, and the Accident and Emergency Department, St Thomas' Hospital, London.

Linda Pearce   MSc RGN SCM OHNc NPDip

Linda Pearce is a respiratory nurse consultant and nurse practitioner. Her interest in respiratory health started while she was an occupational nurse and progressed through her practice nursing. She has considerable involvement in training health professionals in the management of respiratory disease. She researches into many aspects of respiratory disease and has presented her research at national and international respiratory meetings. Linda currently works as a specialist respiratory nurse at West Suffolk Hospital, as a Trainer for the National Asthma and Respiratory Training Centre, and as a coordinator for the University of East Anglia, Suffolk and Norfolk Primary Care Research Network (sunNet). She is a member of the British Thoracic Society Professional Standards committee and is chairperson of the Association of Respiratory Specialist Nurses.

Jill Peters   RGN BSc CMS ENB 393, 93A, 998, 870

Jill Peters is a Dermatology Nurse Practitioner at the Chelsea and Westminster Healthcare Trust. She is also working in partnership with primary care groups in Fulham, South Kensington, Chelsea and Westminster to provide dermatology services in primary care. Jill is involved in teaching dermatology nurses through various universities, is an active member of the British Dermatology Nursing Group and has written extensively for nursing journals and texts.

Claire Pratt   BPhil NPDip BSc(Hons) DPSN SRN ENB 928

Claire Pratt is currently working as a Nurse Advisor for NHS Direct Westcountry. Prior to this she worked for nine years in general practice: seven years as a practice nurse and two as a qualified nurse practitioner. Since qualifying as an SRN in 1979, Claire has worked in a variety of clinical settings, undertaken a number of leadership roles, and been involved in multiprofessional post-registration education. Claire is one of the founder members of the Peninsular Nurse Practitioner Group.

Mary Rawlinson   BSc(Hons) NPDip RGN SCM ONC DN

Mary Rawlinson is a primary care nurse practitioner working in two practices in Berkshire. After qualifying as a registered nurse and midwife, she held a variety of posts in both primary and secondary care including those of sister of an orthopaedic ward and a community nursing sister/midwife in rural Gloucestershire. After a career break to have her children, she returned to primary care, working as a practice nurse. After several years' experience in the field, she decided to extend her role by completing the Nurse Practitioner degree course at the Royal College of Nursing. Mary is also a member of the prescribers group, clinical governance of her local PCT.

Sue Reed   BSc(Hons) NPDip FPCert RGN

Sue Reed is one of a handful of nurse practitioners in East Kent and also runs her own community-based family planning clinic in Margate. She has been a family planning nurse since 1985, when her youngest daughter was six months old. For ten years Sue worked in the Sick Bay at the University of Kent, where she found her family planning skills were much appreciated. During this time, she completed a four-year part-time degree in Health Studies at the Roehampton Institute, where much of her research focused on contraceptive issues and adolescent health. Two years after completing her degree, Sue was appointed to a pilot project as a trainee GP nurse practitioner in Dover. She then undertook the Nurse Practitioner Diploma at the Royal College of Nursing, and is now permanently based at the Dover practice.

Debra Sharu   MSc BA(Hons) PGDEd RGN RSCN CS-FNP

Debra Sharu is currently a Senior Lecturer on the BSc Nurse Practitioner Programme at the Royal College of Nursing Development Centre (RCNDC), South Bank University, London. In addition to educating nurse practitioners, she works as a family nurse practitioner in the Soho Walk-in Centre, London. Before becoming a nurse practitioner, Debra worked with neonates and chronically ill children and she has a particular interest in paediatrics. She actively promotes the role of the British NP both in the United Kingdom and abroad through her work at the RCNDC, publications, conference presentations and continuing professional development workshops. Debra has extensive experience in both the USA and the UK.

Frances Simpson   BA BSc RGN RM NPDip CertEd

Frances Simpson is currently practising as a nurse practitioner in primary care in Charlton, south-east London. She came to general practice from a background as a nurse teacher at King's College Hospital, London and has continued this teaching role amongst practice nurses, nurse practitioners and medical students. As one of the first nurse practitioners from the then IANE course at the RCN, she was involved in setting up The Forum for NPs at the RCN.

Rosie Walsh   BPhil RGN RNT CSP (General Practice Nursing) NP(Dip)

Rosie Walsh is currently employed as Nurse Facilitator at Cornwall and Isles of Scilly Health Authority where one aspect of her role is to facilitate, in partnership with the primary care organisations, continuing professional development opportunities for nurse practitioners, practice nurses and other health professionals. Prior to this, Rosie worked for a number of years in primary care initially as a practice nurse and latterly as a nurse practitioner. Rosie has also worked in a variety of educational settings, her last appointment being Senior Lecturer at the University of Plymouth. With colleagues who studied for the nurse pratitioner degree at the University of Exeter, she co-founded the Peninusla Nurse Practitioner Group more than three years ago.

Morag White   RGN RM MMSC (Educations) BSc(Hons) Dip Prof Studies NP(Dip)

Morag White currently works as a nurse practitioner in a general practice in Belfast, Northern Ireland. She also specialises in asthma/diabetes and cardiovascular disease. She represents both practice nurses and nurse practitioners on various working parties and committees including the Department of Health for Northern Ireland. She is currently United Kingdom Chairperson for the Nurse Practitioner Association practice and policy steering group.

FOREWORD

The early nineties were an exciting time of my professional life. I was teaching the first courses for nurse practitioners at the Royal College of Nursing Institute, and my small classes were made up of energetic, smart and dynamic nurses, who were not afraid of risk and change. Two of these first students are the editors of this book and it is indeed an honour to be invited by them to write this foreword. Of course, students teach their teacher as much as the other way round and, even now, more than 10 years later, I still remember the challenges they set for me in their questioning of both the course and the role of the nurse practitioner. All of us struggled with the role of the nurse in clinical care, where nursing and nurses have always had an uneasy relationship. One of the major criticisms of the nurse practitioner role in those early years was that, because it included advanced clinical skills, the nurse practitioner was no longer a nurse but a kind of second-rate doctor. It was often difficult to respond to those criticisms, usually made by our nursing colleagues, because we *were* asserting that the distinguishing characteristic of the nurse practitioner was that she could assess people presenting with undiagnosed and undifferentiated problems – the traditional medical role. At that time, there could not have been (and was not) a clinical book for nurse practitioners such as this: our textbooks for those first courses came from the USA or were meant for medical doctors. Imagine my pleasure, therefore, at being able to read this book about clinical care, for nurse practitioners, and written by some of those students who also struggled through those early days. It is indeed a landmark.

This book is for those nurses who want to become better informed clinical practitioners. It has always seemed quite obvious to me that nurses have to have, among a large repertoire of skills and competencies, a sound clinical knowledge and judgement. What this does is to make nurses effective, safe practitioners. Who would have confidence in a nurse who didn't understand why chest pain was a symptom to be taken seriously? I use this particular example because my mother, who has been seriously ill, awoke in the night, in hospital, with a sharp pain in her chest and feeling short of breath. Of course, it was a nurse who was the first contact and made the decision about how to deal with her symptom – and made the decision to call a doctor. My mother had a pulmonary embolism – thank goodness the nurse knew her clinical care.

This is also a book for nurses who know how to apply the knowledge it contains. When I was reading it, I was transported back (in my mind!) to sitting with people presenting in general practice, and trying, with them, to make sense of the clues they were giving me. Most people have a history to their current visit to the practice – why today? What made them see the nurse? As I reviewed the 'Top Tips' sections of the chapters (a highly commendable idea), I realised that they almost all begin with an exhortation to consider more than the presenting problem: take a history; find out what your client already knows; don't consider the presenting problem in isolation; do a complete examination. Clinical work is like that – it demands great detective skills, patience and above all the ability to listen well. I am both proud and happy to report that this book emphasises the 'wholism' of clinical work – the importance of getting the whole story in understanding both the nature and the seriousness of the symptoms. In a chapter which I wrote on the search for meaning in advanced nursing (Stilwell 1998) I entitled a section 'The complex whole'. In it, I suggested that it is the total experience of the nursing encounter which is important, not the separate parts of art and science. The advanced practitioner must be able to move seamlessly between scientific knowledge and arts of caring, empathy and advocacy. I said: 'Like the concert pianist, to be an advanced practitioner requires technical brilliance and sensitive interpretation' (p. 47).

As I explored the depths of this book, I became convinced that it will help nurse practitioners towards technical brilliance, as well as influence the sensitivity of the way that clinical findings are both discovered and interpreted. I commend it to you and I am proud to be able to endorse the work of so many of those great students – those early changers in the nurse practitioner world.

Barbara Stilwell

Reference

Stilwell B 1998 The search for meaning in advanced nursing practice. In: Rolfe G, Fulbrook P Advanced Nursing Practice. Oxford, Butterworth Heinemann, 43–49.

HOW TO USE THIS BOOK

The Nurse Practitioner Manual of Clinical Skills is developed around common primary care disorders encountered by nurse practitioners (NPs) practising in their expanded role in various ambulatory care settings. The manual includes sections on related anatomy and physiology. It is assumed that readers have a basic knowledge of anatomy and physiology and, in this manual, these are designed to help readers to apply their knowledge to interpreting symptoms, examining the body and understanding physical signs.

Also included are interviewing techniques for history taking, an overview of usual presenting signs and symptoms, as well as the assessment of mental status, pertinent physical assessment, possible complications and a suggested plan of action for the NP.

Throughout the manual the contributors have tried to emphasise common or important problems, rather than those which are infrequent or obscure. Occasionally a physical sign has been included despite its rarity because it enjoys a solid niche in classic physical diagnosis, or because recognising the abnormality is especially important for the health or even the life of the patient.

This material is augmented with illustrations, tables of medication regimens, 'red flags' (important areas to be aware of, indicated by the symbol ❶) and 'Top Tips' for each chapter.

The scope of problems addressed ranges from those that affect children and adolescents to those found in the aged. A working foundation of knowledge in quality assurance, health maintenance and the new frontiers in nursing and medicine are also presented in this manual. The subject matter has been drawn equally from current resources and from the extensive and diverse experience of our NP colleagues.

It is recognised that standards of care differ according to individual needs, community resources and regional locations and with the emergence of new scientific data and treatment modalities. In conjunction with the above, most instances when the NP must consult the physician or refer to explicit, mutually acceptable written guidelines of care are identified. It is emphasised that legality of practice varies.

This manual is not meant to be the last word in care, but rather a guideline, a springboard from which nurses can utilise their own powers of innovation to focus on health promotion and health maintenance wherever the patient belongs on the health–illness continuum. It is the intent of the editors and contributors to address a comprehensive conceptual framework to assist the nurse with logical and creative problem-solving techniques, with the major focus on patient education.

All nurses – students and practitioners – need a clearly written, well-organised assessment guide. The *Nurse Practitioner Manual of Clinical Skills* is such a resource. Written by and for NPs, the manual describes how to gather data through the nursing health history, physical assessment and laboratory studies, analyse the collected data, formulate appropriate diagnosis, treatment and management options and document findings. Organised in 18 chapters, the manual presents a holistic health-oriented approach to assessment, treatment and management.

Each chapter focuses on assessment skills, describing interviewing the patient, including assessing psychological and cultural influences on health; physical assessment skills; and how to use equipment and perform basic assessment techniques, including inspection, palpation, percussion, auscultation and measurement of vital signs. Chapters follow a standard format. Anatomical illustrations are used where necessary to help the reader visualise the system being assessed. The chapter continues with a health history, health promotion and protection patterns, and role and relationship patterns. Cultural and development considerations are included when appropriate.

Specific assessment procedures are described, illustrating various steps and techniques and presenting normal findings and important developmental considerations. Certain advanced assessment skills – skills needed by those who have mastered basic techniques and whose practice requires more advanced skills – also are described.

Helpful features are:
■ subjective and objective assessment checklists of important questions the nurse should ask herself before beginning the assessment
■ common laboratory studies and commonly ordered tests, and the normal values or findings for each test
■ diagnostic categories that may apply to each body system being assessed.

Each chapter ends with a list of References, including research articles, and many chapters have a Further Reading section.

The efforts of many clinical experts have produced this current, accurate, easy-to-use reference – a practical assessment guide for NPs in various clinical settings. By using the *Nurse Practitioner Manual of Clinical Skills*, student and practising NPs can increase their ability to perform diagnosis, treatment and management with confidence.

HEALTH PROMOTION

Rosie Walsh

Key Issues

- Health promotion is concerned with raising the health status of individuals and communities (Ewles & Simnett 1992)

- Definitions of health are of two main types: those that view health negatively, referring to the absence of qualities (for example, disease and illness); those that adopt a positive approach centred on the presence of certain qualities (for example, physical and mental fitness)

- Three models of health have been identified: the biomedical, the social and the humanist (Rowe et al 1997)

- The first phase in health promotion planning is assessment of needs. Needs are different to wants and Bradshaw (1972) distinguishes four types of need: normative, felt, expressed and comparative. The NHS, however, defines need as the population's ability to benefit from service

- The client's need for information is often underestimated and there is also a misconception that clients require information in short, simple formats in order to make informed choices but this is not substantiated by research

- Community profiling is a method of assessing the health needs of a neighbourhood using a range of techniques such as rapid participatory appraisal, surveys, routine statistics of morbidity, births and deaths and practice-held information

- Lifestyle change can be effected using the six key stages of the Prochaska and DiClemente cycle of change (1986). These are precontemplation, contemplation, preparation, action, maintenance and relapse

- A number of coping strategies to enable people to persevere with behaviour changes have been identified (Ewles & Simnett 1992):

  - finding a substitute, changing routines and habits closely associated with the behaviour to be changed
  - making it difficult to carry on with the 'problem' behaviour
  - getting support from others in the same situation
  - practising ways of dealing with social pressures
  - adopting a 'one day at a time' approach
  - learning relaxation or other ways of dealing with stress

- Working with teenagers presents particular challenges. Research has shown that over 53% of teenagers had difficulties with consultations in primary care. Concern was expressed over the embarrassment felt when discussing personal concerns, difficulties with obtaining quick appointments and disclosure to parents (Donovan 1998)

- Providing the right kinds of information in the right way for elderly people can help support them at home and make an important contribution to their health and sense of well-being (Tester & Meredith 1987). Generally, face-to-face communication and individualised literature have been found to be most effective

Introduction

Health promotion is about raising the health status of individuals and communities (Ewles & Simnett 1992). It has been defined as 'any activity designed to foster health' (Tones & Tilford 1996). Downie et al (1996) identify health promotion as comprising 'efforts to enhance positive health and reduce the risk of ill-health through the overlapping spheres of health education, prevention and health protection' (Fig. 2.1). Seven domains, identified within this model, demonstrate the wide range of possibilities for health promotion. Empowerment is the central theme identified. Health education seeks to empower people by providing the necessary information, helping them to develop skills and a healthy level of self-esteem so that the amount of control they have over

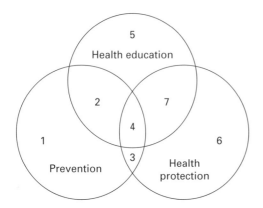

Figure 2.1 *Tannihills's model of health promotion. (Reproduced with permission from Downie et al 1996.)*

what happens to them is increased. The provision of good preventive services and the shaping of a healthful environment through health protection also contribute to this process of empowerment. Raeburn & Rootman (1998) have developed the concept of people-centred health promotion and have encapsulated the key essentials within the mnemonic 'people':

- people-centredness
- empowerment
- organisational and community development
- participation
- life quality
- evaluation.

The World Health Organization in Europe (WHO 1984) identified the following five principles of health promotion:

- it involves the population as a whole
- it is directed towards action on the determinants or causes of health
- it combines diverse but complementary methods or approaches
- it aims particularly at effective and concrete public participation
- health professionals have an important role in nurturing and enabling health promotion.

In 1986, the Ottawa Charter for health promotion was devised. It identifies the purpose and meaning of health promotion as:

- building healthy public policy
- creating a supportive environment
- strengthening community action
- developing personal skills
- reorienting health services.

It should not be forgotten that at government level in the UK there has been a recent shift in balance between public health policy and healthy public policy in line with the Ottawa Charter, with an emphasis on education, employment, housing, homelessness, reducing crime, transport and mobility, nutrition and the fluoridation of water (Department of Health 1999a); however, the main focus of this chapter is on public health and the use of health promotion strategies within the consultation. In recent years, health promotion has also come to be viewed synonymously with the public health agenda.

Health models

Health has been defined in a variety of ways. Two types of official definitions exist: those that define health negatively, referring to the absence of qualities such as disease and illness; and those that adopt a more positive approach, centred on the presence of these qualities (Aggleton 1991). Health has also been seen, by some writers, as a continuum where individual health exists somewhere between a state of absolute health and ill-health (Jones 1994). Seedhouse (1986) has identified a number of different ways of defining health, five of which are particularly important:

1. Health as an ideal state – this relates to the World Health Organization definition of health as 'a state of complete physical, mental and social well-being not just the absence of disease or infirmity'. This definition sets high targets but has been criticised for being idealistic and almost impossible to achieve. Ewles & Simnett (1992), however, propose a more holistic model, also incorporating emotional, spiritual and societal dimensions, whereas Aggleton & Homans (1987) have supplemented this with the inclusion of sensual and sexual aspects. This may be viewed as the social model of health (Rowe et al 1997). In 1984, the WHO refined their definition to incorporate the realisation of ambitions, satisfaction of needs and the ability to adapt to or cope with the environment (Fig. 2.2).

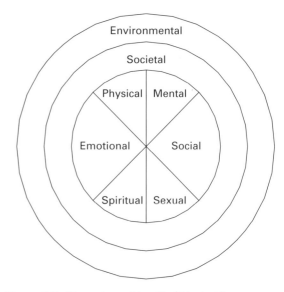

Figure 2.2 *Dimensions of health. (Adapted from Aggleton & Homans 1987 and Ewles & Simnett 1992.)*

2. Health as physical and mental fitness – this statement defines health at an optimum capacity. The emphasis here is on the individual fitting in with society's norms and expectations (normative approach). Parsons (1972) suggested that a high level of health is important for the smooth running of society and anything less is seen as being dysfunctional. This definition can be criticised for ignoring the variations in and degrees of health (Aggleton 1991).

3. Health as a commodity – it has been suggested that this concept relates to the growth of modern medicine and the idea that health can be bought (private health care), sold (health food stores), given (by surgery and medication) and lost (accident and disease). This approach seeks to equate health with a series of clearly definable and measurable qualities, and views restoration of health as little more than a technical matter, in a sense, divorced from the individual (Aggleton 1991). This may be viewed as the biomedical model of health (Rowe et al 1997).

4. Health as a personal strength or ability – these definitions focus on health as physical or mental strength or the ability to resist disease and cope with illness. Dubos (1959) also suggested that it was the ability to adapt to changing circumstances. The nature of these strengths and abilities are rather vague, rarely defined and, as such, difficult to measure other than subjectively, and there is a lack of information about how they may be acquired if lacking (Aggleton 1991).

5. Health as the basis for personal potential – this definition is personally favoured by Seedhouse (1986). Health is composed of a number of factors, foundations for achievements, which enable people to achieve their maximum personal potential. Some foundations are common (basic necessities such as food, water and shelter, or access to information and the ability and confidence to make sense of it), and others are unique, varying according to the individual and the situation within which they find themselves. This definition has been criticised for the lack of clarity of the concept of personal potential and lack of guidance about the range of factors that may count as foundations for achievement (Aggleton 1991). It is difficult to know whether this is any more achievable than the idealistic WHO definition.

It is important to consider that professional and lay beliefs about the nature of health may be different and that concepts of health are also linked with people's social and cultural situations (Richman 1987, Helman 1990, Ewles & Simnett 1992). Townsend (1984) has also recognised that geographical location and gender are major determinants of health as well as social class. There also appears to be a direct correlation between individuals' health status and their level of access to material goods (Rowe et al 1997). Health is usually assessed subjectively by the individual, according to their own norms and expectations, but objectively by

the professional. Blaxter & Patterson (1982) have suggested that the health expectations of elderly people will differ from the young, and those of the poor will differ from the affluent, but that there may be commonality within each social group. For example, studies undertaken with elderly people have shown that health is viewed mainly in the context of being fit to do the jobs expected of them (Williams 1983, Victor 1990). It is also important to recognise that people's ideas of health vary widely and are shaped by their experiences, knowledge, values and expectations and by their view of what they are expected to do and the fitness they need in order to fulfil that role. This lay view may be identified as the humanist model of health (Rowe et al 1997).

The green paper, *Our Healthier Nation* (Department of Health 1998a) has emphasised the need to tackle inequalities in health in order to improve the health of the worst off in society and to narrow the health gap. Two further reports with wide-ranging recommendations for tackling inequalities in health have since been published (Department of Health 1998b, 1999c). In 1997, the Department of Health (1997a) invited bids for the development of health action zones (HAZs). HAZs have been introduced to tackle inequalities in health and as testing grounds for new ideas and innovations to modernise the health services (Evans & Robinson 1999). Currently, 26 exist. A number of researchers have also identified the strong links that exist between deprivation and health (Whitehead 1987; Townsend & Davidson 1990; Blackburn 1992; Doyal 1995).

Assessment of health behaviours

The first phase in health promotion planning is the process of assessing the needs of the individual or population group to enable them to become more healthy (Naidoo & Wills 1995). A need is something that people could benefit from and is different from a demand (Naidoo & Wills 1995). Maslow's hierarchy of needs (1966) identifies the health needs of individuals: these commence with basic physiological needs, which, once satisfied, are followed by safety needs, needs for love and belonging, the need for esteem and, at the pinnacle, the need for self-actualisation. Bradshaw (1972) has distinguished four types of need:

1. Normative needs – these are objective needs, defined by professionals according to a standard, which reflect the judgement of that professional and the resources available. Problems may exist with these value judgements because acceptable standards may vary from one expert to another and may differ from the values and standards of the clients (Ewles & Simnett 1992).

2. Felt needs – these are the needs that clients themselves identify. They may be limited or inflated by people's awareness and knowledge about what might be available. Armstrong (1982) described these as perceived needs.

3. Expressed needs – this is what clients say they need. It is a felt need that has been turned into an expressed request or demand. However, not all felt need is turned into expressed need, either because of lack of opportunity, motivation or assertiveness. It is important to note that lack of demand does not equate with lack of felt need. Expressed need may also conflict with the normative needs identified by the professional.
4. Comparative needs – here comparison is made between similar client groups usually in different geographical areas. Recent examples of this are comparison of provision of services and waiting lists.

It can therefore be seen that the concept of need is a relative one that is influenced by values, attitudes and by other agendas (Naidoo & Wills 1995). Needs are not necessarily objective, observable entities to which interventions are matched.

When identifying needs, it is useful to consider whether the approach is proactive or reactive and whose needs come first – the users or the commissioners. This may be a source of conflict, but recent trends emphasise putting the views and needs of the users at the centre of health promotion provision.

In 1989, the white paper *Working for Patients* (Department of Health 1989) emphasised the need for health authorities to focus on ensuring that the health needs of the population for which they are responsible were met. The NHS defines 'need' as the population's ability to benefit from services. This is seen in the context of health gain, which includes increased life expectancy through a reduction in premature deaths, improved well-being and quality of life. Since the Acheson report (1988), health authorities have also been required to produce an annual report about the health of their population. Tannahill (1992) suggests that one drawback of such a system is that mortality and morbidity data tend to drive the health promotion agenda and the focus for prevention. Within this system, social and psychological health needs may be ignored (despite the inclusion of social indicators) in favour of disease and people's subjective experiences, because health behaviour may not be seen in its social context. There may, therefore, be a tendency to focus on individual responsibility rather than the determinants of health (Naidoo & Wills 1995). The first national strategy for health, *The Health of the Nation*, was published by the Department of Health in 1992. It represented an important milestone in achieving public recognition and commitment to working together to improve health. A more recent white paper (Department of Health 1997b) has focused on the development of local health strategies to provide health improvement targets and 3-year health improvement programmes through partnership working. Primary care organisations will also have a new responsibility for health improvement (Department of Health 1999b). The purpose of assessing health needs has been identified as (Naidoo & Wills 1995):
1. To help in directing interventions appropriately.

2. To identify and respond to specific needs of minority groups, communities or sections of the population whose health needs have not been fully met.
3. To target risk groups – this is a means of directing health promotion activities to people in most need. Normative needs, derived from epidemiological research which identifies groups with poorer than average health, are often used to establish target groups. Comparative need is used to identify at-risk groups with poor uptake rates of services (for example, travellers). This approach may lead to victim-blaming, where the group is seen as responsible through their behaviour for their own ill health. For example, HIV prevention through health promotion campaigns has been targeted at gay men and drug users who inject substances; however, it is not being gay that is a risk, rather it is certain sexual practices. This approach has been rejected by the WHO, which advocates a population rather than a high-risk approach, and many health promoters prefer to work in partnership with groups and communities on the issues that they themselves define as important.
4. Resource allocation.

To enable a systematic approach to the assessment of health promotion needs, Ewles & Simnett (1992) have developed a series of four key questions, the answers to which will help you decide whether to respond to a need and, if so, how:
1. What sort of need is it? Is it a normative, felt, expressed or comparative need?
2. Who decided that there is a need? Was it the health promoter, the client or both?
3. What are the grounds for deciding that there is a need? Is there any objective evidence, such as facts and figures?
4. What are the aims and the appropriate response to the need?

The process of assessing need must therefore involve client participation. This negotiation process and partnership working involves highly developed communication and listening skills. It is important initially to put the client at ease and to build a rapport. This may be achieved through warmth, openness, genuineness, empathy and unconditional positive regard (Rogers 1983). Use of open-ended questions and counselling techniques can help to elicit clients' perceptions about their health and health behaviours (Neighbour 1997). There is a greater emphasis on client-centredness but, despite this, health promoters tend to assess needs in relation to the service they provide (Naidoo & Wills 1995).

Client needs may also be interpreted as the need for information, as this is easy to provide. Health care workers also appear to value information as a vehicle for increasing compliance. Farrant & Russell (1985) identified that clients often require information in greater detail than health promoters provide in order to make informed choices (Fig. 2.3).

Figure 2.3 *Framework for assessing individual health behaviours.*

Topic	Questions that you may consider asking
Health	How healthy do you feel you are? (useful to check here the client's understanding of health) What health problems or worries, if any, do you have or have you had? (e.g. mental or physical, illnesses, diseases, operations) Is there anything you do that you know affects your health? Do any diseases run in your family?
Social situation	Tell me about your family (partner and/or friends) What type of housing do you live in? What leisure activities do you participate in?
Occupation	What do you do for a living? (explore if occupational health risk factors are evident)
Medication/drugs	What medicines do you take that have been prescribed by a doctor? Tell me about any other medicines you take (e.g. over-the-counter medicines, herbal remedies, homeopathic medicines, recreational drugs) A useful question for young people is: A lot of young people take drugs, do your friends, do you?
Disease prevention	What vaccinations have you had and when?
Diet	Tell me about your diet How much fibre do you eat? How much sugar and what sweet things do you eat? How much fat do you have? (saturated, polyunsaturated or monosaturated, junk food) What types of drinks do you have? (water, tea, coffee, fizzy or soft drinks)
Exercise	How much exercise do you take in a week? What type?
Smoking history	Tell me about smoking Have you ever? If so, what age did you start? Do you currently smoke? How many? What type? (important here to ascertain the number of pack-years: 1 pack-year = 20 cigarettes daily for 1 year) Have you ever managed to stop? If so, why did you start again? Are you interested, at all, in stopping now?
Alcohol intake	Tell me about drinking alcohol How much do you drink? What type? Have you ever had a problem controlling drinking? If appropriate, administer the CAGE questionnaire: • Have you ever felt the need to Cut down on your drinking? • Have you ever felt Annoyed by criticism of your drinking? • Have you ever felt Guilty about your drinking? • Have you ever had a drink first thing in the morning (Eye opener) to steady your nerves or cure a hangover?
Sexual history	Tell me about your relationships (but this may not give the required responses and focused questions may be necessary) Do you have a regular sexual partner? (or do you have sex?) Could I just check, is your partner a man or a woman? Do you have sex with anyone else? Is that/are they men, women or both? What contraception do you use? Which variety of condoms do you use? How do you feel about using condoms? Have you had difficulties using condoms? What do you understand by safer sex?

Figure 2.3 *Framework for assessing individual health behaviours.* *(continued)*

Topic	Questions that you may consider asking
	How do you feel about talking about this with...
	Have you any concerns about HIV/STIs/hepatitis infections? (Jewitt 1995, Wetton 1996, Peate 1997, Matthews 1998, Levy 1999)
Further opportunity to share information	Is there anything else that you would like to tell me about yourself/that you think I should know about you?
With older people a full assessment of the activities of daily living, for example, mobility may be necessary (Lorig 1992)	

Young people present a particular health promotion problem. While they are generally seen as one of the healthiest groups in society and 70–90% actually consider themselves to be in excellent health (Dennison 1998), research has shown that 11% of 12–13 year old boys and 14% of girls smoke. This figure increases to 24% for boys and 42% for 15–16 year old girls (Lloyd & Lucas 1998). Also, Miller & Plant (1996) and Goddard (1994) have shown that, in England, the number of 11–15 year olds consuming alcohol in the week previous to their study was 24%. The prevalence of cannabis use in 15 and 16 year olds is 40%, and 9% have used ecstasy (Wright & Pearl 1995, Miller & Plant 1996). The highest recorded rates of drug and alcohol dependency are in 16–19-year-old females but in 20–24-year-old males (Dennison 1998). In a study in 1994, 28% of 16–19 year olds admitted to intercourse by the age of 16 (Johnson et al 1994). Teenage pregnancy rates in the UK are also the highest in Europe (Mawer 1999, Social Exclusion Unit 1999, Wright et al 2000). It is, therefore, apparent that teenagers have a number of risk-taking behaviours (Fig. 2.4) and, consequently, a number of important health needs.

In a recent study, over 53% of 15–16 year olds reported difficulties with primary care consultations (Donovan 1998). The main reasons were:

- embarrassment when talking about personal concerns
- problems with getting an immediate urgent appointment
- concerns over disclosure to parents.

Young people also feel that they have little opportunity to raise the issues that they want during consultation with professionals (Catan et al 1996). In fact, GP consultations with teenagers are on average 2 minutes shorter than consultations with adults (Jacobson & Wilkinson 1994). Studies have also shown that more teenagers would like to discuss health-related areas, such as contraception, sexually transmitted infections and nutrition, with health professionals than actually do so (Epstein et al 1989). These studies hold important lessons for health promoters. These are that (McPherson et al 1996, Dennison 1998):

- There may be ways of making the practice more attractive and welcoming to young people.

- Young people need clear reassurances that their parents will not be told about the content of their consultation.
- Communication with young people requires the same skills as with any client.
- It is important to deal with embarrassment in a way that is not patronising or over-familiar.
- Parents frequently attend consultations with their children and it may be appropriate to ask the parent to leave the consulting room without causing suspicion or offence.
- It is important to allow sufficient consultation time for real problems (felt needs) to emerge and for trust to develop.
- It may be helpful to establish young people's clinics (Donovan & McCarthy 1988) or satellite services in youth centres, or schools. This has the advantage of being in an environment that is familiar and comfortable and, in the teenager's eyes, perceived as more confidential.

It is also worthwhile considering here the health needs of older people. The King's Fund (1988) postulated the following key assumptions about health in old age, very few of which have been substantiated by research:

- Old age is not a disease but a normal stage of life.
- Most people aged over 60 are fit and healthy, but, as they age, they become less likely to recover quickly

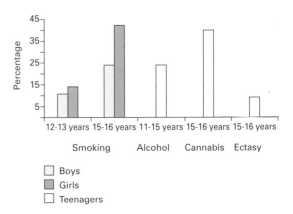

Figure 2.4 *Risk-taking behaviour in young people.*

or completely from illness, more likely to become frail and in need of help to maintain their capacity for self-care.

- Functional capacity in old age can be strengthened through training, stimulation and/or by avoiding factors associated with ill health.
- Elderly people are more diverse socially and psychologically than young people, reflecting the fact that they have been exposed for a longer time to lifelong risks and to varied life experiences. These are reflected in a wide variety of beliefs, values and needs.
- The promotion of health in old age should be directed towards the promotion of good mental, physical and social function as well as the prevention of disease and disability (Ory et al 1992).
- Many measures that affect the health of elderly people lie outside the health sector, but health and social workers are well placed to act as advocates for change outside as well as inside their spheres of work. One such example is transport.

The King's Fund have also made the following recommendations to improve the health of elderly people:

- improved nutrition
- improved housing with higher standards of heating and insulation
- more active participation in exercise (Smith & Jacobson 1989, Grimley Evans et al 1992; Skelton and McLaughlin 1996, Gillies et al 1999, Carter and O'Driscoll 2000)
- more selective and careful prescribing and improved monitoring of medication (this will help to reduce the levels of iatrogenic disease)
- more effective case finding and early diagnosis of preventable disease (where intervention can prevent complication or chronicity)
- substantial reduction in poverty, especially among widows, those living alone and the very old; income-related problems are associated with the prevalence of disease, dysfunction and mortality but also with a person's ability to cope with ill health
- improved support for carers, particularly where these are elderly.

A National Service Framework for older people has just been published by the Department of Health which sets national standards and defines service models (Department of Health 2001). Communication may be particularly difficult with older people who are more likely to suffer from impaired vision, hearing and short-term memory. This may mean that consultations take longer. Research by Tester & Meredith (1987) has shown that providing the right kinds of information in the right way to elderly people can help support them at home and make an important contribution to their health and sense of well-being. Face-to-face consultations have been proven to be more effective than media information. Leaflets about specific aspects of health may help to reinforce health messages and counteract the problems of impaired memory.

The NHS changes of the 1990s and the NHS Plan published in 2000 require that the public are widely consulted about local services at all stages of the commissioning process (Department of Health 2000). The danger is that those voices that are loudest may tend to be the views that are heard and this may not be representative of the entire population. It is important that this is a participative process, with sharing of information, so that felt needs are elicited. Levenson & Joule (cited in Naidoo & Wills 1995) suggest that there are four recognised models of user involvement.

1. 'Tell me you love me', in which a patient satisfaction survey is drawn up by NHS managers.
2. 'Kill them with kindness', the token gesture in which the public are invited to all planning meetings but rarely encouraged to be involved.
3. 'The Godfather', in which a community leader is identified to act as the conduit for black and minority groups.
4. 'Puppet show', in which a group is identified for giving the views of the community.

Community health profiling has been identified as a way of providing a complete picture of needs in a given locality (Shanks et al 1995, Hirst 1997, Hawtin et al 1998). It has been suggested that a mix of assessment methods may provide more information about health needs than one method alone (Murray & Graham 1995). Methods include rapid participatory appraisal where data is collected qualitatively from three differing sources (existing documents about the neighbourhood, interviews with a range of informants and direct observation of the area) (Annett & Rifkin 1988), postal surveys, analysis of routine small-area statistics (such as morbidity, data on births and deaths) and collation of practice-held information (Murray & Graham 1995). A number of guidelines and frameworks have been developed to aid community profiling (Twinn et al 1990, Royal College of Nursing 1993, Rowe et al 1997, Hooper & Longworth 1998, Swage 1999). Healthy alliances will also ensure that the views and experience of local health promoters and professionals are considered. These may include workers in primary care, schools, environmental health, housing, youth workers, police and community workers.

Interventions

Many health promotion interventions in primary care happen opportunistically. Blaxter (1990) has identified four aspects of lifestyle – exercise, diet, smoking and alcohol consumption – around which health promotion activities are often centred. These are usually thought of as the most clearly 'voluntary' and, at least to some extent, the individual's own responsibility. Interventions to effect lifestyle change will be considered in relation to the individual client and small groups. While small-group work is an effective way of working with large numbers of people, it is important to recognise that some people may be reluctant and even embarrassed to

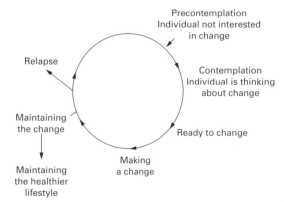

Figure 2.5 *The stages of change model. (After Prochaska &*
DiClemente 1984.)

share information and feelings in front of a large audience. It is therefore particularly important that individuals are offered choices of one-to-one or group sessions within which to participate.

The health education authority provides a national programme, Helping People Change, aimed at health promotion and primary health care staff to enable them to help people effectively change aspects of their lifestyle (Williams et al 1995). The programme advocates the use of the Prochaska and DiClemente's (1986) trans-theoretical model of change. The key stages that people go through in order to change are (Fig. 2.5):

- precontemplation – at this stage the person may be unaware that a problem exists and will often resist pressure to change
- contemplation – at this stage the person begins to be aware and will consider lifestyle change
- preparation – at this stage behaviour change is actively planned and a commitment is made to take action in the near future
- action – existing behaviour is altered as the plan is operationalised
- maintenance – at this point the person continues their efforts to alter existing behaviour
- relapse – the person returns to the old behaviour instead of maintaining the change; this need not be seen as failure if the individual learns from the experience and is able to recommence the change process.

Interestingly, a cluster-randomised controlled trial for smoking prevention and cessation that involved 8352 school students aged 13–14 years found an expert system based on this model to have no effect on the prevalence of regular smoking (Aveyard et al 1999, Velicer et al 1999).

Lifestyle modification involves changes in beliefs, values, attitudes and behaviour (Tones 1995). This model recognises that people cannot be coerced or forced through the change process. However, if health professionals recognise the stage that people are at, they can encourage them to move forward.

Percival (1999) suggests that the role of the health professional is to build the client's belief in their ability to carry out change and to succeed in achieving the goals they have set for themselves while providing support for this process. She also identifies a framework to facilitate motivation, empowerment and decision making:

- find out what the client already knows and believes about their lifestyle and its effect on health
- develop partnerships where the client remains in control of the empowered choices and changes
- recognise that not all clients wish to change and that many may need help to understand the implications of their lifestyle choices
- let the client decide what, when and how to change
- when the client wants to and is ready, jointly formulate an action plan.

Success in habit change is likely when the client (Ewles & Simnett 1992, Percival 1999):

- has thought about the change over a period of time
- has changed when they are ready to and has not been coerced
- understands previous choices and why they now want to change
- is prepared for how they will feel during the change
- has thought of alternative strategies to replace the habit
- has learned how to cope in different ways with tempting situations
- feels in control (which increases self-esteem) and has built a positive self-image of themselves without the habit.

Changing behaviour can mean coping with numerous difficulties until the new behaviour becomes a part of normal life. Self-monitoring, in the form of a diary, can provide precise information about the behaviour pattern, enhance self-awareness and provide a useful starting point for gaining control. The diary can also be used as a baseline against which progress can be checked. The cost of changing behaviour can be considerable, and it is helpful to identify the benefits and devise a system of rewards to encourage perseverance (Watson & Tharp 1985, Kanfer & Goldstein 1986). Targets should be realistic and short term: for example, it is easier to lose 1 kg of weight in 2 weeks than attempting to lose 7 kg in 1 month. If the target is not reached, individuals can feel despondent, disappointed and a failure. This may have a negative effect on motivation. People may adopt a wide variety of coping strategies to ensure success. Ewles and Simnett (1992) have suggested the following strategies:

- finding a substitute – chewing gum or herbal cigarettes for smokers, low calorie foods for those attempting to lose weight
- changing routines and habits closely associated with the behaviour to be changed – for example, drinking tea or fruit juice if coffee is associated with a cigarette

on with the 'problem'
:tting in a nonsmoking
ettes in an inconvenient
ealtimes
in the same situation –
nming or anti-smoking

ı social pressures – for
a cigarette or drink
e' or short time span

ies or other ways of
e the old habit in stress-
find exercise or other

ıccess of health pro-
ency, effectiveness
nce exists for the
atherer et al 1979,
A number of tech-
~sgested (Naidoo &

ıealth promotion and disease prevention programmes

There are divergent views about the nature of health promotion and disease prevention. Nutbeam (1986) has distinguished the two as separate but complementary activities, whereas Downie et al (1996) describe overlapping spheres comprising health education, prevention and health protection. Downie et al (1996) identify four foci for prevention:

1. prevention of the onset or first manifestation of a disease process – this category may include accident prevention and unwanted pregnancy
2. prevention of the progression of a disease process or other unwanted state, through early detection
3. prevention of avoidable complications of an irreversible, manifest disease or some other unwanted state
4. prevention of the recurrence of an illness or other unwanted phenomenon.

Prevention is more usually classified into primary, secondary and tertiary, but Tannahill (1985) admits that there is no consensus for a standard definition of the three levels.

In relation to disease prevention, the concept of health protection makes it more unlikely that people will encounter hazards in the environment. The word environment is used in the broadest sense and is taken to mean political, legislative and social as well as physical. Health protection has been defined as '… comprising legal or fiscal controls, other regulations and policies and voluntary codes of practice, aimed at the enhancement of positive health and the prevention of ill health' (Downie et al 1996). These will include public health

measures, legislation such as banning smoking in the workplace and public places and plans such as the UK National Environmental Action Plan (Department of the Environment & Health 1997). Health protection is about making healthy choices easier choices.

The major causes of mortality and morbidity in modern populations have been identified (Locker 1997) as:

- cardiovascular disease
- cancer
- road traffic accidents
- alcohol-related problems
- suicide
- respiratory disorders
- congenital and genetic disorders
- sexually transmitted disease, including AIDS.

The majority of these are associated with one or two risk factors, which may be modified to prevent disease, disability and death (Locker 1997). *Our Healthier Nation* (Department of Health 1998a) sets clear targets for improvement by the year 2010 in four of these priority areas:

1. Heart disease and stroke – to reduce the death rate from these and related illnesses among people aged under 65 years by at least a further third.
2. Accidents – to reduce these by at least a fifth.
3. Cancer – to reduce the death rate by at least a further fifth. This follows on from the initial recommendations in the *Health of the Nation* (Department of Health 1992).
4. Mental health – to reduce the death rate from suicide and undetermined injury by at least a further sixth.

Saving Lives: Our Healthier Nation (Department of Health 1999c) identifies the action that will be taken to achieve these targets. For example, contracts for health will be implemented in relation to coronary heart disease and stroke, which will identify what the individual citizen, local partnerships and government must do. A major focus within this three-way partnership is on the Healthy Citizens programme which will ensure that people have the knowledge and expertise to better understand health risks and decide on the balance between individual risk and personal freedom. Three strands are identified: NHS Direct and the Health Skills and Expert Patients programmes. For example, in relation to coronary heart disease (CHD) and stroke, the Health Skills programme will include training for members of the public in defibrillator use and the Expert Patients programme will enable people with vascular disease to manage their own condition. The implementation of this contract will be through the National Service Framework for Coronary Heart Disease (Department of Health 1998c) and a high-level task force, accountable to the Chief Medical Officer at the Department of Health, will ensure progress towards achieving the targets that have been set.

Recent research has also identified statistically that being male is a risk factor in itself (Office for National

Statistics 1997). Men have a life expectancy of 73.9 years (women 79.2 years), one in four men will die from a heart attack and one in five men will die prematurely before the age of 75 from heart and circulatory diseases, such as strokes. One in three men will have cancer diagnosed at some point in their lives with one in four eventually dying from it (Imperial Cancer Research Fund 1997). Male health also shows regional variations and men living in the north of England have a premature death rate 38% higher than those in the south-east (British Heart Foundation 1997). Male health can also be related to social class and culture in that the death rate from CHD and strokes for unskilled workers is three times higher than for professionals and 36% higher for South-Asian males (British Heart Foundation 1997). The most significant factor that makes being male such a health risk is lifestyle. Men are more likely to be obese (44% in England), smokers (28%), drink more than the recommended alcohol limit (27%) and take insufficient exercise (only 31% are active enough to provide cardiac protection) (British Heart Foundation 1997).

Traditionally, men have also avoided seeking health advice and are generally unaware of the health promotion activities available in GP practices (Brewer 1998). A new report discusses the issue of men's public health in the light of the green paper, *Our Healthier Nation*, and focuses on employment, crime, the changing social role of men and the educational under-achievement of boys (Men's Health Forum 1999).

Disease prevention is also assisted by national strategies for health which include screening and vaccination programmes. These are both methods of primary prevention. Screening can be defined as the active early diagnosis of disease or risk factors for disease as a prelude to intervention designed to prevent onset or progression (Locker 1997). Screening programmes may be mass ones, such as those for breast and cervical cancer, designed to screen large numbers of the population on a voluntary basis or selective, such as those directed towards a high-risk group. Routine screening also occurs: an example of which is screening of the newborn for congenital abnormalities. Screening may reduce morbidity and mortality by identifying individuals at the earliest stage of the disease process, although some studies show disappointing results for multiphase screening for CHD (Stoate 1989) and there are psychological and other costs which must be weighed against the benefits (Locker 1997).

Revealing previously undiagnosed hypertension resulted in greater absenteeism from work, lower self-esteem and problems in marital relationships (Mossey 1981). Also, evidence of the lasting effect of labelling can be seen in a study where some people had been diagnosed as being hypertensive, then given a clean bill of health following further testing: more depression and a lower level of general health was reported than in a control group (Bloom & Monterossa 1981). A negative result may also have lasting effects, reinforcing unhealthy lifestyles and the idea that the individual is immune to that disease (Tijmstra & Bieleman 1987).

Ethical issues are a particular consideration in immunisation programmes as well as with other health promotion activities. Health promoters have a duty to provide care that respects the rights and individual needs of each of their clients but, in their role as preventive health care workers, they also have a duty to promote and work towards the overall health of the local community (Sampson 1998). This may create ethical conflict when the good of society is at variance with the rights of the individual to make free choice. Seedhouse (1988) has created the 'ethical grid' based on the four ethical principles of beneficence, non-maleficence, justice and respect for autonomy (Beauchamp & Childress 1989), with personal autonomy at its core. He states that autonomy is dependent on the person having sufficient knowledge, understanding and ability to make choices and take decisions based on Mill's utilitarianism (Trusted 1987).

Seedhouse (1988) also states that autonomy should likewise be respected so that, once the decision has been made, the health worker should accept the choice. The two statements at the core of the 'ethical grid' are 'respect persons equally' and 'serve needs before wants'. Kant states that moral behaviour is dependent upon people being treated as ends in themselves and never merely as means (Seedhouse 1988). This suggests that the state must not see herd immunity as paramount, because immunisation of each child, for

---

Top Tips

1 Check what your client already knows and believes about their lifestyle and how it affects their health

2 Provide information to fill knowledge gaps and inaccurate health beliefs

3 Develop partnerships where the client remains in control of choices and changes

4 Recognise that not all clients wish to change

5 A number of clients may need help to understand the implications of their lifestyle choices

6 Let the client decide what, when and how to change

7 Jointly formulate an action plan when the client is ready

8 Remember, success is more likely when the client has thought about the change over a period of time

9 Success is also more likely when the client is prepared for how they will feel during the change

10 It may help to discuss alternative coping strategies for when the client is faced with tempting situations.

example, might be construed as a means only to the end of complete resistance to these diseases in our society (Sampson 1998). Although this may seem a beneficent ideal it would violate the individual's rights as defined by Kant. Dissenting parents would seem to take the consequentialist's view that they accept the risk of infection because they are not prepared to take the risk of immunisation (Sampson 1998). This may pose a dilemma for the health worker, who may be concerned about meeting the child immunisation targets.

Glossary

Consequentialism   Being concerned with ends as well as means
Health gain   Health gain is seen as adding years to life and life to years. This concept includes increasing life expectancy by a reduction in premature deaths and improving well-being and quality of life
Unconditional positive regard   The quality of totally respecting the worth and dignity of a person, irrespective of whether you personally like the person or agree with their views or behaviour
Utilitarianism   The greatest good for the greatest number of people. One of the main problems with this approach is that, if the aim of all actions is to achieve the greatest good, does this justify harm or injustice to a few if society benefits?

References

Acheson D 1982 Public health in England: Report of the Committee of Inquiry into the Future Development of the Public Health Function. HMSO, London

Aggleton P 1991 Health. Routledge, London

Aggleton P, Homans H 1987 Educating about AIDS. National Health Services Training Authority, Bristol

Annett H, Rifkin S 1988 Guidelines for rapid appraisal to assess community health needs. World Health Organization (WHO), Geneva.

Armstrong P 1982 The myth of meeting needs in adult education and community development. Critical Social Policy 2(2):24–37.

Aveyard P, Cheng K K, Almond J, Sherratt E et al 1999 Cluster randomised controlled trial of expert system based on the transtheoretical ('stages of change') model for smoking prevention and cessation in schools. British Medical Journal 319:948–953.

Beauchamp T L, Childress J F 1989 Principles of biomedical ethics. Oxford University Press, Oxford.

Bell J, Billington D R, Macdonald M, Drummond N, Thompson G 1985 Annotated bibliography of health education research completed in Britain from 1948–1978 and 1979–1983. Scottish Health Education Group, Edinburgh.

Blackburn C 1992 Improving health and welfare work with families in poverty. Open University Press, Buckingham.

Blaxter M 1990 Health & lifestyles. Tavistock/Routledge, London.

Blaxter M, Patterson E 1982 Mothers and daughters: a three generational study of health attitudes and health behaviour. Heinneman, London.

Bloom J, Monterossa S 1981 Hypertension labelling and sense of well-being. American Journal of Public Health 71:1228–1232.

Bradshaw J 1972 The concept of social need. New Society 19:640–643.

Brewer S 1998 Promoting male health. Practice Nursing 9(9):25–27.

British Heart Foundation 1997 Coronary heart disease statistics. BHF, London.

Carter N, O'Driscoll M L 2000 Life begins at forty! Should the route to promoting exercise in elderly people also start in their forties? Physiotherapy 86(2):85–93.

Catan L, Dennison C, Coleman J 1996 Getting through: effective communication in the teenage years. BT Forum, London.

Dennison C 1998 Get through to the young. Practice Nurse 16:549–553.

Department of Health (DoH) 1989 Working for patients. HMSO, London.

Department of Health (DoH) 1992 The health of the nation. HMSO, London.

Department of Health (DoH) 1997a Health action zones: invitation to bid. HMSO, London.

Department of Health (DoH) 1997b The new NHS: modern, dependable. HMSO, London.

Department of Health (DoH) 1998a Our healthier nation: a contract for health. HMSO, London.

Department of Health (DoH) 1998b The Report of the Independent Inquiry into Inequalities in Health (the Acheson Inquiry). HMSO, London.

Department of Health (DoH) 1998c A first class service – quality in the new NHS. HMSO, London.

Department of Health (DoH) 1999a Reducing health inequalities: an action report. Our Healthier Nation. DoH, London.

Department of Health (DoH) 1999b CMO's Update 23: a communication to all doctors from the Chief Medical Officer. DoH, London.

Department of Health (DoH) 1999c Saving lives: our healthier nation. HMSO, London.

Department of Health (DoH) 2000 The NHS plan. The Stationery Office, London.

Department of Health (DoH) 2001 National service framework for older people. Modern standards and service models. The Stationery Office, London.

Department of the Environment & Health 1997 The UK National Environmental Action Plan. HMSO, London.

Donovan C 1998 Teenagers views on the general practice consultation and provision of contraception. British Journal of General Practice 47:715–718.

Donovan C, McCarthy S 1988 Is there a place for adolescent screening in general practice? Health Trends 20:64.

Downie R S, Tannahill C, Tannahill A 1996 Health promotion: models and values, 2nd edn. Oxford University Press, Oxford.

Doyal L 1995 What makes women sick: gender and the political economy of health. Macmillan Press, Hampshire.

Dubos R 1959 The mirage of health. Harper & Row, New York.

Epstein R, Rice P, Wallace P 1989 Teenagers' health concerns: implications for primary health care professionals. Journal of the Royal College of General Practitioners 39:247–249.

Evans S, Robinson M 1999 Take action to tackle health inequalities. Practice Nurse 17:218–222.

Ewles L, Simnett I 1992 Promoting health: a practical guide, 2nd edn. Scutari Press, London.

Farrant W, Russell J 1985 Health Education Council Publications: a case study in the production, distribution and use of health information. HEC, London.

Gatherer A, Parfit J, Porter E, Vessey M 1979 Is health education effective? Health Education Council, London.

Gillies E, Aitchison T, Macdonald J, Grant S 1999 Outcomes of a 12 week functional exercise programme for institutionalised elderly people. Physiotherapy 85(7):349–357.

Goddard E 1994 Teenage drinking in London. HMSO, London.

Green I W, Lewis F M 1986 Measurement and evaluation in health education and health promotion. Mayfield, California.

Grimley Evans J, Goldacre M J, Hodkinson M, Lamb S, Savory M 1992 Health: abilities and wellbeing in the third age. Carnegie UK Trust, Dunfermline.

Hawtin M, Hughes G, Percy-Smith J 1998 Community profiling: auditing social needs. Open University Press, Buckingham.

Helman C G 1990 Culture, health and illness, 2nd edn. Wright, London.

Hirst T 1997 Local health needs assessment for general practice patient populations. Practice Nurse 14(9):566–568.

Hooper J, Longworth P 1998 Health needs assessment in primary health care: a workbook for primary care teams. Department of Health (DoH), Leeds.

Imperial Cancer Research Fund (ICRF) 1997 Cancer statistics fact sheet. ICRF, London.

Jacobson L D, Wilkinson C E 1994 Review of teenage health: time for a new direction. British Journal of General Practice 44:420–424.

Jewitt C 1995 Sexual history taking in general practice. The HIV Project, London.

Johnson A, Wadsworth J, Wellings K, Field J 1994 Sexual attitudes and lifestyles. Blackwell, Oxford.

Jones L J 1994 The social context of health and health work. Macmillan Publications, London.

Kanfer F H, Goldstein A P 1986 Helping people change. Pergamon Press, Oxford.

King's Fund 1988 Promoting health among elderly people. King's Fund, London.

Levy L 1999 Taking a patient's sexual history. Practice Nursing 10(2):34–36.

Lloyd B, Lucas K 1998 Smoking in adolescence. Routledge, London.

Locker D 1997 Prevention and health promotion. In: Scrambler G (ed) Sociology as applied to medicine, 4th edn. W B Saunders, London.

Lorig K 1992 Patient education: a practical approach. Mosby – Year Book, St. Louis.

McPherson A, Macfarlane A, Donovan C 1996 The health of adolescents in primary care: how to promote adolescent health in your practice. Royal College of General Practitioners & National Adolescent & Student Health Unit, London.

Maslow A H 1966 Motivation and personality. Harper & Row, New York.

Matthews P 1998 Sexual history taking in primary care. In: Carter Y, Moss C, Weyman A (eds) RCGP handbook of sexual health in primary care. RCGP, London.

Mawer C 1999 Preventing teenage pregnancy, supporting teenage mothers. British Medical Journal 7200:1713–1714.

Men's Health Forum 1999 Men's health – a public health review. Men's Health Review, London.

Miller P, Plant M 1996 Drinking, smoking and illicit drug use among 15 and 16 year olds in the UK. British Medical Journal 313:394–397.

Mossey J 1981 Psychosocial consequences of labelling. Clinical Investigative Medicine 4:201–207.

Murray S A, Graham L J C 1995 Practice based health needs assessment: use of four methods in a small neighbourhood. British Medical Journal 310:1443–1448.

Naidoo J, Wills J 1995 Health promotion: foundations for practice. Baillière Tindall, London.

Neighbour R 1997 The inner consultation. Petroc Press, Newbury.

Nutbeam D 1986 Health Promotion Glossary 1(1):113–126.

Office for National Statistics 1997 Population trends. HMSO, London.

Ory M G, Abeles R P, Lipman P D (eds) 1992 Aging, health and behavior. Sage Publications, Newbury Park.

Parsons T 1972 The social system. Free Press, Glencoe, Illinois. In: Jaco E, Gartley E (eds) Patients physicians and illness: a sourcebook in behavioural science and health. Collier-Macmillan, London, 117.

Peate I 1997 Taking a sexual health history: the role of the practice nurse. British Journal of Nursing 6(17):978–983.

Percival J 1999 Health promotion. In: Royal College of Nursing (RCN) Practice Nurse Association Handbook. RCN, London.

Prochaska J O, DiClemente C C 1984 Towards a comprehensive model of change: treating addictive behaviours. Plenum Press, New York.

Raeburn J, Rootman I 1998 People-centred health promotion. John Wiley, Chichester.

Richman J 1987 Medicine and health. Longman, London.

Rogers C R 1983 Freedom to learn for the eighties. Charles E Mervil, Ohio.

Rowe A, Mitchinson S, Morgan M, Carey L 1997 Health profiling: all you need to know. John Moores University & Premier Health NHS Trust, Liverpool.

Royal College of Nursing (RCN) 1993 The GP practice population profile: a framework for every member of the primary health care team. RCN, London.

Sampson D 1998 Immunisation: identifying and resolving the ethical issues. Community Practitioner 71(4):133–135.

Seedhouse D 1986 Health: the foundations for achievement. John Wiley, Chichester.

Seedhouse D 1988 Ethics: the heart of health care. John Wiley, Chichester.

Shanks J, Kheraj S, Fish S 1995 Better way of assessing health needs in primary care. British Medical Journal 310:480–481.

Skelton D A, McLaughlin A W 1996 Training functional ability in old age. Physiotherapy 82(3):159–167.

Smith A, Jacobson B (eds) 1989 The nation's health: a strategy for the 1990s. King's Fund, London.

Smith G, Cantley C 1985 Assessing health care: a study in organisational evaluation. Open University Press, Milton Keynes.

Social Exclusion Unit 1999 Teenage pregnancy (Cm 4342). Department of Health, London.

Stoate H 1989 Can health screening damage your health? Journal of the Royal College of General Practitioners 39:193–195.

Swage T 1999 Skills to assess the nation's health needs. Practice Nurse 17:79–82.

Tannahill A 1985 Reclassifying prevention. Public Health 99:364–366.

Tannahill A 1992 Epidemiology and health promotion. In: Bunton R, Macdonald G (eds) Health promotion: disciplines and diversity. Routledge, London.

Tester S, Meredith B 1987 Ill-informed? Policy Studies Institute, London.

Tijmstra T, Bieleman B 1987 The psychological impact of mass screening for cardiovascular risk factors. Family Practitioner 4:287–290.

Tones K 1995 Health education as empowerment. In: Health promotion today. Health Education Authority, London.

Tones K, Tilford S 1996 Health education: effectiveness, efficiency and equity, 2nd edn. Chapman and Hall, London.

Townsend P 1984 Inequalities in the city of Bristol: a preliminary review of statistical evidence. University of Bristol, Bristol.

Townsend P, Davidson N 1990 Inequalities in health: the Black Report. Penguin, London.

Trusted J 1987 Moral principles and social values. Routledge & Kegan Paul, London.

Twinn S, Dauncey J, Carnell J 1990 The process of health profiling. Health Visitors Association, London.

Velicer W, Norman G J, Fava J L, Prochaska J O et al 1999 Testing 40 predictions from the transtheoretical model. Addictive Behaviour 24:455–469.

Victor C R 1990 What is health? A study of the lay beliefs of older people. Journal of the Institute of Health Education 28(1):10–15.

Watson D L, Tharp R G 1985 Self-directed behavior: self-modification for personal adjustment. Wadsworth, Stamford, CT.

Wetton T 1996 Suggestions for discussing sexual health. In: Practice makes perfect: a sexual health resource for primary care. Bexley & Greenwich Health, London.

Whitehead M 1987 The health divide: inequalities in health in the 1980's. Health Education Authority, London.

Williams J, Harvey J, Jacobson B 1995 Local application of national strategy. In: Health promotion today. Health Education Authority, London.

Williams R 1983 Concepts of health: an analysis of lay logic. Sociology 17: 185–204.

WHO 1984 Health promotion: a discussion document on the concepts and principles. World Health Organization, Copenhagen.

WHO 1986 Ottawa Charter for Health Promotion. World Health Organization, Geneva.

Wright D, Henderson M, Raab G et al 2000 Extent of regretted sexual intercourse among young teenagers in Scotland: a cross sectional survey. British Medical Journal 7244:1243–1244.

Wright J, Pearl L 1995 Knowledge and experience of young people regarding drug misuse 1969–1994. British Medical Journal 310:20–24.

Further reading

Ewles L, Simnett I 1999 Promoting health: a practical guide, 4th edn. Scutari Press, Harrow.

Naidoo J, Wills J 1995 Health promotion: foundations for practice. Baillière Tindall, London.

McPherson A, Macfarlane A, Donovan C 1996 The health of adolescents in primary care: how to promote adolescent health in your practice. Royal College of General Practitioners & National Adolescent & Student Health Unit, London.

Rowe A, Mitchinson S, Morgan M, Carey L 1997 Health profiling, all you need to know. John Moores University & Premier Health NHS Trust, Liverpool.

3

BLOOD DISORDERS

Frances Simpson

Key Issues

■ Blood disorders are relatively common, and careful history taking and assessment is needed

■ Patients with blood disorders may present with seemingly unrelated symptoms

■ Blood disorders, and particularly anaemia in the elderly, can be easily missed and the cause remain undiagnosed

■ Anaemia is not a diagnosis. It is an abnormal clinical finding requiring an explanation for its cause

Introduction

This chapter, which is devoted to blood disorders, explains terminology and discusses common conditions. We all know blood is essential for life and is one of the most examined substances in terms of diagnosis of ill health and disease.

Blood composition

Erythrocytes (red blood cells) form 45% of a blood sample and are known as the haematocrit. Leucocytes (white blood cells) and platelets form less than 1% of blood volume. Plasma forms the remaining 55% of whole blood. The blood's colour varies from scarlet (rich with O_2) to dark red (O_2 poor). The pH is between 7.35 and 7.45. The volume of blood in healthy males is 5–6 litres and in healthy females is 4–5 litres.

Plasma

Plasma is 90% water; 8% by weight of plasma volume = plasma proteins, of which 60% is albumin, acting as a carrier.

Formed elements of blood

Erythrocytes or red blood cells (RBCs) are 7.5–8.0 μm in diameter. They are, biconcave discs with no nucleus and are described as 'little bags' of the specialised protein haemoglobin.

Normoblasts (nucleated red cells) appear in the blood if erythropoiesis is occurring outside the marrow (extramedullary erythropoiesis) and also with some marrow diseases (reticulocyte cell count will give a rough index of the rate of RBC formation).

Erythropoietin production will be stimulated if blood oxygen levels are lower than normal:
■ in haemorrhage or excess RBC destruction
■ if reduced availability of oxygen to the blood, e.g. at higher altitude or pneumonia
■ if increased tissue demands for oxygen, e.g. aerobic exercise.

Conversely, erythropoietin production will be low in severe renal disease despite anaemia being present. This is due to inadequate production of the hormone erythropoietin, 90% of which is produced in the kidney, the other 10% in the liver.

Erythropoietin therapy is used intravenously (IV) or subcutaneously (SC) for end-stage renal disease. It is also under trial for post-chemotherapy or bone marrow transplantation; and in anaemia of chronic disorders, e.g. cancer, rheumatoid arthritis.

Approximately 65% of the body's iron supply is in haemoglobin. The remainder is stored in the liver, spleen and bone marrow. Iron, being toxic, is stored inside cells as protein–iron complexes such as ferritin and haemosiderin. In the blood, iron binds to the transport protein transferrin from where developing erythrocytes take up iron as needed. As we know, anaemias occur with iron, vitamin B_{12} or folate deficiencies, and in renal disease, with deficiency of erythropoietin. Anaemias also occur with amino acid, thyroxine or androgen deficiency, but these are possibly due to lower tissue oxygen consumption rather than directly due to the effect of these deficiencies on erythropoiesis.

Anaemia also occurs in vitamin C deficiency and in vitamin E and riboflavin deficiencies but it is not yet known whether this is due to the effect of these deficiencies on erythropoiesis. Iron in small amounts is lost each day in faeces, perspiration and urine. In women, loss is increased by menstrual flow. The average daily loss of iron is 0.9 mg in men and 1.7 mg in women.

Anaemia

Anaemia is normally defined as haemoglobin (Hb) concentration in the blood of less than 13.5 g/dl in adult males and less than 11.5 g/dl in adult females (levels of 14.09 g/dl and 12.0 g/dl are sometimes used).

From the age of 3 months to puberty, less than 11.0 g/dl haemoglobin concentration indicates anaemia.

❶ Taking a careful history in patients with blood disorders is particularly important, as mild anaemia will often reveal no symptoms or signs whereas these will usually be present with a Hb of below 9–10 g/dl. Bear in mind that severe anaemia (Hb 6.0 g/dl) of gradual onset can produce few symptoms in a healthy young adult whereas some people with mild anaemia may be severely incapacitated.

Clinically, adaptations to anaemia will occur in the cardiovascular system, with increased stroke volume and tachycardia:

- If anaemia is rapid there are likely to be more symptoms as the cardiovascular system will have less time to adapt.
- In the elderly, anaemia will be less well tolerated due to the lack of oxygen in organs as a result of increased cardiac output and tachycardia.
- Babies may suffer from anaemia after about 4–6 months of age when neonatal iron stores are declining. This can be prevented by the addition of iron-fortified cereal and other solid foods to the diet at 6 months of age (Nathan & Oski 1992).

Assessment

Subjective assessment

Taking a careful history gives you the chance to build up a relationship with the patient so that a trusting partnership is established. This may be particularly helpful when patients, who tend to get anxious over blood tests and results, return to see you for further investigations and possibly treatment.

Using open-ended questions you will need to discover whether the patient is experiencing:

1. Shortness of breath, particularly when exercising.
2. Feelings of weakness, tiredness or lethargy.
3. Swollen ankles.
4. Any changes with bowel habits.
5. Haemorrhoids.
6. Weight loss.
7. Headache, chest pain or palpitations.
8. In pre-menopausal women ask if pregnant, possibly pregnant or postnatal.
9. It will be necessary in these women to ask about their menstrual cycle and any menorrhagia. This can be difficult to assess. Ask about clots, use of pads and tampons and whether periods are prolonged.
10. Family history may reveal inherited haematological disorders, e.g. sickle cell or thalassaemia.
11. Past and present medical history, noting particularly if Crohn's disease or coeliac disease present.
12. Past surgery, particularly partial or total gastrectomy – also splenectomy.
13. Symptoms of peripheral neuropathy.

14. Current drug therapy should be ascertained, including over-the-counter (OTC) medicines and the use of aspirin or nonsteroidal anti-inflammatory drugs (NSAIDs) noted.
15. Dietary intake, e.g. whether vegan.
16. Alcohol consumption.
17. Smoking history.
18. Whether blood donor and, if so, how often.

Following travel abroad:

1. ask if travel taken in area where malaria exists.
2. consider possibility of HIV infection.
3. possible hookworm infection.

In the elderly:

1. ask about chest pain or, if already suffering from angina, whether it has worsened
2. vision may have worsened as a result of retinal haemorrhages (in severe anaemia)
3. intermittent claudication is a possibility.

In the psychiatrically disturbed, consider the possibility of self-induced haemorrhage.

Objective assessment

The history will provide you with a guide as to the physical examination required. This in its turn will lead you to possible diagnoses.

General approach

- Observe general appearance, noting pallor and whether cyanosis present.
- Also notice if jaundiced.
- Pallor of mucous membranes may be present but this usually only occurs if the haemoglobin level is less than 9–10 g/dl.
- Check weight, height, blood pressure and pulse rate. Check temperature if history reveals possible presence of fever.

Physical assessment

- Inspect the conjunctival mucosa for pallor.
- Examine the mouth for ulcers, any sepsis and the tongue for a red beefy inflamed looking appearance which may be painful (glossitis).
- Examine the corners of the mouth for any fissuring or ulceration (angular cheilosis).
- Examine the nails for any spoon shape. The nail beds may be pale but only in severe anaemia.
- Observe the skin for any rashes or purpura.
- Check respiratory rate.
- Examine chest and heart (see Chapters 7 and 8 for examination techniques). This is of particular importance with the elderly when signs of congestive cardiac failure may be present.
- When examining the chest also include palpation of lymph nodes for tenderness and/or enlargement. If nodes are enlarged or tender it will be important to assess whether enlargement of lymph nodes is

widespread or in one area only. Using the pads of index and middle fingers, palpate gently with light pressure which can gradually be increased. Starting with the head and neck, palpate the preauricular; parotid and mastoid nodes (postauricular). Continue to the occipital, submandibular, submental and anterior cervical nodes. Ask the patient to relax in order to drop the clavicles, then feel for and palpate the supraclavicular nodes lateral to the sternomastoid muscle. Then find the infraclavicular nodes below the clavicles and palpate them. Axillary nodes can be assessed by palpating high in the patients axilla and pressing against the axillary muscles and the chest wall.

- Abdominal examination, including assessment of liver and spleen (see Chapter 9 for examination technique).
- After carrying out the abdominal examination, while the patient is lying supine, palpate the inferior superficial inguinal (femoral) lymph nodes. Press gently below the junction of the saphenous and femoral veins (vertical group). To palpate the superior superficial inguinal lymph nodes, follow the course of the saphenous veins from the inguinal area to the abdomen (horizontal group) (Bates 1987).
- Examine for ankle oedema.

The history and physical assessment should be documented.

Diagnostic tests

Once you have taken the history and carried out the physical assessment it will be necessary to decide on appropriate tests.

If anaemia is suspected:

- The full blood count (FBC), which will include white cell differential, will give an indication as to the type of anaemia if present, plus other useful information (Table 3A).

If the history suggests:

- Urine should be checked for haematuria and, if positive, sent to the laboratory for microscopy.
- Stools should be checked for occult blood from the digestive tract. Three consecutive stool specimens should be sent to the laboratory together.
- If hookworm infection (patients from tropical or subtropical areas) is a possibility, check stool sample by sending to the laboratory for microscopy to look for ova.

Plan

If necessary, referral of patients for other investigations may be required, including:

Table 3A *Normal values*

Test	Males	Females	Males and females
Haemoglobin	13.5–17.5 g/dl	11.5–15.5 g/dl	
Red cells (erythrocytes)	$4.5-6.5 \times 10^{12}/l$	$3.9-5.6 \times 10^{12}/l$	
PCV (haematocrit)	40–52%	36–48%	
MCV			80–95 fl
MCH			27–34 pg
MCHC			20–35 g/dl
White cells (leukocytes)			
total			$4.0-11.0 \times 10^9/l$
neutrophils			$2.5-7.5 \times 10^9/l$
lymphocytes			$1.5-3.5 \times 10^9/l$
monocytes			$0.2-0.8 \times 10^9/l$
eosinophils			$0.04-0.44 \times 10^9/l$
basophils			$0.01-0.1 \times 10^9/l$
Platelets			$150-400 \times 10^9/l$
Red cells mass	30 ± 5 ml/kg	25 ± 5 ml/kg	
Plasma volume	45 ± 5 ml/kg	45 ± 5 ml/kg	
Serum iron			10–30 µmol/l
Total iron-binding capacity			40–75 µmol/l (2.0–4.0 g/l as transferrin)
Serum ferritin*	40–340 µg/l	14–150 µg/l	
Serum vitamin B_{12}*			160–925 ng/l
Serum folate*			3.0–15.0 µg/l
Red cell folate*			160–640 µg/l

* Normal ranges differ with different commercial kits.
MCH, mean corpuscular haemoglobin; MCHC, mean corpuscular haemoglobin concentration; MCV, mean corpuscular volume; PCV, packed cell volume.

- if bleeding from the gastrointestinal (GI) tract is suspected, oesophagogastroduodenoscopy (OGD), proctoscopy, sigmoidoscopy and colonoscopy should be performed.
- chest X-ray.

Differential diagnoses

Many forms of anaemia will present in primary care. It is important to remember that, although not covered in this chapter, you may see patients in your surgery with one of the following haematological malignancies. This could be:

1. (a) Acute lymphoblastic leukaemia (ALL) in a child aged usually between 2 and 10 years. The child may be suffering from easy bruising, purpura and mucous membrane bleeding with fatigue and obvious pallor. Alternatively, the child may present with fever and infection, such as sinusitis or purulent otitis, which has not responded to oral antibiotics. Bone pain may also feature when you take the child's history (Friebert & Shurin 1998). On examination, swollen lymph nodes and enlarged liver and spleen are likely. The child may be acutely ill and, in all cases, will need urgent referral to specialist care.

(b) Acute myeloid leukaemia (AML), which is a common form of leukaemia seen in adults and the elderly. Again, the patient is likely to be acutely ill and needing urgent referral to secondary care.

(c) (i) Chronic myeloid leukaemia (CML), mainly seen in patients between 40 and 60 years but also occurring in babies, children and the very elderly. The patient may be asymptomatic or may complain of:
- night sweats, weight loss, anorexia and fatigue
- dyspnoea
- bruising, epistaxis or menorrhagia.

An urgent blood screen will be essential and may show anaemia with leucocytosis $> 50 \times 10^9$/dl and may be $> 500 \times 10^9$/dl.

(c) (ii) Chronic lymphatic leukaemia, which occurs mainly in the elderly. It is rare in the under-40s age group. It may be found on routine FBC. However, the patient may present to you with:
- herpes zoster
- anaemia causing dyspnoea
- bruising or purpura.

FBC will show
- lymphocytes raised to 300×10^9/dl or more
- 70–90% white cells appearing as small lymphocytes
- thrombocytopenia.

If the patient is acutely ill, specialist care will be needed urgently.

2. Malignant lymphomas, e.g. Hodgkin's disease, which peaks in young adults age 20–30 years and again after age 50 years. It is rare in children. There is a 2:1 male predominance. A patient might present to you with:
- painless non-tender asymmetrical, firm, discrete and rubbery enlargement of the superficial lymph nodes.
- cervical predominance in 60–70% of cases.
  axillary   10–15%
  inguinal   6–12%

FBC will show normochromic, normocytic anaemia. ESR will be raised. Diagnosis will normally be made by lymph node biopsy.

Classification of anaemia

❶ The full blood count (FBC) will give an indication as to the type of anaemia present plus other useful information. Thus:

- The type of anaemia from the size of red cells and the haemoglobin content can be ascertained as to the likely nature of underlying detect (Table 3.1). The mean corpuscular volume (MCV) and mean corpuscular haemoglobin (MCH) are measured.
- Abnormal red cell indices may suggest an abnormality before anaemia has developed: macrocytosis (large red cells) with early vitamin B_{12} or folate deficiency or alcohol excess.
- Abnormal indices may indicate a disorder in which anaemia does not occur, e.g. thalassaemia trait, where

Table 3.1 *Classification of anaemia (From Hoffbrand & Pettit 1999, with permission of Blackwell Science.)*

Microcytic, hypochromic	Normocytic, normochromic	Macrocytic
MCV < 80 fl	MCV 80–95 fl	MCV > 95 fl
MCV < 27 pg	MCH > 26 pg	
Iron deficiency	Many haemolytic anaemias	Megaloblastic: vitamin B_{12} or folate deficiency
Thalassaemia	Secondary anaemia	
Anaemia of chronic diseases (some cases)	After acute blood loss	Non-megaloblastic: alcohol, liver disease, myelodysplasia, aplastic anaemia, etc.
Lead poisoning	Mixed deficiencies	
Sideroblastic anaemia (some cases)	Bone marrow failure, e.g. post-chemotherapy, infiltration by carcinoma, etc. Renal disease	

red cells are small (microcytic) but due to increase in their numbers haemoglobin is within normal range.

- Mean corpuscular volume may be high: in newborn babies it drops and rises throughout childhood to normal adult range.
- In normal pregnancy there is a rise in MCV even in the absence of other causes of macrocytosis, e.g. folate deficiency.
- Leucocyte and platelet count may aid diagnosis

Measurement will help in ascertaining whether anaemia is 'pure' or due to lowering in red cells, granulocytes and platelets, which could indicate a marrow defect. In haemorrhage or haemolysis, neutrophil and platelet counts may be raised. In infections, but also in leukaemias, leucocytes may be raised.

In anaemia a blood film will be examined for any other abnormality of cells flagged up by the FBC and will aid diagnosis by assessing the presence or absence of abnormal cells.

Specific disorders

Let us look now at *iron deficiency* and other *hypochromic anaemias*. Iron deficiency is the most common cause of anaemia throughout the world. It causes microcytic, hypochromic, anaemia in which the MCV, MCH and mean corpuscular haemoglobin concentration (MCHC) are reduced – the thalassaemias will be considered later. Iron is a common element, but the body has a limited ability to absorb iron and loss of iron due to haemorrhage is frequent.

Haemoglobin, which contains approximately two-thirds of the body's iron, is absorbed into developing erythroblasts in the bone marrow and into reticulocytes. A small amount of plasma iron comes from dietary iron absorbed through the duodenum and jejunum. When red cells are finally broken down their iron is released into the plasma. Some of the iron is also stored in the reticuloendothelial system as haemosiderin and ferritin, the amount dependent on the overall body iron status.

Dietary iron.   In general, meat, particularly liver, is a better source than vegetables, eggs or dairy foods. The Western diet contains on average 10–15 mg of iron from which only 5–10% is normally absorbed. The proportion can be increased by 20–30% in iron deficiency or pregnancy, but most dietary iron remains unabsorbed. Iron absorption occurs through the duodenum and less through the jejunum.

Internal iron exchange is mainly concerned with providing iron for erythropoiesis. Estimated daily iron requirements vary according to age and sex; it is highest in pregnancy, adolescence and menstruating females. If the history leads you to suspect iron deficiency anaemia, the physical assessment will support the diagnosis (Table 3.2).

Table 3.2 *Causes of iron deficiency (From Hoffbrand & Pettit 1999, with permission of Blackwell Science.)*

Chronic blood loss
- uterine
- gastrointestinal, e.g. oesophageal varices, hiatus hernia, peptic ulcer, aspirin (or other nonsteroidal anti-inflammatory drugs (NSAIDs)) ingestion, partial gastrectomy, carcinoma of the stomach, caecum, colon or rectum, hookworm, angiodysplasia, colitis, haemorrhoids, diverticulosis, etc.
- rarely haematuria, haemoglobinuria, pulmonary haemosiderosis, self-inflicted blood loss

Increased demands
- prematurity
- growth
- child-bearing

Malabsorption
- for example, gastrectomy, coeliac disease

Poor diet
- A contributory factor in many countries but rarely the sole cause

Diagnostic tests

- Take blood or order FBC (minimum).
- If anaemia is confirmed by the FBC result (see Table 3.1) but the cause is not obvious, it will be necessary to check the serum ferritin. In iron deficiency anaemia this may be very low (see Table 3A). However, serum ferritin will be normal or raised in the anaemia of chronic disorders.
- If iron deficiency anaemia is confirmed, providing the laboratory does not flag up the need for further testing, locating and treating the cause and giving an iron supplement should replenish iron stores.

Treatment plan

Review patient's diet with them.

❶ Treat the located cause of the anaemia (Table 3.2) e.g. uterine bleeding.

First-line line treatment

- Give prescription for oral ferrous sulphate: 67 mg iron in 200 mg 6-hourly doses for maximum absorption in the duodenum.

Patient education

Advising how to take the iron is very important. Taking it on an empty stomach produces the best results. However, taking it after food will help to reduce gastrointestinal side effects, which can be a problem (Table 3.3).

Vitamin C will improve the uptake of oral iron, so that patients can be advised to increase their intake of

Table 3.3 *Iron absorption (From Hoffbrand & Pettit 1999, with permission of Blackwell Science.)*

Factors favouring absorption	Factors reducing absorption
1. Ferrous form	1. Ferric form
2. Inorganic iron	2. Organic iron
3. Acids – HCl, vitamin C	3. Alkalis – antacids, pancreatic secretions
4. Solublizing agents, e.g. sugars, amino acids	4. Precipitating agents – phytates, phosphates
5. Iron deficiency	5. Iron excess
6. Increased erythropoiesis	6. Decreased erythropoiesis
7. Pregnancy	7. Infection
8. Primary haemochromatosis	8. Tea
	9. Desferrioxamine

Table 3.4 *Failure of response to oral iron (From Hoffbrand & Pettit 1999, with permission of Blackwell Science.)*

- Continuing haemorrhage
- Failure to take tablets
- Wrong diagnosis – especially thalassaemia trait, sideroblastic anaemia
- Mixed deficiency – associated folate or vitamin B_{12} deficiency
- Another cause for anaemia – e.g. malignancy, inflammation
- Malabsorption – this is a rare cause
- Use of slow-release preparation

vitamin C with orange juice, for example. Conversely, antacids will reduce the uptake of oral iron.

Remember to warn patients that their stools may change colour and darken or look black. Constipation can be a problem in the elderly, so careful monitoring will be necessary as faecal impaction can occur (BNF 1999).

Second-line treatment

- If nausea, abdominal pain, constipation or diarrhoea are experienced with ferrous sulphate, try ferrous gluconate (less iron): 37 mg per 300 mg tablet
- If problems with both these preparations are encountered, try ferrous succinate, lactate or fumarate, which may be better but are more expensive
- Elixir is available for children
- Combinations of iron with vitamins are not recommended, except for iron/folic acid combinations in pregnancy
- Note. Slow-release preparations give up most of their iron in the lower intestine, where it cannot be absorbed.

Parenteral iron

- Intramuscular injections of Imferon or Jectofer
- There may be hypersensitive or anaphylactic-type reactions, so only use if urgent requirement, e.g. in late pregnancy
- Note. Haemoglobin will rise no faster than with oral iron, but iron stores are replenished much faster
- Dosage will be estimated according to weight of patient; if unsure, discuss with haematologist
- Always check *British National Formulary (BNF)*, which has an entire chapter dedicated to drugs affecting nutrition and blood (Chapter 9, BNF 1999)
- Iron should be given for 4–6 months in order to correct anaemia and replenish iron stores
- The haemoglobin should rise 2 g/dl every 3–4 weeks.

Review patient at regular intervals and repeat FBC after 3 months (after 1 month, if anaemia is severe). If there is failure of response to iron, consider other possible reasons (Table 3.4). If the cause of continuing anaemia is unclear, refer to GP for further advice.

Anaemia of chronic disorders

❶ This form of anaemia is related to reduced release of iron from macrophages to plasma, reduced cell lifespan and inadequate erythropoietic response. The anaemia will only be corrected by successful treatment of the underlying disease and does not respond to oral iron.

It is found in patients with chronic inflammatory and malignant disease, such as:

- infections, e.g. tuberculosis, osteomyelitis, pneumonia, bacterial endocarditis
- rheumatoid arthritis, systemic lupus erythematosus (SLE), sarcoidosis, Crohn's disease
- carcinoma, lymphoma, sarcoma.

Diagnostic tests

FBC, erythrocyte sedimentation rate (ESR), vitamin B_{12} serum folate, serum iron and total iron-binding capacity (TIBC) should be ordered.

Results

- haemoglobin range 7–10.0 g/dl
- MCV normal or reduced
- ferritin usually normal but may be raised
- serum iron and TIBC normal or reduced.

Diagnosis

Diagnosis may be drug related:

- side effects from e.g. azathioprine and methotrexate
- secondary to gold therapy in rheumatoid arthritis.

If the history and physical assessment leads you to consider chronic blood loss due to, e.g. nonsteroidal anti-inflammatory drugs (NSAIDs), the following *investigations* will be necessary:

Investigations

- check stools for blood
- referral for OGD (gastroscopy)
- if haematuria on urinalysis, send specimen to laboratory for microscopy

- if positive for blood cells, renal scan needs to be carried out and *referral* to renal surgeon for cystoscopy must be made.

Megaloblastic anaemias and macrocytic anaemias

In this group of anaemias deoxyribonucleic acid (DNA) synthesis is impaired, giving rise to the appearance of abnormal erythroblasts in the bone marrow. Megaloblasts are abnormally developing RBCs which are large with nuclei and which fail to mature. Macrocytes will also show up on blood film; these are large cells, which may be round or oval. Thus, macrocytic anaemias caused by megaloblastic haemopoiesis are referred to as megaloblastic anaemias and are usually due to deficiency of vitamin B_{12} or folate.

Vitamin B_{12} (with folic acid) is necessary for DNA synthesis and vitamin B_{12} for neurological functioning. Vitamin B_{12} is absorbed in the terminal ileum after binding to intrinsic factor produced by gastric parietal cells. The body stores of 2–3 mg vitamin B_{12} are sufficient for 3 years; it is available in meats, fish, eggs and dairy produce.

Vegan diets are low in vitamin B_{12}, but not all vegans develop clinical evidence of deficiency.

Causes of vitamin B_{12} deficiency

- Pernicious anaemia – gastric atrophy, probably autoimmune, leading to loss of intrinsic factor production necessary for absorption of vitamin B_{12}.

Incidence is usually in people of over 40 years of age and the condition is associated with other autoimmune problems, e.g. hypothyroidism, Hashimoto's disease, thyrotoxicosis, coeliac disease. It is more common in females than males (ratio 1.6:1), peaking at 60 years. The disease is most common in North Europeans, but is found in all races. It may be familial (e.g. blood group A, blue eyes and early greying of the hair). Ninety per cent of patients will have parietal cell antibodies.

If vitamin B_{12} deficiency is severe, neuropathy affecting peripheral sensory nerves may be evident. Patients, mostly male, report tingling in the feet, difficulty in walking and falling over. Optic atrophy may also occur. The connection between deficiency and neuropathy is not so far understood.

Subjective assessment

When taking the patient's history:

- note any neuropathy as described above
- establish in particular whether total or partial gastrectomy has been carried out
- whether resection of ileum, or Crohn's disease
- any history of diverticulae or inflammatory bowel changes causing competition for available vitamin B_{12}
- tropical sprue, coeliac disease
- vegans, i.e. dietary deficiency.

Investigations

Many patients will be diagnosed when an FBC is carried out when anaemia is suspected. This is because the laboratory will flag up the need for further testing if the original FBC sample shows reduced reticulocyte and white blood count (WBC):

- the blood film may show poikilocytosis (abnormally pencil-shaped RBCs)
- basophilic stippling (denatured ribonucleic acid (RNA)) may be seen.

As a result, the laboratory will request further blood testing, including:

- serum vitamin B_{12} (which will be reduced)
- serum red cell folate, which is likely to be normal or raised
- autoantibody screen, which may show gastric parietal cell antibodies.

Alternatively, if the patient presents to you and the history includes sensory neuropathy, look also for:

- pallor of mucous membranes
- mild jaundice due to excess breakdown of haemoglobin due to inadequate erythrocytosis in bone marrow.

If present:

- order or take blood urgently for FBC when haemoglobin may be less than 6.0/dl, MCV > 95–110 fl although may be normal.
- leucopenia and thrombocytopenia may be seen.

Management

Following blood testing, referral will need to be made to the haemotologist. Unless anaemia is severe, when admission to hospital is indicated, the haematologist will normally establish a treatment protocol immediately. Ideally, test of vitamin B_{12} absorption will be carried out before treatment, e.g. Schilling test. Gastroscopy or barium meal with follow through will be necessary in order to demonstrate possible gastric atrophy and exclude carcinoma of the stomach. However, with long waiting lists and depending on local policy, treatment is often initiated immediately.

Treatment

Intramuscular (IM) injections of hydroxocobalamin, 1 mg, and sometimes folic acid orally, 5 mg once daily, will be started. A response is likely within 24 hours.

- The dose of the vitamin B_{12} replacement hydroxocobalamin 1 mg IM will be between 5 and 10 doses on alternate days in the first 2 weeks.

Patient education

- Patients will need explanation of the cause of their problems but can be reassured that they will normally start to feel much better after a few days of treatment.
- Patients should be warned that they may have some pain at the injection site following administration.
- They may also feel feverish, dizzy or nauseated.

- Patients with any cardiac conditions may suffer with arrhythmias, These patients should be kept at the surgery for a period of approximately 30 min after the initial injection. They should also be warned to be in touch with the surgery immediately if they feel unwell.

Patients will need to be educated as to the need for follow-up doses of vitamin B_{12} at 3-monthly intervals. They will also need explanation of the fact that once well they will need annual blood checks of FBC and thyroid function.

Note. Gastric cancer is twice as high in these patients compared with the normal population.

Folate deficiency

Folate is essential for DNA and RNA synthesis and without it haemopoiesis will be impaired, usually due to inadequate intake of folate in the diet alone or in combination with increased folate utilisation or malabsorption. Any excess cell turnover including pregnancy increases the need for folate (Table 3.5).

Subjective findings

Take a full history, noting in particular the following:
- a sore beefy-red tongue (glossitis)

Table 3.5 *Causes of folate deficiency (From Hoffbrand & Pettit 1999, with permission of Blackwell Science.)*

Nutritional
Especially old age, institutions, poverty, famine, special diets, goat's milk anaemia, etc.

Malabsorption
Tropical sprue, coeliac disease (adult or child). Possible contributory factor to folate deficiency in some patients with partial gastrectomy, extensive jejunal resection or Crohn's disease

Excess utilization
Physiological
- Pregnancy and lactation, prematurity
Pathological
- Haematological diseases, haemolytic anaemias, myelosclerosis
- Malignant disease; carcinoma, lymphoma, myeloma
- Inflammatory diseases; Crohn's disease, tuberculosis, rheumatoid arthritis, psoriasis, exfoliative dermatitis, malaria.

Excess urinary folate loss
Active liver disease, congestive heart failure

Drugs
Anticonvulsants, sulphasalazine

Mixed
Liver disease, alcoholism, intensive care

- cracks in the corners of the mouth, which may be fissured and ulcerated (angular cheilosis)
- easy bruising of the skin.

Objective findings
- Notice pallor, and inspect the mouth carefully for glossitis.
- Inspect corners of the mouth for angular cheilosis.
- Inspect the skin for purpura due to thrombocytopenia (platelet count reduced).

Investigations
Take blood or order (Table 3.6):
- FBC
- serum vitamin B_{12}
- serum folate
- red cell folate.

Results are likely to show:
- macrocytic anaemia MCV > 95 fl (120–140 fl in severe cases) with oval macrocytes
- serum iron and ferritin normal or raised.
  It may be difficult to ascertain combined deficiencies.

Referral
If in doubt, refer to haematologist, as macrocytosis not caused by vitamin B_{12} or folate deficiency will need referral for bone marrow examination.

Therapeutic intervention

Prophylaxis
Folic acid in pregnancy, 400 µg daily preconception and for 12 weeks thereafter. In patients where previous pregnancy resulted in a fetus with a neural tube defect, folic acid 4 mg daily preconception and for first 12 weeks of pregnancy.

Note. Vitamin B_6 hypochromic microcytic anaemia: give vitamin B_6 to patients taking isoniazid for tuberculosis therapy.

Haemolytic anaemias

In severe haemolysis, red cells may survive for only a few days in contrast to the normal 120 days. There are various causes, two of which are described below. On blood testing:
- reticulocyte count will be raised
- folate deficiency usually present.

Specific red cell studies will be necessary.

1. Hereditary haemolytic anaemia: G6PD (glucose-6-phosphate dehydrogenase) deficiency

This occurs due to congenital abnormality of the enzyme system. The red cell membrane requires energy in order to operate, including maintenance of

Table 3.6 *Laboratory tests for vitamin B₁₂ and folate deficiency (From Hoffbrand and Pettit 1999, with permission of Blackwell Science.)*

Test	Normal value*	Result in	
		Vitamin B$_{12}$ deficiency	Folate deficiency
Serum vitamin B$_{12}$	160–925 ng/l	Low	Normal or borderline
Serum folate	3.0–15.0 µg/l	Normal or raised	Low
Red cell folate	160–640 µg/l	Normal or low	Low

*Normal values differ slightly with different commercial kits.

shape and flexibility. In G6PD deficiency, synthesis is impaired probably due to deficiency of the enzyme protein or functional disorder of the enzyme.

Four hundred variants of the enzyme (G6PD) have been described which are abnormal, the commonest being Type B Western and Type A in Africans. It seems that 200 million people worldwide are deficient in the enzyme. It is usually asymptomatic, but problems can occur with certain drugs.

The inheritance is sex-linked: affects males, carried by females. These females have resistance to falciparum malaria, which occurs in West African races and in Mediterranean peoples, and which is occasionally severe in Caucasians.

Haemolysis may occur following infection and fever. It may also occur after ingestion of certain drugs; fava (broad) beans are also implicated. Haemolysis will begin in 1–3 days after ingestion of the drug or 1–2 days after onset of fever and may begin only hours after ingestion of fava beans (Table 3.7).

Table 3.7 *Agents which may cause haemolytic anaemias in G6PD deficiency (From Hoffbrand & Pettit 1999, with permission of Blackwell Science.)*

1. Infections and other acute illnesses, e.g. diabetic ketoacidosis
2. Drugs
   - antimalarials, e.g. primaquine, pamaquine, chloroquine, Fansidar, Maloprim
   - sulphonamides and sulphones, e.g. co-trimoxazole, sulphanilamide, dapsone, Salazopyrin
   - other antibacterial agents, e.g. nitrofurans, chloramphenicol
   - analgesics, e.g. aspirin (moderate doses are safe), phenacetin
   - antihelminths, e.g. beta-naphthol, stibophen, nitrodazole
   - miscellaneous, e.g. vitamin K analogues, naphthalene (moth balls), probenecid
3. Fava beans (possibly other vegetables).

Note. Many common drugs have been reported to precipitate haemolysis in G6PD deficiency, e.g. aspirin, quinine, penicillin, but not at conventional doses.

Subjective assessment

- Patient will describe low back and abdominal pain
- They may notice that their urine is dark red (black sometimes)
- Following fava bean ingestion, severe shock may develop which can be fatal
- History taking will reveal if patient is known to be G6PD deficient
- If G6PD deficient, history taking must focus on discovering the cause, if drug ingestion or fava beans
- If fever and infection are suspected, a description of the possible infection the patient may be suffering from must be elicited.

Objective assessment

- Vital signs: the temperature is likely to be raised if infection is present
- Check for pallor of mucous membranes
- Examine the abdomen, checking in particular for an enlarged spleen
- Check urine, which may look dark/black, but which is unlikely to contain bile
- Send urine for microscopy, as haemoglobin may be present in the urine.

Plan

- Referral to hospital
- In acute phase the deficiency can be difficult to diagnose from blood tests.

Blood tests will show normal between crises. In the Mediterranean population, haemolysis is less likely to be self-limiting.

2. Drug-induced haemolytic anaemia

Some drugs interfere with the lipid component of the RBC membrane (as already stated in G6PD subjects) in normal individuals if drugs are given or taken in large doses, e.g. dapsone or sulfasalazine.

Some drugs may form immune complexes with antibody which then become attached to the RBC membrane when RBC destruction occurs, e.g. quinine, quinidine, rifampicin, antihistamines, chlorpromazine, tetracycline and probenecid. Methyldopa can produce an autoimmune haemolytic anaemia, although the mechanism is not clear.

Treatment

Stop taking the drug.

Genetic defects of haemoglobin: the haemoglobinopathies

Genetic defects of haemoglobin that result in morbidity and mortality worldwide are also the most common genetic disorders worldwide. As well as presenting from known areas of the world, i.e. tropical and subtropical areas, patients will also present in Northern Europe, including the UK, particularly among Greek, Italian, Afro-Caribbean, Asian and Chinese populations (Rochester-Peart 1997).

Haemoglobin molecules in fetal and postnatal life are made up of four globin chains, two α and two non-α chains. Normal adult blood contains haemoglobin A (HbA), which contains two α and two β chains ($\alpha_2 \beta_2$), HbA2 ($\alpha_2 \delta_2$) and a small amount of HbF (fetal) ($\alpha_2 \gamma_2$). Genes for the globin chains appear on chromosome 11 (β globin) and 16 (α globin).

Haemoglobin abnormalities fall into two groups; (a) haemoglobin disorders arising from imbalanced globin chain production – globins produced are structurally normal but their relative amounts are incorrect and lead to the thalassaemias; (b) structural abnormalities of haemoglobin due to alterations in DNA coding for the globin protein, leading to an abnormal amino acid in the globin molecule, and resulting in sickle cell anaemia. As already stated, the switch from fetal to adult haemoglobin takes place at 3–6 months of age although the mechanism is still unclear.

(a) Thalassaemias

In *α-thalassaemia* the α globin gene is altered so α globin synthesis (a$^+$), or abolished (a^0) from red blood cells.

Alpha–thalassaemia traits

In *silent alpha thalassaemia* (–a/aa) only one gene is deleted:

- patients are unlikely to have any symptoms.
- on routine FBC, e.g. during pregnancy or preoperatively, the MCV and MCH may be found to be reduced in a minority of patients.
- haemoglobin electrophoresis will be normal in these patients.
- further studies or DNA analysis will be needed to be certain of the diagnosis.
- patients can be reassured; there is a tendency for the β-thalassaemia trait to be confused with other forms of thalassaemia, producing intense anxiety.

In α-thalassaemia trait (aa/– – or –a/–a) – deletion of one or two genes but asymptomatic:

- in these patients haemoglobin may be normal or minimally reduced
- MCV and MCH are likely to be reduced
- if on routine FBC, a patient is found to have mild anaemia and reduced MCV and MCH, it will be necessary to exclude other causes of anaemia, e.g. iron deficiency.

In haemoglobin H disease (– –/–a) – deletion of three genes:

- In these patients with only one functioning copy of α globin gene/cell, moderate anaemia is common.

Subjective assessment

There is a possibility that these patients, who will be of Afro-Caribbean, Mediterranean or of Far-Eastern origin, will present to you complaining of:

- symptoms of anaemia, made worse for example by pregnancy
- infection
- chronic leg ulceration.

Focus on family history, looking for haematological disorders.

Objective assessment

- Vital signs, including temperature, if infection is present
- Observe whether jaundice is present
- Abdominal examination should be carried out to check for possibility of enlarged spleen.

Investigations

These should include:

- FBC and ESR
- haemoglobin electrophoresis.

Results

These will probably show

- moderate anaemia, with Hb 7–11 g/dl
- MCV and MCH reduced
- haemoglobin electrophoresis may be normal.

Referral

Referral for α/β synthesis studies or DNA analysis may be needed to confirm diagnosis.

Treatment plan

- treat infection
- treat ulceration
- if the patient is pregnant, ensure regular folic acid is taken.

These patients will need to be referred to secondary care, as splenectomy and blood transfusion may be necessary.

Follow up

Monitoring will be necessary, as anaemia is likely to recur.

(b) Beta-thalassaemia syndromes

There are two copies of the β-globin gene normally per cell. An abnormality in one β globin gene results in β-thalassaemia trait (minor). This is normally symptomless but it may be found on routine FBC in an antenatal or a preoperative patient.

Investigation

Findings will show:
- mild or no anaemia, with Hb 10–15 g/dl
- MCV and MCH reduced
- serum iron and ferritin are normal (indicating anaemia not due to iron deficiency). Referral for further blood tests may be required to aid diagnosis.

Treatment plan

None is usually required.

Education

Education and advice to the patient however is vital.

❶ If the β-thalassaemia trait (minor) is found, potential parents need to be informed of the necessity for preconception screening of partner. This is because if both parents carry the β-thalassaemia trait, there is a 25% chance that their child will be born with thalassaemia major (see below).
- Many areas now have genetic counsellors to refer patients to and who also produce leaflets to help educate patients (see Useful Addresses).
- *Pregnancy*. If a diagnosis of a haemoglobin defect is made in a pregnant woman, then her partner will need testing. If he proves positive to β-thalassaemia it will be important to offer antenatal diagnosis.
- Referral for fetal blood sampling in mid-second trimester is relatively safe but late for diagnosis if abortion is to be performed.
- Amniotic fluid cells can be obtained in the first or second trimester when DNA can be analysed (at certain centres).

Beta-thalassaemia intermedia

This is a thalassaemia of moderate severity, inheritance of mild β-thalassaemia mutations, which may be mixed with α-thalassaemia trait, may increase the level of anaemia.

Subjective assessment

- patients may have few symptoms or be severely anaemic
- history taking may reveal symptoms of possible mild or severe anaemia
- physical examination may appear normal or reveal severely abnormal findings.

Investigations

For the patient with mild anaemia:
- FBC may show mild anaemia with Hb 10.0–12.0 g/dl.
- The laboratory will flag up need for further investigations such as electrophoresis.

For the patient with severe anaemia, history taking will reveal symptoms of severe anaemia.

Physical assessment

- Chronic leg ulceration
- Enlarged liver and spleen
- In children, growth and development may be reduced
- Skeletal deformities may be evident.

Investigations

- FBC will show anaemia (Hb 7.0–10.0 g/dl but Hb may be as low as 6.0 g/dl).

Referral

Referral will be necessary for supervision in secondary care, although blood transfusions are not normally necessary.

Beta-thalassaemia major (Cooley's anaemia)

If parents are both carriers of the β-thalassaemia trait, their child has a one-in-four chance of being affected. It will be seen in babies, when severe, at 3–6 months, when the switch from fetal to adult blood takes place. Recurrent bacterial infections are likely to occur.

Subjective assessment

- History from patients, especially their haematological history – looking for possibility of abnormal haemoglobins – is essential.
- Whether infections are recurrent.

Objective assessment

- Vital signs will be checked, as fever is likely to be present
- Check for infection, which may be severe
- Child likely to be severely anaemic and thus very unwell.

Urgent referral to secondary care will be necessary.

Investigations

- FBC and haemoglobin electrophoresis
- Moderate-to-severe anaemia, with Hb 3–9.0 g/dl
- MCV and MCH reduced
- reticulocytes raised
- haemoglobin electrophoresis shows absence or almost total absence of HbA, with almost all haemoglobin being HbF (fetal).

Treatment

These children are likely to develop an enlarged liver and spleen and skeletal deformities due to excessive red cell destruction and later iron overload. The enlarged spleen increases blood requirements by increasing RBC destruction and pooling and causing increase in the plasma volume. Facial abnormalities occur due to marrow hyperplasia.

Iron overload occurs due to repeated blood transfusions. Each 500 ml of blood contains approximately 250 mg of iron. Iron damages the liver and endocrine organs, resulting in failure of growth and delayed or absence of puberty. Diabetes mellitus, hypothyroidism, hypoparathyroidism and damage to the myocardium may result.

Death may occur between the ages of 10 and 30 from congestive heart failure or cardiac arrythmias unless iron overload has been prevented by iron chelation therapy. Skin pigmentation, giving a slate-grey appearance due to iron overload, will occur. Administration of desferrioxamine IV, which reduces iron overload by promoting iron secretion in the stool and urine, can prevent this (though not without side effects, e.g. retinal damage).

Bone marrow transplantation has an 80% success.

Lack of compliance with attendance for desferrioxamine IV is a problem, particularly as children grow into adolescence. Trials are ongoing with oral iron chelation therapy.

Infections due to anaemia, including pneumococcal and meningococcal infections, are likely if splenectomy is carried out. Antibiotic (penicillin), 250 mg twice a day orally, must be taken; the dose is titrated to age in babies.

Liver disease can be due to viral hepatitis from blood transfusion (hepatitis B and C infections are common); HIV has been transmitted by blood transfusion.

Pneumococcal vaccine and hepatitis B immunisation should be given and regular folic acid e.g. 5 mg daily.

Note. Children should be given the usual immunisations.

Beta-thalassaemia trait with other haemoglobinapathies

Combinations of conditions, e.g. β-thalassaemia trait and sickle cell haemoglobin S, will produce sickle cell anaemia rather than thalassaemia.

Sickle Cell anaemia

Haemoglobin S is a haemoglobin variant which comes about due to a substitution in the DNA coding for an amino acid in the β-globin chain; as a result, an amino acid change from glutamic acid to valine occurs. When oxygen tension is low, crystals form, which distort the cells into the characteristic sickle (crescent) shape.

Clinically, the disease follows a very variable course, with some patients leading near normal lives, whereas others have frequent crises as infants and may die in childhood or as young adults.

In the UK, amongst the Afro-Caribbean population, the sickle cell gene is present in a ratio of approximately 1:10.

Homozygous disease

Patients will have parents who are both carriers of β S gene, i.e. sickle cell trait, producing sickle cell anaemia (HbSS) in the child.

Subjective assessment

- Symptoms of anaemia may not be present, as anaemia is often mild
- Severe pain in bones and joints may be described (hips, shoulders and vertebrae most affected) due to vascular-occlusive crises
- Abdominal pain may be a feature
- Swollen, painful hands and feet may be present, due to infarcts of small bones (dactylitis)
- Chest pain, suggestive of pleurisy, with shortness of breath may be described
- Ulcers of lower legs are common, due to vascular stasis and local ischaemia
- Urinary output must be assessed, as there may be a failure to concentrate urine leading to:
  - dehydration
  - nocturnal enuresis
  - in women, urinary tract infections are common.

Objective assessment

- Assess patient's general demeanour
- Look for vital signs likely to be abnormal, with fever, tachycardia and increased heart rate especially in children. The blood pressure (BP) may be low
- Observe for signs of dehydration, skin turgor and moistness of mucous membranes
- Examine joints for swelling and range of movement; levels of pain should be assessed using a pain scale
- Examine chest for any signs of infection or pleurisy
- Carry out urinalysis to look for evidence of possible urinary tract infection
- Examine abdomen to include palpation of liver and spleen, which may be enlarged.

Plan

The acutely ill child or adult will need referral to hospital urgently for IV fluids, antibiotics, analgesia and, sometimes, blood transfusion.

Investigations

Blood for FBC and ESR, sickle cell tests and electrophoresis.

Results

Results are likely to show:

- Hb 6–9 g/dl.
- blood film will show sickle cells
- reticulocytes will be raised
- sickle cell tests positive (tests for sickling when blood deoxygenated)
- electrophoresis: HbSS, no normal HbA; HbF variable, normally 5–15%; larger amounts usually associated with a milder disorder, e.g. 'benign sickle cell anaemia' in Saudi Arabia.

Education

Preconceptual screening for haemoglobinopathies in primary care is vital. Screening should be built into new patient checks, family planning, clinic history taking and chocks on healthy men and women. Also, checks should be carried out opportunistically, when patients present to you (McIntyre 1995, Eboh & Van Den Akker 1997).

Thus, preconceptual screening for the sickle cell trait should be discussed if status is unknown by patient or partner.

If already pregnant, focus on the importance of screening for patient and partner (father of the child) in early pregnancy. The tests will consist of fetal blood sampling (as for thalassaemia) in midsecond trimester from the umbilical cord or amniotic fluid sampling in the second trimester. DNA sampling may be carried out during the first trimester by chorionic villus biopsy, usually at a specialist centre

As already stated, patients with *sickle cell anaemia* have a wide variation in the severity of the disease. This can range from a few symptoms to severe and frequent crises:

- sickle cell anaemia tends to be diagnosed by the age of 1 year as HbF (fetal haemoglobin) is replaced by HbSS
- infection, whether bacterial or viral, will tend to be severe and life threatening, e.g. streptococcal pneumonia
- crises can be triggered by infection, dehydration and cold and temperature changes and, in adults, by drinking alcohol and menstruation in women.

As a result of the sickle cells, the spleen undergoes enlargement in infancy and childhood but becomes smaller in adults due to infarcts:

- damage to the liver will occur
- gallstones will be frequent
- kidneys are vulnerable to infarcts
- growth retardation is likely in children.

Treatment

- Avoidance of the factors known to cause crises.
- Folic acid, usually 5 mg daily.
- Good general nutrition and hygiene.
- Babies should have all the usual immunisations.

- Pneumococcal vaccination (increased risk of pneumonia).
- Hepatitis B vaccination (to protect against possible infection from blood transfusion) (Zimmerman et al 1997).
- Penicillin daily to prevent infections
- Rest and rehydration in crises with antibiotics and adequate analgesia.

Education

This is a very important area where you can help mothers to understand the importance of avoidance of crises:

- This means they must act fast if they think their child has an infection by keeping up the child's fluid intake and bringing the child in to the practice for a checkup and possible referral for antibiotics.
- Pain must be kept under control with adequate analgesia given regularly if crises occur, NSAIDs can be useful here.
- Make sure the mother understands the importance of giving the daily dose of penicillin (orally 250 mg twice a day, 125 mg twice a day for young children) and folic acid. There is a need here for close cooperation so that prescriptions are always available.
- Ensure that a good mixed diet is taken.
- Hygiene should be discussed in order to help prevent infections.

Many of these children will be admitted to hospital when sickle cell crises occur. Research shows, however, that some children who are encouraged to live active lives by their parents and have a positive self-image may manage their pain at home, whereas other children come to rely on hospital care in all crises (Maxwell & Streetly 1998). As primary care providers, we should – as part of the team – make sure that we are adequately trained to support and treat these patients (Miller 1997).

Blood transfusions can sometimes be given repeatedly when iron overload may become a problem.

Hopefully, gene therapy will be possible, in the future.

Sickle cell trait

Patients with known sickle cell trait may present to you with a severe infection that can precipitate a crisis. Haematuria is a common symptom.

History taking, assessment and *treatment* will be as for sickle cell anaemia.

Sickle cell anaemia may be combined with *β-thalassaemia*, e.g. S/β-thalassaemia. Patients will present and be treated as for sickle cell anaemia.

Aplastic anaemia

This anaemia is due to aplasia of the bone marrow. The peak age is 30 years, and slightly higher incidence occurs in males than in females. The anaemia is described as pancytopenia (anaemia, leucopenia and thrombocytopenia). It may be congenital (Fanconi's

Table 3.8 *Causes of aplastic anaemia (From Hoffbrand and Pettit 1999 with permission of Blackwell Science.)*

Primary	Secondary
Congenital (Fanconi anaemia and non-Fanconi types)	Ionizing radiations: accidental exposure (radiotherapy, radioactive isotopes, nuclear power stations)
Idiopathic acquired	Chemicals: benzene and other organic solvents, TNT, insecticides, hair dyes, chlordane, DDT
	Drugs that regularly cause marrow depression (e.g. busulphan, cyclophosphamide, anthracyclines, nitrosoureas)
	Drugs that occasionally or rarely cause marrow depression, (e.g. chloramphenicol, sulphonamides, phenylbutazone, gold and others)
	Infection: viral hepatitis (A or non-A, non-B).

anaemia) or a form which develops with no known cause. Other causes of aplastic anaemia given as reasons for the illness include industrial, drug induced and infections (Table 3.8).

Subjective assessment

Adults and children aged between 5 and 10 years (when Fanconi's anaemia usually diagnosed) are likely to present with severe infection of the mouth and throat. Take the history, focussing on the presence of:
- sore mouth
- bleeding gums
- sore throat
- ask if any epistaxis
- in female patients, enquire if menorrhagia present.

Objective assessment

Examine as for anaemia but paying especial attention to:
- mouth for bleeding gums and/or infection
- throat for infection
- nose for any obvious bleeding point
- examine skin for evidence of bruising
- examine abdomen, including lymph nodes, which may be enlarged, and liver and spleen, which are not usually enlarged.

Treatment

Depending on severity of infection and bleeding, patients will usually need to be referred urgently to hospital. Treatment will be instigated and diagnosis made by bone marrow aspirate and trephine.

Laboratory tests

- FBC will show anaemia
- MCV often 95–110 fl
- Reticulocyte will be reduced or very low
- lymphocyte count may be low.

Treatment

- Treatment in hospital will consist of blood transfusion, removing cause if drug induced.

- Antibiotics and antifungals will be given.
- Some patients undergo spontaneous recovery. For others, particularly after viral hepatitis, the prognosis is poor.
- Chemotherapy and bone marrow transplant may be carried out.

White blood cells (WBCs) – leucocytes

A WBC count of over 11,000/l, i.e. leucocytosis, may be seen in response to bacterial or viral invasion of the body. *Granulocytes* include neutrophils, eosinophils and basophils, which, with monocytes, comprise the phagocytes and account for half or more of the WBC population. Their lifespan in the blood is approximately 10 hours, after which they move into the tissues to perform their phagocytic function.

The blood count will pick up granulocytes and monocytes circulating in the bloodstream (half the number) but not those in the tissues.

Neutrophil leucocytosis

An increase in circulating neutrophils is very commonly seen on blood counts (Table 3.9).

Eosinophilic leucocytosis (eosinophilia)

Eosinophilic leucocytosis is seen in allergic diseases, e.g. bronchial asthma, hayfever, urticaria, food sensitivity or during recovery from acute infection. It is also seen in certain skin diseases, e.g. psoriasis.

Basophilic leucocytosis (basophilia)

An increase in basophils is uncommon. If present, it is probably due to chronic myeloid leukaemia or polycythaemia vera. Can be found in myxoedema, chicken pox infection and ulcerative colitis.

Table 3.9 *Causes of neutrophil leucocytosis (From Hoffbrand and Pettit 1999, with permission of Blackwell Science.)*

1. Bacterial infections (especially pyogenic bacterial, localised or generalised)
2. Inflammation and tissue necrosis, e.g. myositis, vasculitis, cardiac infarct, trauma
3. Metabolic disorders, e.g. uraemia, eclampsia, acidosis, gout
4. Neoplasms of all types, e.g. carcinoma, lymphoma, melanoma
5. Acute haemorrhage or haemolysis
6. Corticosteroid therapy (inhibits margination)
7. Myeloproliferative disease, e.g. chronic myeloid leukaemia, polycythaemia vera, myelosclerosis
8. Treatment with myeloid growth factors, e.g. G-CSF, GM-CSF

G-CSF, granulocyte colony-stimulating factor; GM-CSF, granulocyte-macrophage, colony-stimulating factor.

Table 3.10 *Causes of lymphocytosis (From Hoffbrand and Pettit 1999, with permission of Blackwell Science.)*

1. Infections
   - Acute: infectious mononucleosis, rubella, pertussis, mumps, acute infectious lymphocytosis, infectious hepatitis, cytomegalovirus, HIV, herpes simplex or zoster
   - Chronic: tuberculosis, toxoplasmosis, brucellosis, syphilis
2. Thyrotoxicosis
3. Chronic lymphocytic leukaemia and polylymphocytic leukaemia (B- and T-cell types)
4. Acute lymphoblastic leukaemia
5. Non-Hodgkin's lymphoma (some)
6. Hairy cell leukaemia

Neutropenia

- The lower limit of the normal neutrophil count is $2.5 \times 10^9/l$, except in the Middle East, where $1.5 \times 10^9/l$ is normal. With a low count, recurrent infections are common.
- Clinical features will include severe infections of the mouth and throat with intractable ulcers.
- Septicaemia is common and patients will need referral for bone marrow examination and treatment.

Lymphocytes (part of WBC population)

- Lymphocytes are involved in immune responses, which assist phagocytes to overcome infections in the body
- Lymphoid cells are mainly found in lymphoid tissue but may be seen in blood
- Lymphocytosis occurs in infants and children as a response to an infection that would produce a neutrophil reaction in adults (Table 3.10).

Infectious mononucleosis (glandular fever)

This is most commonly caused by infection with the Epstein–Barr virus (EBV) and tends to occur in the 15–40 age group, although children under 10 years are seen with the disease.

Subjective assessment

- The patient will complain of a sore throat
- Symptoms of fever may be described
- Headache may be a feature
- A feeling of lethargy is often described
- It will be necessary to ask if they have a stiff neck
- Establish if they have a cough, which is usually dry.

Objective assessment

- Signs of anaemia unlikely to be present
- Check mouth and throat, which may have inflamed oral and pharyngeal surfaces
- Follicular tonsillitis may be seen
- Check cervical lymph nodes: lymphadenopathy is present in 75% of cases
- Check vital signs: fever may be present and can be severe
- Check whether photophobic or any conjunctivitis present
- Examine the abdomen for enlargement of spleen (occurs in over 50% of cases) and enlargement of liver (occurs in approximately 15% of cases)
- Examine for jaundice (may occur in 5% of cases).

Investigations

- Take blood or order FBC
- Paul–Bunnell test
- Liver function tests (LFTs) if liver enlarged.

Diagnosis

If infectious mononucleosis, blood result will show:

- Lymphocytosis: atypical lymphocytes on blood film between the 7th and 10th day of illness, and cells may persist in blood for 1–2 months.
- Paul–Bunnell/monospot test will be positive, the highest levels during 2–3 weeks after the start of the illness and usually persisting for 6 weeks.
- WBC raised (e.g. $10–20 \times 10^9/l$).

Treatment

- Rest
- Analgesia for headache and sore throat.
- ❶ If antibiotics given for treatment of tonsillitis initially, avoid penicillin as a rash is likely to develop.

Top Tips ✓

1 Remember to take a very careful history and try to uncover problems, e.g. lack of compliance with iron therapy

2 Physical examination is very important; the signs and symptoms of anaemia can be difficult to detect

3 Order relevant blood tests only, not an entire battery without justification

4 Scrutinise results and, if in doubt as to interpretation, the laboratory is there as a resource – likewise, the haematologist

5 Order repeat blood tests if warranted as false-positives/negatives do occur

6 Do give the laboratory the clinical picture, as they are likely to be more helpful if they know what they may be looking for!

7 Normal values are usually printed on blood results: so do not think you have to remember them all

8 Always be very alert for ethnic/mixed race abnormalities, e.g. thalassaemia

9 Listen very closely to mothers of small children – they know their child best

10 Anaemia is not a diagnosis: it is an abnormal clinical finding that requires an explanation for its cause.

Course and prognosis

■ Recovery usually about 4–6 weeks after initial symptoms
■ Slow convalescence and relapse can occur
■ Chronic fatigue syndrome may develop
■ Depression can occur
■ Rarely, encephalitis can occur with convulsions and coma; oedema of the glottis; also splenic rupture (Mead 1995).
■ Mesenteric nodes may mimic appendicitis.
■ In immunosuppressed patients, e.g. following renal, bone marrow or cardiac transplant and in those suffering from AIDS, lymphoma may develop (see Table 3.10).

Glossary

ALL　Acute lymphoblastic leukaemia
AML　Acute myeloid leukaemia
CML　Chronic myeloid leukaemia
DNA　Deoxyribonucleic acid
Epstein–Barr virus (EBV)　Atypical lymphocytes infected with EBV and causing infectious mononucleosis. Immunosuppressed patients, e.g. following renal or cardiac trans-plantation or with acquired immune deficiency syndrome (AIDS), who are carriers of EBV may develop malignant lymphoma
ESR　The rate at which red blood cells (RBCs, erythrocytes) settle out of suspension in blood plasma, measured under standardised conditions. The ESR rises in the presence of chronic infection rheumatic disease and malignant disease
HbF　Haemoglobin F (fetal Hb)
Heterozygous　An individual in whom the members of a pair of genes determining a particular characteristic are dissimilar, e.g. β-thalassaemic trait
Homozygous　An individual in whom the members of a pair of genes determining a particular characteristic are identical.
Poikilocytosis　Abnormally pencil-shaped RBCs
RNA　Ribonucleic acid
Schilling test　It may be used to confirm vitamin B_{12} anaemia. An oral dose of radioactive vitamin B_{12} is given to the patient, who then saves a 24-hour sample of urine for assessment of vitamin B_{12} content. It is contraindicated in pregnant or breast-feeding women
SLE　Systemic lupus erythematosus

Useful addresses

Leukaemia Research Fund (LRF), 43 Great Portland Street, London WC1N 3JJ. Tel: 0207 405 0101. Fax: 0207 242 1488. *Booklets are available on the acute and chronic leukaemias, lymphomas including Hodgkin's disease suitable for patients and their carers.*

United Kingdom Thalassaemia Society, 19 The Broadway, Southgate Circus, London N14 6PH. Tel: 0208 882 0011. Fax: 0208 882 8618.

National Sickle Cell Programme, PO Box 322, London SE25 4BW. Tel: 0208 771 4365.

References

Bates B 1987 A Guide to physical examination and history taking. Lippincott, Philadelphia.

British National Formulary (BNF) 40 1999 British Medical Association, London.

Eboh W, Van Den Akker O 1997 Antenatal screening for couples at risk of having children with sickle cell disorders. Midwives 110(1309):26–27.

Friebert S, Shurin S 1998 Contemporary Paediatrics 15(2):124–127.

Hoffbrand A, Pettit J 1999 Essential haematology, 3rd edn. Blackwell Science, Oxford.

McIntyre A 1995. Haemoglobinopathies – a condition for life. Healthlines 27:14–16.

Maxwell K, Streetly A 1998 Living with sickle cell pain. Nursing Standard 13(9):33.

Mead M 1995 Glandular fever. Practice Nurse 10(4):278–279.

Miller B 1997 Cell out. Health Service Journal 107(5540):12.

Nathan D, Oski F 1992 Haematology of infancy and childhood, 4th edn. WB Saunders, Philadelphia, 415–422.

Rochester-Peart C 1997 Specialist nurse support for clients with blood disorders. Nursing Times 93(41):52–54.

Zimmerman S, Ware R, Kinney T 1997 Gaining ground in the fight against sickle cell disease. Contemporary Paediatrics 14(10):158–162.

Further reading

Hoffbrand A, Pettit J 1999. Essential haematology, 3rd edn. Blackwell Science, Oxford.

Hughes-Jones N, Wickramasinghe S 1996 Lecture notes on haematology, 6th edn. Blackwell Science, Oxford.

Martin P 1990 Nurses clinical guide to health assessment. Springhouse, Pennsylvania.

Provan D, Chisholm M, Duncombe A, Singer C, Smith A 1998 Oxford handbook of clinical haematology. Oxford University Press, Oxford.

Weatherall D, Ledingham J, Warrell D 1996 Oxford text book of medicine, 3rd edn. Oxford University Press, Oxford.

4

DERMATOLOGY

Jill Peters

Key Issues

■ Use of senses when carrying out an examination – listen, look, touch, smell

■ Be aware of your facial expression when examining skin: you do not have to say something to offend or reject a human being

■ Opportunity to promote skin care with every patient you see, no matter what their chief complaint is

■ Good lighting and a full skin examination

■ Use of a body graph to illustrate severity and clinical signs

Introduction

There are over 2000 different skin conditions, and this chapter will cover the most common presenting conditions. It will build on the history-taking skills you already have and enable you to make a differential diagnosis, carry out investigations and plan a package of care that leads to improved control of the skin condition.

Assessment

The environment

A warm room with good natural lighting or artificial lighting that will not change the natural colour of the skin is essential (Lawton 1998). A magnified lamp is useful when assessing lesions; this allows the use of perpendicular lighting when looking for subtle skin changes. In the patient's home, use natural lighting where possible; otherwise, take a small portable light with a magnifying lens with you.

The assessment should start at the onset of consultation. Consider the patient's physical bearing and posture; it could indicate how she feels about herself. The skin is the window into the patient's inner feelings and is often reflected through her facial expression (Mairis 1992) before she first speaks.

❶ It is essential for safe practice to examine and compare all the skin; no lesion/rash should be looked at in isolation (Epstein 1985, Peters 1998). The chance of detecting a melanoma is 6.4 times greater with a complete skin examination than with a partial examination of just-exposed skin (Rigel et al 1996).

Thus, it is important to explain to the patient why you require her to undress down to her underclothes. Be aware of cultural and religious differences, as well as embarrassment, especially if the patient perceives it to be a local problem, e.g. mole on the face (Epstein 1985).

Subjective data

Ask the patient to tell you about her skin complaint, record it in her own words, but also guide her to describe how and when it started? What is the rash like? Explore any symptoms: this will give you insight into her perceptions and expectations of the consultation. This is important, as the skin takes time to reveal itself and you often have to see the patient a couple of times as the condition may not have evolved when she first presents.

Here are some questions that you may like to ask patients:

■ What is their main problem?

■ How and when did it start?

■ What did it look like at first, compared with now?

■ What time lapse has occurred since the onset of the rash – hours, days or months?

■ How long was the lesion present on the skin? e.g. hours (urticaria).

■ Where is the site of initial lesion (target lesion) and, then, had the rash spread over the body and in what kind of distribution?

■ What symptoms have you experienced? (see Box 4.1)

Using analogue scales to check out severity of symptoms is a method that can be used on reviewing the

Box 4.1 *PQRST scale of symptomology*

P Palliative relief/provocative cause

Q Quality/quantity

R Region/radiation

S Severity/scale 0–10

T Timing

patient at subsequent consultations to indicate remission or exacerbation of symptoms. The scale 0–10, where 0 = the best their skin has been and 10 = the worst, can be used for measuring intensity of itching, scaling, soreness or erythema.

More questions to ask patients:

- Has this ever occurred previously and what was the outcome?
- Had anything occurred prior to this acting as the trigger or precursor (e.g. tingling, pruritus, tenderness, trauma-localised increase in temperature) or systemic symptoms (febrile or joint soreness or throat infection).
- Does the rash improve at the weekends or when on holiday?
- Have they travelled abroad recently?
- Any new activity, hobby or job?
- Any activities they can no longer do?
- Any new medication or anything taken that was bought over the counter or any recreational drugs?
- Sun exposure – have they lived abroad? What sun protection factor do they use? Does the sun influence the skin condition in any way? Sexuality – HIV infection can exacerbate psoriasis and seborrhoeic dermatitis.
- Any family history of 'atopy', 'psoriasis' or 'skin cancer', depending on the presenting complaint.
- Have they had any time off work or can relate it to the workplace.

- Ask what initiated their enquiry: any fears or anxieties.
- What do they think is wrong with them and their expected outcomes?

Objective review

Although the patient has presented with a skin problem, consider a complete holistic review of all systems; however, as you become more experienced, you may focus on certain ones. A skin condition may be a symptom of systemic disease, e.g. tiredness and itching could be hypothyroidism. Or a patient may be too embarrassed to mention the real problem unless specific questions are asked, e.g. vulva itching may be a symptom of lichen sclerosus rather than a sexually transmitted disease.

❶ An holistic review also needs to consider the psychological impact of skin diseases; questionnaires are a useful tool to measure impact, such as the Dermatology Quality of Life Index (Finlay & Khan 1994) or disease-specific, such as the acne scoring system (Cunliffe 1994). It is useful if the same practitioner sees the patient on subsequent visits and carries out the scoring.

When carrying out the physical examination remember that skin condition can be uncomfortable and hurt, so be gentle but sure in your movements. Use your senses when examining the skin, e.g. look, touch and smell. Use a systematic approach to your examination (Table 4.1).

Table 4.1 *Physical examination*

Examination procedure	Action
Carry out the examination from the right side of the couch using the skill of touch	This light surface palpation allows you to assess the texture and extent of the lesions
Start from the nails, up the fingertips to finger webs, then palms and dorsum up, moving up both arms	Are the cuticles intact? Any pitting, onycholysis, or extra lines? Check for signs of lesions or damage, both flexural and extensor sides into the axilla
Check the scalp	Parting the hair to examine the hair shaft, feel the texture of the hair. Note the pattern of thinning around the hairline and behind the ears. Any bald patches?
Examine the face	Note, not only any obvious lesions but pay attention to the eyes, including lashes and eyebrow. Around the nasolabial folds and also the oral mucosa and tongue, it is important not to miss the primary lesion or initial symptom
Work your way down the trunk	Start from under the chin, into both axillas, down the chest wall across the abdomen to the pelvic area. This ensures no area is missed
Start again at the nails on the feet, and work your way up the front of the legs	Ensure to check in between the toes and soles of the feet for moles. Raise the patient's awareness for monitoring
Ask the patient to turn over or stand, so you can examine from the nape of the neck to the feet	Be methodological, ensuring that no skin is left unexamined
When examining the genitalia area, be respectful and gentle	Ask the patient to manoeuvre and to point to the areas of concern. For close examination, gloves should be worn if the skin is ulcerated or broken (universal precautions)

Use a body map to record the location and distribution of lesions. Label the diagram, including length and diameter of lesions if necessary (Fig. 4.1). Closer examination of the lesions occurs after the general survey. This gives a picture of the patient's skin, extent of the condition and any particular landmarks, scars, tattoos and any signs of knobnerisation or atrophy. Questions can be asked during this time: i.e. 'Had a lesion changed pigment, or was it larger now?' The patient often volunteers information that she had not thought important.

Remember, the skin does not lie, but it can mimic different rashes. Patients often deny scratching but excoriations are evidence that one cannot dismiss. Question them closely. Do they scratch more at night? Anyone else scratching, e.g. scabies? Making a diagnosis is a process of elimination through history taking and clinical presentation.

Distribution

What is the distribution of the present condition and does this give us any clue to the diagnosis. Identify the primary lesion and its anatomical position. Is it generalised or a localised rash (see Box 4.2)? Endogenous rashes are usually symmetrical, e.g. psoriasis. Exogenous rashes may result in only one side of the body being affected, e.g. tinea. Herpes zoster (see Plate 1) is restricted to a dermatome (Ashton 1998). Sun-exposed areas of the skin affected, e.g. photosensitivity, check for areas of sparing where shaded, e.g. under the chin, under the eyebrows. Is there a demarked line/border to indicate contact dermatitis, e.g. just above the wrists indicating allergy to rubber gloves? Does it affect the body and the mucosa of the mouth? e.g. lichen planus or pemphigus.

When considering your findings you will have to relate to the age of your patient and what expected

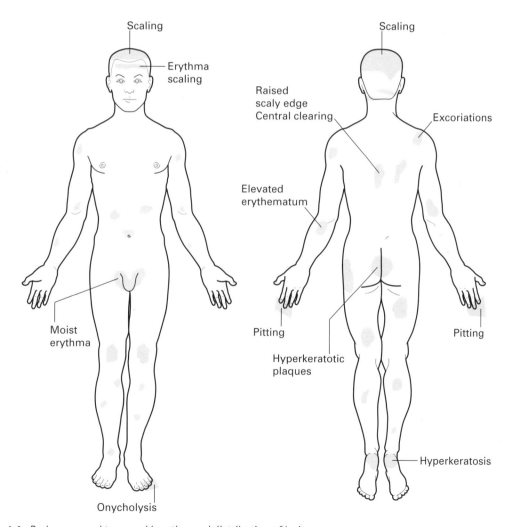

Scaling

Erythma scaling

Moist erythma

Onycholysis

Scaling

Raised scaly edge
Central clearing

Excoriations

Elevated erythematum

Pitting

Hyperkeratotic plaques

Pitting

Hyperkeratosis

Figure 4.1 *Body map used to record location and distribution of lesions.*

Box 4.2 *Labelling of lesions by configuration and distribution (Hill 1998)*

Configuration	The arrangement or pattern of lesions in relation to other lesions
Distribution	The arrangement of lesions over an area of skin
Annular	Ring shaped
Iris lesion	Concentric rings 'bulls eye'
Gyrate	Ring spiral shape
Linear	In a line
Nummular or discoid	Coin-like shape
Polymorphous	Occurring in several form's
Punctate	Marked by points or dots
Serpiginous	Snake-like
Solitary	Single lesion
Satellite	Single lesion in close proximity to a larger group
Grouped	Cluster of lesions
Confluent	Merging together
Diffuse	Widely distributed, spreading
Discrete	Separate from other lesions
Generalised	Distributed diffusely
Localised	Limited areas of involvement that are clearly defined
Symmetrical or asymmetrical	Distributed bilaterally or unilaterally
Zosteriform	Band-like distribution along a dermatome

Box 4.3 *Skin phototypes based on a person's own estimate of sunburning and tanning (Fitzpatrick et al 1997)*

Skin type I	Always burns, never tans
Skin type II	Sometimes burns, always tans
Skin type III	Always tans, never burns
Skin type IV	Mediterranean skin
Skin type V	Brown skin
Skin type VI	Black skin

physiological changes will have occurred naturally. Learn to recognise what is normal across the age spectrum: this will come with experience.

Pigment

It is also important to be aware of the range of colour (differences in pigmentation) of the skin belonging to

Table 4.2 *Assessment of pigmented skin*

Aetiology	Changes in pigmented skin
Pallor	Ashen grey in black skin, yellow-brown in brown skin, they are both dull looking
Inflammation	Hyperpigmentation in black or brown skin but lighter on tips of noses, in front and behind ears. Use of palpation – for increased warmth
Erythema	Purplish tinge, difficult to see dark area, macular or diffuse. Palpate for increased warmth with inflammation, for taut skin and hardening of deep tissue.
Purpura	Jet-black in lighter negroid
Oedema	Lightens the skin, weals appear pale. Palpation – slick tight skin. Palpate for warmth of oedema
Cyanosis	Ashen-grey on lips or check nail beds, only severe cyanosis apparent in skin
Jaundice	Yellowing of the sclera of the eyes, junction of hard and soft palate and also in palms

the human race. Depigmentation can occur following inflammatory changes and is often seen after herpes zoster and eczema in those with skin types – VI (Box 4.3) An understanding of the normal pigmentation allows detection of change; palpation is often useful in darker pigmented skins (Baxter 1993) (Table 4.2). Inflammation in black skin can lead to colour changes; the skin is prone to be more papular (raised and spotty) and follicular (focus around a hair follicle). There is an increased risk of scarring.

The skin itself can tell its own story and often takes time to reveal itself, which is why you may have to see the patient several times before making a final diagnosis. The skin has the ability to mimic different skin diseases. If misdiagnosed and treated, it can change its clinical appearance and be incognito. The presenting skin condition can be a symptom of systemic disease and, thus, the assessment process should be more than skin deep, i.e. acquired ichthyosis = lymphoma (T cell).

Describing the lesion/rash

Questions to ask yourself when touching the skin:
- Is the skin smooth, uneven or rough to touch?
- Has the skin lost turgor or elasticity – lift a fold of skin and release. Note if it was easy and the ease with which it returned.
- Are the skin lines accentuated? Has the skin become lichenified, (dirty or shiny nails are often the signs of a scratcher) or is it very dry and looks like crazy paving (eczema craquelé) (see Plate 2)?
- What colour pigment is seen? Assess what is normal for that patient and what is abnormal – erythema,

jaundice, blanching, pallor. If hyperpigmented, you need to identify the normal skin colour of the patient.

- Any sensitivity to touch, tingling or pain?
- Is the skin moist or dry, sweaty or oily?
- Is the skin hot or cold to the touch (touch the lesion and compare it to the surrounding skin that is not involved: note the difference).
- Is there excessive scaling in between the skin creases – possible fungal infection. Consider skin scraping.
- Have the skin lesions been changed through trauma of scratching, rubbing or the application of topical preparations?
- Inspect a lesions that has not been altered – what does it look and feel like?
- What is the surrounding skin like? Is the margin smudged or excoriated?
- Are there signs of pricking or rubbing?
- Is there any scale, crusting or weeping? Consider skin scrapings or swabs for laboratory tests?
- Does the skin smell? Is the smell distinguishable from the smell of old skin or is it indicative of infection?
- Colour of the lesion, i.e. yellow – xanthoma (lipid deposit) or sebaceous gland. Pigment lesions, i.e. blue-black for cellular blue naevus or red in strawberry naevus? Has the lesion changed in the last weeks rather than months (Box 4.4)?

Palpation

- Use deep palpation by compressing the lesion between finger and thumb. How thick is it and how deep?
- A soft lesion can be compressed easily and feels like your lips. A normal lesions is just like squeezing your own cheek.
- A firm lesion can only just be compressed; it has a certain degree of infiltrate, like urticaria weals.
- A hard lesion cannot be compressed, as it contains fibrous tissue, like a histocytoma.
- Induration of the lesion is palpable thickening in the lesion itself, like squamous cell carcinoma.

Characteristics affecting nails

Observation of the nails starts with the colour and shape. To check the capillary return, apply pressure to the nail. This blanches the nail bed underneath. Note the length of time it takes blood to return by the change in colour. Look for changes to the surface of the nail. They can give clues of skin disease, e.g. psoriasis causes pitting of the nails and onycholysis (lifting of the nail plate from the bed). Tinea can also cause hyperkeratosis (build up of keratin cells) of the nail plate and onycholysis. Onycholysis can also be caused by repeated pressure trauma, like jogging. To assist with confirmation of diagnosis, nail clippings should be sent for mycology prior to any treatment being commenced.

Pigment in the nail bed can be caused by trauma, but if it extends into the surrounding skin consider referral

Box 4.4	*Suspicious symptoms and signs in a naevus*

Major
    Change in colour
    Irregular shape of the margin
    Irregular pigment within the naevus
    New mole (in those over the age of 30)

Minor
    Over 7 mm in diameter
    Inflamed
    Oozing or bleeding
    Itch

to a dermatologist with a possible differential of malignant melanoma (acral-lentiginous melanoma). White spots within the nails usually follow trauma to the nail and grow out slowly with the nail. They also can be caused by over-vigorous repeated manicuring.

Paronychia is inflammation of the proximal and lateral nail folds; the cuticles may have disappeared and the folds are swollen and sore. People who immerse their hands in hot water are susceptible to this developing. Candida infections can cause painful paronychia; it is also associated with HIV disease and mucosal candidiasis.

Beau's lines (Fig. 4.2) are transverse depressions in the nails associated with acute severe illness. The lines emerge from the proximal nail folds weeks later and grow out with the nail.

Mees' lines are transverse white lines associated with acute or severe illness, seen in arsenic poisoning. The lines emerge from the proximal nail folds and grow out with the nails.

Periungual telangiectasia occurs when the capillary loops of the proximal nail folds becomes tortuous and dilated. There are degrees of severity. It can be caused by repeated injury from infection but is also a characteristic of dermatomyositis.

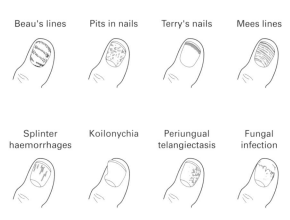

Beau's lines   Pits in nails   Terry's nails   Mees lines

Splinter haemorrhages   Koilonychia   Periungual telangiectasis   Fungal infection

Figure 4.2 *Characteristics affecting nails.*

Characteristics affecting hair

The scalp and hairline should always be examined, as many skin disorders affect either the scalp or the hair. Check for any lesions that may also be present but invisible with a search through the hair by parting the hair in sections around the scalp to examine the underlining skin.

When examining the scalp and other body hair you need to consider the pattern of the hair. Is the texture correct for the position of hair on the body? Does the hair shaft break easy. Has the colour greyed prematurely? Are there signs of scarring from the hair loss or erythema, which could mean inflammatory disease at work? Signs of skin scale along the shaft that often breaks the hair due to the weight and any underlying inflammatory disease may be identified, e.g. seborrhoeic dermatitis.

Androgenetic alopecia is the normal progressive balding that occurs through the combined effect of a genetic predisposition and the action of androgen on the hair follicles in the scalp; this is normal in men. Observe for normal presentation of hair and then observe the abnormal.

The increase of hair in abnormal places, i.e. hair on a woman across both breasts and down the umbilicus to the groin, could indicate hirsutism. Loss of hair from the normal area either in the form of bald patches in alopecia or to a general thinning across the scalp is abnormal. In a woman, following the male pattern of baldness, investigate for reduced ferritin levels (needs to be 15–200 µmol/l to promote hair growth). In these cases the patient is distressed by the presentation of the disease.

Patients often bring hair that has been shed prior to their visit to support their story. If infection were present, then investigation of the debris or hair shaft would need to be sent to the laboratories (mycology). Changes might be linked to other ongoing medical conditions or medication, so the history should always be thorough.

Stress or following an acute illness or pregnancy after a time delay in which the increase shedding of club hair (telogen) from resting scalp follicles, secondary shift of anagen (growth phase) into catagen and telogen (resting phase), sees an increase in daily loss of hair and, if severe, generalised thinning. Following chemotherapy, anagen effluvium can occur, which is generalised loss of hair involving the whole scalp. There are many drugs that can induce an alopecia of this type, e.g. ACE (argiotensin-converting enzyme) inhibitors, heavy metal poisoning.

❶ Examination tips

1. Undress the patient totally. Never look at a lesion in isolation. If you have not seen it, it does not exist!
2. The blanche test is a test of erythema. Apply firm pressure then release, if redness turns white (blanches) it indicates erythema. This is due to dilated blood vessels.
3. If a lesion has a covering of a crust, then it should be removed to examine what is underneath.
4. If the skin does not look scaly initially, stretch the skin and release repeatedly two or three times between thumb and index fingers and then observe closely. If scaling occurs, then consider pityriasis versicolor.
5. If trying to make a differential diagnosis on a scaly rash, then pick the scale off. If profuse scale detaches or bleeding occurs, then it is likely to be psoriasis.
6. Koebner or isomorphic phenomenon (see Plate 3) is the occurrences of an inflammatory skin condition on the site of a previous trauma, i.e. a surgical scar. This is particularly characteristic in psoriasis, lichen planus and active eczema.
7. When examining bullae, try dislodging the epidermis by finger pressure in the area of a lesion, leading to erosion of the blister. This is known as the Nikolsky sign, i.e. positive for pemphigus and erythema multiforme but negative for pemphigoid.

Investigations

Investigations assist with the process of elimination or act as supporting evidence for a working diagnosis. Decide whether the inconvenience to the patient or the usage of resources gives you evidence on which to act.

What investigation should you send your skin swabs for and what should be the indicators?

- Primary infection such as staphylococcus may be the trigger factor in atopic eczema; β-haemolytic streptococcal may be the trigger factor in guttate psoriasis or cause of scalded skin infection.
- Secondary infection such as staphylococcus imposed on top of eczema such as impetigo.
- Distinguishing between colonisation and infection is essential, as wounds colonised by bacteria will heal without antibiotics (Collier 1994), whereas infected skin will require antibiotics. Identification of growth sensitisation is just as important as known allergies when making the treatment choice.
- Bacterial investigation – looking for either primary or secondary bacterial infection to support clinical presentation of a host response: erythema, heat, oedema. (In some skin conditions the pus is sterile in some disease, i.e. pustular psoriasis.)

How to take a skin swab

1. Ensure that the swab tip is moist, either with normal saline (Rudensky et al 1992) or transport medium (Committee Members of the Wound Care Society 1993), so that you pick up the bacterial cells.
2. Rotating the swab between the fingers in a zigzag motion across the wound/skin lesion (Cooper &

Lawrence 1996): this collects cells from an adequate depth and ensures maximum coverage of the swab tip. If pus is present, then swab that.

3. Put the swab into the transport medium and indicate where the swab was taken from. Results are available within 24 hours. However, methicillin resistance takes longer to clarify.

Viral investigation – looking for primary or secondary infection. Use the virology specimen pots with pink liquid medium to send to serology for herpes simplex virus (HSV) culture. If a vesicle is present, pierce the roof and swab the content.

Primary infection – herpes zoster or shingles. Secondary infection such as herpes simplex on top of eczema, results in eczema herpeticum (see Plate 4); look for the characteristic disseminated punched-out vesicles.

Mycology: the investigation for fungal or yeast infection

Mycology investigation supports clinical findings in some cases or gives a definite diagnosis. In others, it ensures the correct systemic or topical therapy. The most common reason for treatment failure is misdiagnosis (Goodfield 1998); thus, skin scrapings or nail clippings or hair debris should be sent:

- Skin scrapping – use a blunt blade at 45° angle to remove skin cells, without cutting the patient's skin, onto a black filter paper. Do not seal with adhesive tape, as the specimen may be lost when the technician struggles to undo it.
- Nail clippings – use nail clippers; put the specimen of the nail in a black filter paper.
- Hair debris – use a stiff toothbrush to collect skin, exudate and hair.

Mycology culture takes 1 month, as dermatophytes are slower than bacteria in growth. However, microscopic examination takes 2 weeks and can identify yeast infections and indicate a possible positive culture.

| Box 4.5 | *Wood's light examination* |

Erythrasma: fluorescence coral red; bacterial infection caused by *Corynebacterium minutissimum*

Pityriasis versicolor: fluorescence blue-green of scales of Pityrosporum ovale yeast infection

Tinea capitis: fluorescence greenish on hair infected with *Microsporum*

Elevated porphyrin in urine: fluorescence orange-red

Wood's light examination

This is often carried out to identify bacterial, fungal or yeast infections (Box. 4.5). You need a Wood's light (UVL handset) and a room that you can completely darken with a patient in a place of safety while you fluoresce the skin with the UVL light.

The Wood's light can also be used to measure the depth of the melanin in the skin, since variations in the epidermal pigmentation are more apparent under Wood's light than under visible light (as in vitiligo) (Champion et al 1992).

Common blood tests within dermatology

This list will not be exhaustive but we try and indicate the most relevant tests to be carried out when considering a dermatological diagnosis or related systemic disease (Table 4.3).

Diagnostic biopsy

The decision regarding the need for a biopsy is dependent on the differential diagnosis. Without this you are unable to decide if surgery is necessary or the type of procedure required. Lawrence (1996) states that the correct interpretation of histological changes in the skin are dependent on the operator choosing the right

Table 4.3 *Common diseases and blood tests*

Test	Pruritus	Atopic Eczema	Alopecia	Urticaria	Erythroderma
FBC	*	*	*	*	
Albumin					*
U & E	*			*	*
ESR	*			*	*
IgE		*			
LFT	*			*	
Thyroxine, TSH	*		*	*	
Ferritin	*		*		*
Antinuclear factor	*			*	

ESR, erythrocyte sedimentation rate; FBC, full blood count; IgE, immunoglobulin E; LFT, liver function test; TSH, thyroid-stimulating hormone; U & E, urea and electrolytes

biopsy site and obtaining an adequate specimen along with the differential diagnosis.

Punch biopsy provides a full-thickness excision of the skin down to the fat. It can be used to send samples of possible tumours for diagnosis and decision about the treatment or surgical removal. It is very useful for inflammatory rashes or skin infiltrates when multiple biopsy can be taken with ease. It is common practice to biopsy both affected and unaffected skin for comparison.

An elliptical biopsy can be useful to remove a sample of skin across the margin/junction between affected and non-affected skin. The skin sample can also be divided for different investigations. Skin samples can sent for:

- *histological* interpretation or *culture* for bacterial infections
- *immunofluorescence* (detecting the presence and positioning of substances, e.g. antigens, antibodies, cell components for diagnostic purpose for blistering conditions).

Other dermatological investigations to aid differential diagnosis

Dermographism

It was found that 4.2% of the general population has a positive dermographic response (Fitzpatrick et al 1997). Stroke the skin firmly with a wooden stick; after 5 min urticaria pink wheals will appear, which should last about 30 min. This is a positive diagnostic test for urticaria or for symptomatic urticaria.

Diascopy

Using a glass microscopic slide, press firmly over a skin lesion. This will enable the practitioner to determine whether the redness in a macule or papule is due to erythema (capillary dilation) or to purpura (extravasation of blood) or a haemolytic rash of meningitis.

Acarus hunt

Patients with persistent itch should be closely examined for evidence of burrows. The search for mites in burrows is difficult because they are in the stratum corneum. Once you have found a likely burrow add a few drop of 5% potassium hydroxide; this will dissolve the keratin and expose the mite and its debris. Then scrape the cells onto a microscopic slide and examine under a microscope for positive identification. You can clearly see the mite or its larvae on the slide.

Patch testing

Allergy patch testing is one of the investigations carried out to detect contact allergy of the delayed sensitivity type. This is a type IV delayed type of hypersensitivity. The investigation is quite time consuming for the patient

with several appointments. Patch tests are usually read after 48–72 hours and up to 1 week later. Contact urticaria reactions can be read at 0.5 hours. Patients are often convinced that they have an allergy, looking to blame something for the condition of their skin.

IgE antibodies

Immunoglobin E (IgE) is the classical anaphylactic antibody of man, and mediates most anaphylactic (immediate type I hypersensitivity) actions. IgE, which is present in normal serum in very small quantities (10–70 µg/100 ml), is the antibody formed by atopic persons to a wide number of common allergens. Non-atopic persons also form IgE antibody as a result of vaccinations, e.g. tetanus.

Radioallergosorbent test (RAST)

This blood test measures the amount of specific IgE produced against a suspect allergen. Some amounts of IgE are too small to be detected by conventional techniques but can be detected using antibody reagents with radioisotopes. This gives a definite answer regarding allergy for those allergic to cat and dog dander, house dust mite, peanuts, milk, egg white, etc. In the case of skin prick tests, there is sometimes a danger of anaphylaxis to foods but, as this is a blood test, there is no danger of anaphylaxis.

Erythrocyte sedimentation rate (ESR)

The mechanism of this blood test is not fully understood but it is useful as a non-specific indicator of systemic disease. In dermatology it is helpful when considering whether more extensive investigation is required in a patient with pruritus of unknown cause. An ESR above 50 mm/h is nearly always associated with some significant illness, i.e. vasculitis, systemic lupus erythematosus (SLE).

Ovasites and parasites sellotape test This is a simple but sometimes awkward investigation. The aim is to try and capture the worm on a piece of Sellotape for identification in the laboratories. A piece of Sellotape is stuck across the anal orifice overnight so that when the worm emerges it sticks to the Sellotape.

Differential diagnoses

There are many different skin diseases that can present in primary care; some are non-specific, as a reaction to an infection, but many others are chronic and frustrating for patients who have to care for their skin everyday. The most common diseases will be discussed in the next section: the majority are not age-specific, and severity can differ from one day to the next. Intervention depends on the needs of individual patients and, depends on the psychological impact the disease has on them and their carers.

SPECIFIC SKIN DISEASES

Atopic eczema

Definition: Atopy implies a genetic predisposition to asthma, hayfever and eczema. More than one-third of children with eczema develop both or either of the other two conditions over their lifetime. Eczema is an inflammatory disorder; the precise aetiology is unknown. There is an immunological component, with 80% of children with eczema demonstrating a raised immunoglobulin E (IgE) level (Higgins & du Vivier 1996). Atopic eczema (see Plate 5) is an acute, subacute but usually chronic pruritic inflammation of the epidermis and dermis (Fitzpatrick et al 1997).

Diagnosis is based on the criteria developed by a working party of the Royal College of Physicians 1995 (McHenry et al 1995):
Must have:
An itchy skin condition
Plus three of the following:
1. A history of itchy rash. Infants: on the cheeks. Others; skin creases (elbows, knees and front of ankles or under neck)
2. History of asthma or hayfever. Under 4: family history in first-degree relatives
3. Generalised dry skin in the past year
4. Visible eczema. Under 4: over convexities (cheeks, forehead, outer arms). Over 4: in skin creases (as in 1 above)
5. Onset in first 2 years of life.

Subjective findings

The patient/carer will often give a history of:
- skin is very dry, itchy and scaly
- skin is very red and itchy, hot to the touch
- skin texture has changed, lumpy under the surface
- disturbed nights sleep from the itch, with blood on the sheets
- exudate seen and feels unwell in themselves
- cannot stop scratching
- feels embarrassed, unable to socialise, has stopped sports activities
- rash developed after weaning from the breast (close questioning regarding food products in relation to reactions within the skin).

Objective findings

Examine all of the skin:
- Acute: excoriations with serous exudate with erythematous papules and vesicles (see Plate 6). Exfoliation seen.
- Sub-acute: erythematous, excoriated papules or plaques that are either grouped or scattered. Signs of lichenification.
- Chronic: lichenification, excoriated fibrotic papules and nodules. Signs of post-inflammatory hyperpigmentation or hypopigmentation. Painful fissures.
- Infected: any of the above plus pyrexial, exudate and crusting, inflammation, vesicles and bullae seen. Erythema or excessive scaling in skin creases/flexures.
- Cover their skin with clothing and have poor eye contact.
- Nappy area is spared.

Differential diagnosis/assessment

Infected atopic eczema, eczema herpeticum, contact dermatitis, varicose eczema, pompholyx.

Investigations

Investigations that may be required to clarify diagnosis are FBC, ESR, IgE, RAST, patch testing and bacterial or viral swab.

Management plan

1. Patient/carer education
   - Introduction to the disease (concept of control rather than cure). The course of the disease will be exacerbations and remissions: that for some children, they may grow out of it only for it to flare when life events occur, e.g. exams; that they will always have tendency for dry skin and that emollient therapy will be lifelong, as part of their everyday skin hygiene.
   - Discuss possible triggers (infection, food, infection, animals).
   - Explain the role of secondary infection and avoidance of people with cold sores (herpes).
   - The itch–scratch–itch cycle; distraction in children; pinching of the skin rather than rub or scratch. The use of cotton clothing next to the skin.
   - Environment factors (house dust mite, central heating/air conditioning, changes in the weather).
   - Explain the role of therapies and give practical advice on application of therapies (balance the affects versus side effects).
   - Introduction to the patient support group, National Eczema Society, who provide excellent written information.
2. Pharmacotherapeutics
   - Antibiotics: if sure of clinical presentation. Bacterial swab to confirm sensitivities. Oral if generalised and feeling unwell or topical (combined with steroids) if localised.
   - Antivirals: oral. Virology swab to confirm. (For severe cases involving the face, urgent same day referral to a dermatologist.)
   - Bath oil: recommend daily bath or wash to cleanse and hydrate the skin, using tepid water.
   - Soap substitute: to cleanse and hydrate the skin (small tubes at all sinks).
   - Antiseptic/oxidiser (potassium permanganate) soaks are helpful on weeping moist skin for 10 min twice a day for 3–5 days; stop once the skin is dry (light pink solution).

- Emollient (moisturiser): patient preference, frequent thin smooth applications going in the direction of the hair (do not rub or apply heavily). If very dry, then apply hourly – reduce frequency as skin improves. Use oil-based emollient if the skin is very dry, but creams if the skin is sore or moist. If applying in a hot room, then the body temperature will increase with the occlusion of the skin and cause the skin to become itchy, so keep the room temperature cool.
- Topical steroid: potency depends on severity of the condition and location; review after 5–7 days with a view to reduce potency (mild-to-moderate potency steroids can be used for longer but must be regularly reviewed, Greaves & Gatti 1999). Explaining how they work should help to relieve worries about their use; eczema is often under-treated, due to underuse of topical steroids.
- Antihistamines: helpful at night with the sedating effect (if hungover the next day, take it early evening rather than just prior to bed; a good night's sleep for all the family).
3. Communication
   - Involve the health visitor or school nurse to ensure the family and child are fully supported. The community paediatric team could participate in the home care, supervising wet wrapping and relieving the workload on the parents (Mitchell et al 1998) to keep the family unit together. The school nurse can assist with the administration of emollients at school and observe for name calling or bullying.

Third-line treatments that may be considered which would involve regular reviewing

- Impregnated bandages: (if free of infection) useful for lichenified itchy patches (ankles, wrists, flexural areas), mild-to-moderate potency steroid to be used as potency is increased when occluded.
- Occlusive dressings (DuoDERM): (if free of infection) useful for lichenified patches; acts as a barrier for up to 5–7 days; no steroid should be used underneath (unless at dermatologist's request).
- When having an acute onset, intense emollient therapy plus topical steroids. Take a couple of days off school/work to concentrate on skin care.
- Occlusive wet wraps: if erythematous and intensely itchy, with no signs of infection, then discuss with local dermatologist for potency strength to be used under the moist Tubifast. Supervision of application of wet wrap essential; review every 48 hours, make sure that the wrap does not prevent social development of the child. Wet wraps should only be used for short periods of time, 3–7 days (Mitchell et al 1998).
- If history indicates diet, then exclusion diet only under direct supervision of dietician.

Indications for referral

- Urgent: eczema herpeticum or severely infected eczema (febrile) to consultant dermatologist
- Immediate: infected eczema should be reviewed after 72 hours and further review dates arranged
- Chronic: if first line management fails, referral for patch testing if indicated by history; phototherapy; behaviour modification or systemic therapies.

Complications

- Wet wrapping on top of infected skin
- Permanent atrophy damage due to incorrect potency of steroid used under wet wrap or any other occlusive dressing
- Eczema herpeticum in erythrodermic (90% body surface red) eczema, especially around the eyes
- Nutritional deficit due to unsupervised occlusion diet
- Social isolation, loss of self-esteem and low spirits
- Breakdown of the family unit.

Varicose eczema

Definition: Gravitational statis eczema of the lower leg (see Plate 7), often accompanied with venous insufficiency, a chronic eczematous condition of the lower legs, which can on occasions become acute with infection. Williams (1997) cited the NHANES study (prevalence of significant skin pathology among 20,749 US persons aged 1–74 years) that suggested that around 1% of the population had a clinically significant eczema that was not atopic eczema or contact dermatitis. Thus, the combination of statis eczema and ulceration can be complicated by itch, infection and superimposed contact dermatitis.

Subjective findings

The patient will often give a history of:
- skin is very dry, itchy and scaly
- skin is very red and itchy, feels hot to the touch
- skin texture has changed and is discoloured.

Objective findings

Examine all of the skin, check for signs of secondary spread of the eczema:
- Acute: excoriations with serous exudate with erythematous papules and vesicles. Exfoliation seen and pitting oedema of the ankles.
- Sub-acute: erythematous, excoriated papules or plaques that are either grouped or scattered. Signs of lichenification and oedema at the ankles.
- Chronic: lichenification, excoriated fibrotic papules and nodules. Signs of post-inflammatory hyperpigmentation or hypopigmentation. Pigment staining from haemoglobin breakdown. Xeroderma seen.
- Infected: any of the above plus pyrexial, exudate and crusting, inflammation, vesicles and bullae seen.

- Inflammatory skin correlated to dressing used (note demarked margins).
- If ulceration present, then confirm venous ulceration with assessment of ankle brachial pressure index (Stubbing et al 1997).

Differential diagnosis/assessment

Infected varicose eczema, cellulitis, superimposed contact dermatitis.

Investigations

Investigations that may be required to clarify diagnosis are bacterial swab and patch testing.

Management plan

1. Patient/carer education
   - Introduction to the disease (concept of control rather than cure); progression of exacerbations and remissions; that emollient therapy will be part of everyday skin care.
   - Discuss probable cause and possible triggers (infection, allergy, poor venous circulation).
   - Explain the role of secondary infection.
   - The itch–scratch–itch cycle; pinching of the skin rather than rub or scratch. The use of cotton clothing next to the skin.
   - Environmental factors (central heating/air conditioning, changes in weather).
   - Need to promote circulation and prevent oedema through passive exercises and elevation of the legs when sitting or in bed.
   - Explain the role of the therapies and give practical advice on application.
2. Pharmacotherapeutics
   - Antibiotics: if sure of clinical presentation. Bacterial swab to confirm sensitivities. Avoid topical antibiotic creams if an ulcer is present to reduce possibility of sensitisation; neomycin and framycetin remain the most common sensitisers in leg ulcers (Cameron 1998).
   - Soap substitute: recommended daily wash to cleanse and rehydrate the skin, using tepid water rather than hot to avoid causing vasodilation and dehydration.
   - Emollient (moisturiser): patient preference, frequent thin smooth applications going in the direction of the hair (do not rub or apply heavily) several times a day. If the skin is especially itchy and hot at night, add menthol to one of the emollient creams. Use oil-based emollient if skin very dry, but creams if the skin is sore or moist. If applying in a hot room, then the body temperature will increase with the occlusion of the skin and cause the skin to become itchy, so keep the room temperature cool.
   - Topical steroid: potency depends on severity of the condition and location; review after 5–7 days with a view to reduce potency (mild-to-moderate potency steroids can be used for longer but must be regularly reviewed, Greaves & Gatti 1999). Explaining how they work should help to relieve worries about their use; eczema is often under-treated due to under use of topical steroids.
   - Impregnated bandages (if free from infection) are effective for hydration and cool the skin; they can act as a physical barrier to reduce damage to fragile skin from scratching.
   - If this occurs while a patient is having compression bandaging then it is worth reassessing and altering the regime so that the eczema is treated on a daily basis, taking priority over the ulcer.
3. Communication
   - Involve the practice nurse or district nurse to ensure the patient is supported in the community and plan intervention with them if the patient requires.

Indications for referral

- Urgent: if the varicose eczema becomes severely infected and cellulitis develops with the patient being febrile, refer to a consultant dermatologist
- Immediate: if the varicose eczema becomes widespread or infected, a review of the patient should occur after 72 hours and further review dates should be arranged.

Complications

- Use of impregnated bandages on top of infected skin
- Allergy to any component in the topical therapies
- Atrophy in the skin of the elderly from potent steroids
- Social isolation, loss of self-esteem and low spirits, especially if the patient also has a leg ulcer.

Allergic contact dermatitis

Definition: Contact dermatitis (see Plate 8) is a generic term applied to acute or chronic inflammatory reactions to substances that come into contact with the skin (Fitzpatrick et al 1997). This can be spilt into two types: contact irritant dermatitis caused by a chemical irritant or contact allergic dermatitis caused by an antigen that elicits type IV delayed hypersensitivity.

Contact allergic dermatitis is a delayed cell-mediated hypersensitivity response to an antigen to which you would have been exposed previously. The presentation can vary from severe pruritus to erythema, papules and vesicles, which initially occur on the site of contact and which may give clues to possible causes, e.g. demarked cut-off margin above the wrists indicates rubber gloves. In chronic irritant dermatitis, the epidermis barrier is disturbed and hyperkeratosis, fissuring and maceration can occur.

Subjective findings

The patient/carer will often:

- give a family history of atopy
- say that the condition improves at weekends or when on holiday
- have identified a possible cause related to specific activities, e.g. hair dye, perfume, cheap jewellery
- have skin that is red, dry and itchy
- have had blisters and weeping skin
- have noted skin texture changes related to scratching; ask what it first presented like.

Objective findings

Examine all the skin and the affected areas:

- Acute: background erythema with papules or vesicles. Crusting from exudate and scaling. Area affected has a demarked edge, location could be help for differential diagnosis and there may be some secondary erythema.
- Chronic: erythematous plaques with papules, fissures, scaling and crusts; the edge is more blurred with some generalised involvement. Signs of lichenification.

Differential diagnosis/assessment

Irritant contact dermatitis, infected allergic contact dermatitis, atopic eczema, pompholyx, pustular psoriasis, fungal infection.

Investigations

Investigations that may be required to clarify diagnosis are IgE, patch testing, bacterial swab and skin scraping.

Management plan

1. Patient/carer education
   - Introduction to the disease.
   - Identification of cause (rubber, hair dye, perfume, nickel, etc.) where possible and discussion on avoidance and how that might impact on their life (hairdresser – hair dye). The role of the allergen in daily life, e.g. perfume found in shampoo, airfreshers, food, etc.
   - Explain role of secondary infection with the epidermal barrier impaired.
   - Explain the role of the topical and systemic therapies and give practical advice on application.
   - Explain the procedure for referral to a dermatologist for patch testing.
2. Pharmacotherapeutics
   - Antibiotics: if sure of clinical presentation. Bacterial swab to confirm sensitivities. Oral if generalised and feeling unwell, or topical (combined with steroids) if localised.
   - Bath oil: recommend daily bath or wash to cleanse and hydrate the skin, using tepid water.
   - Soap substitute: to cleanse and hydrate skin (small tubes at all sinks) (essential in hand dermatitis).
   - Antiseptic/oxidiser (potassium permanganate) soaks are helpful on weeping moist skin for 10 min twice a day for 3–5 days; stop once the skin is dry (light pink solution).
   - Emollient (moisturiser): patient preference, frequent thin smooth applications going in the direction of the hair (do not rub or apply heavily). If very dry, then apply hourly – reduce frequency as skin improves. Use oil-based emollient if skin very dry, but creams if the skin is sore or moist.
   - Topical steroid: potency depends on severity of the condition and location, review after 5–7 days with a view to reduce potency (mild-to-moderate potency steroids can be used for longer but must be regularly reviewed). Explaining how they work should help to relieve worries about their use.
   - First-generation antihistamines: helpful at night with the sedating effect.
3. Communication
   - Ensure that the known allergen is well documented and the patient understands the importance of telling other health professionals. (Latex allergy can alter from type IV to type I hypersensitivity.)
   - Check all the patient's topical and systemic medication once allergens have been identified following patch testing (also check dressings that may be in use).

Indications for referral

- Urgent: acute inflammatory response with bulla and angio-oedema to consultant dermatologist
- Immediate/chronic: referral for patch testing and advice on further management.

Complications

- Sensitisation from patch testing
- Type I hypersensitivity
- Cellulitis.

Psoriasis

Definition: A chronic, non-infectious, inflammatory disease with several clinical expressions, but the most common are characterised by well-defined erythematous plaques bearing large adherent silvery scales (see Plate 9). There is a genetic predisposition that affects 1.5–2% of the population in the Western world (Fitzpatrick et al 1997). A child with one affected parent has a 25% chance of developing the disease and this rises to 60% if both parents are affected (Hunter et al 1995).

Precipitating factors

- Trauma – psoriasis appears on skin damaged by scratching, surgical scars, or tattoos, etc. (Koebner phenomenon).
- Infection – β-haemolytic streptococcal throat or upper respiratory infections often trigger guttate psoriasis.
- Sunlight – most psoriatic patients improve, but 10% get worse.

- Drugs – antimalarials, β-blockers and lithium worsen the condition. Rebound if systemic or potent topical steroids have been used.
- Emotion – emotional upset can cause some exacerbations.
- Disease – HIV can exacerbate the disease. Joint pain – arthritis (incidence is 5–8%) more common in pustular or erythrodermic psoriasis (see Plate 10) (Fitzpatrick et al 1997). Using the Vancouver criteria 8% of all cases of childhood arthritis are diagnosed as psoriatic arthritis (Pringle 1999).

Types of psoriatic arthritis (Pringle 1999)

Asymmetrical	Occurs in approximately 70% of cases
Oligoarticular	Involves one or more joints, especially the knees, fingers and toes, which may show sausage-like swelling
Symmetrical rheumatoid-like	Affects approximately 5% of psoriatic arthritis sufferers
Distal interphalangeal (DIP)	Involves the last small joint of the fingers or toes, nail changes are common
Arthritis mutilans	Severe, deforming arthritis that involves multiple small joints of the hands, feet and spine
Spondylitis	Inflammation of the spine and sacroiliac joints

Subjective findings

The patient will often give a history of:
- skin is very scaly, with raised red patches on their body (and scalp)
- skin is very itchy and uncomfortable (including groin and flexural areas)
- white pus spots
- nail changes
- skin fissures
- skin is very red and they feel cold
- feels embarrassed; in low spirits and withdrawn from socialising
- fatigue and joint stiffness.

Objective findings

Examine all the skin:
- macular/papular hyperkeratotic rash
- lesions are well demarcated – ranging in diameter from a few millimetres to several centimetres
- plaques are raised pink to salmon red, with silvery scales on top
- excoriations, fissures with signs of bleeding on plaques

- pitting of the nails and hyperkeratosis of the nail bed
- pityriasis amianteciea (scale along the hair shaft), some hair loss from scratching
- wearing clothes warmer than climate requires – skin erythrodermic
- pustules seen
- in the submammary, axillary and angential folds, well-demarcated glistening plaques, little scale
- swollen, painful single large joint or a few interphalangeal joints.

The physical assessment tool may be useful to assess distribution and severity of the condition when deciding on the management required.

The psoriasis area and severity index (PASI)

Four main anatomic sites are assessed:
  (i)   Head (h)
  (ii) Upper extremities (u)
  (iii) Trunk (t)
  (iv) Lower extremities (l)
They roughly correspond to 10, 20, 30 and 40% of the body surface area (BSA), respectively. Each BSA is then assessed using a 4-point scale, where
  0 = no symptoms
  1 = slight
  2 = moderate
  3 = marked
  4 = very marked
for the following:
  E = Erythema
  I = Induration
  D = Desquamation
  A = Area
The score varies in steps of units from 0.0 to 72.0. The highest score represents complete erythroderma. (From McKenna & Stern 1997, cited by Watts 1999.)

Although rarely life-threatening, psoriasis can be disabling and have a significant impact on quality of life, making it a potentially psychologically debilitating disease. Thus, a tool which measures quality of life may be useful when considering intervention management.

Dermatology life quality index (DLQI)

The aim of creating the DLQI was to meet the need for a short, simple and validated questionnaire to measure the impact of skin disease on patients' quality of life (Finlay & Khan 1994).

Each question was designed to refer to the experience of the previous week. The question topics of the DLQI are given in Box 4.6. The scoring is based on each question having four alternative responses, scored from 0 to 3. The maximum score is 30, representing maximum handicap.

For use with children there is the Children's Dermatology Life Quality Index (CDLQI); the authors of this are now working on a cartoon version. The scoring is the same as for the adults.

Differential diagnosis/assessment

Erythrodermic psoriasis, guttate psoriasis, pustular psoriasis, fungal or bacterial infection.

Investigations

Investigations that may be required are skin scrapings, nail clippings, throat swab and rheumatoid factor.

Management plan

1. Patient/carer education:
   - Introduction to the disease. Treatment is suppression rather than curative and the progress of the disease is recurrences and remissions.
   - Discuss possible triggers (infection, psychological).
   - Discuss exacerbating factors (smoking, alcohol, drugs).
   - Explain the role of topical therapies and practical advice about application (balance the affects against the side effects).
   - Discuss ways of maintaining joint mobility.
2. Pharmacotherapeutics:
   - Bath oil: recommend daily bath or wash to cleanse and hydrate the skin, using tepid water.
   - Soap substitute: to cleanse and hydrate the skin (small tubes at all sinks).
   - Emollient (moisturiser): patient preference, frequent thin smooth applications going in the direction of the hair (do not rub or apply heavily). If very dry, then apply hourly – reduce frequency as skin improves. Use oil-based emollient if the skin is very dry, but creams if the skin is sore or moist. Moisturising removes the scale on the surface that would otherwise block penetration by the therapeutic medications. If the patient has arthritis, suggest an emollient that has a pump dispenser delivery.
   - Topical steroid: moderate to mild steroids used to reduce inflammation (flexural areas and scalps); liquid form may be useful for nails.
   - Topical steroids and coal tar solution reduces inflammation and acts as an antipruritic (yellow and greasy – glisten on the plaques, useful in widespread superficial small plaques and guttate psoriasis).
   - Shampoo for the scalp with tar.
   - Oil preparation to the scalp lesion to remove the scale (coconut oil) – part the hair every half-inch and apply directly to the scalp. If very scaly, then occlude with a shower cap over night.
   - Preparations for the scalp combining steroid and tar to treat the plaques.
   - Vitamin D analogues: apply precisely to the plaques up to the edge but avoid surrounding skin as they can cause irritation; they clear scale and make the plaques redder. Lotion can be useful for hyperkeratosis under the nail plate.
   - Short-contact anthralin requires precise application to plaques to avoid burning surrounding skin, and care in handling and removal to avoid staining skin and household materials; it is only applied for maximum of 30 min.
   - Retinoid therapies, which are useful in those with large-scale plaques (no more than 20% body surface), can cause irritation of the plaques and surrounding skin as it is easy to apply; avoid going on to surrounding skin.
   - Analgesia to control joint pain and enable joint mobility.
3. Communication
   - Involve the district nurses/home care teams to assist patients to carry out the applications at home, especially if they have arthritis.
   - Paediatric community team and school nurse for children/teenagers to prevent bullying and encourage mobility of painful joints.

Indications for referral

- Urgent: 90% surface areas involved are erythematous with pustulation.
- Immediate: referral for phototherapy for guttate psoriasis.
- Chronic: referral for consideration for day care topical therapies and/or phototherapy. Poorly motivated patients who need extra support.

Complications

- Erythrodermic – loss of body heat, protein and dysfunction of lipid barrier
- Generalised pustulation
- Secondary infection
- Psoriasis unstable due to use of potent/very potent steroids
- Social isolation and breakdown of interpersonal relationships
- Severe arthritis; skin condition takes second place while pain management is adjusted

Impetigo

Definition: *Staphylococcus aureus* and *Streptococcus pyogenes* are capable of causing superficial infection of the epidermis characterised by yellow crusting erosions (see Plate 11) (Fitzpatrick et al 1997). It can be a primary infection of a small traumatised area of skin or a secondary infection of pre-existing dermatoses.

Subjective findings

The patient/carer will often give a history of:
- eruptions suddenly appearing
- erosions that are weepy
- yellow crusting on the surface and feels unwell
- lesions are itchy
- febrile.

Objective findings

Examine all of the skin:
- Clinical signs of infection – heat, erythema, swelling and pain (streptococcal infections are usually painful)
- Excoriations
- Background dermatoses exacerbated
- Superficial small vesicles or pustules, scattered discrete lesions variable in size
- Distribution on face, arms, legs and buttocks (bullous trunk, face, hands, intertriginous sites)
- Erosions with a yellow crusting on surface
- Bullae may be present and contain yellow fluid that easily erupts with no surrounding erythema
- Lymphadenopathy may occur
- Check temperature.

Differential diagnosis/assessment

Infected atopic eczema, bullous impetigo.

Investigations

Investigations that may be required to clarify diagnosis: bacterial swabs and nasal swab. Culture or use Gram's staining, so that sensitivities can identify group of antibiotics necessary.

Management plan

1. Patient/carer education
   - Introduction to the role of infection and cross-infection within the family setting.
   - Arrange to check other family members (20–25% of individuals are carriers of nasal staphylococcus).
   - Identify portal of entry – trauma or underlying dermatoses.
   - Explain the importance of completing the course of oral medication and how to use an emollient. What to do if side effects/intolerance occurs.
   - Identify if occurrence is due to treatment failure.
   - Organise management plan of underlying dermatoses.

2. Pharmacotherapeutics
   - Antibiotics: if sure of clinical presentation, commence broad-spectrum antibiotics until sensitivities are identified, and alter if necessary
   - Consult with a local microbiologist before prescribing topical therapy (Mupirocin).
   - Personal hygiene is essential to clearance of infection. Introduce a soap substitute with an antiseptic to cleanse the skin surface.
   - Separate bathing flannel and towel to reduce cross-infection from other family members.
   - Use emollient therapy to restore epidermal barrier.
3. Communication
   - Contact school nurse for incidence at school.

Indications for referral

- Urgent: cellulitis or erysipelas or suppurative lymphadenitis or septicaemia to consultant dermatologist or to Accident & Emergency Department
- Immediate: localised cellulitis, scarlet fever.

Complications

- Systemic illness following impetigo
- Scarring of the lesions
- Management of the underlying dermatosis.

Herpes simplex

Definition: Herpes virus hominis is the cause: type I is extragenital; type II occurs mainly on the genitals.

Primary occurrence in children is nongenital herpes simplex virus (HSV), an acute gingivostomatitis accompanied by malaise, fever, headaches and enlarged cervical nodes. The route of infection may be through mucous membranes or broken skin and the incubation period is between 2 and 20 days (average 6 days) for primary infection (Fitzpatrick et al 1997). Recurrent infection may occur in the same place and may be triggered by respiratory tract infection, ultraviolet (UV) light, menstruation, underlying immunosuppression, and stress. An attack usually lasts 1 week.

Subjective findings

The patient/carer will often report:
- tingling/painful (burning) sensation lasting several hours
- a red lesion with blisters that becomes crusty
- underlying eczema flares.

Objective findings

Examination of all the skin:
- clusters of tense vesicles (commonly on the face), with an erythematous base on keratinized skin

- erythema and oedema of the gingiva
- crusting of lesions occur within 48 hours, with erosions underneath
- the skin, in general, is erythematous, dry and scaly
- check the patient's temperature
- lymphadenopathy may occur.

Differential diagnosis/assessment

Eczema herpeticum, erythema multiformis.

Investigations

A viral swab investigation may be required to clarify diagnosis.

Management plan

1. Patient/carer education
   - Introduction of the condition.
   - Discuss possible triggers.
   - Identify if anyone at home is atopic. Mention concerns about cross-infection.
   - Skin-to-skin contact should be avoided to prevent further cross-infection.
   - If triggered by UV light, discuss future sun behaviour to reduce possibility of recurrence.
   - Give advice on how to apply topical therapies and how to cleanse the skin.
2. Pharmacotherapeutics
   - Antivirals – for localised non-atopic patient, antiviral cream is applied 5 or 6 times a day to the crop of vesicles for 5 days. If more widespread, systemically unwell or atopic, then oral antiviral tablets are given for 5 days.
   - Normal saline soaks are helpful to soften the crusts.
   - Greasy emollient softens crusts and hydrates the skin surface.
3. Communication
   - Contact school nurse to inform her of the outbreak. Identify possible contacts.

Indications for referral

- Urgent: generalised, with atopic eczema, or localised to eyes, refer to dermatologist/ophthalmologist for intravenous (IV) antiviral therapy
- Immediate: if resistant to topical therapy, review for oral antivirals and investigate for possible immunosuppression
- Chronic: refer for advice as regards prophylactic antiviral therapy and investigate for possible immunosuppression.

Complications

- Eczema herpeticum on the face, leading to cornea ulcers and scarring
- Resistance to first-line oral antivirals may require IV antivirals
- Re-occurrence in immunosuppressed patients.

Herpes zoster

Definition: An acute dermatomal infection with reactivation of the varicella-zoster virus, characterised by unilateral pain and vesicular or bullous eruption limited to a dermatome innervated by a corresponding ganglion (Fitzpatrick et al 1997) since an earlier episode of chickenpox (varicella). Post-zoster neuralgia can last for over 18 months.

Most common factor is diminishing immunity to the varicella-zoster virus with advancing age, with 66% of over 50s becoming infected. Immunosuppressed, post-radiotherapy and HIV-infected individuals have an eight-fold increased incidence of zoster (Fitzpatrick et al 1997).

Subjective findings

The patient may report:
- stabbing, shooting or sharp pain and/or itching, burning, tingling or freeze-burning occurs 3–5 days prior to cutaneous eruptions
- blisters/vesicles then erupt for 3–5 days before crusting occurs over the following 3 weeks
- complaining of malaise, fever or headaches in the early stages
- post-neuralgia pain then occurs, lasting months to years, which make the patient depressed; little relief is gained with analgesia.

Objective findings

Examine all of the skin:
- Prodromal stage: malaise, headaches, check temperature, pain in the skin, heightened sensitivity to stimuli.
- Active vesiculation: neuritic pain, papules – vesicles/bullae occur between 24 and 48 hours with erythematous bases, superimposed clear vesicles. If traumatised, then haemorrhagic.
- Clusters occur along a dermatome unilaterally: can involve one or two dermatomes, but does not cross the midline.
- Depending on the dermatome, affect check on the mucous membranes (mouth, vagina and bladder) for vesicular eruptions.
- Lymphadenopathy can occur.
- Check temperature for low-grade pyrexia.
- Involvement of nasociliary VI of the trigeminal nerve – clusters on the side and the tip of the nose.
- Isolated vesicular/crusty lesions found outside of the involved dermatome.
- Localised inflammation, as possible secondary infection, could be present.

Differential diagnosis/assessment

Myocardial infarction, acute abdomen, migraine, contact dermatitis, photoallergy (poison ivy), bullous impetigo.

Investigations

Investigations that may be required to clarify diagnosis are electrocardiogram (ECG), imaging, blister fluid, and viral swab.

Management plan

1. Patient/carer education
   - Introduction to the disease.
   - Discuss possible contact. Identify other family members who have not had chicken pox before.
   - Explain the role of infection and cross-infection.
   - Demonstrate how to apply wet dressings.
   - Discuss the importance of completing courses of systemic therapies.
   - Discuss management of pain and the possible duration.
2. Pharmacotherapeutics
   - Antivirals systemic in the first 72 hours can be effective in accelerating healing and decreasing pain (7–10 day course).
   - IV antivirals for ophthalmic zoster or in an immunosuppressed patient.
   - Oral corticosteroids can reduce the likelihood and severity of post-neuralgic pain.
   - Pain management is crucial to prevent sleep loss, fatigue and depression. Narcotic analgesia may be needed initially. Topical local anaesthetic creams may be useful, as may nerve block or acupuncture. Tricyclic drugs may be useful for treating pain and low spirits.
   - Moist dressings (water or saline) to the dermatome may relieve irritation and pain.
3. Communication
   - Regular review of pain control is required, depending on the patient's circumstance, either by the nurse practitioner (NP) or district nurse or shared care.

Indications for referral

- Urgent: ophthalmic zoster or dissemination beyond two dermatomes or an immunosuppressed patient for IV antiviral therapy
- Immediate: review every day initially to manage pain and monitor progress of the disease or if there is any temporary paralysis of an upper or lower limb
- Chronic: referral to pain management team if unstable post-neuralgic pain.

Complications

- Cornea ulcers and scarring
- Underlying cause if there is widespread involvement
- Depression.

Pediculosis

Definition: Infestation of scalp or bodily hair. Pediculosis capitis is an infestation of the head louse, which feeds on the scalp and neck, it lays eggs on the hair shaft, causing little discomfort. Pediculosis pubis is an infestation of hair-bearing regions, most commonly the public area, but they can include hairy upper chests, axilla and eyebrows. This usually causes some pruritus.

Pediculosis capitis is more common in young children; pediculosis pubis can affect all ages, but more extensive infestation occurs in men.

Subjective findings

The patient/carer will often report:
- itchy scalp or nape of neck
- itchy in pubic areas or in other hairy places
- children can be distracted or restless in school
- debris found when brushing hair (dry lice faeces – black gritty powder) or in white underwear
- carer is often angry or distressed about this possible infestation, looking to blame someone
- has had a previous infestation.

Objective findings

Examine the scalp by parting the hair every half-inch and looking closely at the hair shaft or all bodily hairy areas (depending on history):
- wet comb the hair to identify live lice, faecal matter, eggs attached to hair shafts (wet the hair, part it into sections and comb through with a plastic detection comb and then wipe onto a dry tissue and observe as the lice move as they become dry again).
- excoriations, lichenification and secondary infection (swab) due to excess scratching in the affected hairy area
- small erythematous papules on the surrounding skin (feeding sites)
- white-grey specks (beads) along the hair/skin junction (eggs) are signs of active infestation
- serous crusting and oedema of the eyelids, if infested
- lymphadenopathy, if secondary infected.

Differential diagnosis/assessment

Eczema, seborrhoeic dermatitis, impetigo, lichen simplex chronicus, dandruff.

Investigations

Investigations that may be required to clarify diagnosis are wet hair combing for debris and taking a bacterial swab (secondary infection).

Management plan

1. Patient/carer education
   - Assurance to relieve embarrassment.
   - Modes of transmission (close head-to-head contact with a temperature of 30°C before the lice passes from hair to hair). Close bodily contact, sharing of hats, sleeping in the same bed. Head lice can survive off the scalp for up to 55 hours (Fitzpatrick et al 1997).

- Identify any possible contacts (in the last 4 weeks) so that they may receive treatment at the same time and prevent re-infection.
- Identify the family's responsibility to prevent, detect, treat and monitor for head lice.
- Explain fully how to use the topical preparations (identify safety issues), use of hair conditioner and the technique of wet combing.
- Pediculosis pubis – decontamination of environment, machine wash bedding and clothing or remove from bodily contact for at least 72 hours.

2. Pharmacotherapeutics
- Three groups of insecticides are available, but there is little evidence on the comparative effectiveness of these products (Simmons 1999). However, a course of two treatments 7 days apart is generally recommended; it takes the lice 5 days to die and they become more visible on the scalp, which is often seen as a sign of failed treatment. For pediculosis capitis, apply to the scalp and leave on for 12 hours/overnight and then wash out. For pediculosis pubis, apply and leave on for 1–12 hours before washing off. The treatment of choice should be in line with local policy, and length of time the treatment is left in contact with the hair varies with different preparations.
- Systemic antibiotics may be required to treat the host response – choice depending on sensitivities.
- Sexual partners in the last month should be treated (Fitzpatrick et al 1997).
- Occlusive ophthalmic ointment should be applied to the eyelid margins twice a day for 10 days.

3. Communication
- Contact school nurse to inform her, so that notification of other parents can occur. Check what support is available for the families.
- Tracing contacts is an important part of prevention and guidance may be required for those people contacted by the family or the school nurse.

Indications for referral

- Chronic: monitoring of patient/carer who has complied with all instructions yet still has persistent pruritus; then, review for re-diagnosis.

Complications

- Misdiagnosis; skin more exacerbated from topical insecticides.

Scabies

Definition: Scabies is an infestation by the mite *Sarcoptes scabiei* (see Plate 12). It usually spreads by skin-to-skin contact and is characterised by a generalised intolerable pruritus, with often minimal cutaneous findings. A healthy adult with scabies has on average 6–10 mites infesting his body. The mite can remain alive over 2 days and thus can be transmitted in shared clothing.

Subjective findings

The patient will report:
- generalised intolerable itching for several weeks
- itchiness is worse at night or when hot
- red scaly rash (known atopy) occurred several weeks after the pruritus
- lumps or spots in the axilla
- scaly lesions on the penis
- crusty lesions, not that itchy, and a history of immunosuppression
- previous infestation, and has had a known contact.

Objective findings

Examine all of the skin:
- Observe closely for intradermal burrows (grey or skin-coloured ridges), 0.5–1.0 mm in length, either linear or wavy, with a minute papule or vesicle at the end of the tunnel (see Plate 13). Burrows average 5–10 mm in length. The blind end of the burrow, where the mite resides, may be slightly elevated with a halo of erythema around it. No cutaneous signs are found.
- Examine areas that have few or little hair follicles, where the stratum corneum is thin and soft (e.g. in the toe/finger webs, flexural areas, axilla, wrists, elbows, shaft of penis, genitalia). In babies, it can occur anywhere. In the elderly, the burrows can be numerous when the host response is modified, e.g. in dementia the perception of itch may be different to normal or with severe arthritis it is difficult to scratch.
- Excoriations and lichenification as a result of scratching.
- Erythematous, scaly dry dermatitis at sites of heaviest infestation.
- Well-demarcated plaque covered with a thick crust that has been present for some months–years.
- Small urticarial papules, mainly on anterior trunk, thighs, buttocks, as an 'id' or autosensitisation-type reaction.
- Impetiginised excoriations – inflammation from secondary infection.

Differential diagnosis

Atopic eczema, metabolic pruritus, adverse cutaneous drug eruption, papular urticaria (insect bites), crusted scabies and impetigo.

Investigations

Investigations that may be required to clarify diagnosis are microscopy of mites' bodies, their eggs and their faecal pellets and taking a bacterial swab.

Management plan

1. Patient/carer education
- Introduction to the condition and reassurance.
- Discuss possible mode of transmission and identify contacts who may have been in skin-to-skin contact in the last month (family members,

Table 4.4 *Causative agents of tinea*

Organism	Tinea pedis	Tinea corporis	Tinea capitis	Tinea unguium
Trichophyton rubrum	✓	✓		✓
Epidermophyton floccosum	✓			
Microsporum canis		✓		
Trichophyton verrucosum		✓	✓	
Microsporum audouinii			✓	
Trichophyton tonsurans			✓	
Trichophyton mentagrophytes				✓

sexual partners, children playing or health care professional) and the importance of carrying out the treatments simultaneously to prevent re-cross-infection. Everyone at risk should be treated, regardless of whether they are showing any symptoms, because there is a latent period of 4–6 weeks after scabies is acquired and itching develops (Burns 1999).

- Discuss how the topical therapies should be carried out: the importance of soaking every little skin fold and the duration of the itch which will continue for several weeks after successful treatment.
- Decontaminate the environment, machine wash bedding and clothing or remove from bodily contact for at least 72 hours.

2. Pharmacotherapeutics
- Scabicides applied to the skin of all those involved (avoiding the eyes) and left on for 12 hours prior to washing off; instruction will vary depending on the product used. The scabicides used will depend on local policies, as will the option of a second application within 7 days. In small children, application may include the head. Safety issues apply with some products, e.g. do not apply following a bath or shower.
- Systemic therapy (named patient only) could be an alternative to several applications of topical scabicides.
- Antihistamines, oral or topically, for symptomatic relief of itch (be aware of sedating effects).
- Oral corticosteroids may be given if there is a severe hypersensitivity to the mite.
- Mild-to-moderate potency steroids reduce the inflammatory response to scratching, especially for those with atopic eczema.
- Systemic antibiotics may be required for secondary infection, depending on the host response and sensitivities.
- Topical emollient therapy may be of use to smooth the skin; certain products have an antipruitic effect.

3. Communication
- Assistance may be required if a nursing/residential patient is involved. Treat all patients, health care professionals, visitors and families.

- Contact the school nurse if a school aged child is affected to organise treatment of classmates and their families.

Indications for referral
- Urgent: referral for consideration of systemic steroids for severe hypersensitivity reaction
- Chronic: review and consider alternative diagnosis if pruritus is persistent; diagnosis not confirmed by successful treatment.

Complications
- Misdiagnosis
- Resistance to topical therapies
- Scabietic nodules.

Tinea

Definition: Fungal infections are usually described according to the site they affect. The term fungal is used to describe a group of infections caused by the following: dermatophytes (ringworm), non-dermatophytes moulds (aspergillus, scopulariopsis) and yeasts, (candida and pityrosporum) (Table 4.4). Fungal infections are usually unilateral, whereas yeast infections are bilateral (except in the groin). A dermatophyte can be identified by scaly erythema-defined edge plaques with central clearing, excessive scaling in the skin creases or, if by stretching the skin between two fingers (5 cm apart), fine scaling is seen. Yeast infections are often moist with pustules along the periphery and on nearby healthy skin or macerated in between skin webs. It can be intensely itchy – scratching can cause secondary infection and spread. Confirmation from the mycology of a fungal infection is important, so that the most effective treatment can be given.

Tinea corporis: affecting skin surface
Tinea capitis: affecting the scalp
Tinea pedis: affecting the feet
Tinea unguium: affecting the nail.

Subjective findings

Patients may report:
- skin is irritated and itchy between the toes
- skin is red, flaky and itchy with some pus-like spots on their body or in the groin or flexures

- loss of hair, scaling and irritation
- nails look unslightly, discoloured or thickened.

Objective findings

Examine the entire skin surface, as a secondary lesion may be present; compare healthy nails to affected nails. Examine the scalp by parting the hair every half-inch and looking at the hair shaft:

- Skin is flaking and fissuring has occurred. Maceration and inflammation of surrounding tissue. Nails and palms can also be involved.
- Pustules or vesicles may be seen periphery to the scaling edge.
- Large scaling-demarcated edged plaques with central clearing. Pustules present at the edge.
- Dull red, tan or brown hyperpigmentation, depending on the pigment of the skin.
- Signs of lichenification from scratching.
- Inflammation and crusting of secondary infection.
- Severity of scaling ranges from mild to diffused with possible alopecia.
- Erythematous lesions or formation of kerion with pus exuding under pressure.
- Yellow crusting and malodorous scalp.
- Hyperkeratosis and onycholysis of the nail bed at the distal end of the nail.

Differential diagnosis

Erythrasma, impetigo, eczema, contact dermatitis, intertrigo or psoriasis.

Investigations

Investigations that may be required to confirm diagnosis are skin scrapping, nail clippings, hair debris for mycology, Wood's light examination, and a bacterial swab.

Management plan

1. Patient/carer education
   - Give an explanation of what a fungal infection is and reassure (especially if there is hair loss).
   - Discuss possible contact and mode of transmission and cross-infection.
   - Explain about secondary infection.
   - Discourage the sharing of towels, hats, bedding and personal items.
   - Shoe/inner sole hygiene, wearing of shoes in communal area, open footwear to reduce sweating of the feet as chronicity can occur.
   - Explain how to apply and the duration of the medication to be used or the course of tablets to be completed, especially for children, as the course should be 8 weeks in length. If nail involvement identify how long it would be for a clear nail to grow out (9 months).
2. Pharmacotherapeutics
   - Systemic antifungals should be prescribed for nails and hair; mycology results are important to identify the causative agent, so that the most effective treatment may be given. Liver function/renal blood tests may be required for baseline values to monitor for adverse effects of azoles drugs. If there is chronic re-infection of the skin or several areas of the skin are involved, then systemic therapy is effective.
   - Topical antifungals should be applied to the affected skin twice a day after cleaning and drying the skin. Duration depends on the product prescribed, but warn the patient about stopping too soon once the skin has improved.
   - Topical antifungal powders may be helpful to powder the inside of shoes.
   - Systemic antibiotics for host response to secondary infection; choice of drug depends on sensitivities.
3. Communication
   - Involvement of other agencies if there is permanent hair loss (hairpieces).
   - Referral to plastic surgeon once clear of disease for tissue expansion, for revision of scarred alopecia areas of the scalp.
   - Contact school nurse or nurseries so that the contact can be traced.

Indications for referral

- Urgent: scarring alopecia with kerion formation needs systemic therapy to reduce permanent hair loss; if clinical signs significant, refer immediately – do not await mycology results
- Immediate: if mycology positive but has a history of hepatic/renal impairment, consider systemic therapy but half-dose levels and repeat bloods
- Chronic: reoccurrence of tinea considered failure of topical treatment; refer for systemic therapy.

Complications

- Misdiagnosis
- Permanent hair loss
- Hepatic/renal impairment.

Pityriasis versicolor

Definition: This is a chronic itchy, scaling dermatosis associated with the yeast *Pityrosporum ovale*, which is present in the hair follicles; an overgrowth in the yeast is associated with a host response. Pityriasis versicolor appears mainly on the front and back of the upper trunk and is characterised by fine scaling and post-inflammatory hyperpigmentation, illustrating the hypopigmentation of the normal skin tone (see Plate 14).

Subjective findings

Patients may report that:

- a rash that has been present for months
- a rash has appeared on their trunk that is more noticeable since being on holiday (tanned skin)

- the skin has lost pigment and is scaly in patients with skin type III–VI (see Box 4.3)
- there is a scaly pink rash present on the skin in patients with skin type I–II (see Box 4.3)
- the skin is irritable and itchy.

Objective findings

Examine all of the skin:
- hypopigmented, well-demarcated macules or follicular macules usually found on the trunk but can involve the limbs
- pink-tan scaly macules – scaling can appear once the skin has been stretched back and forth between two fingers to visualise it
- lichenification from scratching but little excoriation
- Wood's light examination would be positive with a blue-green fluorescence of the scale unless the patient had just had a bath or shower.

Differential diagnosis/assessment

Vitiligo, post-inflammatory pigmentation, guttate psoriasis, discoid eczema, tinea corporis.

Investigations

Skin scrapping and Wood's light examination are investigations that may be carried out to clarify diagnosis.

Management plan

1. Patient/carer education
   - Introduction to the condition and possible causative factors (heat, humidity, excessive sebum production, occlusive creams (coconut cream).
   - Reassurance regarding cross-infection.
   - Discuss the pattern of presentation. Discuss how control of the condition is managed through specific skin hygiene and how to use the antiyeast shampoos as a body wash and the frequency of use.
   - Reassure the patient that the pigment will settle and normal skin tone will return.
2. Pharmacotherapeutics
   - Topical antiyeast shampoo used as a body lotion is left on the skin for a minimum of 20 min before washing off. This would need to be repeated to clean the skin of yeast initially daily for 2 weeks and then allowing recolonisation. Maintainance may be required of once every 6 weeks in a physically active person from April to October in the case of reoccurrence.
   - Topical antiyeast preparations (creams or sprays) may also be helpful in removing the yeast and easing the irritation of the skin: application twice a day for 2 weeks.
   - Systemic azoles may be useful in a chronic case. Dosage and course depend on the drug of choice.
3. Communication
   - Contact the school nurse to give diagnosis and reassurance that it is not contagious.

Indications for referral

- Chronic: referral for consideration of systemic therapy if topical therapy fails.

Complications

- Misdiagnosis.

Pityriasis rosea

Definition: It is an acute, self-limiting disease, probably infective in origin that affects mainly children and young adults. Pityriasis rosea is characterised by the formation of a single lesion (herald patch), followed by an erythematous eruption (see Plate 15), often longitudinal in pattern, like a Christmas tree pattern on the trunk. The eruption usually lasts between 2 and 10 weeks. Question about any recent illness.

Subjective findings

Patient/carer will report:
- pink scaly rash on the trunk and limbs
- may mention an original lesion that appeared prior to the rash developing
- itchy skin that is slightly scaly.

Objective findings

Examine all of the skin:
- identify herald patch larger in size (2–5 cm), usually sited on the trunk, thigh or arms. Has a defined demarcated margin, erythematous scaly plaque?
- erythematous (pink) papules on the trunk, neck and extremities with light scaling on the periphery of the lesions
- lichenoid papular lesions more common in African skin
- longitudinal pattern
- severe: numerous erythematous follicular papules
- examine the mucous membranes: should be normal.

Differential diagnosis/assessment

Guttate psoriasis, pityriasis versicolor, secondary syphilis, drug eruptions.

Investigations

Blood serology for syphilis may be required to clarify diagnosis.

Management plan

1. Patient/carer education
   - Discuss possible infective agent – that it is self-limiting – duration of the condition and severity of symptoms
   - Discuss whether itching or appearance is distressing and treat those explaining how to carry out the different treatments.
2. Pharmacotherapeutics
   - Oral antihistamines to relieve the itch. Product choice depends on age, severity, and time when worse.

- Topical emollients applied lightly but frequently to the skin in smooth downward stroke may relieve itching and scaling.
- Topical mild-to-moderate potency steroids help to reduce the erythema and discomfort.
- UV light therapy may hasten resolution.
3. Communication
   - School nurse to be informed of diagnosis.

Indications for referral

- Immediate: if resolution does not start within 6 weeks, consider diagnostic punch biopsy
- Chronic: if itching persists over 3 months, reconsider diagnosis.

Complications

- Misdiagnosis.

Acne

Definition: An inflammation of the pilosebaceous units of certain bodily areas (face and trunk – see Plate 16) that occurs more frequently in adolescence and manifests itself in several different forms: comedones (open – blackheads and closed – whiteheads); papules; pustules; nodules; cysts; pitting and hypertrophic scars (see Plate 17). It is more severe in males than in females. Exacerbation can be caused by topical or oral corticosteroids, oral contraceptives, lithium and greasy cosmetics. Peak onset in females is 16–17 years and 17–19 years in males. Late onset occurs more frequently in women and can be related to polycystic ovaries: 5% of women and 1% of men require treatment into their 30s and 40s.

Assessment tool

Assessment of psychological and social effects of acne – APSEA (Cuncliffe 1994).

Subjective findings

Patient reports that:
- reoccurring painful red spots (squeezing releases pressure)
- have lots of blackheads and spots under the skin
- skin is very greasy
- have altered their diet with no success
- impact on lifestyle, withdrawn from social events
- worried about scarring or has raised ugly scars
- spots are worse prior to menstruation.

Objective findings

Examine the face, chest and back (insist, despite embarrassment):
- lack of direct eye contact
- inflammatory papules: severity is based on redness and damage to surrounding skin
- pustules

- closed and open comedones
- nodules that are very inflamed and painful to the touch
- excoriations and inflammation
- hypertrophic scars (keloid)
- greasy skin.

Differential diagnosis/assessment

Folliculitis; rosacea.

Investigations

Investigations that may be carried out to clarify diagnosis: total testosterone and free testosterone.

Management plan

1. Patient education
   - Discuss the myths about the disease and identify the possible cause, how the different treatments work and the need for regular review every 3 months. Response to treatment does not occur immediately (6 weeks to see a response to oral antibiotics and the course should be a minimum of 3 months).
   - If the patient is atopic, then discuss the dryness that might occur when using acne treatments.
   - Discuss the healing process and how scratching and picking delays the healing process and increases the possibility of scarring.
   - The severity of the condition, inflammation and scarring may indicate the level of treatment that is commenced.
2. Pharmacotherapeutics
   - Topical acne preparations depend on severity of the condition and can be used in combination with each other as well as systemic therapies. Some are used as keratolytics and abrasives to peel and unblock the pilosebaceous follicular openings; some are combined with antibiotics to reduce inflammation and bacterial load on the skin surface or just as antibiotics. Vitamin A preparations increase epidermal turnover, reducing keratinous plug formation and increasing sebum drainage. Dryness and irritation/inflammation may occur initially, but reduction in frequency and use of a light emollient should ease the situation.
   - Systemic antibiotics have an antibacterial action against propionibacterium acnes, anti-inflammatory properties, and reduce keratin in pilosebaceous ducts. For patients who are sexually active, discuss extra protection for the initial month. Finding which one of the antibiotics is most effective may take several courses, which is why regular review is necessary (3 months).
   - Manipulation of hormonal levels can be obtained through using certain contraceptive products that lower testosterone, which leads to a reduction in sebum secretion – monitoring should occur as if it was for contraceptive use.

- Silcone gel dressing used to debulk keloid scars is cut to size and applied directly to the skin for at least 12 hours a day. Each piece of silcone gel should last 7–10 days and the course of treatment should be 3 months.
3. Communication
  - If school age, contact the school nurse to discuss diagnosis and awareness of bullying and the possibility of skin care/medication that may occur when at school.

Indications for referral

- Urgent: active scarring and inflammation – to consultant dermatologist for Roaccutane
- Immediate: failing oral antibiotics – consideration for Roaccutane (isotretinoin), camouflage techniques, treatment of keloid scars – to consultant dermatologist
- Chronic: once suppression is achieved with topical or oral therapies, the need for repeat prescription may continue for several years but review is still necessary.

Complications

- Scarring for life
- Depression/low self-esteem
- Suicide.

Urticaria

Definition: Urticaria (see Plate 18) is a transient eruption consisting of areas of erythema and weals that lasts less than 24 hours and is extremely itchy. It is defined as acute if lesions reoccur for less than 1 month and chronic if lasting over 30 days (Box 4.7). Acute urticaria may be due to drugs (NSAIDs and ACE inhibitors), food or infections or thyroid/collagen vascular disease but for most patients with chronic idiopathic urticaria there is no identifiable cause. To rule out any possible precipitating factors aids diagnosis and this should be reflected in questioning the patient.

Subjective findings

The patient may report:
- severe itch prior to any skin weal appearing
- nettle rash that is extremely itchy

Box 4.7	*Urticaria*

Causes of chronic urticaria	Types of physical urticaria
Chronic idiopathic 75%	Cold
Physical 16%	Solar
Allergic (IgE mediated) 5%	Heat
Vasculitis 5%	Cholinergic
Hereditary angioedema 3%	Dermographism
	Delayed pressure

- red swellings in the skin surface in areas of tight clothing, on back of thighs having been seated for a while
- swelling around the eyes, mouth or genital areas
- pain on walking
- flushing or burning sensation of the skin
- may feel uncomfortable with abdominal pain.

Objective findings

Examine the skin surface:
- Pink-white central papular weal with a peripheral erythema. Weals are of variable size: papular weal (1.0–2.0 m) or weal plaques (1–8 cm), lasting less than 24 hours anywhere on the skin.
- Angiooedema (swelling of the subcutaneous tissue) less pronounced than weals; enlargement around the eyes, lips, and tongue.
- Physical examination for lymphadenopathy.
- Pattern may be annular or linear and can be localised, regional or generalised.
- Light stroking of the skin invokes a weal with itching.

Differential diagnosis/assessment

Insect bites, adverse drug eruptions, urticaria contact dermatitis, underlying systemic disease (SLE), vasculitis.

Investigations

Investigations that may be carried out to clarify diagnosis are FBC, U&E (urea and electrolytes), ESR, LFTs (liver function tests), thyroxine, antinuclear factor, complement, abdominal ultrasound, chest X-ray and dermographism.

Management plan

1. Patient education
  - Explain the role of released histamine and how antihistamines work to prevent attacks by taking one every day for at least 6 months before having a trial without.
  - Identify any possible causative agents and suggest avoidance of aspirin. Ask patients to check their own medication for those that are known to induce urticaria.
  - Patients should keep a food diary if there is concern about an item in their diet; once identified, then avoid it.
  - Avoidance of the causative agent is not always straightforward but it is the only way to eliminate it; e.g. avoidance of heat, cold (ice cream and swimming), sun exposure, etc.
2. Pharmacotherapeutics
  - Systemic antihistamines on a daily basis for at least 6 months, before a trial without; product prescribed depends on local policy, but combination between fast-acting and sustained-release medicines should blunt any peaks or troughs, and

histamine activity is blocked through the night. Advise the patient about safety factors when using machinery or driving.

- Manipulation of the dose may be required.
- Systemic corticosteroids may be used if severe, cause is known and there are no contraindications.

3. Communication
- May need supporting letter for work if dealing with machinery.

Indications for referral

- Urgent: angiooedema affecting the airways
- Immediate: weals present for more than 24 hours; abnormal blood results with failure to respond to anti-histamine therapy; review diagnosis.

Complications

- Misdiagnosis – vascular urticaria.

Napkin dermatitis

Definition: It is a primary irritant contact dermatitis (see Plate 19). Napkin dermatitis is caused by exposure to the irritating effects of urine (ammonia) and faecal matter and can lead to a severe reaction if contact is prolonged (occluded by thick rubber nappy pants).

Superinfection by *Candida albicans* is common in napkin dermatitis that has been present for over 72 hours. This leads to erythematous papules or vesico-pustules that appear around the main erythematous, moist, glazed, sore epidermis, except in the skin folds (Higgins & du Vivier 1996). The presence of *Staphylococcus aureus* within a warm moist nappy can lead to bacterial infections.

Since the introduction of the super-absorbent dispos-able nappy, which keeps the skin drier, the incidence of napkin dermatitis since the 1980s has fallen. If, however, the nappy (cloth or disposable) is not changed frequently enough or the skin is overwashed with soaps and detergents, then these substances also act as a primary irritant by breaking the lipid barrier.

Subjective findings

The carer will report:
- well-defined, red sore-looking skin in the napkin area
- red spots and a whitish appearance on the red skin
- a child that is distressed and cries a lot during nappy changing.

Objective findings

Examine all the skin, including the mucosa:
- defined erythematous, moist, glazed rash in the shape of a nappy
- sparring of the skin fold areas
- erythematous papules or vesicopustules periphery to the rash
- no signs of scaling (napkin psoriasis) or excoriations (eczema)

- check oral cavity for whitish plaques.

Differential diagnosis/assessment

Seborrhoeic dermatitis, atopic eczema, psoriasis, irritant napkin rash.

Investigations

No investigations are usually needed to clarify diagnosis.

Management plan

1. Carer education
- Identify the possible causes of napkin dermatitis and discuss present skin cleansing and nappy-changing routine and give reassurance.
- Discuss the need for checking and changing nappies frequently (cost element), immediately after defecation or 2 hourly when awake. Use super-absorbent nappies during this time to keep the skin drier and avoid rubber nappy pants.
- At each nappy change, wash the skin with tap water with or without a soap substitute, avoiding the wet wipes.
- Make sure the skin is dry and apply a barrier cream (do not use a warm hair dryer as this can cause burning of the skin).
- When possible, leave the nappy off to let the skin enjoy a warm environment (but do not expose to direct sunlight to prevent sunburn).

2. Pharmacotherapeutics
- Soap substitute for all washing of the baby's skin and ensuring the skin is patted dry.
- Topical antiyeast cream to the affected skin twice a day for 2 weeks.
- Topical antibiotic/steroid cream may be required depending, on sensitivities and host response twice a day for 2 weeks.
- Topical antiyeast for the mouth everyday for 5 days. Nystatin liquid given by mouth but is in contact with the mucosa, thus it is topical not sys-temic.

3. Communications
- Contact health visitor to support the mother at home to manage this condition with confidence.

Indications for referral

- Not responsive to treatment: review for diagnostic purposes.

Complications

- Misdiagnosis.

Seborrhoeic dermatitis

Definition: Seborrhoeic dermatitis is a chronic dermato-sis characterised by redness, itchiness and scaling that occurs in areas where sebaceous glands are most active, e.g. face and scalp and skin folds (Plate 21). If this occurs in the first months of life, it is known as 'cradle cap' thick yellow scales adherent on the scalp. It is more common in males (see Plate 20), with an incidence of 2–5% of the population (Fitzpatrick et al 1997). It is often a genetic state, but is also more common in patients with an HIV infection.

Subjective findings

The patient/carer will report:
- excessively scaly itchy red skin
- yellow crusts in scalp, eyebrows and other hairy places
- spots also found on the skin
- facial redness, which involves the skin around the nose and mouth area
- very bad dandruff.

Objective findings

Examine all of the skin:
- facial erythema (flushing) in a butterfly pattern across the nose and cheeks (baby unconcerned)
- yellowish erythema in the hairline, eyebrows, hairy chest with scaling, crusting within the hair; chronic blepharitis
- involvement in skin folds (groin, axilla, napkin area)
- discrete erythematous macules on the face and trunk
- diffuse involvement in the scalp; excoriations present and some loss of hair
- scaling – yellow crusts across the scalp.

Differential diagnosis/assessment

Psoriasis, impetigo, tinea corporis/capitis, pityriasis versicolor, lupus erythematosus.

Investigations

No investigations are usually needed to clarify diagnosis.

Management plan

1. Patient/carer education
   - Caused possibly by an overproduction of Pityrosporum yeasts.
   - Management is suppressive rather than curative. Infantile and adolescent seborrhoeic dermatitis disappear with age (Fitzpatrick et al 1997).
   - Condition usually improves in the summer (UV light beneficial) but the progression of the disease is that of recurrences and remissions. Thus it requires initial treatment and then maintainance.
   - Explain the roles of therapies, demonstrate application techniques and give practical advice.
2. Pharmacotherapeutics
   - Use shampoo containing an antifungal element or an imidazole or tar to wash the scalp; can also be used to wash face and trunk (avoid eyes), daily, initially, and then less frequently for control. Soap substitute can be used on baby's scalp.

- To remove sticky scales, apply olive oil followed by gentle teasing of the scale from the scalp; this may be repeated over 1 week until the scalp is clear and then used to maintain clearance.
- Topical antifungal/yeast creams are used if very inflamed, or in flexural areas a combination antiyeast/corticosteroid or antibacterial/corticosteroid cream can be used. Apply twice a day for an initial period and then reduce application to keep clear. Stop the corticosteroid cream once inflammation has cleared and just use antiyeast cream.
3. Communication
   - Involve health visitor to support a mother and supervise response to therapy and maintainance.

Indications for referral

- Urgent: in a baby, failure to thrive, diarrhoea and chronic seborrhoeic dermatitis – refer to consultant dermatologist/paediatrician for further investigations (generate C5a chemotactic factor – Leiner's disease).
- Immediate: review severe florid exacerbation to consider systemic antiyeast drugs.
- Routine: review after 1 week to ensure topical steroid creams are stopped and therapy is altered. Observe for signs of atrophy.

Complications

- Misdiagnosis and failure to respond.

Generalised pruritus

Definition: A generalised itchy skin that causes great distresss, sleeplessness, fatigue and even pain for the patient, is difficult to control, and is usually a symptom of a cutaneous disease or a symptom of an underlying systemic disease (liver, lymphoma, thyroid). Physiological changes do occur with age and, thus, the skin is drier and itchy and emollient therapy may be introduced with good effect, but a full investigation should be pursued initially to rule out an organic cause. Management may be directed to control and relief of symptoms but the itch is very subjective to each patient. The patient may not have any cutaneous lesions, but physiological changes may have occurred in response to scratching and rubbing; a complete physical examination should still be carried out.

Subjective findings

The patient may report:
- generalised itch, with little relief – 'have tried everything'
- drier skin
- sleepless nights from itching
- fatigue
- holes appearing in the skin after scratching – 'infection coming out'
- there are no skin lesions
- feels in low spirits because the itching will not stop.

Objective findings

Carry out a complete physical and skin examination:
- recognise any non-specific skin changes induced by scratching (rather than the cause of itching)
- xerosis or ichthyosis seen (visually dry scaly skin)
- baseline observations, weight (loss), urinalysis (diabetes, renal), temperature (febrile)
- lymphadenopathy
- palpate the thyroid (hyper/hypothyroidism)
- check dermographism.

Differential diagnosis/assessment

Atopic eczema, xeroderma, lichen simplex, iron deficiency, liver or thyroid disturbances, lymphomas, eczema craquelé, scabies, chronic renal failure, diabetes mellitus, delusion of parasitosis.

Investigations

Investigations that may be carried out to clarify diagnosis: FBC, U&Es, ESR, LFTs, thyroid, fasting glucose, antinuclear factor, complement, hepatitis antigens, abdominal ultrasound, chest X-ray, stool specimen for parasites.

Management plan

This depends on the diagnosis and the patient may require several consultations to explore all possible outcomes or will need referral to a dermatologist after the initial consultation.
1. Patient education
   - Explore all external possible causes for body itch – primary skin condition (eczema, scabies, etc.), age, weather, overwashing with soap, rough clothing, avoidance of causing vasodilatation from overheating or alcohol consumption
   - Symptom relief through antihistamines and emollient therapy.
2. Pharmacotherapeutics
   - Topical emollient therapy preferable with preparations that have an antipruritic effect (check *MIMS (Monthly Index of Medical Specialities)* or *BNF (British National Formulary)*) as found in bath oils and topical moisturisers. Some emollient creams may have menthol added to cool the skin as well as hydrate. Stop the use of soap and replace with a soap substitute. Frequent application may give more relief.
   - Systemic antihistamines: non-sedating for during the day but, if having disturbed nights, then those with a sedating effect are useful (beware of hung-over effect in the morning). Topical antihistamine preparations can be effective but be careful of the amounts used as they can still cause drowsiness.
   - Low-dose systemic antidepressants (also have an antipruritic effect and can be helpful in assisting with sleep and lifting low spirits).

3. Communication
   - Involve the district nurse or home care team if there is difficulty in the patient's ability to bath or to apply topical emollient therapy.

Indications for referral

- Urgent: if physical examination revealed ichthyosis (excessive accumulation of cutaneous scale – fish-like scale pattern on the skin) or pruritus is associated with weight loss
- Immediate: review after 2 weeks with results if no metabolic or endocrine disorders identified and if no improvement then referral to dermatologist
- Chronic: review after 3 months and revisit diagnosis.

Complications

- T cell lymphoma
- depression
- misdiagnosis.

Viral warts

Definition: Human papillomaviruses (HPV) cause subclinical infection or a variety of benign clinical skin lesions on the skin or mucous membranes (see Plate 22). Common viral warts represent 70% of all cutaneous warts and occur in 20% of all school age children (Fitzpatrick et al 1997), and planter warts are common in older children, accounting for 30% of cutaneous warts.

The HPV virus enters the epidermis through sites of trauma or when the skin has been softened, e.g. after swimming. Autoinoculation from picking at existing lesions or nail biting or shaving is common. The incubation period varies from 1 month to 1 year and seems to be influenced by the patient's immune response and skin resistance status. Classification is based on appearance or anatomical location (Box 4.8).

Box 4.8	*Classification of warts*
Common warts	Skin-coloured, hyperkeratotic, roughened, excrescent papules – hands and other parts of the body
Planter warts	Involve soles of feet, slightly protuberant, hyperkeratotic – causing pain on weight-bearing areas
Plain warts	Smooth flat-topped papules on the face and hands: often follows a scratch or trauma line
Mosaic warts	Cluster of lesions found on the soles or palms
Filiform warts	Hyperkeratotic lesion with filiform protrusions
Periungual warts	Painful, and may bleed clusters of hyperkeratotic lesions around the interphalangeal joints; more common in nail biters

Subjective findings

The patient/carer will report:

- disfiguration by warts or verruca
- painful lesions when knocked
- thick hard skin
- pain on walking
- have tried everything and nothing works
- has been there for years.

Objective findings

Examination of the patient may be restricted to just the affected areas if the patient has been questioned closely about any other possible lesions:

- elevated circumscribed hyperkeratotic lesion
- rough surface with papillary projections
- villi extensions may be seen
- black capillaries visible after paring down the surface.

Differential diagnosis/assessment

Seborrhoeic keratosis, corn, angiogential wart, squamous cell carcinoma.

Investigation

Investigation is not required but do pare the skin to remove thickened skin and expose the thrombosed vessels (black dots).

Management plan

1. Patient/carer education
   - Describe what a wart is, how it is infected, and set parameters on the possible outcome of treatment.
   - Limit the exposure of the infected skin in wet environments, e.g. occlusive dressings when swimming.
   - Treatment must be sustained over many weeks for it to be successful.
   - Paring the skin with a disposable nail file to remove dead skin, which might block the absorption of the treatment solution, or using a sharp blade, technique is important. Do not try and cut it out, as you end up with a scar and possible reoccurrence of the wart.
2. Pharmacotherapeutics
   - Chemical agents such as salicylic acid and lactic acid are used in a film-forming preparation that can be applied to the wart after paring down daily without a secondary dressing. Salicylic acid and lactic acid also come in solutions that require secondary dressing: together they soften and remove the hyperkeratotic skin under which the wart virus hides. Care in application should be taken to protect the surrounding skin from irritation. This form of treatment is effective on common, periungual, mosaic and planter warts.
   - Cryotherapy, which is the use of liquid nitrogen (strict health and safety rules are involved in storage and handling), is applied directly to the wart after paring down. It is important to be aware of the underlying structure, which could be damaged when forming an ice ball and completing a freeze–thaw–freeze cycle. Exposure time for freezing is critical: too little, and the wart is not removed; too much, and there is a risk of increased scarring and post-exposure pain. Cryotherapy can be used in combination with chemical agents for common warts or on its own for plain, filiform and periungual warts.
3. Communication
   - Contact the school nurse so that she can ensure that schoolage children with planter warts over their lesion prior to going swimming with either occlusive film or dressing. Swimming shoes can be worn but may encourage bullying because they are more visual. Avoidance of walking around barefoot in wet areas is advised.

Indications for referral

- Immediate: misdiagnosis, review or referral to consultant dermatologist for treatment of facial warts if concerned about diagnosis or competence for cryotherapy. Mosaic warts are more difficult to treat; some centres will use cytotoxic drugs.
- Chronic: review monthly if receiving cryotherapy. This allows time for the skin to recover from the inflammatory response, which may include blistering, further paring and chemical treatment.

Complications

- Misdiagnosis
- Scarring and post-exposure pain.

Sun damage and pigmented lesions

Definition: Skin changed either directly due to sun exposure and pigmented lesions that occur or change due to exposure to UV radiation. This is not a definitive section and will not cover all pigmented skin lesions or all those conditions in which UV radiation plays a contributing factor (Box 4.9).

Subjective findings

The patient will often report that:

- a partner noticed the lesion on their person
- they noticed a new lesion
- a change in size
- a change in colour – darker or lighter
- the margin of the lesion was now irregular
- that the lesion sometimes bled and was itchy.

Objective findings

A full skin examination is required, including soles of feet and in between toe webs:

- examine all the skin and pigmented lesions first before you examine the lesion identified by the patient

Box 4.9 *Sun-damaged skin lesions*

Dermatoheliosis (photoageing) (see Plate 23)

Results from excessive/prolonged exposure of the skin to UV radiation before the age of 35. The syndrome consists of severe wrinkling, leathery appearance of skin, 'premature' ageing. Development of solar lentigines, solar keratosis, solar elastosis (fine nodularity and inelasticity), yellow dermal papules and basal cell carcinoma

Chronic actinic dermatitis (CAD)

Photoallergic dermatitis can persist for months – years. May be triggered by a drug-induced photoallergy but continues despite the discontinuation of the photoallergen with every new UV radiation exposure. Chronic eczematous lichenified and itchy confluent plaques result on the skin exposed to UV radiation, so there is a cut-off area, e.g. V-neckline, nape of neck

Solar lentigo

Proliferation of melanocytes due to UV radiation exposure resulting in circumscribed 1.0–3.0 cm brown macules on sun-exposed skin, usually resulting from sunburn in skin type I–II

Solar keratosis

Discrete rough-surfaced scaly lesions, which may have a pink/grey base, occur on sun-damaged skin; they are rarely larger than 1.0 cm in diameter. It is caused by the cumulative effects of UV radiation on skin type I–II, who do not have the protection of melanin. Running the tip of your finger over the skin, you can feel the 'catch' of the rough surface. These lesions are precancerous and rarely turn into a squamous cell carcinoma

Basal cell carcinoma (BCC) (see Plate 24)

This form of skin cancer has a limited ability to metastasise but is aggressive locally, causing ulceration. It is often first noticed as a lesion that crusts, bleeds and crusts again and is non-healing. It is a solitary oval/round smooth shiny demarcated lesion with a pearly appearance; telangiectatic vessels present and it is firm on palpation. The centre may be umbilicated.

If ulceration has occurred, then there is a crusted central necrotic area. Dermatoheliosis will be noticeable on the surrounding skin. A pigmented BCC may be brown – blue-black in appearance.

Superficial spreading BCC are flat well-demarcated plaques with a rolled edge, and can bleed easily when scratched.

They are caused by the accumulative effects of UV radiation exposure, especially before the age of 14 in skin type I–II; X-ray therapy for facial acne; and ingestion of arsenic 30–40 years previously in any skin type. There is less urgency to excise these lesions, except if ulcerating; if lesions are facial you may want to refer to a plastic surgeon or to carry out Mohs' technique

Squamous cell carcinoma (SCC) (see Plate 25)

This is a malignant tumour of epithelial keratinocytes (skin and mucous membranes) of which there are two types:

1. Highly differentiated SCCs – show signs of keratinization either within or on the surface. These are firm or hard on palpation.

2. Poorly differentiated SCCs – clinically appear freshly, granulomatous and thus soft on palpation. They have the ability to metastasise.

SCCs are caused by accumulative UV radiation in skin types I–II, ingestion of arsenic, exposure to ionising radiation (X-rays and γ-rays, PUVA for psoriasis), industrial carcinogens (pitch, tar, crude paraffin oil). Thus, they can occur in all skin types. May be in situ in Bowen's disease, slowly enlarging erythematous plaque with a sharp border, slight scaling but little infiltration, or in situ in erythroplasia of Queyrat in the vulva area or on the glans as a well-demarcated, erythematous glistening plaque.

They require excision, are sometimes referred to general surgeons or plastic surgeons or are excised using Mohs' technique based on site and diameter

Malignant melanoma (MM)

There are several types of this malignant skin cancer. It is aggressive and metastasises. It is rare before puberty and in skin type IV–V but has a higher incidence in skin types I, especially those who are Celtic in origin.

About 30% of melanomas arise from pre-existing naevus, but 70% are in normal skin. The site of melanomas is not restricted to sun-exposed skin, but both incidence and mortality increases with decreasing latitude.

Lesions vary in appearance, depending on type and location, so in some cases definitive diagnosis may only be made on histological excision rather than on clinical appearance.

History should include details about sun exposure, living abroad and sun behaviour and family history.

Most melanomas represent proliferating malignant melanocytes that in most melanomas produce melanin pigment; thus, presentation is due to change in colour. Prognostic difference between clinical types relates mainly to the duration of the radial growth phase, which may last from years to decades in lentigo maligna melanoma; from months to 2 years in superficial spreading melanoma; and even shorter (6 months or less) in nodular melanoma (Fitzpatrick et al 1997).

Types of malignant melanomas:

1. lentigo maligna
2. lentigo maligna melanoma
3. superficial spreading melanoma in situ
4. superficial spreading melanoma
5. acral-lentiginous melanoma in situ
6. acral-lentiginous melanoma
7. nodular melanoma.

Early detection increases survival rates; thus, the thinner the lesion according to the Breslow scale, the better the prognosis.

Immediate excision is essential; this may be followed by a further excision to ensure clear margins and may be done by a general surgeon or a plastic surgeon. Depending on the Breslow scale, referral on to an oncologist may be required. The patient will require the support of the Macmillan nurses

---

- comment on the range of colour seen within the pigment lesions and then on the lesion concerned
- often, the lesion identified by the patient is not the one that you notice as being different
- note the skin changes – dermatoheliosis, freckles, lentigenes

- complete a full body chart of all findings
- check for lymphadenopathy.

❶ Only a medical professional is covered under medical-legal terms to give assurances about benign lesions. All patients should be referred to a doctor or a dermatologist.

Investigations

Investigations that may be required to clarify diagnosis: diagnostic biopsy of pre/non-malignant lesion or full excision with a 1 mm clear margin of possible malignant lesion for histological review. Use photography to record mole distribution of colour, shape or diameter for comparison 3–6–12 months later.

Management plan

1. Patient education
   - Discuss current sun exposure and reasons for tanning (sexual, healthy, feel good, peer pressure).
   - Discuss how patients should enjoy the sun without burning or prematurely ageing their skin (avoid direct sunbathing between 11 a.m. and 3 p.m.; use of clothing/hats to cover and protect the skin; seek the shade; use sunscreens SPF15 or above); check if sunscreens used all the time, not just on holiday (advise on regular reapplication if sunscreens are to be relied on).
   - Instruct on how patients should skin type their own skin (see Box 4.3); raise patients awareness that their skin type may change as they get older.
   - Give instruction on how patients should survey their skin so that they get to know what their moles look like and even how to fill out a body chart. They will be able to notice change over weeks rather than months: sudden rapid growth in size, appearance of new moles, changes in pigment (darker or lighter) or border. Self-examination should never replace a screening check by an NP or dermatologist. The more sun exposure they receive, the more likely they will develop more moles, freckles, lentigenes and solar keratosis (seborrhoeic keratosis is a benign lesion that first presents as a yellow-tanned flat plaque which, over time, develops into a brown-black raised hyperkeratotic plaque that looks greasy and stuck on; these are hereditary and can be either frozen or undergo curettage – they are often a cosmetic problem, although they can become traumatised under clothing).
   - Prepare the patient that, if referred to a dermatologist, a full skin examination will be carried out even if the lesion is on the face and that she will be expected to undress down to her underwear. The lesion will not always be excised on a first visit unless the patient is attending a pigmented lesion clinic or see and treat clinic that offers a one-stop visit.

Top Tips

1 Never examine a lesion on its own
2 Always undress the patient and examine the skin
3 Touch lightly with tips of fingers when palpating
4 Check the hair, nails and mucosa
5 Good lighting and privacy
6 Support clinical finding with investigation results
7 Remove any crusts and check underneath
8 If in doubt ask for a second opinion
9 The skin will always reveal itself
10 Think systemic

3. Communication
   - Involve different support agencies for the patient and family, especially if the diagnosis is malignant melanoma (Marc's line: see Useful Addresses for this helpline for melanoma and related cancers of the skin set up by Polly Buchanan following the death of a 19-year-old boy, whose family needed support and information.

Indications for referral

- Urgent: a changing mole or possible malignant melanoma (including if already excised, but histology indicates MM) referral via the phone to a dermatologist, who will make arrangement for the patient to be seen immediately.
- Immediate: refer if concerned about a lesion that is related to the sun (if patient should be seen urgently, include telephone number so that the patient can be contacted by the hospital if sending a referral letter) or send the patient to a local pigment lesion clinic (check with a local dermatologist what kind of clinics are held and when) with a letter (responsibility is given to the patient to access the hospital).
- Chronic: some skin lesions can be treated or excised (all specimens excised should be sent for histopathology).

Complications

- Misdiagnosis
- Delayed treatment and poor prognosis.

Glossary

Primary lesions		Examples
Abscess	(> 1 cm), pus-filled lesion	Pseudocyst
Blister	(> 1 cm), fluid-filled lesion	Pompholyx

Bulla   (< 1 cm), fluid-filled lesion, circumscribed elevation, over 0.5 cm in diameter containing a liquid

Macule   stain (<1 cm), change in colour only, surface is flat and does not blanche

Nodule   (>1 cm), rounded elevated solid lesion, i.e. thickness = diameter

Patch   (>1 cm), change in colour only, surface is always normal, a large macule

Papule   (<1 cm), any raised lesion or scaly, crusted, keratinized or macerated surface

Plaque   (>1 cm), raised flat-topped lesion, i.e. diameter » thickness

Pustule   (<1 cm), pus-filled lesion

Vesicle   (<1 cm), clear fluid-filled.

Herpes zoster
Pemphigoid
Pemphigus
Bullous impetigo
Brown lentigo
Café-au-lait
Drug rash
Secondary syphilis
Hypopigmented (vitiligo)
Purpura
Erythema nodosum
Rheumatoid nodules
Kaposi's
Lipoma
Cancer
Mycosis fungoides (stage 1)

Skin colour or white, pink, yellow skin tags or warts; brown colour – melanoma, nevus; seborrhoea

Secondary lesions

Atrophy   A diminution of tissue

Erosion   Superficial or total loss of epidermis or mucous membrane; heals without scarring

Fissuring   Slits through the whole thickness of skin due to excessive dryness or inflammation

Ulcer   Full-thickness loss of epidermis and upper dermis; heals with scarring

General glossary

Acantholysis   The separation of keratinocytes of the epidermis by loss of intercellular connections, permitting the cells to become round and hyaline

Allergen   An external substance which stimulates an immunological response

Alopecia   Fox mange – a fall of hair

Annular   Round or ring-shaped

Asymmetrical   One side more involved than the other

Atopy   'No (without) place'. An inheritable clinical state associated with eczema, asthma and hayfever

Burrow   Linear lesion caused by parasites 3–5 mm long

Callus   Hyperplasia of the stratum corneum due to physical pressure (keratoderma)

Carbuncle   A necrotizing infection of the skin and subcutaneous tissue comprising a group of furuncles (boils)

Cellulitis   An inflammation of cellular tissue

Coalescing   Lesions merge into one another

Comedones   Papule plugging sebaceous follicles, containing sebum and cellular debris: closed comedones, whitehead; open comedones = blackhead

Cream   Water preparation

Crust   Outer layer consisting of dead cells and serum

Cutaneous   Appertaining to the skin

Cyst   A closed cavity or sac lined with epithelium containing fluid, pus or keratin

Dermatome   Cutaneous nerve distribution on one side of the body

Discoid   Disc shape

Discrete   Separate lesions

Disseminated   Discrete lesions scattered over a wide area

Emollient   Moisturiser that stays on the skin, reducing scaling and water loss

Erosion   Loss of epidermis, which heals without scaring

Erythema   Redness of the skin caused by vascular congestion or perfusion

Erythrodermic   A generalised redness of the skin, at least 90% of total surface, associated with desquamation

Excoriation   Any loss of substance of skin produced by scratching

Exfoliation   The splitting off or separation of keratin and epidermal skin surface in scales or sheets

Fibrosis   The formation of excessive fibrous collagen

Fissure   Any linear gap or slit in the skin surface

Fistula   An abnormal passage from a deep structure to the skin surface

Flexural   Area of skin against skin, e.g. axilla, groin

Furuncle   A localised pyogenic infection originating in a hair follicle

Gangrene   Death of tissue, associated with the loss of blood

Gel   Semi-solid colloidal solution

Generalised   Widespread eruption covering at least 50% of body surface

Granuloma   Chronic inflammatory tissue composed of macrophages, fibroblasts and granulation tissue

Guttate   Drop-like

Haematoma   Localised tumour-like collection of blood

Horn   A keratosis which is taller than broad

Infarct   An area of coagulation necrosis due to localised ischaemia

Keloid   Elevated progressive scar formation without regression

Keratoderma   Hyperplasia of the stratum corneum

Kerion   A nodular inflammatory, pustular lesion due to a fungal infection

Lichenification   A chronic thickening of the epidermis with exaggeration of its normal markings, often as a result of rubbing or scratching

Lesion   Any area of skin with changed colour, elevation or texture that is surrounded by normal skin

Milia   A tiny white cyst containing lamellated keratin

Necrobiosis   Partial degeneration of tissue, such as swelling and degeneration of collagen

Necrosis   Death of tissue or cells

Ointment   Oil-based preparation – emollient

Onycholysis   Nail separation from nail bed

Papilloma   Nipple-like projection from the surface of the skin

Petechia   A punctate haemorrhagic spot 1–2 mm in diameter

Poikiloderma   Dermatosis characterised by variegated cutaneous pigmentation, atrophy and telangiectasia

Pruritus   An irritating skin sensation which elicits the scratch response

Purpura   Discoloration of the skin or mucosa due to extravasation

Pus   Yellowish viscid fluid formed by the liquefaction of dead tissue

Pyoderma   Any purulent skin disease either bacterial or non-bacterial in origin

Rash   A collection of many lesions, some of which are coalescing

Regionalised   Local to any one area of the body, e.g. face

Scale   A flat plate or flake of stratum corneum

Scar   Fibrous tissue replacing normal tissue destroyed by injury or disease

Sclerosis   Induration or hardening of the skin

Sinus   A cavity or channel that permits the escape of fluid

Stria   A streak or band of linear, atrophic, pink, purple or white lesions of the skin due to changes in the connective tissue

Symmetrical   Both sides involved to a similar extent

Telangiectasia   A visible vascular lesion formed by dilation of small cutaneous blood vessels

Tumour   An enlargement of the tissue by normal or pathogenic material or cells that form mass

Turgor   Rigidity due to the uptake of water into living cells or tissues

Vegetation   A growth of pathological tissue consisting of multiple closely set papillary masses

Verruca   An epidermal tumour caused by a papilloma virus

Vibex   A narrow linear mark, usually haemorrhage from scratching

Weal   An elevated white compressible, evanescent area produced by dermal oedema

Xeroderma   Wrinkled, freckled dry skin

Useful addresses

Psoriatic Athropathy Alliance
PO Box 111,
St Albans
Al2 3JQ
Tel: 01923 672837
Email: *info@paalliance.org*
http://www.paalliance.org

National Eczema Society
Association (SPHERE)
163 Eversholt Street
London NW1 1BU
Tel: 020 7388 4097
Email: *http://www.eczema.org*

British Dermatology Nursing Group
BAD House
19 Fitzroy Square
London W1P 5HQ
Tel: 020 7383 0266

The Vitiligo Society
19 Fitzroy Square
London W1P 5HQ
Tel: 0800 0182631
Email: *all@vitiligosociety.org.uk*
http://www.vitiligosociety.org.uk

The Psoriasis Association
7 Milton Street
Northampton NN2 7DG
Tel: 01604 711129

The Wessex Cancer Trust's Marc's Line
Marc's Line Resource Centre
Level 3, Salisbury District Hospital
Salisbury SP2 8BJ
Tel: 01722 415071
Email: *http://www.k-web.co.uk/charity/wct/wct.hml*

Acne Support Group
1st Floor, Howard House
South Ruislip
Middlesex HA4 6SE
Tel: 020 8561 6868
Email *alison@the-asg.demon.co.uk*
http://www.m2w3.com/acne

Herpes Viruses
and Shingles Support Society
41 North Road
London N7 9DP
Tel: 020 7607 9661

Ichthyosis Support Group
16 Cambridge Court
Cambridge Avenue
London NW6 5AB
Tel: 020 7461 0356 (after 8 pm)

References

Ashton R 1998 The art of describing skin lesions. Dermatology in Practice 6(2):11–14.

Baxter C 1993 Observing the skin. Community Outlook Jan: 19–20.

Burns T 1999 Scabies in the elderly. Dermatology in Practice 7(5):12–13.

Cameron J 1998 Contact sensitivity in patients with venous leg ulcers. British Journal of Dermatology Nursing 2(4):5–7.

Champion R H, Burton J L, Ebling F J G (eds) 1992 Rook, Wilkinson and Ebling. Textbook of dermatology, 5th edn. Blackwell Scientific Publications, Oxford.

Collier M 1994 Assessing a wound. Nursing standard (RCN Update) 8(49):3–8.

Committee Members of the Wound Care Society 1993 Wound care procedures. Journal of Wound Care 2(2):7–70.

Cooper R, Lawrence J 1996 The isolation of bacteria from wounds. Journal of Wound Care 5(7): 335–340.

Cunliffe W J 1994 New approaches to acne treatment. Martin Dunitz, London.

Epstein E 1985 Crucial importance of the complete skin examination. J Am Acad Dermatol 13(1):150–153.

Finlay A Y, Khan G K 1994 Dermatology Quality of Life Index. Clin Exp Dermatol 19:310–316.

Fitzpatrick T B, Johnson R A, Wolff K, Polano M K, Suurmond D 1997 Colour atlas and synopsis of clinical dermatology, 3rd edn. McGraw-Hill, New York.

Goodfield M 1998 Superficial infections. Prescriber J 38:183–189.

Greeves M W, Gatti S 1999 The use of glucorticocoids in dermatology. Journal of Dermatological Treatment, 10(2):83–91

Higgins E, du Vivier A 1996 Skin diseases in childhood and adolescence. Blackwell Science, Oxford.

Hill M J (ed) 1998 Dermatology nursing essentials: a care curriculum. Anthony J Janntte, New Jersey.

Hunter J A A, Savin J A, Dahl 1995 Clinical dermatology, 2nd edn. Blackwell Scientific, London.

Lawton S 1998 Assessing the skin. Professional Nurse 13(4):S5–7.

McHenry P M, Williams H C, Bingham E A 1995 Management of atopic eczema. British Medical Journal 310:843–847.

Mairis E 1992 Four senses for a full skin assessment: observation and assessment of the skin. Professional Nurse 7(6):376–380.

Mitchell T, Paige D, Spowart K 1998 Eczema and your child. Class, London.

Peters J 1998 Assessment of patients with a skin condition. Practice Nurse 15(9): 525–530.

Pringle F 1999 Psoriatic arthritis. British Journal of Dermatology Nursing 3(2): 10–12.

Rigel D S, Freidman R J, Kopf A W, et al 1986 Importance of complete cutaneous examination for the detection of malignant melanoma. J Am Acad Dermatol, 144(5):857–860.

Rudensky B, Lipschits M, Issacsohn M, Sonnenblick M 1992 Infected pressure sores: comparison of methods for bacterial identification. Southern Medical Journal 85(9):901–903.

Simmons R 1999 Nitwit. Nursing Times Skin Care (Suppl) Sept. 15:15–16.

Stubbing N J, Bailey P, Poole M 1997 Protocol for accurate assessment of ABPI in patients with leg ulcers. J Wound Care 6(9):417–418.

Watts J 1999 Psoriasis. Professional Nurse 14(9):623–626.

Williams H 1997 Dermatology Health Care Needs Assessment. Radcliffe Medical Press, Oxford.

Further reading

Mitchell T, Paige D, Spowart K 1998 Eczema and your child. Class, London

Papadopoulos L, Bor R 1999 Psychological approaches to dermatology. ISBN 1–85433–292–9.

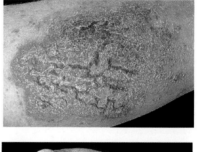

Plate 4 Eczema herpeticum – punched-out individual vesicles, required hospitalisation. (Reproduced with permission of the Medical Illustration Department, Chelsea and Westminster Healthcare Trust and Imperial College.)

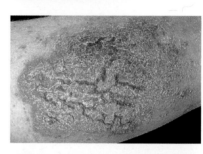

Plate 8 Contact dermatitis to perfume – localised, inflamed dry skin at site of contact. (Reproduced with permission of the Medical Illustration Department, Chelsea and Westminster Healthcare Trust and Imperial College.)

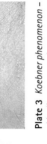

Plate 3 Koebner phenomenon – skin disease occurring on previously undamaged epidermis (e.g. psoriasis). (Reproduced with permission of the Medical Illustration Department, Chelsea and Westminster Healthcare Trust and Imperial College.)

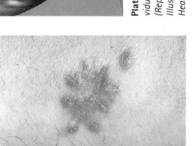

Plate 2 Asteatotic dermatitis (eczema craquelatum) – elderly skin which has been over-washed with soap. (Reproduced with permission of the Medical Illustration Department, Chelsea and Westminster Healthcare Trust and Imperial College.)

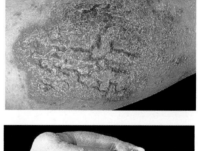

Plate 7 Chronic varicose eczema – inflamed, fissured and lichenified. (Reproduced with permission of the Medical Illustration Department, Chelsea and Westminster Healthcare Trust and Imperial College.)

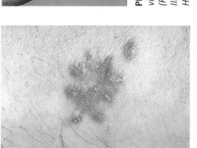

Plate 1 Herpes zoster (shingles) – unilateral pain and vesicular eruption along a dermatome. (Reproduced with permission of the Medical Illustration Department, Chelsea and Westminster Healthcare Trust and Imperial College.)

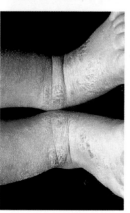

Plate 6 Acute atopic eczema – widespread, inflamed and excoriated. (Reproduced with permission of the Medical Illustration Department, Chelsea and Westminster Healthcare Trust and Imperial College.)

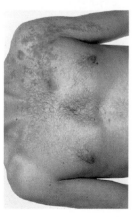

Plate 5 Atopic eczema – dry and scaly, early signs of lichenification. (Reproduced with permission of the Medical Illustration Department, Chelsea and Westminster Healthcare Trust and Imperial College.)

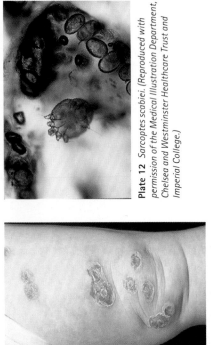

Plate 12 *Sarcoptes scabiei. (Reproduced with permission of the Medical Illustration Department, Chelsea and Westminster Healthcare Trust and Imperial College.)*

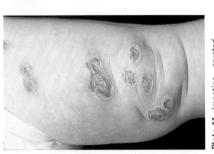

Plate 11 *Impetigo – crusted papular lesion, superficial epidermis infection by either Staphylococcus aureus or Streptococcus pyogenes confirmed by microbiology result. (Reproduced with permission of the Medical Illustration Department, Chelsea and Westminster Healthcare Trust and Imperial College.)*

Plate 10 *Erythrodermic psoriasis – 90% of body surface red, exfoliating, poor body temperature control, loss of protein, would require hospitalisation. (Reproduced with permission of the Medical Illustration Department, Chelsea and Westminster Healthcare Trust and Imperial College.)*

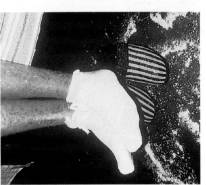

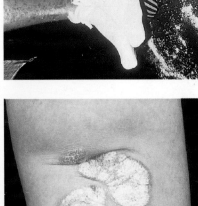

Plate 9 *Chronic plaque psoriasis – salmon-pink plaques with silvery scales. (Reproduced with permission of the Medical Illustration Department, Chelsea and Westminster Healthcare Trust and Imperial College.)*

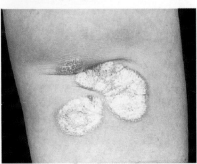

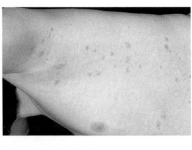
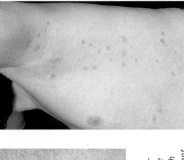
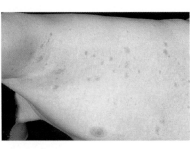

Plate 16 *Acne – papules and pustules (always check the chest and back). (Reproduced with permission of the Medical Illustration Department, Chelsea and Westminster Healthcare Trust and Imperial College.)*

Plate 15 *Pityriasis rosea – acute eruption which has a first lesion (herald plaque) develop on the trunk 1 or 2 weeks before a generalised secondary eruption occurs. (Reproduced with permission of the Medical Illustration Department, Chelsea and Westminster Healthcare Trust and Imperial College.)*

Plate 14 *Pityriasis versicolor – overgrowth of Pityrosporum ovale, variable pigment with well-demarcated scaly lesions, gentle abrasion of the surface accentuates the scale. (Reproduced with permission of the Medical Illustration Department, Chelsea and Westminster Healthcare Trust and Imperial College.)*

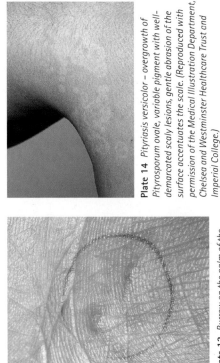

Plate 13 *Burrow on the palm of the hand. (Reproduced with permission of the Medical Illustration Department, Chelsea and Westminster Healthcare Trust and Imperial College.)*

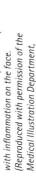

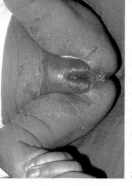

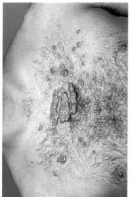

Plate 17 Acne – papules causing immediate scarring in the inflammatory stage called keloid scarring. (Reproduced with permission of the Medical Illustration Department, Chelsea and Westminster Healthcare Trust and Imperial College.)

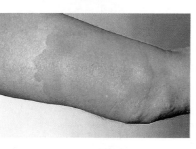

Plate 18 Urticaria – elevated, erythematous transient wheals. (Reproduced with permission of the Medical Illustration Department, Chelsea and Westminster Healthcare Trust and Imperial College.)

Plate 19 Candida infection in the nappy region. (Reproduced with permission of the Medical Illustration Department, Chelsea and Westminster Healthcare Trust and Imperial College.)

Plate 20 Seborrhoeic dermatitis – associated with cradle cap and scaly with inflammation on the face. (Reproduced with permission of the Medical Illustration Department, Chelsea and Westminster Healthcare Trust and Imperial College.)

Plate 21 Seborrhoeic dermatitis – inflamed and scaly; also involving other areas where sebaceous glands are most active. (Reproduced with permission of the Medical Illustration Department, Chelsea and Westminster Healthcare Trust and Imperial College.)

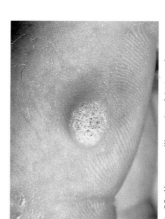

Plate 22 Human papillomavirus (viral wart) – elevated hyperkeratotic papules with thrombosed capillaries (brown–black dots). (Reproduced with permission of the Medical Illustration Department, Chelsea and Westminster Healthcare Trust and Imperial College.)

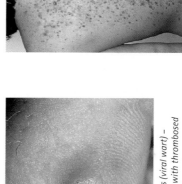

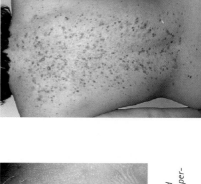

Plate 23 Sun-damaged skin (under 30 years old), freckles and lentigenes. (Reproduced with permission of the Medical Illustration Department, Chelsea and Westminster Healthcare Trust and Imperial College.)

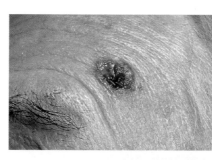

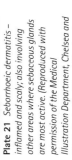

Plate 24 Basal cell carcinoma – history of a non-healing lesion on sun-exposed skin. (Reproduced with permission of the Medical Illustration Department, Chelsea and Westminster Healthcare Trust and Imperial College.)

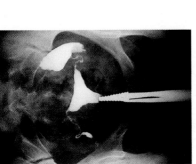

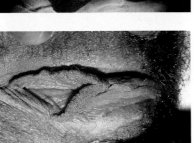

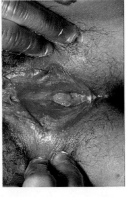

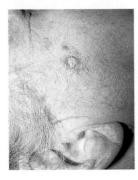

Plate 25 Squamous cell carcinoma – erythema margin with keratinisation on top. (Reproduced with permission of the Medical Illustration Department, Chelsea and Westminster Healthcare Trust and Imperial College.)

Plate 26 Acute candidiasis infection (female) showing redness of labia with watery white discharge. (Reproduced with permission of Dr Gillian George, Barnstaple, North Devon.)

Plate 27 Chronic candidiasis infection (female) showing lichenification due to itchiness. (Reproduced with permission of Dr Gillian George, Barnstaple, North Devon.)

Plate 28 Hysterosalpinogram (HSG) showing narrowing of the fallopian tubes as a result of chlamydia infection (female). (Reproduced with permission of Dr Gillian George, Barnstaple, North Devon.)

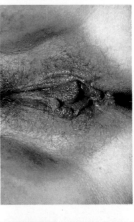

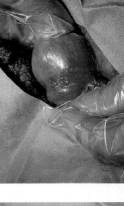

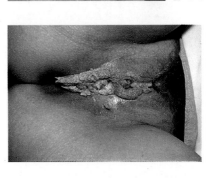

Plate 29 Genital warts (female) showing both single warts and groups of warts. (Reproduced with permission of Dr Gillian George, Barnstaple, North Devon.)

Plate 30 Genital warts with balinitis (male) showing warts on corneal sulcus. (Reproduced with permission of Dr Gillian George, Barnstaple, North Devon.)

Plate 31 Genital herpes (male) showing ulcerated lesion. (Reproduced with permission of Dr Gillian George, Barnstaple, North Devon.)

Plate 32 Trichomoniasis (female) with intertrigo of surrounding skin. (Reproduced with permission of Dr Gillian George, Barnstaple, North Devon.)

5

THE EYE AND EXTERNAL ADENEXA

Anna Hunter

Key Issues

- History taking is a major component of ocular examination and, together with assessment, leads to a diagnosis and management

- Systemic pathology, diagnosed and undiagnosed, can manifest itself through ocular symptoms

- Six cranial nerves are involved with the eye and external adenexa: CNII, CNIII, CNIV, CNV, CNVI and CNVII

- Visual acuity tests the function of the optic nerve (CNII)

- The visual acuity test and documentation is important in ocular trauma and has legal implications in a battle for compensation

- Ocular examination can be divided into six main parts: general, pupils, acuity, ocular motility, fields and fundi

- ❶ Ocular emergencies: sight-threatening conditions due to trauma, unexplained sudden loss of vision and acute glaucoma (closed angled) are ophthalmic emergencies and must be seen and treated by an ophthalmologist to ensure the optimum outcome for the patient

Introduction

To present the eye and external adenexa, which are the eyelids, eyebrows, lacrimal system, conjunctiva and extraocular muscles, it is necessary to review the properties of light, revisit the anatomy and physiology of the globe and check out the part of the brain responsible for interpreting what we see.

The eye has two main purposes: an optical function, whereby the ocular structures, mainly the cornea and the lens, refract light on to the retina; and neurosensory function, whereby the retina transforms light into electrical impulses, which are transmitted through the optic nerve into the optic tract, to the cerebral cortex of the brain for interpretation – and this is how we see. The

external adenexa – the eyebrows, eyelids, eyelashes and lacrimal apparatus – in the main acts as protection for that sight, and prevents dust particles and sweat from getting into the eyes. The extraocular muscles attached to the eye are responsible for the balance and the alignment of the eyes, which is important for binocular vision, essential for three-dimensional eyesight. The extraocular muscles are the superior, inferior, lateral and medial rectus muscles, and superior and inferior oblique muscles which are innervated by the occulomotor (CNIII), trochlea (CNIV) and abducens (CNVI) nerves.

Light

Light is radiation energy from the sun and takes approximately 8 min to travel from the sun to the eye (Johnson 1996). This energy travels in waves and is measured in metres. Each type of energy has a different wavelength, e.g. *γ-rays* have short wavelengths and *radio* waves have long wavelengths. The full electromagnetic spectrum is the collective term for all these light waves of energy. Only a proportion of the full electromagnetic spectrum is visible to the naked eye; this is known as the visible spectrum. The colours that can be seen are red, orange, yellow, green, blue, indigo and violet and can be seen in a rainbow when droplets of rain act as a prism reflecting the light. These light waves vary in wavelength from 400 nm to 700 nm and can be reflected, diffracted and refracted, which is important in relation to how light progresses through the structure of the eyeball to the retina.

The eye

The eye is hollow, spherical, about 2.5 cm in diameter and sits in the bony orbit of the skull, in adipose tissue, with only the anterior part in view. The eyelids open and shut over the eyeball.

The structure of the eye consists of three layers: sclera and cornea, choroid and retina. The outer layer of the eyeball is the sclera and cornea. The *sclera* surrounds 78% of the globe and is a dense and avascular structure that gives support to the internal contents of the eye. The anterior part of the sclera is visible as the white of the eye. The remaining 22% of the outer layer is the *cornea*. This is the transparent anterior part of the eye and is continuous with the sclera. The diameter of the cornea is 11.5 mm, it is approximately 0.5 mm thick at the centre and 1 mm thick at the periphery. The cornea is richly innervated by the cilliary branches of the ophthalmic division of the trigeminal nerve (CNV) and continuously bathed in a tear film.

The middle layer of the eye is known as the *uvea*. This is the pigmented and vascular part of the eye. It is composed of three parts: the *choroid*, the *cilliary body* and the *iris*. The blood supply to the choroid comes from the ciliary arteries, a branch of the ophthalmic artery, that is a meshwork of arteries and veins which supplies the blood to the outer layer of the retina. The ciliary body has two main functions: the secretion of aqueous humour by the ciliary processes and the movement of the intraocular lens, which involves the ciliary muscle. The iris is a circular muscular disc – a diaphragm containing pigmented cells that produce the colour of the eye. The central part of the iris is a circular hole, which is the pupil through which light passes to the retina. The iris controls the amount of light entering the eye by dilating and contracting the *pupil* of the eye. The size of the pupil is regulated by the circular and smooth muscle fibres of the iris and depends on the balance between the parasympathetic and sympathetic nervous system. The parasympathetic nerve fibres constrict the pupil and relate to the CNIII, and the sympathetic fibres which arise from the thoracic segment by way of the superior cervical ganglion, dilate the pupil.

The *retina* is the innermost layer and is the sensory part of the eye. The main landmarks on the retina are the optic disc, which is the head of the optic nerve; the macula, which is the site of central and colour vision; and the blood vessels of the central retinal artery and vein. The internal components of the eye are the *aqueous humour, lens* and *vitreous humour*. The interior anterior segment of the eye is divided into two: the anterior and posterior chambers. The anterior chamber is the aqueous humour filled space between the posterior part of the cornea and the anterior surface of the iris and lens. The posterior chamber refers to those structures behind the lens; i.e. the vitreous humour, the retina and the neurosensory part of the eye follows.

The *aqueous humour* is a clear fluid that is secreted by the ciliary processes into the posterior chamber; it flows through the pupil into the anterior chamber and drains through the trabecular meshwork into the canal of Schlemm on the inner surface of the sclera. The function of the aqueous humour is to nourish the lens and cornea. When the peripheral edge of the iris comes into contact with the peripheral edge of the cornea, it stops the flow of aqueous humour and causes the intraocular pressure to rise. The angle between the iris and cornea is important in acute glaucoma, otherwise known as closed-angled glaucoma, and requires emergency referral and treatment from an ophthalmologist. The *lens*, which is situated behind the iris, is biconvex in shape, highly elastic and transparent. The thickness of the lens

changes with contraction and relaxation of the cilliary processes and is part of the process involved in accommodation of the eye. Accommodation occurs when the eye is focused on an object that is near; the curvature of the lens increases and light rays are refracted onto the macula. The eyeballs rotate slightly inwards and the pupils constrict to complete the accommodation process. To focus onto an object in the distance, the lens elongates and becomes flatter. This elasticity of the lens decreases as we age and affects the ability of the lens to accommodate, as in reading – e.g. presbyopia (old sight) – and is why people need reading glasses in middle age.

Vitreous humour is a transparent avascular gel-like substance and fills the area of the globe behind the lens.

The eye socket is pyramidal in shape, with the apex situated behind, and is composed of seven bones: the ethmoid, frontal, lacrimal, maxillary, palantine, sphenoid and zygomatic bones. This bony socket protects the eye and can be fractured in severe blunt trauma to that area.

The *eyelids* are composed of two movable skin folds that cover the anterior surface of the eye when closed. The *conjunctiva* lines the eyelids: the frame of each eyelid is formed by fibrous tissue, i.e. the tarsal plate and orbital septum. The conjunctiva is a thin translucent mucous membrane which has two parts: the palpebral conjunctiva and bulbar conjunctiva. The conjunctiva protects the eye from foreign bodies and dessication. The main muscles of the eyelid are the levator palpebrae, which are innervated by the occulomotor (CNIII), and the obicularis oculi, a muscle of facial expression that is innervated by the facial nerve (CNVII). The purposes of the eyelids are to protect the eye and to distribute the tear film over the surface of the eye. The eyelids also aid in limiting the amount of light let into the eye. The distal end of the eyelid, known as the lid margins, exhibits a fine grey line. In front of the grey line are the eyelashes and behind are the tarsal glands (meibomian glands) and other sudoferous glands.

The *blood supply* to the eye is from the ophthalmic artery, which is a branch of the internal carotid artery. The artery emerges from the cavernous sinus and passes through to the optic canal below and lateral to the optic nerve, then crosses over to reach the medial wall of the orbit. It crosses the optic nerve and nasociliary nerve. The ophthalmic artery enters the retina through the centre of the optic disc and divides into four retinal arteries. These four central retinal artery branches are visible when the fundus is inspected using an ophthalmoscope. Other arterial branches of the ophthalmic artery are muscular, ciliary, lacrimal, supratrochlear and supraorbital. The ophthalmic veins are the superior and inferior veins; they pass backwards and drain into the cavernous sinus. There are no lymphatic vessels or nodes in the orbital socket.

The *lacrimal apparatus* consists of the lacrimal gland, lacrimal canaliculi, the lacrimal sac and the nasolacrimal duct. The lacrimal gland is situated in the upper eyelid, below the eyebrow on the lateral side towards the temple. This gland is responsible for tear production, which moistens the eye. *Tears* are then wiped across the ocular surface by blinking and drawn into the lacrimal punctum, from where they drain into the nasal meatus. The tear film consists of the lipid, aqueous and mucin layers. The lipid layer, which is the outermost layer, is exposed to the air and is produced by the meibomian glands. The aqueous layer is in the middle and is produced by the lacrimal gland and accessory gland. The mucin layer sits directly on the surface of the conjunctiva and is produced by the goblet cells in the conjunctiva. The normal tear film provides a smooth optical surface for the refraction of light rays. It lubricates the eyelids and has a protective function, in that tears contain a bactericidal enzyme, immunoglobulins IgA, IgG, enkephalins and other substances. The presence of enkephalins may explain the reason why we sometimes feel better after a good cry (Marieb 1995).

Assessment

Ocular problems can be classified under the headings of trauma, infection, inflammatory, degenerative and miscellaneous others.

Subjective assessment

This is what the patient tells you is the problem and reason for attending. Careful history taking is paramount and utilising a framework for symptom analysis can help to keep you focused, e.g. the mnemonic OLD-CARTSS: **O**nset, **L**ocation, **D**uration, **C**haracteristics, **A**ssociated symptoms, **R**elieving or aggravating factors, **T**reatment, **S**equence, **S**ummarise. Use open-ended questions to allow the patient to tell you what happened.

Types of questions to ask

1. What happened to your eye?
2. When did it happen? How long have you had this for?
3. How did it happen?
   - sporting activities
   - allergies
   - infection
   - sudden, no reason.
4. Is it related to the type of work that you do?
   - industrial, chemical exposure, welding, other factors influencing work environment: was safety equipment available and worn?
5. What were you doing at the time?
   - How much force?
6. When did you first notice any problem/visual/pain/discharge?
7. Is pain/discharge/redness/visual disturbance there all the time, intermittent, occassional?
8. How is your eyesight affected?
9. What colour is the discharge?
   - watery
   - sticky and gummed up.
10. Can you describe the pain/visual disturbance?
11. How much can you see?
12. What makes it better or worse?
    - wearing sunglasses because of photophobia.
13. Have you treated this yourself at all?
14. What did you use?
    - prescription medicine
    - over-the-counter (OTC) medicine, herbal preparation
    - homeopathic cure.
15. Do you wear glasses, contact lenses?
    - reading glasses
    - distance glasses
    - bifocals, varifocals
    - contact lenses.
16. Tell me what happened first of all and how did it all progress to this stage?
17. Let me just recap on what you have said and tell me if I've got it right?

Objective assessment

All four principles of physical examination are used in ocular assessment and a light gentle touch is essential as many people tell you that they are '*squeamish about eyes*'. The order for assessment is:
- *inspection* – a general inspection of the eye using the other eye for comparison, and a more focused inspection using a pen light and ophthalmoscope.
- *palpation*, e.g. lesions, tender areas and digital assessment of intraocular pressure, swollen pre-auricular and neck glands.
- *auscultation* is used to assess the state of the arteries, e.g. bruits of the carotid.
- *percussion* is used to determine a reflex, such as direct percussion, to elicit the glabellar reflex.

General approach

- Observe the general demeanour of the patient. Note whether the patient is afraid or in pain? Did he or she need help to walk in to see you? Other clues such as the wearing of sunglasses would indicate a degree of photophobia or hiding a blemish considered ugly by the patient.
- Check blood pressure and urinalysis in patients who present with visual disturbance or loss of eyesight who have no history of trauma.
- Check temperature and pulse if ocular cellulitis is observed.
- Test visual acuity and document.
- A drawing clarifies documentation.

Physical assessment

Ocular inspection is usually carried out and documented in this sequence; however, dependent on presenting symptoms, not all may be required:
- general overview

- face
- eyelids
- test visual acuity
- conjunctiva
- cornea
- pupil
- anterior chamber (AC)
- fundus
- ocular motility
- fields to confrontation
- colour vision.

General overview. Note the general impression that the patient makes on you, such as age, gait and dress, which can indicate occupation, etc.

Face. Inspect the face and observe symmetry of facial expression; note complexion, lesions and lacerations or scarring. Note the alignment of the eyes, the head posture of the patient and whether the blink reflex is normal.

Eyelids. Inspect the eyelids for erythema, oedema and lesions; take notice of the opening and closing of the eyelids and whether there is any disturbance along the eyelid margins, e.g. *entropion, ectropion lesions*. Look at the eyebrows and eyelashes: observe growth, distribution and direction of growth. Note whether there is any dandruff or oily type particles in the eyebrows and eyelashes and check out the quantity. Notice the colour of the eyelid rims. It may be more convenient at this stage to gently palpate any eyelid lesions and examine in accordance with the principles of a dermatological examination. Check out the area around the lacrimal punctum, especially in the lower eyelid, and note the alignment of the punctum with the upper eyelid. If a foreign body is suspected, evert the upper eyelid and remove with a wetted cotton bud so as not to leave any cotton fibres behind.

Conjunctiva. Use the pen light, and gently pull down the eyelid to examine the conjunctiva. Check out the state of the conjunctiva in the lower fornix of the eyelid and note the colour and any discharge from that area e.g. *hyperaemia, mucous strands, foreign body*. Observe the bulbar conjunctiva, which normally allows the white of the sclera to show through. Note any redness and dilatation of the blood vessels and do they extend to the area around the limbus of the cornea: this, with photophobia, can indicate a degree of intraocular inflammation.

Cornea. Observe the cornea for clarity and smoothness of the surface of the eye. Check out the corneal light reflex. Check for the presence of a foreign body and, if found, document, using the times of the clock to show its position in the eye.

Pupil. Observe pupils, shape, size and equality in comparison with the other eye. Use a pen light to inspect the reflex reaction to light, i.e. *light reflex*, and note direct and the consensual response of fellow pupil, i.e. *consensual reflex*.

Anterior chamber. The depth of the anterior chamber should be assessed prior to the instillation of mydriatic eye drops. This is done by shining the pen torch from the temple side of the eye tangentially at the conjunctival scleral limbus and asking the patient to look at an object in the distance. Inspect the nasal aspect of the iris and note whether it is illuminated, or in part shadow: the latter would show that it is a shallow angle between the cornea and iris periphery. This patient is at risk of acute angle closure glaucoma and mydriatic drops should not be used without access to an ophthalmologist and specialist ophthalmic department.

Fundus. Examine the fundus in a darkened room and shine the light from the ophthalmoscope onto the pupil and note the red reflex. Before proceeding to examine the fundus, inform the patient that you will need to get close, as you will be in their personal space; this is disconcerting for some people, and their instinctive reaction is to back away.

Then, follow the red reflex with the light and move in to inspect the fundus. The patient should still be focused on a distant object even though you will obscure their view. Inspection of the fundus is easier if the pupil has been dilated with mydriatic eye drops. The patient's right eye is examined with your right eye, as you view through the ophthalmoscope and vice versa. When the fundus is in view, observe the general background and note the overall colour of the retina, and remember that the fundus is darker in dark-skinned people due to more melanin pigmentation. Observe and note the colour, shape and margins of the optic nerve and check out the cup-to-disc ratio. Note the retinal blood vessels and observe how they emanate from the optic disc. Follow the length of the paired artery and vein in each quadrant of the eye towards the periphery and note contour and whether there is any tortuosity of the vessels to the edge of the fundus.

You will require the patient to look in different directions to get a good view. The artery is recognisable by the strip of light in the centre of the vessel. As you inspect the fundus, check the junctions where the arteries and veins cross over each other and note whether there is any nipping of the vessels, and whether the vessels are flat or tortuous. Check out the macula, the area approximately two disc diameters away from the optic disc towards the temple side of the patient's eye, the area without blood vessels. The fovea is a minute pit at the centre of the macula and in young people behaves as a concave mirror. It is seen as a small shimmering spot of reflected light, the *foveal reflex*, and dazzles the examiner inspecting the fundus with the ophthalmoscope.

Special manoeuvres: to evert the upper lid to remove a subtarsal foreign body

- Ensure good lighting
- Dampen cotton bud with saline solution
- Stand behind the patient
- Ask the patient to look downwards towards toes
- Place dry end of cotton bud on to lid
- Gently take hold of upper eye lid rim and lashes between thumb and fore finger
- Evert eye lid and with wetted end of cotton bud wipe tarsal conjunctiva which should remove the foreign body.

Corneal light reflex

Corneal light reflex checks out alignment of the eyes:
- position yourself and sit directly in front of the patient, so that you are at the same eye level
- ask the patient to look straight ahead into the distance; if this is a young child, use a toy to attract their attention and gently hold the child's chin to keep head posture straight
- using the pen light, shine the light into the patient's eyes from a distance of approximately 30 cm towards the bridge of the nose
- flick the pen light on and off so as not to be confused with other reflected light sources within the room
- note where the light from the pen torch is reflected in the cornea, this should be symmetrical in each cornea.

Cover test

Ocular fixation is essential for binocular vision. The normal response is for each eye to remain focused on the image in front:
- position yourself sitting directly in front of the patient with your eyes level with the patient if possible
- hold the picture end of the occluder in front of the patient at approximately 30 cm away (or an eraser toy that can be stuck on the end of a pencil)
- ask the patient to keep his eyes focused on the picture on the occluder
- cover one eye with a card or the fingers of the dorsal aspect of your hand
- observe the uncovered eye, i.e. does the eye stay fixed on the image in front
- repeat the process with the other eye.

Accommodation

The eyes converge and pupils constrict and the lens constricts and thickens inside the eye:
- instruct the patient to focus on an object in the distance – the pupils will dilate slightly; hold a pen or finger close to and ask the patient to look at it – the pupil will constrict and the eyeballs will rotate slightly towards the nose.

Ocular motility

Ocular motility assesses movement of extraocular muscles (Fig. 5.1):
- you may have to hold the patient's chin gently to stop head movement
- position yourself sitting directly in front of the patient, your eyes level with his eyes
- use an object that is easily visible, such as a pen
- instruct the patient to follow the direction of the pen as you move it along:

from

Left to right	→
Right to left	← *tests movement of the left and right rectus muscles*
Up towards the forehead	↑
Down towards toes	↓ *tests movement of superior and inferior rectus muscles*

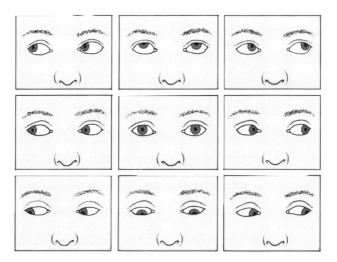

Figure 5.1 Testing of ocular movements. (Reproduced with permission from Battersby & Bowling 1999.)

Up and outward to right — *tests movement of*
Down and outward to left — *superior and inferior*
Up and outward to left — *obliques muscles*
Down and outward to right
Move pen towards the nose — *tests movement of rectus*
and observe eyes converge — *muscles*

Fields to confrontation

This assumes that the examiner's peripheral vision is normal and makes use of this to test patients' peripheral field of vision for assessment which can detect hemianopias. Further specialised tests will be required to detect subtle changes in the peripheral vision associated with chronic open-angle glaucoma or neurologic causes. To examine:

- Position yourself directly opposite and in front of the patient, with your eyes on a level with those of the patient.
- Cover your left eye and ask the patient to cover his right eye.
- Place your finger at the edge at the periphery of your visual field, asking the patient to tell you when the finger is within sight of his visual field. Ask the patient to count your fingers. Assess all quadrants within the field of vision on that side.
- Follow the same procedure for the other eye, covering your right eye and the patient his left eye.

Pupil reaction to light

- Assess the direct and consensual pupil response to the light from the pen torch. Note size, shape and whether pupils are equal when they react to light.

Diagnostic tests

Diagnostic tests are dependent on the result of your history taking and subjective and objective assessment findings. They can include blood tests for haemotology and biochemistry, microbiology, X-rays, brain scans, ultrasound, and a host of other investigations in relation to the specialities of orthoptics and optometry:

- Full blood count (FBC) and white cell differential: these will indicate anaemia, chronic inflammation, infection or leukocytosis.
- Rheumatoid factor in relation to arthritis.
- Erythrocyte sedimentation rate (ESR) as an indicator of generalised inflammation.
- Urea and electrolytes, to establish renal function.
- Blood pressure, to check out whether the patient has underlying hypertension.
- Urinalysis, as routine, in patients presenting with sudden and intermittent loss of vision.
- Fluorescein staining: use fluorescein drops or strips to examine the cornea and conjunctiva with a blue filter on the pen torch if an abrasion is suspected. This will show up as a fluorescent green stain.
- pH of tear fluid: useful in chemical injury to the eye to check on whether the chemical is acid-or alkaline-based and the amount of chemical remaining around

the ocular surface of the eye before and after irrigation. Instil a topical anaesthetic if the eye is painful. Fold over small amount of pH strip, approximately 5 mm, and ask the patient to look up toward the eyebrows. Place the pH strip into the lower fornix, ask the patient to close his eyes and leave the strip for approximately 20 seconds. Remove the strip and check the pH against the pH colour indicator. Continue irrigation of the eye with normal saline, check the pH and record. Trauma involving an alkaline-based chemical which seeps into the eye and can damage the interior eye, needs copious irrigation. The result of the pH test is documented in the notes.

- Digital testing for raised intraocular pressure can be done in the absence of equipment that measures intraocular pressure, i.e. tonometry. Ask the patient to close their eyelids and gently palpate the ocular surface of both eyes. Compare the tension of both eyes. The eye with a very high intraocular pressure will feel tense and hard in comparison with the other eye. *Digital palpation would not be useful for checking out intraocular pressure that is slight or moderately raised.*
- Palpation of the eyeball must not be done when the globe has been traumatised by injury or is too painful to touch.
- Schirmer's test is one of the tests used to establish wetness of tear fluid in patients with dry eyes.
- X-ray of the orbital skull may be done to establish the presence of a metal foreign body in the eye, or to investigate whether there is any systemic disease or fractures to the skull.

COMMON EYE PROBLEMS

The acute red eye

Acute red eye can be classified under the following headings:

- trauma
- (infection)
- (inflammation).

Specific disorders will now be considered.

Trauma: corneal foreign body

Particles such as metal, glass or material of organic origin get into the eye and become either superficially attached or embedded in the cornea. The cornea, which is responsible for 60% of the optical focusing power of the eye, is composed of five layers. The *epithelium*, the outermost layer, is continuous with the conjunctiva. It is composed of several epithelial layers, which become flatter as they get nearer to the surface. Damage to this epithelial layer has fast regeneration properties; it is the only layer of the cornea to heal without scarring.

The second layer of the cornea is the *Bowman's membrane*, which is the smooth surface of the third layer, the *stroma*. The stroma is the thickest part of the cornea and is made up of connective tissue. Collagen fibres are layered in parallel to the surface of the eye, which helps to maintain the transparency of the eye. This layer is continuous with the sclera at the limbus. *Descemet's membrane* is the clear elastic layer underneath the stroma.

The *endothelium,* the innermost layer of the cornea, is composed of a single cellular layer that extends over the trabecular mesh works of the angle of the anterior chamber. The cornea is an avascular structure, and blood supply is restricted to the periphery. Nerve supply to the cornea is from the ophthalmic branch of the trigeminal nerve (CNV), which is why injury to the cornea is painful.

Subjective findings

- The patient will usually present with a history of something going into the eye.
- On questioning, the patient might give a history of e.g. welding or drilling, while working in the garden or that the foreign body was blown into the eye by a gust of wind.
- You will need to establish exactly what the patient was doing at the time and how much force was involved.
- You will need to check what attempts at treatment have been instigated by the patient or by other people.

Equipment: pen light, magnifying glass, Snellen's test chart or equivalent.

❶ Ask the patient to keep both eyes open while you are examining the affected eye. Explain that the eyes work in synchrony, as some patients will close the unaffected eye in the belief that this will facilitate examination of the injured eye.

Objective findings

Inspect the patient and observe the patient's demeanour with regard to how painful the affected eye is:

- Note blink reflex, and any erythema or swelling around the eyelids, and or epiphoria.
- If the eye is painful, instil topical anaesthetic to facilitate the examination.
- With a pen light examine the conjunctiva, the upper and lower fornix and bulbar conjunctiva. Evert the upper eyelid to ensure that there are no unknown foreign particles tucked away in the upper fornix.
- Note and document that you have examined this area and your findings. Note and document any hyperaemia or mucous strands, or floating foreign particles in the conjunctival fornixes; the latter can be removed at this stage with a damp tipped cotton bud. Note the extent of any redness of the bulbar conjunctiva and document.
- Expose the cornea by gently lifting the upper eyelid and asking the patient to look downwards. Inspect the upper cornea with a pen light for any foreign particle. Release the upper eyelid gently. Now examine the lower part of the cornea, by asking the patient to look upward while holding the lower eye-lid down. Ask the patient to move his eyes to the left and right to ensure good scrutiny of the cornea.
- When the foreign body has been seen on the cornea, document its whereabouts on the cornea by using the clock method of sign posting.
- Examine the pupil for direct and consensual response.
- Test the patients eyesight using Snellen's Test chart or equivalent and document. *If glasses are normally worn for distance vision, test visual acuity with them on and document.*
- Test with the pin hole if the letters or numbers that the patient can see are limited to those above the red line on the Snellen's chart and document.

Treatment

Removal of the foreign body should be carried out by a health professional skilled in this task:

- If you are refering the patient for removal of the foreign body, commence treatment with chloramphenicol 1% ointment, three times a day, or some other suitable antibiotic eye ointment. This will help to prevent infection and will soften up the area around the foreign body, and can make it easier to remove. If you have removed the foreign particle, commence treatment with an appropriate antibiotic such as chloramphenicol 1% ointment or chloramphenicol 0.5% eye drops. Apply a pad over the affected eye, ensuring that the eyelids are closed underneath the dressing, and secure with Sellotape for approximately 24 hours. The patient should continue to use chloramphenicol, either in drop form or ointment, for 1 week.
- Instruct the patient to return or seek treatment from the Ophthalmic Department in a hospital if there is no improvement.
- If the patient is driving, leave the dressing off, as stereoscopic vision is affected and perception of distance and depth will be impaired. Instruct the patient on how to apply the dressing at home.
- There is some debate as to whether it is necessary to pad the injured eye after treatment. My own experience would say that it is dependant on how much the cornea has been injured. A small superficial abrasion may not cause the patient any pain at all, whereas a small but deep abrasion that affects the stroma will be more painful.

Health education

If the injury is a work injury, then explore health and safety issues, such as protective eye wear.

Complications

- *Incomplete removal of foreign body*
- *Iritis*: intraocular inflammation – the immune response to foreign body toxicity

■ *Hypopyon*: an intracorneal abscess.
Complications are referred to an ophthalmologist for urgent treatment.

Conjunctivitis can be due to:
■ Infection: viral or bacterial.
■ Trauma: usually chemical or exposure to ultraviolet radiation.
■ Allergic: grass pollen.
■ Degenerative or multi-causal: dry eyes. Sjögren's syndrome, an autoimmune disease, involves the following three symptoms: dry eyes, dry mouth and rheumatoid arthritis.

Conjunctivitis: bacterial

Subjective findings

The patient may complain of:
■ red, sore, gritty eyes over the past day or two
■ eyelids are stuck together and are especially 'gummed up' on waking
■ eyelids can be swollen, either from the patient constantly rubbing the eye, or oedema
■ eyesight is unaffected, although the patient may have a degree of photophobia.

Objective findings

■ Observe the patient generally and inspect both eyes with a pen light.
■ Check for any dried crusty discharge on the eyelids and eye lashes.
■ Pull the lower eye-lid down gently and ask the patient to look upward and examine the conjunctiva in the lower fornix. Note any mucous discharge and hyperaemia on the bulbar conjunctiva.
■ Examine the upper eyelid and, by asking the patient to look downwards and evert the upper eyelid, inspect the upper fornix of the conjunctiva.
■ Note whether the patient is photophobic.
■ Test visual acuity.
■ Document findings.

Investigations

■ Microbiology culture and sensitivity of conjunctival discharge
■ Viral culture, if chlamydial infection suspected
■ Schirmer's test, if dry eye is suspected
■ In the infant that is only a few weeks old, consider ophthalmia neonatorum, or viral conjunctivitis such as *Chlamydia*.

Inflammation: uveitis

Uveitis is defined by Kanski (1989) as inflammation of the uveal tract within the globe. The type of uveitis is described according to which segment of the uveal tract is involved, i.e. anterior uveitis, intermediate uveitis or

posterior uveitis. If inflammation of all three segments occurs, it is called pan uveitis. Uveitis can be acute or chronic.

Acute uveitis

Subjective findings

■ The patient complains of a painful, red eye with varying degrees of photophobia, and worsening eyesight.

Objective findings

Examination may be difficult if the patient is very photophobio. Darkening the room may help to facilitate the examination:
■ Test visual acuity.
■ Gently inspect the conjunctiva. It will have a very red appearance over the bulbar conjunctiva and the blood vessels will be visible around and up to the edge of the cornea.
■ Inspect the pupil for size, shape and reaction to light, e.g. *miotic pupil is characteristic of acute uveitis*.

Investigations

FBC, rheumatoid factor.

Treatment

Refer to an ophthalmologist for treatment which will involve mydriatic and steroid medication, either topical eye drops or via subconjunctival injection.

Chronic uveitis

Subjective findings

■ The patient will complain of minimal symptoms but will have a past history of uveitis
■ The conjunctiva may be white.

Objective findings

■ Slit lamp biomicroscopy will show inflammatory cells in the anterior chamber of the eye.

Treatment

As above, and refer to ophthalmologist.

Allergic conjunctivitis

Subjective findings

The patient usually presents for treatment, anxious and in a state of panic. The eyes are watery, the white of the eye is swollen, called chemosis, which can have the appearance of the swelling of an egg when first put in to the hot fat of a frying pan. There is a history of being around grass pollens. A calm and professional manner will reduce the patient's anxiety and the information that it is an allergic response to grass pollen.

Objective findings

- Inspect the eyelids – note whether there is any redness or swelling, which usually occurs as a consequence of rubbing
- Gently inspect the conjunctiva and note how much chemosis is present
- Check visual acuity, if necessary.

Treatment

- Avoid the causative allergen
- Reassure the patient that swelling will resolve over the next few hours, once he is removed from the allergen
- Application of a cold compress over the eyelids will help
- Give oral antihistamine.

Eye-lid pathology can also be classified according to trauma, infection and inflammation.

Trauma

Lacerations of the eyelid that affect the eyelid rims or tear ducts need to be sutured by an ophthalmologist. Deep lacerations involving the eyelid muscles and tarsal tendons will also need repair by an ophthalmologist.

Infection: external hordeolum (stye)

An acute bacterial infection of the eyelids, mainly the eyelid margin around an eyelash follicle, due to *Staphylococcus aureus*.

Subjective findings

- The patient complains of a sore, swollen eyelid, which may or may not have a discharge. He may have tried an OTC preparation.

Objective findings

Inspect with good lighting:
- Examine the affected eyelid; note any erythema and/or swelling
- Note whether there is an abscess around an eyelash follicle
- Note whether there is any crusty discharge along the eyelid margins and eyelashes.

Treatment

- The eye can be bathed to remove crusts and a hot compress applied to the affected eyelid
- Apply antibiotic ointment such as chloramphenicol 1% three times daily for 1 week to 10 days.

Complications

Consider diabetes in patients with chronic persistent styes.

Inflammation: blepharitis

Definition: Chronic inflammation of the lid margins. The meibomian glands in the eyelid secrete fluid that makes up the oily part of the tear film. Microscopic dried meibomian fluid makes waxy particles that adhere to the bottom of the eyelashes and eyelid margins can cause inflammation and infection. Blepharitis is often associated with the skin condition Rosacea.

Subjective findings

The patient complains of sore, itchy eyes, with a history that these symptoms have been going on for a long period of time.

Objective findings

Inspect:
- the face for reddened areas of skin, or telangectasia, paying attention to the cheeks, nose and forehead, indicative of rosacea
- check out the eyelid rims and note any redness
- with a magnifying glass, check eyelashes for the presence of dandruff-type particles
- note any infected, or ulcerated lesions along the eyelid rims.

Treatment

- An antibiotic ointment applied to the eyelid edges, if infected or ulcerated eyelid lesions are present, e.g. chloramphenicol 1%, three times daily for 1 week, or Fucithalmic 1%, twice daily for 1 week.
- Lid hygiene: the patient must clean the eyelid rims daily. There are three methods and choice depends on the patient's lifestyle and finances:
- Method 1 – a solution of 1 teaspoon of soda bicarbonate to one pint of water that has been boiled and cooled.
- Method 2 – a solution of diluted baby shampoo: half a teaspoon to an egg cup of warm water.
- Method 3 – ask the patient to buy an OTC eyelid care lotion, which is available from most chemists. This product comes as a lotion or in individual sachets.

Health education

Instruct the patient to clean eyelid margins daily and that this problem is controllable and is not a curable condition. If regular eyelid hygiene is stopped the symptoms will return. Instruct the patient to clean eyelid rims gently.

Complications

- Blepharo keratoconjunctivitis, internal hordeolum (meibomian cyst).
- Consider pediculosis. If pediculosis is found in a child, consider abuse.
- Over a long period of time, chronic low-grade inflammation distorts the growth of the eyelashes and can cause trichiasis.

MISCELLANEOUS

Dry eyes

There are many factors that affect the production of tears or affect the stability of the tear film which can cause symptoms of dry eyes.

Subjective findings

- The patient tells you that his eyes feel dry and gritty. This has usually been going on over a lengthy period of time. He may feel that this affects his work, e.g. on computers, which involves staring at a monitor for long periods of the day.

Objective findings

Inspection:
- Examine and check out the eyelids and observe that they open and close efficiently. Note whether there is any deficiency in the movement of the eyelids.
- Examine the ocular surface of the eye with a pen light and check for any lesions, e.g. conjunctival erythema.

Diagnostic tests

- Schirmer's test
- Slit lamp biomicroscopy examination of the tear film and the evaporation time of the tear film.

Treatment

- Correction of any mechanical problem that affects the function of the eyelids, e.g. ectropion
- Some people will have to stop wearing contact lenses due to an insufficient tear film
- Artificial tear film supplements are available OTC in drop and ointment form and can be used as often as required
- The patient will need to be aware of the environmental factors that cause rapid evaporation of their remaining tear film, e.g. anything that blows hot or cold air around, such as air conditioning and hot air central heating, the air blower in the car to demist the windscreen, a smoky atmosphere, etc.

Health education

There are many factors that can cause the problem of dry eyes to a greater or lesser degree. Apart from those pathologies that affect the mechanical production of the tear film, the commonest causes for dry eyes are the ageing process, hormonal changes, some other pathology such as arthritis and some drug therapies such as beta blockers, etc. There is no cure for dry eyes and the treatment is ongoing, which is a disappointment to many people who suffer. Learning to avoid or control the environmental factors that worsen the symptoms of dry eyes is important and makes the condition more bearable.

Subconjunctival haemorrhage

Definition: bleeding which can be due to trauma or occur spontaneously. Traumatic subconjunctival haemorrhage must be referred to an ophthalmologist for ocular examination, as it can be indicative of a skull fracture.

Subjective findings

The spontaneous subconjunctival haemorrhage often occurs without the patient knowing when it happened, or occasionally a minor twinge was felt and ignored. It is often unnoticed until pointed out by someone or the patient sees himself in a mirror. It can be caused by sneezing, coughing or straining. The effect can be quite dramatic and alarming to the patient.

Objective findings

Inspection:
- examine the eye and conjunctiva; note and document the extent of the haemorrhage.

Health education

Explain and reassure the patient that although the eye may look alarming, the condition is not serious. Explain that as the anterior eyeball is heavily oxygenated, the haemorrhage will remain bright red. As it is reabsorbed by the eye, the haemorrhage will change colour in the same way that a bruise in the skin is absorbed.

Consider whether the patient is on anticoagulant therapy and check out the patient's blood pressure.

Floaters

Floaters can often be seen by the patient on a bright sunny day against a plain background such as a white wall. As we age, strands of the vitreous humour, a gel-type substance in the eyeball, thicken and shrink, which causes shadows on the retina; this is seen by the person as a floater or several floaters. The shrinkage of the vitreous humour can cause pulling on the retina, which is seen as flashing lights and can cause a posterior vitreous detachment, which in some cases can tear the retinal layer of the eye.

Subjective findings

- The patient attends the surgery worried about floating specks or blobs that affect his vision.

Objective findings

Check visual acuity and document.

Treatment

Explain what a floater is.

Health education

Ensure that the patient understands when urgent referral to an ophthalmologist is required. The ophthalmologist will examine the eye for retinal tears or detachment, if the following symptoms arise:

- if more floaters suddenly appear that affect his vision
- flashing lights suddenly appear, which would indicate a retinal disturbance
- either partial or whole loss of vision occurs in the affected eye.

Open-angle glaucoma

Open-angle glaucoma is commonly picked up by the optometrist, when a person decides to have their eyes checked as they feel the need to wear glasses. The progress of this type of glaucoma is gradual and slow. Glaucoma as a result of optic nerve degeneration causes a slow loss of peripheral vision that goes unnoticed by the affected person. There is an hereditary factor involved, and if a parent has this type of glaucoma, so too may the offspring when they get to middle age. From the age of 40 years, it is advisable for people to have an annual eye check with their optometrist. This will ensure that early changes in the vision or the fundus are detected, which will require referral to an ophthalmologist for further assessment and treatment. Treatment may include careful observation and monitoring with ocular therapeutics, or surgery.

Cataract

Cataract means an opacity of the lens inside the eye. Although some children may have congenital cataracts, or cataracts caused by trauma, cataracts occur mainly as a result of the ageing process, which affects the eye, in this case the lens, as it does other organs of the body. Cataracts cause gradual loss of vision and can be a problem for car drivers, where they affect the refraction of light rays, which can cause glare from oncoming car headlights. Some systemic pathology, such as diabetes, increases the risk of cataracts and some drugs such as steroid use. Treatment is by surgery.

Top Tips ✔

1. When testing visual acuity using Snellen's chart, check that glasses for distance vision are worn. Most people want to put their reading glasses on to read the chart

2. Explain that the Snellen's test is to test what the patient can see. Some people automatically react to the chart as a memory test

3. Encourage patients to see if they can read any more letters on the next line down. There is a tendency for some people to stop reading when they can only read a completed line

4. When instilling topical eye drops ask the patient to look upwards towards their eyebrows, getting the cornea out of the way, while the lower lid is gently pulled to create a small space for the drop in the lower fornix of the eyelid

5. When instilling topical eye ointment the same as the above, but after installation ask the patient to look downward, then to close their eyes. Although ointment causes blurring of vision for a brief moment, this procedure lessens the gumming up of the eyelashes

6. A complaint of a gritty sensation in the eye usually indicates ocular surface irritation; a complaint of a pain from within the patient's eye usually indicates intraocular problems

7. An easy way to irrigate the eyes as a result of chemical injury, when there is no irrigation equipment available: fill the sink up with tap water, ask the patient to submerge his face in the water, and open and shut his eyes under water in the same way as swimming under water in a swimming pool

8. When the patient presents with the symptom of pain in his eye and he holds his head on that same side, it is usually an indicator of severe pain and requires attention urgently or referral to ophthalmic unit rather than a lengthy wait in a general Accident and Emergency Department

9. If the treatment decided upon consists of a dressing pad over the affected eye, ensure that this eye is closed underneath by using two pads. One pad is folded over to fill the eye socket and the second pad is secured over the top with Sellotape. A badly applied eye dressing (a) does nothing or (b) can add further injury through bits of cotton filament getting in that same eye

10. As a general rule, do not apply eye pad dressings to the under 6-year-old child as (a) it can be traumatic and (b) it can cause supression of vision in the affected eye after the injury has healed, e.g. a superficial abrasion of the cornea

Glossary

Anterior chamber   The inner eye is divided into two compartments: the anterior and posterior chambers. The anterior chamber is from the posterior corneal layer of the eye to the anterior part of the iris and includes the aqueous humour. The posterior chamber is from the posterior part of the iris to the fundus and includes the vitreous humour

Aqueous humour   A watery fluid that flows through the anterior and posterior chambers. The aqeuous humour supplies nutrient to the lens and cornea and removes waste products.

Chemosis   Oedema of the conjunctiva that is excessive

Chlamydia   Sexually transmitted infections caused by the bacterium *Chlamydia trachomatis* which can manifest as urethritis, epididymis and proctitis in men and cervicitis, salpingitis, urethritis and proctitis in women. In relation to ocular symptoms, this bacterium can cause conjunctivitis. See also *http://www.bact.wisc.edu/Bact330/lecturchlamydia*

Dessication   Dried out

Diplopia   Double vision. The person complaining of diplopia is seeing two images

Ectropion   The eyelid margin is turned outwards. It can be congenital or occur through trauma or loss of elasticity of the obicularis oculi muscle

Erythema   Tissue redness due to inflammation

Entropion   The eyelid margin is turned inward towards the eyeball. It can be congenital, or due to trauma or loss of elasticity of the obicularis oculi muscle. Eyelashes cause trauma – they prick and scratch the eyeball

Hemianopias   Blindness or defective vision within half the field of vision in one or both eyes. Examples are:
- **absolute hemianopia**   Blind to light colour and shape in half the field of vision
- **altitudinal hemianopia**   Blind in the upper or lower half of the field of vision
- **bilateral hemianopia**   Blindness that affects the visual field in both eyes
- **binasal hemianopia**   Blindness that affects the visual field on the nasal aspect of both eyes
- **bitemporal hemianopia**   Blindness that affects the vision in both eyes on the temporal aspect of both eyes
- **complete hemianopia**   Blindness that affects half the vision in one eye

Hypereamia: Excess blood, engorgement

OTC   Refers to over-the-counter drugs that can be purchased without a prescription

Orthoptist   A qualified health professional who is educated and trained to assess and treat defective binocular vision as a result of extraocular muscle imbalance. An orthoptist works in conjunction with an ophthalmologist

Ophthalmia neonatorum   Purulent conjunctivitis in the newborn contracted at birth as a result of a vaginal infection of the mother

Optometrist   A qualified health professional who deals with the improvement of vision by the prescription of spectacles and contact lenses and detects eye pathology

Ophthalmologist   A medical practitioner, a surgeon that specialises in the pathology of the eye

Photophobia   Abnormal intolerance to light

Pin hole test   The pin hole test works on the same principle as a pin hole camera and works by focusing the light rays onto the retina of the eye. It can be made easily from a piece of card large enough to occlude the eye. Pierce a hole in the centre of the card the size of the shaft of a dressmaker's sewing pin. Ask the patient to read the Snellen's chart, holding the card close to the eye being tested, and read the Snellen's chart through the pin hole with the other eye occluded. The letters on the Snellen's chart may sharpen up the letters seen. If there is an improvement in the vision of several lines of letters on the Snellen's chart this can indicate that there is a refractive error and the patient may benefit from wearing corrective glasses. Refer to an optometrist for full eye examination if there is no obvious pathology of the eye.

Schirmer's test   Used to assess the quantity of tears in relation to dry eyes

Snellen's test   A visual acuity (VA) assessment that tests distance vision. RVA, right visual acuity; LVA, left visual acuity; PH, pin hole. Each eye is tested separately. An example of documentation;
- RVA. 6/9 unaided LVA 6/6
- RVA 6/9 with glasses LVA 6/6
- RVA 6/18 unaided 6/12 LVA 6/9 with PH 6/6

If patients are not able to see the letters, then counting fingers (CF) would be the next step to obtain visual acuity assessment taken from 6 m away initially, moving in to 3 m and finally 1 m away from the patient. It can be documented as:
- RVA 3/CF unaided LVA 6/6

A patient who could only see hand movements (HM) would be documented as
- RVA. HM unaided LVA 6/9

Spectacles
- Distance: corrects distance vision
- Bifocal: corrects distance and presbyopic vision
- Varifocal: corrects distance and middle distance and presbyopic vision.

Telangectasia   Dilation of existing blood vessels

Trichiasis   Inward-growing eyelashes that can scratch the eye globe

References

Battersby M, Bowling B 1999 Ophthalmology. Churchill Livingstone, Edinburgh.

Johnson K 1996 Physics for you. New National Curriculum edition by GCSE, 2nd edn. Stanley Thornes, Cheltenham.

Kanski J 1989 Clinical ophthalmology, 3rd edn. Butterworth-Heinemann, Oxford.

Marieb E N 1995 Human anatomy and physiology, 3rd edn. Benjamin Cummings, California.

Further reading

Battersby M, Bowling B 1999 Ophthalmology. Churchill Livingstone, Edinburgh.

Berkovitz B K B, Moxham B J 1988 A textbook of head and neck anatomy. Wolfe Publishing, London.

Chawla H B 1999 Ophthalmology: a symptom based approach, 3rd edn. Butterworth Heinemann, Oxford.

Foss M, Farine T 2000 Science in nursing and health care. Prentice Hall, London.

Jarvis C 1996 Physical examination and health assessment, 2nd edn. W B Saunders, Philadelphia.

6

HEAD AND NECK

Wendy Johnson

Key Issues

- Conditions of the head and neck system are very common

- Many are self-limiting and require merely self-care advice

- There has been a major trend away from antibiotic use for these conditions

- Seasonal factors are important in causation

- Allergy is implicated in several ENT disorders

- Health promotion issues include simple self-help measures to manage infections, allergen avoidance, and smoking cessation

Introduction

Diseases of the ear, nose and throat will form a major part of the workload of primary care nurse practitioners (NPs). These conditions constitute 23% of primary care consultations and often require urgent appointments, especially for children. It is therefore important to have a clear understanding of such problems.

- Many are short-lived and self-limiting infections, some of the most common in the community, and require simple self-help advice or over-the-counter (OTC) remedies. However, dealing with these conditions can present a challenge to the NP.

- Overdiagnosis and overtreatment is widespread.

- The current focus on antibiotic overuse, and concerns regarding antibiotic resistance are of particular relevance to these conditions: current evidence suggests that antibiotics offer little or no benefit in most respiratory tract symptoms – indeed, adverse effects of treatment are fairly common.

- There is often patient demand and expectation for prescriptions. However, the medicalising effect of prescribing encourages reattendance (Little et al 1997) and reinforces help-seeking behaviour (Audit Commission 1994).

- An important part of the NP role will be advising patients on the rationale for management; NPs will need to recognise and explore patients' understanding of the nature and cause of their illness, its likely clinical course and treatment options. Patients whose expectations are addressed are more likely to accept a treatment plan, even if it does not fulfill their initial expectations (Eisenthal & Lazare 1976).

- Advice on self-care, together with interventions that encourage patient empowerment should form an important part of the NP role for dealing with these conditions (Kai 1996). Patient leaflets are a useful adjunct to verbal advice. Changes to both practitioner and patient behaviour, with avoidance of inappropriate treatment, and emphasis on enhancing self-care abilities, are required.

- Future management is likely to focus on identifying clinical predictors of who will benefit most from treatment.

- Health promotion strategies are important regarding the role of allergens and smoking in the causation of certain conditions. Passive smoking is implicated in a causal relationship in children with both acute and chronic middle ear disease (Strachan & Cook 1998).

- Allergens are a major factor in many conditions, and the incidence of atopy is rising in industralised societies. Allergy sufferers are more prone to bacterial secondary infection.

- Smoking has an adjuvant effect in increasing the risk of developing an allergic response, and is implicated in some mouth and throat disorders.

- Heavy alcohol consumption may also play a part in mouth and throat disease.

- Socioeconomic factors, e.g. damp accommodation, poor ventilation and overcrowding, are implicated in respiratory disease.

- Seasonal factors are relevant: upper respiratory infections are much commoner in winter months, while allergies are more common in spring, summer and autumn.

- A healthy mouth and teeth are important both to quality of life and nutrition.

- Immunocompromised patients are at special risk of infections in this region.

Common signs and symptoms

Symptoms in this area may occur in combination or singly: commonly, these include pain, discharge, obstruction, general malaise, fever, sensory disturbance, i.e. smell, taste or hearing impairment, balance disturbance, dryness or soreness of the mouth, itching of the throat and ears (in allergy), dysphagia and lymphadenopathy. Referred pain is common: the ear shares sensory innervation with the oropharynx cranial nerve (CNIX), laryngopharynx CNX, upper molars, temporomandibular joint, parotid gland CNV and cervical spine (C2 and C3 vertebrae).

There is a complex interrelationship between the systems, i.e. nose, throat, ear and chest; therefore, assessment usually includes them all.

General approach

Diagnosis is usually based solely on history and physical examination signs without recourse to further investigations. However, the predictive value of clinical signs is not always accurate, thus emphasising the importance of careful history taking. There is an ongoing search for more robust diagnostic criteria and predictors of which groups are at higher risk of more serious illness, and who will clearly benefit from treatment with antibiotics (Butler et al 1998).

Intervention, therefore, consists of a thorough history, consideration of whether the patient is systemically unwell, and whether their symptoms are getting better or worse.

General survey

This begins as the client enters the room. Consider general malaise, hearing, voice or swallowing abnormality noticed in conversation.

Examination techniques

1. The patient should be examined with good lighting (powerful pen torch, auriscope, head mirror or head lamp).
2. Conduct the examination in the sitting position.
3. Inspect and palpate (where appropriate).
4. Follow a systematic approach that includes the entire ear, nose and throat system, lymph nodes of the head and neck, with chest examination also if appropriate. The nasopharynx and larynx are not accessible to view with standard primary care equipment.
5. Examining small children often presents a challenge – balance what is essential with what is possible.
6. Distinguish regional and generalised lymphadenopathy.

History taking

1. History of present illness.

2. Is it getting worse or better?
3. Generalised symptoms, malaise, severity.
4. What have you done to help yourself? Use of medication, oral and topical, including sprays and drops.
5. Explore symptoms using symptom analysis, e.g. 'pqrst' (Gonce Morton 1990).
6. Is there a history of symptoms of this region: hearing disturbance, use of hearing aid, tinnitus, vertigo, earache, discharge, frequent colds, nasal congestion, discharge, itching, hayfever, nosebleeds, sinus problems, sore or dry mouth, frequent sore throats, hoarseness, pain, lumps or swelling of the neck?

EXAMINATION

Ear

The ear is the sensory organ for hearing and maintaining equilibrium. It comprises three parts: the external, middle and inner ear. The outer ear consists of the pinna and external auditory meatus. The canal curves inwards and is approximately 2.5 cm long. The outer portion is surrounded by cartilage. The canal is lined with skin and is thus susceptible to most systemic dermatological conditions. In the outer portion, the skin is hairy and contains glands that produce cerumen. The canal's squamous epithelium lining has the unique property of being migratory, so that dead cells and cerumen are carried out of the canal. It is innervated by the vagus nerve (CNX); this explains the cough reflex often initiated on examination of the ear. The inner portion of canal is surrounded by bone (the mastoid process of the temporal bone) and lined by thin hairless skin.

The tympanic membrane separates the middle and outer ear (Fig. 6.1). It has three layers: an outer squamous, middle fibrous, and an inner columnar epithelial layer continuous with the middle ear space. The membrane lies obliquely and is held inward at its centre by the tip of the malleus. It has a pearly grey

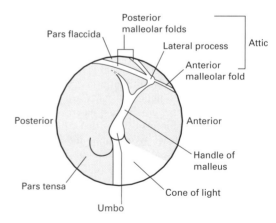

Figure 6.1 *Anatomy of normal tympanic membrane.*

colour, and a cone of light reflects downward and anteriorly. The umbo, short process and manubrium of the malleus are all visible through the drum. The pars flaccida is a small slack portion superiorly, while the pars tensa constitutes the remainder of drum; it is taut and thicker. A tough outer fibrous annulus forms the rim of the eardrum. The middle ear lies within the temporal bone. The cavity is lined by columnar epithelium, and is continuous with the mastoid air cell system. It is connected to the nasopharynx by the eustachian tube that allows passage of air. It opens on yawning or swallowing to allow equalisation of air pressure on either side of the tympanic membrane.

The middle ear space contains three ossicles – the malleus, incus and stapes – which transmit sound to the inner ear. It is innervated by the facial nerve (CNVII). The inner ear contains the bony labyrinth, in which the organs of hearing and balance lie. The cochlea receives transmission of sound energy from the stapes via the oval window, while the semicircular canals, utricle and saccule compose the vestibular apparatus. Head position and acceleration cause movement of equilibrium receptors, feeding information to the cerebellum concerning position in space, so that equilibrium is maintained. The hearing pathway begins as vibrations travelling through the air of the external ear; these pass through the eardrum, to the ossicles, then on to the cochlea (conductive phase). Nerve impulses leave via the auditory nerve (CNVIII) to the brain (sensorineural phase).

Ear examination technique

Only the outer ear and part of the middle ear are accessible to direct examination. Inspect the auricle and surrounding tissue for masses, lesions and skin changes. If pain, discharge or inflammation are present, apply traction to the pinna, and pressure on tragus and mastoid process, assessing whether this causes discomfort. Inspect the canal and eardrum using an auriscope with the largest speculum that fits the ear. Position the patient appropriately, then gently pull the auricle upwards, backwards and laterally; this straightens the curved canal. In small children under 3 years, pull the pinna straight down, to match the slope of the ear canal. Bracing your hand against the patient's face enables you to follow unexpected movements. Insert the auriscope gently in a downward and forward direction. Inspect the canal for discharge, inflammation and cerumen quality, the tympanic membrane for colour, contour, cone of light, the usual landmarks (handle of malleus and its position, short process of malleus), all of the tympanic membrane, its margins and intactness. Scars from previous perforation may be visible.

The mobility of the tympanic membrane may be assessed by the Valsalva manoevre: ask the patient to pinch the nostrils and blow air into the nose, while you observe the tympanic membrane. Slight movement is normal, indicating air pressure change (this checks the patency of the eustachian tube).

Testing of auditory function allows inferences about the function of the middle and inner ear, which are not open to direct examination. Tests should be conducted in a quiet room. Gross hearing may be assessed by occlusion of one ear at a time, and whispering from a short distance away; ensure the patient is not lip-reading. Air conduction is the normal first phase of hearing; tests of bone conduction may be carried out to bypass the external and middle ear, instead directly stimulating the cochlea with a vibrating tuning fork. Air and bone conduction should be tested with a 512 Hz tuning fork, which is in the range of human speech. Set the fork into light vibration: the Weber test for lateralisation is performed by placing the tuning fork midline on top of the head or forehead, and asking where the sound is heard. The normal response is midline, or in both ears. The Rinne test compares air and bone conduction. Place the vibrating tuning fork base on the mastoid process; when the client can no longer hear a sound, quickly place its vibrating end close to the ear canal, and assess if it is still audible. Normally air conduction is greater than bone conduction (Fig. 6.2).

Special techniques for the ear

Head mirror or head light. A valuable tool that enables both hands free for instrumentation.

Aural toilet. Dry mopping technique, with cotton wool mounted on Jobson Horne probe, valuable in treating otitis external and otitis media with perforation.

Pneumatic bulb attachment to auriscope. Allows a puff of air to be directed toward the tympanic membrane to assess its mobility.

Tympanometry. Measurement of compliance and resistance of the middle ear mechanism. Valuable in assessing young children with glue ear.

Positional testing. The Hallpike manoeuvre, used to differentiate vertigo caused by otological and central pathology; from an erect position on a couch, lie the patient flat with the head over the top edge, turned to one side. Ask the patient to report vertigo, and observe for nystagmus. If present, allow these to settle before sitting the patient upright. Repeat with the head turned to the other side.

Mouth and pharynx

The lips form the anterior border of the oral cavity, which is lined by buccal mucosa, rich in mucous glands. Gingiva [gums] are firmly attached to the teeth, with scalloped margins and pointed interdental papillae. Each lip is connected to the gingiva by a labial frenulum. Thirty-two adult teeth lie in bony sockets with their enamel-covered crowns visible. The tongue is a large mobile structure composed of several muscles covered by mucous membrane. Its dorsal surface is covered

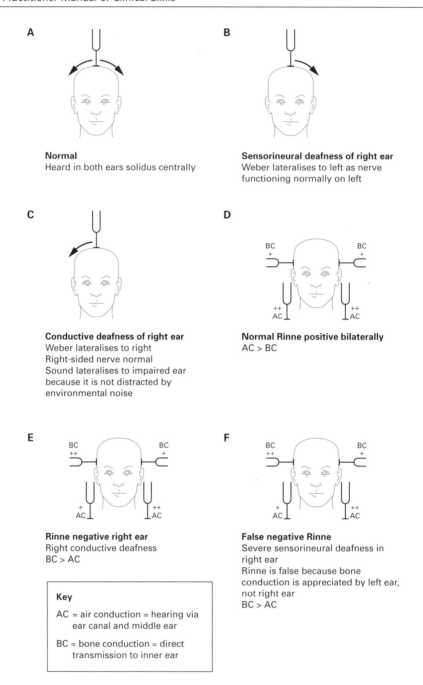

A

Normal
Heard in both ears solidus centrally

B

Sensorineural deafness of right ear
Weber lateralises to left as nerve
functioning normally on left

C

Conductive deafness of right ear
Weber lateralises to right
Right-sided nerve normal
Sound lateralises to impaired ear
because it is not distracted by
environmental noise

D

BC
+
BC
+
++
AC
++
AC

Normal Rinne positive bilaterally
AC > BC

E

BC
++
BC
+
+
AC
++
AC

Rinne negative right ear
Right conductive deafness
BC > AC

F

BC
++
BC
+
+
AC
++
AC

False negative Rinne
Severe sensorineural deafness in
right ear
Rinne is false because bone
conduction is appreciated by left ear,
not right ear
BC > AC

Key

AC = air conduction = hearing via
       ear canal and middle ear

BC = bone conduction = direct
       transmission to inner ear

Figure 6.2 *The interpretation of tuning fork tests. A–C Weber test; D–E Rinne test. These tests are invalidated if the ear canals are not free of wax debris.*

with papillae, making its surface rough. It is connected to the floor of the mouth by a lingual frenulum. Two pairs of salivary glands empty via the submandibular ducts (opening at either side of the lingual frenulum) and parotid ducts (opening close to the second upper molar). These secrete saliva, keeping the oral cavity moist and aiding in swallowing. Above and behind the

tongue an arch is formed by the anterior and posterior pillars, soft palate and uvula.

Tonsils lie in fossae between the anterior and posterior pillars. On their surface are 10–15 crypts into which mucous glands open. The nasopharynx and buccal cavity are encircled by a ring of lymphoid tissue, known as Waldeyer's ring: this is composed of the adenoids in

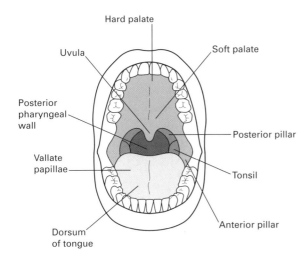

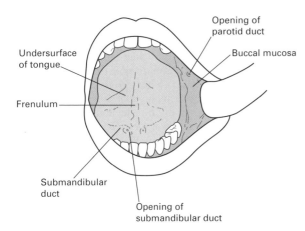

Figure 6.3 *Examination of the mouth and throat.*

the postnasal space, pharyngeal tonsils and lingual tonsil (situated on the posterior one-third of the tongue). (The size is age-related, as lymphoid tissue becomes gradually smaller after age 5: Chapter 17). Tonsils vary in size and the extent to which they are visible within the pharynx because they vary in their relation to the pillars of the fauces. A grading system exists:

1+ visible
2+ halfway between tonsillar pillars and uvula
3+ touching the uvula
4+ touching each other.

Examination technique

Inspect with a bright light, examining in a systematic fashion from anterior to posterior (Fig. 6.3). Examine the lips for symmetry, colour, pigmentation, ulcers, and cracks, especially at the corners of the mouth. Ask the patient to open and close the mouth to check jaw mobility and occlusion of the teeth. Palpate the temporo-mandibular joint for crepitus, tenderness or referred ear

pain, with the mouth opened wide then closed. Inspect the anterioinferior area between the lower lip and gum, the buccal mucosa, roof, palate, pharynx and Stensen's ducts (the openings of the parotid glands, opposite the upper second molars), using a tongue depressor to retract structures. Note mucosal colour, normally light pink, and moisture: hydration is assessed from the state of the tongue and mucous membranes, as well as from skin turgor. If dentures are worn, ask the patient to remove these before examination of the mouth.

Examine the dorsum of the tongue, for colour, coating or ulceration, then its undersurface, floor of mouth and Wharton's ducts (the openings of the submandibular glands, opening on either side of the frenulum). Ask the patient to protrude the tongue, and assess for mobility and tremor. Ask the patient to say 'ah' and note rising of the soft palate and uvula in the midline (testing CNX), and the appearance of the posterior oropharynx. The gag reflex (testing CNIX and CNX) is elicited by touching the posterior wall with a tongue spatula (see Chapter 11). Inspect the gums for swelling, redness, bleeding or pigmentation. Gross assessment of the teeth only is required, assessing general condition, hygiene, caries and missing teeth. Palpate the lips and inside of the mouth with a gloved finger if any lesions are detected. Throughout your assessment, notice any odours.

Nose

The upper third of the nose consists of bone, while the lower two-thirds is composed of cartilage. The entrance is a widened vestibule lined by skin with hair, above which a narrow passage leads to the nasopharynx. Medially, the passages are divided by the nasal septum of cartilage and bone. Extending inward from the lateral wall are three turbinates – inferior, middle and superior – which are curved bony protuberances extending along the cavity. A groove lies beneath each one, into which drainage occurs. The nasolacrimal duct drains under the inferior meatus, and the sinuses drain beneath the middle meatus. The nasal cavity is lined by mucous membrane with a good blood supply. It has an air-conditioning function, and its large surface area ensures cleansing, humidification and warming of inspired air. Specialised olfactory mucosa high in the nasal vault provide the function of smell.

The paranasal sinuses, four paired air-filled cavities – frontal, maxillary, ethmoidal and sphenoidal – lie within the skull bone. Like the nose, they are lined with a mucous membrane of ciliated pseudostratified columnar epithelium. Each sinus has a narrow ostium that opens into the nasal cavity. A mucous blanket covers these cilia and envelopes bacteria and other irritants. It is moved constantly towards the ostia (Evans 1994).

Examination technique

Inspect the outer nose, for shape and symmetry, and linearity. Check patency of the nostrils – close one nostril

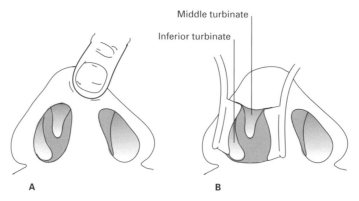

Figure 6.4 *Anterior rhinoscopy using (a) digital pressure and (b) thudicum speculum.*

with finger pressure, then ask the client to sniff. For children, hold a mirror beneath the nares and observe it for steaming up (for testing of sense of smell see Chapter 11). Inspection of the internal nose through the anterior nares is limited to a partial view of the vestibule, anterior septum, lower and middle turbinates. Tilt the head back slightly. Apply gentle pressure on the tip of the nose to widen nostrils, then inspect with torch or auriscope, with the short wide speculum attached. A thudicum speculum will facilitate viewing by opening the vestibule (Fig. 6.4). Initial inspection is carried out with a direction of view along the floor of the nose, later tilting the head to view the upper part. Assess whether cavities are approximately equal and the colour of the mucosa, which should be smooth, pink and glisten with a thin mucus coating. Check for evidence of swelling, bleeding or exudate.

Inspect the septum for position, deviation, inflammation, evidence of obstruction and the presence of polyps or ulcers. Little's area (an aggregation of blood vessels on the anterior part of the septum, a frequent source of bleeding) is visible on tilting the tip upwards. Assess turbinate size, shape, colour and hydration; the lower turbinate is most visible. Secretions are normally clear and mucoid. Only the frontal and maxillary sinuses are accessible to examination. Palpate the frontal sinuses under the eyebrows, and the maxillary just below the cheekbones, for tenderness; apply pressure using the thumbs.

Transillumination may be applied if inflammation is suspected: in a completely darkened room, shine a bright light through the frontal or maxillary sinus, and observe the amount of light transmitted through the palate. A diffuse red glow occurs in normal subjects, whereas a fluid-filled sinus fails to transilluminate; however, the value of this technique is questionable, as poor consistency and poor correlation with the presence of fluid has been reported.

Skin prick testing using the four most common allergens – house dust mite, cat, dog and grass pollen – may be helpful to confirm atopic status of patients giving a clear history of allergy.

Neck

The sternomastoid muscle divides the neck into the anterior and posterior triangles. The mandible lies above, and the clavicle below. The carotid artery lies in a groove between the trachea and sternomastoid muscle. There are two jugular veins: the larger internal jugular lies deep and medial to the sternomastoid muscle, while the external jugular vein is more superficial and lies lateral to the sternomastoid muscle, running diagonally across it (see Chapter 8 for further discussion). The trachea is 10–11 cm long and begins at the cricoid cartilage in the neck.

The thyroid gland consists of two lobes connected by a narrow isthmus. The isthmus lies over the second and third tracheal rings, with the lobes curving backwards between the trachea and sternomastoid muscles.

The lymphatic system of the neck is extensive, and drains the mouth, throat, face and head. Pre and posterior auricular nodes, occipital, posterior cervical, superficial cervical, deep cervical chain, submental, submandibular, tonsillar and supraclavicular nodes are all lymph nodes of the head and neck (Fig. 6.5; see also Chapter 17).

Examination technique of lymph nodes

Palpate using a systematic approach to ensure full coverage. Ensure the patient is relaxed with a slightly flexed neck. Use fingers pads, moving the skin over underlying tissue in each area, examining both sides concurrently. Note the size, consistency, mobility, whether discrete or matted together, and if tender. Normal lymph nodes are round, smooth, soft and non-tender, and are not usually palpable. If enlarged or tender nodes are present, seek the source of this abnormality, by examining the area drained by that node (Fig. 6.5). Infection often results in tender nodes; hard nodes may be present in malignancy. Check for regional lymph node involvement and general lymphadenopathy if local abnormality is found. Always review in a few weeks.

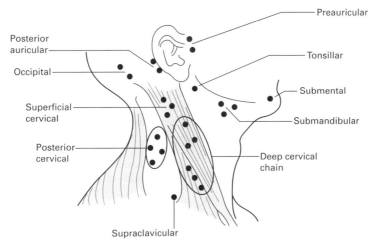

Figure 6.5 *Lymph nodes of the head and neck.*

Ear symptoms

Ear symptoms comprise otalgia, ear pressure sensation, swelling, otorrhoea, referred pain, hearing loss, disturbance of balance (dizziness, vertigo) and tinnitus.

Nasal symptoms

Nasal symptoms include obstruction, which may be anatomical, due to mucous membrane abnormality, or an autonomic abnormality that causes increased swelling and secretion. This may result in mouth breathing and snoring.

Discharge may be thin and watery, thick, purulent or mucopurulent. Dryness and crusting may occur in atrophic rhinitis. Unilateral discharge suggests the presence of a foreign body. Other symptoms are sneezing, bleeding and disturbance of the sense of smell.

Mouth and throat symptoms

Any of the structures of the mouth may be involved in local disease or may exhibit lesions as part of a systemic disorder. Certain symptoms may be features of systemic disease and should not be considered in isolation:

- dry mouth (xerostomia) may be due to drugs, emotion or salivary gland dysfunction, disease or mouth breathing, when associated with thirst may indicate diabetes
- bad taste and halitosis may be due to mouth and respiratory tract infections but often no cause is elicited
- tongue or mouth soreness may be due to haematological, allergic or systemic disease
- ulceration, lumps, red, white, or pigmented lesions should be carefully assessed to exclude malignancy
- speech quality may be affected
- infections may affect the mucosa of the whole of the nasopharynx and oropharynx or may be localised to the lymphoid tissue

- gum and teeth disorders, e.g. gingivitis and dental abscess, present as swelling, redness, easy bleeding and pain.

Common cold

The common cold is a mild, self-limiting viral syndrome involving the upper respiratory tract mucosa. Colds are the most common acute illnesses in the industrialised world. On average, adults suffer 2–4 colds per year, while children suffer 6–8 (Mossad 1998). Colds are highly contagious, transmitted by direct physical contact, from nasal mucosa to the hand to another person, or by droplets released at a cough or sneeze. The commonest cause is the rhinovirus; other viruses implicated include coronavirus and, parainfluenza, respiratory syncytial and influenza viruses.

Subjective findings

The patient will complain of variable degrees of:
- sneezing
- nasal discharge (initially clear, then thicker after 4–7 days) and blockage
- dry or sore throat
- cough and malaise
- low-grade fever
- hoarseness.

Symptoms tend to be more pronounced in smokers. Infants may present with non-specific symptoms of poor feeding, anorexia, lethargy, diarrhoea and earache. Patients may give a history of recent exposure to others with cold symptoms.

Objective findings

- Temperature – mildly elevated
- Pulse and respiratory rate – may be mildly elevated
- Tympanic membranes may be inflamed in children
- Nose – red, oedematous mucosa, clear thin discharge initially, mucoid or purulent later

- Throat – mild erythema
- Cervical lymph nodes – no lymphadenopathy
- Chest – breathing sounds normal
- Check for hydration in children

Assessment

Differential diagnosis:
- Influenza
- Allergic rhinitis
- Pharyngitis.

Plan

Diagnostics. Nil.

Management. Since colds are generally self-limiting and benign, symptomatic treatment only is recommended.

Pharmacotherapeutics. Simple analgesia may be given to relieve aches and fever, and enhance excretion of the virus. First-generation antihistamines, e.g. chlorphenamine (chlorpheniramine), reduce nasal discharge and sneezing, and their side effect of drowsiness can aid sleep (Howard et al 1979). Alpha-adrenergic agonists, e.g. xylometazoline, are potent decongestants, suitable for short-term use only, but must be used with caution in hypertensives (Mossad 1998). Intranasal anticholinergics, e.g. ipratropium, reduce sneezing and nasal drainage (Diamond et al 1995). Normal saline nose drops are useful for infants where nasal congestion inhibits feeding. Vitamin C has a modest effect on duration and severity of symptoms; large doses are most effective.

Behavioural. Steam inhalations help liquefy nasal secretions and ease discomfort (Tyrell et al 1989). Encourage fluid intake, especially in febrile children.

Patient education. Advise to wash hands after sneezing or blowing the nose, to cover the mouth during sneezing or coughing and to avoid crowds.

Advise against using nasal decongestants for more than 5 days to avoid rebound congestion. Encourage simple home remedies and self-management for future episodes.

Patient leaflets
Fighting Colds and Flu (Doctor: Patient Partnership).
Ebenezer Sneezers Guide to Colds and Flu (Consumer Health Information Centre).

Indications for referral

Rarely required. Apnoea attacks in infants.

Follow up

Advise patients to return for review if worsening symptoms or difficulty in breathing occurs. Otherwise, none is required.

Complications

- Otitis media in young children

- Infants and the elderly may be at greater risk of pneumonia
- Exacerbation of existing complaints, e.g. asthma.

Otitis externa

Definition: An inflammatory condition of the external auditory canal, which may be diffuse or local, i.e. furuncle, a tender swelling of the outer canal. Acute diffuse 'swimmers ear' is the commonest. Susceptible individuals may have recurrent attacks or chronic inflammation. Ten per cent of the population will suffer this condition at some point in their lives (Raza et al 1995). It is five times more common in swimmers, and has a 10–20-fold incidence in hot weather.

Causes may be infective or reactive. Recognition of predisposing and precipitating factors is important: trauma from scratching, ear syringing, following bathing or swimming, hot humid conditions, allergy, chronic skin disease, psychological, congenital narrow ear canals. Bacterial infection is commonly due to *Staphylococcus aureus*, occasionally *Pseudomonas*. Fungal superinfection may occur following prolonged use of topical antibiotics, in diabetics or immuno-compromised clients.

Subjective findings

- Otalgia
- Pruritus
- Severe tenderness of outer ear
- Hearing loss (if meatus obstructed)
- Discharge, which may be thick or scanty
- History of previous episodes
- Systemic illness – mild.

Objective findings

- Pinna may be inflamed
- Pain on movement of pinna
- Exquisite superficial tenderness on application of tragus pressure
- Auditory canal – erythematous, inflamed and containing moist or flaky debris
- Otorrhoea – moderate
- Furuncle may be visible as localised swelling of outer canal
- Canal may be occluded by oedema or debris in severe cases
- Tympanic membrane (eardrum) normal (though otitis media sometimes coexists) – the tympanic membrane may be difficult to visualise
- Lymphadenopathy of preauricular/postauricular nodes may be present
- No mastoid tenderness
- Fungal infection – black-topped filaments and hyphae.

Assessment

Differential diagnosis:
- foreign body

- wax
- otitis media
- perforated tympanic membrane
- folliculitis
- malignant otitis externa (rare, mainly in diabetics and immunocompromised)
- mastoiditis – pain and swelling over mastoid process, severe systemic disturbance
- chronic dermatides, e.g. eczema, psoriasis, seborrhoeic dermatitis
- cholesteatoma – foul-smelling discharge, due to eroding epithelial tissue in the middle ear/mastoid cavity
- herpes zoster – vesicles on canal, eardrum, pinna, oropharynx; may be accompanied by facial nerve palsy or deafness (Ramsey Hunt syndrome).

Plan

Diagnostics:　nil for acute episode. If recurrent or treatment failure: microbiological swab; urinalysis for glucose.

Management

Pharmacotherapeutics:　Eardrops containing antibacterial or antibiotic and steroid combination, to cure infection and reduce irritation. There is no difference in therapeutic efficacy between preparations, but a 20-fold price difference; therefore, the cheapest preparations should be selected, e.g. flumetasone/clioquinol 1%, prednisolone/neomycin, betamethasone/neomycin, gentamicin/hydrocortisone (listed in order of expense) for 7–10 days for mild cases. Aminoglycosides (neomycin, framycetin, gentamicin) and polymyxins should be avoided in tympanic membrane perforation because of possible ototoxicity. Oral antibiotics are indicated in more severe cases, with surrounding cellulitis, systemic illness, lymphadenitis, or if underlying otitis media is suspected, e.g. flucloxacillin 250 mg qds or erythromycin 250 mg qds for 5 days.

Fungal infection – topical antifungal, e.g. clotrimazole, oral itraconazole in resistant cases. Continue treatment for 2 weeks after symptom resolution.

Analgesia may be required; nonsteroidal anti-inflammatory drugs (NSAIDs) are most effective.

Aural toilet.　Dry mopping to remove debris prior to instillation of drops, or gentle syringing. This allows effective penetration of topical treatment (Raza et al 1995). In chronic cases, careful repeated cleaning and ear care advice, aiming to restore normal cerumen production. A wick inserted into the ear if the canal is very swollen allows the drops to travel to the other end of the canal: it is inserted with alligator forceps; drops are then applied into the wick, which is left in place for 3–4 days. Furunculosis is treated symptomatically with analgesia and local heat; if accompanied by severe pain it may require incision and drainage of the abscess.

Patient education.　Advice on hygeine, keeping the ear dry, avoid blocking drainage with cotton wool left in the ear, avoidance of trauma, e.g. from dirty finger nails, cotton buds.

Technique for instillation of drops: lie with the affected ear upwards, put several drops in the ear and lie in this position for 1–2 min.

Avoid water in the ears immediately following infection. For atopic dermatitis, avoid irritants, e.g. cosmetics and shampoo.

If recurrent attacks, advise to keep dry during washing by inserting cotton wool smeared with vaseline; use of silicone ear plugs for swimming.

Indications for referral

- Failure to respond to treatment
- Doubt concerning diagnosis
- Severe pain
- Possible malignant otitis externa or mastoiditis (urgent)
- Stenosis and scarring of canal
- Severe infection occluding the canal and making aural toilet impossible
- Chronic otitis externa may indicate underlying pathology.

Follow up

Only if persistent symptoms.

❶ Severe otitis externa can progress to osteomyelitis of the base of the skull and intracranial infection. This presents as severe pain out of proportion with signs. Malignant necrotising otitis externa is a deep bacterial invasion, usually with *Pseudomonas*, leading to progressive destruction of the temporal bone (Ruddy & Bickerton 1992).

❶ Risk of sensorineural deafness with topical aminoglycosides in diabetics or the immunocompromised; otitis externa can have life-threatening complications.

Acute otitis media

Definition: Inflammation of the middle ear, which becomes filled with pus and fluid, resulting in pain and bulging of the tympanic membrane. It is one of the commonest complaints in children, but occurs less frequently in adults.

Peak incidence occurs under 8 years, and two-thirds of all children will have at least one attack before age 2 (Seller 1996). It may be of bacterial or viral origin though differentiating the two is difficult. Although often attributed to bacteria such as *Haemophilus influenzae* and *Pneumococcus*, these organisms have been isolated from very few cases. Most attacks are viral in origin and self-limiting. Acute otitis media nearly always follows an upper respiratory tract infection (URTI): the eustachian tube becomes blocked as a result of negative pressure, resulting in middle ear effusion. It is now a benign condition of childhood, though in the past, when *Streptococcus* was prevalent, and poor social factors existed, complications such as mastoiditis were common. Otitis media has been one of the commonest reasons for giving antibiotics to children. However, recent evidence shows that early use of antibiotics is of only modest benefit: most children are pain-free within 24 hours, regardless of treatment. Eighty per cent of acute otitis media resolves in 2–3 days, though dullness/pinkness of the eardrum and deafness may take 2–3 weeks to clear (Del Mar et al 1997). Risk factors include season, with most cases occurring in winter, parental smoking, allergy, bottle-feeding, and craniofacial abnormality. One of the challenges of management is to identify clinical predictors of who will benefit from treatment.

Eustachian tube dysfunction may occur, especially with an URTI, causing pain particularly in children.

Perforation of the eardrum may occur, when a blood-stained mucopurulent discharge will be seen. If discharge is present, the perforation must be located, its size and position described, and a careful follow up made. Central perforations are considered 'safe', and are rarely associated with serious disease. Management is as otitis externa, with very frequent mopping, and they usually heal quickly. Chronic suppurative otitis media occurs if inflammation persists and healing fails: surgical repair may be necessary. Attic or annulus perforation in contrast is considered 'unsafe', and is associated with progressive destructive disease: it may be related to cholesteatoma. This should be referred.

Subjective findings

- Rapid onset
- History of URTI
- Pain
- Fever
- Hearing loss
- General malaise
- Loss of appetite.
- History of previous ear disease?
- Discharge if perforation.

Objective findings

- Erythematous tympanic membrane, pink, red, yellow if pus or fluid in middle ear
- May be bulging, injected, opaque, loss of landmarks
- If effusion present, tympanic membrane mobility will be reduced
- If perforated tympanic membrane: discharge in canal, profuse and mucopurulent or purulent.

Objective assessment

- Temperature, pulse, respirations
- Ear, nose, throat and chest examination.

Differential diagnosis

- Otitis externa

- Cellulitis
- Sinusitis
- Pharyngitis (causing referred ear pain)
- Eustachian tube dysfunction.

Plan

Diagnostics.   Nil.

Management: pharmacotherapeutics.   Initially analgesia, e.g. paracetamol for 12–24 hours.

- Most children require symptomatic treatment only.
- Withhold antibiotic – explain rationale.
- Persisting symptoms – amoxicillin, erythromycin.
- Perforation: no antibiotic, ear mop and review: perforation heals spontaneously. Advise to keep dry, review in 1 month.
- There is contradictory advice regarding the use of aminoglycoside drops in chronic otitis media. The Committee on Safety of Medicines warn of the danger of ototoxicity; however, antibiotic ear drops are more effective than oral preparations.

Behavioural.   Avoid allowing ear to become wet if perforated eardrum. Eustachian tube dysfunction – Valsalva manoeuvre to reinflate.

Referral

- Recurrent acute otitis media causing concern, hearing loss, speech delay
- Margin/pars flaccida perforation
- Chronic perforation
- Offensive discharge
- Mastoiditis, labyrinthitis, meningitis (rare).

Secretory otitis media (glue ear/otitis media with effusion)

Definition: The presence of fluid in the middle ear cavity for 3 months or more, behind an intact tympanic membrane without signs or symptoms of infection. This causes conductive deafness. Various theories of causation exist: anatomical, where the eustachian tube function is poor, resulting in insufficient aeration of the middle ear. This causes negative pressure in the middle ear, drawing in thick and glue-like fluid from mucosal glands. Newer theories are a microbiological causation, following infection, or part of an allergic or immunological process. In children 10–50% develop residual effusion following acute otitis media. There is a high prevalence of coexisting allergic disorders, e.g. rhinitis, asthma. Secretory otitis media is the commonest cause for childhood hearing impairment and elective surgery.

Subjective findings

Stuffy, uncomfortable ear, otalgia from retracted tympanic membrane (eardrum), conductive deafness fluctuates.

Objective findings

- Eardrum dull and retracted
- Honey-coloured or blue
- Absent light reflex
- Air bubbles or fluid levels may be seen
- Visible blood vessels on the periphery and radially
- Eardrum mobility reduced
- Tympanometry flat trace.

Plan

Watchful waiting, since 50% resolve in 3 months, and 95% within 12 months without treatment. Resolution is more likely in children over 6 years of age.

Maintenance of eustachian tube function: auto-inflation – opening of the eustachian tube by blowing up a balloon with the nose. There is a suggested benefit but few studies.

Medical management (Scadding et al 1993): treatment of allergies, steroid nasal spray, e.g. beclometasone aqueous.

Antibiotic therapy is highly controversial, and the evidence is contradictory. Although antibiotics are usually not required, children with a history of recurrent acute otitis media may benefit (Paradise 1995). If hearing loss – review 2-monthly since hearing fluctuates.

Referral

- If 3 months persistent hearing loss
- Persistent severe pain
- Speech delay, behavioural or cognitive disturbance thought to be a consequence
- Parental concern management.

Acute labyrinthitis

Acute labyrinthitis presents as vertigo (severe dizziness in which there is a sensation of gross rotational movement) of abrupt onset, occurring first thing on waking. Symptoms may be severe for 1–3 days, are minimised by keeping the head still, and provoked by any head movement. The condition is often associated with nausea and vomiting. A gradual resolution of symptoms occurs over a few weeks, although mild symptoms may still be provoked by sudden head movements for several months but will fully resolve. Older people take longer to recover from vestibular upset. Up to half of all sufferers have had an URTI or other viral infection just before the onset of symptoms; thus, labyrinthitis is regarded as a viral syndrome, with symptoms resulting from infection causing labyrinthine irritation. However, there appears to be no evidence base for this assumption.

Subjective assessment

- Severe dizziness with sensation of rotation.
- Provoked by head movement.
- Relieved by keeping head immobile.
- History of URTI or other viral infection.
- Nausea and vomiting.

Objective assessment

- Blood pressure lying and standing.
- Extraocular movements – complete range of movements, conjugacy.
- Presence of nystagmus, which may occur on forward gaze or lateral gaze only.
- Gait and Romberg sign.
- Tympanic membranes.
- Rinne and Weber tests should be normal (eliminate Meniere's disease). Hallpike manoevre/positional testing.

Plan

Diagnostics: Nil.

Pharmacotherapeutics.   May be required in the acute stage for a few days, such as labyrinthine sedatives, e.g. prochlorperazine, cinnarizine.

Behavioural.   Rest from normal activities.

Patient education.   Reassure that the condition is self-limiting in a few weeks.

Differential diagnosis

- Other causes of dizziness: cochlear symptoms?
- Meniere's disease – deafness
- Benign positional vertigo
- Loose particulate matter in semicircular canals
- Multiple sclerosis
- Cardiovascular causes
- Vascular occlusion
- Brain stem lesion.

Indications for referral

More than 6-week history.
❶ Sudden deafness

Sore throat

Definition: A common symptom seen in general practice (RCGP/OPCS 1995), which peaks around ages 5–10 and 15–25 years, and is rare in young children and the elderly. The spectrum includes pharyngitis (predominantly inflammation of the oropharynx but not the tonsils), laryngitis (few signs of visible infection but complaint of soreness lower down the throat, often with hoarse voice), with a minority acute tonsillitis (tonsils particularly inflamed). Cases occur mainly between September and May, and are spread by droplet infection from oral, nasal and respiratory secretions.

- 50% are viral infections (caused by organisms similar to the common cold)

- 20% are bacterial – group A beta-haemolytic strepto-coccus (GABHS) being the commonest
- in 30% no cause can be found: symptoms may be related to environmental factors, allergies and mouth breathing.

In immunocompromised patients, thrush, cytomega-lovirus and herpes simplex are involved. Non-infective causes of sore throat include blood dyscrasia, gastro-oesophageal reflux, allergic rhinitis, post nasal drip and mouth breathing.

Chronic sore throat may be related to the irritant effects of smoking and excessive alcohol intake; malignancy should be excluded.

Differentiating bacterial from viral infections can be difficult. A scoring system has been developed to assist (Dobbs 1996), based on symptoms, duration and clinical features. Fever, tonsillar exudate, anterior cervi-cal lymphadenopathy, odour, absence of cough, and duration of greater than 3 days are significant features. Diagnostic tests are problematic – a rapid antigen test is costly and not widely available in primary care, and throat swabs mean a 2–3 day delay before treatment decision. The use of antibiotics is questionable, though they reduce the duration of symptoms. In GABHS-positive patients only, after 1 week there is no difference in outcome between treated and untreated patients (Dagnelie et al 1996). Nevertheless, up to 95% of patients may be prescribed antibiotics. Little et al (1997) showed that prescribing antibiotics made marginal dif-ference to symptoms, but increased patient belief in antibiotics and intention to consult for future attacks. Historical reasons for treating sore throats included the prevention of rheumatic fever (now very rare), and to prevent spread of infection and epidemics. Although penicillin eradicates bacteria in 24–48 hours, no reduc-tion in spread has been demonstrated. Treatment is therefore only necessary for imminent complications and patients at risk of serious complications, e.g. quinsy.

Subjective findings

- Sore throat
- Dysphagia
- Malaise, fever
- Other manifestations of URTI – runny nose, cough.

Objective findings

- Pharynx inflamed
- Exudate
- Cervical lymphadenopathy
- Scarlatina rash in young child (streptococcal infection)
- Halitosis.

Plan

- Symptomatic – simple analgesia, fluids
- Diagnostics: usually none; glandular fever test, full blood count may be indicated. Antistreptolysin (ASO) titre – serological test for streptococcal infection

- Antibiotic if indicated – penicillin V or erythromycin, 10-day course required to eradicate streptococcus.

Referral

- Quinsy (peritonsillar abscess).
- Epiglottitis (child dysphagia, change in voice characteristic like 'plum in throat', inspiratory stridor)
- Dysphagia
- Hoarseness prolonged
- Recurrent throat infection (at least seven in pre-ceeding year) for consideration of tonsillectomy.

❶ Hoarseness more than 2 weeks (to exclude neo-plasm, nodules, polyps, vocal) epiglottitis: high fever, drooling, inspiratory stridor: hospitalise (risk of sudden fatal airway obstruction) do not examine
- dysphagia
- ulceration: consider blood dyscrasia, agranulocytosis
- unusual presentations: consider human immuno-deficiency virus (HIV)
- abscess
- otitis media
- quinsy
- systemic diseases occurring as an immunological response to beta-haemolytic streptococcus – rheu-matic fever, acute glomerulonephritis (rare).

Patient leaflet. *Antibiotics, not a miracle cure* [Doctor Patient Partnership].

Sinusitis (rhinosinusitis)

Definition: Inflammation of the mucous membrane linings of paranasal sinuses resulting in obstruction of the normal sinus mucociliary transport of secretions. It is usually caused by viruses, bacteria, allergens and irri-tants, e.g. smoke. Prolonged colds, smoking, allergies and anatomical abnormalities such as deviated septum and polyps all predispose to infection. Chronic, recur-rent attacks may occur. Poor drainage and secretion retention also occur in those with anatomical variation. Mucociliary transport is impaired by hypersecretion of mucus and inflammatory mediator release.

Symptoms occur in 0.5–5% of those suffering a common cold. It is often difficult to distinguish between a viral common cold and bacterial sinusitis, and there is evidence of overdiagnosis.

Differential diagnosis

- Bacterial
- Viral
- URTI
- Chronic allergic rhinitis.

Subjective assessment

- History of preceeding URTI
- Mucupurulent nasal discharge
- Postnasal drip

- Malaise
- Ache/pressure behind eyes
- Facial pain above/below eyes, increased on leaning forward
- Toothache-like pain
- Headache
- Congestion
- Reduced sense of smell
- Chronic sinusitis: similar but less specific
- Chronic dry cough
- Persistent laryngitis
- Foul taste
- Mucopurulent rhinorrhoea with acute exacerbations
- Headache at maximum 3–4 hours after getting up, which slowly improves.

Objective assessment

- Nasal airway reduced
- Hyperaemic mucosa
- Purulent secretions, dry forming crusts
- Polyps if prolonged inflammation
- Pale oedematous mucosa (suggests allergy)
- May be pus in middle meatus
- Turbinates inflamed, hyperaemic
- Sinus tenderness
- Fever
- Failure to transilluminate.

Plan

Diagnostics:
- Skin prick testing
- CT scan if failure of maximum medical therapy
- X-ray not helpful – mucosal thickening.

Pharmacotherapeutics:
- Aim to eradicate infection, reduce inflammation, restoration of ventilation of sinuses allowing return of normal mucociliary function.
- Analgesia.
- Topical decongestants and vasoconstrictors, e.g. xylometazoline, ephedrine, for a maximum of 1 week to relieve symptoms.
- Topical steroid may be helpful in atopic patients, e.g. beclometasone aqueous nasal spray
- Antibiotic use is controversial: Stalman et al (1997) report they have no effect if used.
  However, the SMAC guidelines (1998) advise a short course of amoxicillin or erythromycin for 3 days only.

Behavioural: Steam inhalation to relieve symptoms.

Patient education: Drops applied in the 'mecca position' for 2 min; sprays applied head down/left hand to right nostril.
- Chronic: identify predisposing factors – physiological, anatomical
- Antibiotic 2–6 week course
- Antihistamine.

Referral

Chronic sinusitis in which medical treatment fails (consider surgery)
- ❶ Periorbital swelling
- Orbital abscess
- Meningitis – rare complications requiring urgent hospital treatment.

Rhinitis including allergic rhinitis/hayfever

Definition: A symptom complex of two or more symptoms of nasal blockage, nasal discharge, sneezing and nasal itching lasting for more than 1 hour on most days (Lund et al 1994). It is a common condition and can have numerous causes. The most commonly seen condition in primary care is infective: acute – usually due to viral infection – the common cold; bacterial; allergic – the commonest of all allergic disorders affect 15–20% of the population, and accounting for 3% of all GP consultations (seasonal, perennial, occupational); structural; and others, including vasomotor, iatrogenic, hormonal (hypothyroidism). Allergic rhinitis is increasing in prevalence in developed countries despite declining pollen levels. Common allergens include grass and tree pollens, moulds (seasonal), house dust mites (perennial). Peak prevalence is in adolescence and early adulthood. Rhinitis can severely disrupt quality of life and cause impaired work and academic performance. Management guidelines are available.

Subjective assessment

The most important part of an initial assessment:
- sneezing; itching of nose, eyes and palate; rhinorrhoea
- nasal blockage, nasal discharge, postnasal catarrh
- history of exacerbating seasons, sites, factors
- age of onset
- impact on lifestyle
- presence of other atopic disorders, family history of atopy
- use of OTC products and their efficacy.

Objective assessment

- Always conduct examination of nasal passages
- Structure: septum displacement
- Turbinates – enlarged if long-standing condition, pink, purple, sensitive
- Polyps – pale, insensitive
- Mucosa – inflamed, oedematous, pale blue in allergic rhinitis
- Nature of nasal secretions (watery, clear, mucopurulent, bloody)
- Posterior rhinorhoea (post-nasal drip) may be visible
- Eyes – allergic conjunctivitis
- Chest – be aware of the coexistence of asthma (check peak expiratory flow rate (PEFR)).

Plan

Diagnostics: Skin prick testing – to identify specific causative allergens
- RAST (radioallergosorbent test) for specific immunoglobulin (IgE)
- Allergen avoidance where possible.

Pharmacotherapeutics. Follow management guidelines (British Society of Allergy and Clinical Immunology 1998) – treatment is usually highly effective: choice depends on predominant symptoms.
- oral antihistamines relieve sneezing, nasal itching, rhinorrhoea, eye symptoms. Second-generation antihistamines are preferred, e.g. cetirizine, loratadine. They are available OTC.
- nasal blockage, short-term use of decongestant, which enhances penetration of other medication; decongestant, e.g. xylometazoline, for thick nasal secretions short term only, risk rebound (rhinitis medicamentosa)
- new nasal sprays – evidence awaited: cromolyns, nedocromil
- topical steroids for moderate to severe symptoms, e.g. beclometasone aqueous nasal spray, fluticasone
- short-course oral steroid for 5 days in very severe exacerbations
- avoid depot steroid injections (Drugs and Therapeutics Bulletin 1999)
- anticholinergic, e.g. ipratropium for vasomotor
- immunotherapy – for severe seasonal allergic rhinitis not controlled by allergen avoidance/pharmacotherapy; specialist units
- structural, may need referral.

Patient education. Allergen avoidance most important:
- listen to the pollen forecast and plan the day accordingly
- avoid cutting grass, picnics, camping
- if out in the countryside, shower and wash hair on return
- wear wrap-around sunglasses when outside
- before evening (when pollen descends as air cools) bring in washing and close bedroom windows
- keep car windows closed; consider buying an air filter for the car
- avoid smoking and other irritants such as fresh paint
- avoid other allergens that affect you
- how to use nasal sprays/drops
- disease course and expected outcome.

Referral

- Structural nasal problems.
- Severe allergic rhinitis uncontrolled by pharmacotherapy: to allergy specialists for consideration of immunotherapy.
- Unilateral blockage, especially if with blood-stained discharge or facial pain or unilateral deafness.

Infectious mononucleosis ('glandular fever')

Definition: a viral syndrome caused by Epstein–Barr virus (EBV) infection. It is a disease of adolescence: peak incidence in males is 16–18 years and females between 14 and 16 years. It is commonly in higher socioeconomic groups and students.

By adulthood, most people have been infected by EBV, but young children have subclinical infection (this occurs mainly in lower socioeconomic groups). The virus has a low level of contagion; transmission is by direct intimate contact with another shedding EBV from the oropharynx (fresh secretions also genital – may be sexually transmitted). The suggested link with chronic fatigue has been disproved.

Subjective assessment

- Fever
- Severe sore throat
- Unusual presentations also common – headache, anorexia, abdominal pain, jaundice
- Prolonged course residual fatigue
- Young child fairly asymptomatic.

Objective assessment

- General appearance
- Temperature, pulse, respirations
- Exudative pharyngitis, erythematous
- Palantine petechiae
- Significant cervical lymphadenopathy
- Epitrochlear lymphadenopathy
- Hepatomegaly in 50%
- Splenomegaly in 75%.

Differential diagnosis

- Streptococcal pharyngitis
- Measles
- Viral exanthema
- Viral hepatitis
- Cytomegalovirus (CMV)
- HIV
- Leukaemia
- Thyroiditis.

Plan

Diagnostics. A laboratory test is essential as unusual presentations are common:
- full blood count (FBC) and differential: lymphocytes > 50% with atypical lymphocytes and monocytes
- glandular fever test, if symptoms suggestive; may be negative in young child, takes 7–10 days to become positive
- liver function tests.

Management. Symptomatic only.

Pharmacotherapeutic.   Usually nil. Concurrent strepto-coccal infection coexists in 26% of cases and these may require penicillin.

Behavioural.   Rest, fluids, gargles.

Patient education.   Avoid strenuous exercise or contact sport for 1 month, because of risk of splenic rupture.

Influenza

Definition: an acute contagious viral URTI spread by airborne droplets shed by those with symptoms. There are three influenza virus types: A, B and C. Most patients do not develop complications and symptoms subside within 3–5 days. However, severity tends to increase with age, and the elderly, people with chronic disease and women in the third trimester of pregnancy are particularly at risk. Influenza can have devastating morbidity and mortality, particularly in those aged over 75 with underlying medical conditions. Complications, if they occur, are mainly respiratory, i.e. otitis media, influenza pneumonitis, secondary bacterial pneumonia, exacerbations of chronic respiratory disease, croup and bronchiolitis in children; also febrile convulsions, toxic shock syndrome, Reye's syndrome, myositis and myocarditis; and neurological sequelae, e.g. Guillain–Barré syndrome, encephalitis, meningococcal infection (Wiselka 1994). Influenza can occur in unpre-dictable epidemics (defined as 400 cases per 100 000 GP consultations), the last occurring in England and Wales in 1989–90. There are periodic worldwide pandemics, occurring at intervals of 11–42 years, caused by sudden mutations in the virus, producing new antigenic strains. Weekly surveillance and reporting gives important infor-mation regarding the timing and potential impact of out-breaks to enable a public health response.

Subjective assessment

- Fever – median duration 3 days
- Malaise
- Myalgia
- Headache
- Respiratory symptoms, harsh dry cough which often persists 1–2 weeks. Airway hyperreactivity may persist for several weeks
- Clinical features are often indistinguishable from other respiratory viruses currently circulating in the community
- Sometimes prostration.

Objective assessment

- Looks unwell
- Fever, usually
- Tachypnoea
- Chest wheezes, crackles
- Clinical severity variable
- Complicated: purulent sputum, pleurisy, breathless-ness

Differential diagnosis

- Other viral infections
- Bacterial pneumonia
- Other acute infectious illness.

Plan

Diagnostics.   Nil.

Pharmacotherapeutics.   There are three types – relief of symptoms, treatment of complications and specific antiviral treatment.

Most uncomplicated cases require symptomatic treatment only: paracetamol or aspirin. Specific anti-viral agents include amantidine, an anti-influenza drug that inhibits type A strain but has little action on B or C strains or other respiratory viruses. It can be used for treatment of influenza A infection, reducing viral shedding and shortening duration of symptoms by one-third if started within 48 hours of onset. As pro-phylaxis, it is highly effective, providing protection for 50% and preventing symptoms in more than 70% of people. It is indicated for unvaccinated high-risk groups at the start of an epidemic. Zanamivir, a new antiviral, reduces the duration of illness by 1 day if started within 48 hours of onset. Because of insuffi-cient trials in high-risk groups, current guidance advises it should not be prescribed; further trials are underway (NICE 1999).

Complications.   Treatment should be considered for high-risk groups who develop symptoms during an outbreak. The British Thoracic Society recommends that an antibiotic against *Staphylococcus* should be included when there is evidence of pneumonia during influenza epidemics (Jones et al 1991).

Behavioural.   Increase fluid intake, stay at home, rest. There is a 20–40% impairment of reaction times even in a mild attack (Smith et al 1993); this has implications for those who continue to work.

Role of immunisation.   Prophylaxis for at-risk groups should be the basis of management. Immunisation is the most effective approach to preventing serious morbidity and mortality of those at highest risk. The Department of Health publishes guidelines annually. Those at most risk include people of all ages, but especially the elderly, who are at increased risk of influenza-related complications or exacerbations of their underlying disease, e.g. those with chronic respira-tory disease including asthma, chronic heart disease, chronic renal failure, diabetes and other endocrine dis-orders, immunosuppression due to disease or treat-ment, and residents of nursing homes, old peoples homes and other long-stay facilities where rapid spread is likely to follow introduction of infection. The rate of uptake in high-risk groups remains poor despite evi-dence of efficacy, which is thought to be due to poor perceptions of disease severity, concerns over vaccine

Top Tips ✓

1 There is a close interrelationship between organs of the head and neck; therefore a complete examination should include all of them

2 Many conditions are self-limiting. However, overdiagnosis and overtreatment of problems is widespread. Encourage self-management, and a 'wait and watch' policy

3 Certain groups at particular risk need more aggressive therapy

4 Use of symptom-scoring systems to best-guess diagnosis may be helpful

5 Hearing loss has major functional effects: children and the elderly may be greatly disadvantaged in daily activities

6 Allergy has an important role in many disorders

7 Distinguish lymphadenopathy as regional or generalised, and follow-up if unexplained

8 Seasonal factors may indicate causation

9 Referred pain is common; consider distant sites

10 Mouth disorders may represent systemic or local disease; beware of immunosuppression

efficacy and possible adverse effects. There are logistical difficulties in identifying and targeting high-risk groups, but it is likely that a future focus will be on improving strategies for targeting these groups.

- ❶ Elderly, pregnant, severely ill
- Respiratory distress

Patient leaflet. *What Should I Do about Flu* [Department of Health]

Glossary

Audiometry: Pure tone audiogram, which is a standard means of recording hearing level. Using headphones, each ear is tested individually for air conduction and, if necessary, bone conduction thresholds. Results are measured in decibels and plotted on a graph

Eustachian tube dysfunction Disturbance of normal ventilation of the middle ear. Obstruction causes negative pressure in middle ear. Seen as retracted eardrum and prominent landmarks

Furuncle Infected hair follicle of ear canal; presents as exquisitely tender inflamed swelling with regional lymphadenopathy

Hallpike manoeuvre Positional testing for vertigo. The patient is seated on a couch with head turned to watch the examiners's forehead. The head and body are swung backwards so that the head is below the horizontal. The eyes are watched

for 30 seconds. The test is repeated on the other side. In benign positional vertigo the manoeuvre causes violent vertigo accompanied by nystagmus; characteristically, a latent period of a few seconds, a rotatory beat towards the underlying ear, subsiding after a few seconds. Positional nystagmus lacking any of these features may be caused by brainstem or cerebellar disease

Nystagmus Repetitive involuntary eye movement to and fro, caused by vestibular dysfunction. Direction determines origin – peripheral vestibular disease causes horizontal movement, while central disease results in movement in other directions

Presbycusis Hearing loss associated with ageing; due to wear and tear of cochlear hair cells

RAST (radioallergosorbent test) for specific IgE Blood test, less accurate than skin prick test

Referred pain Pain that is felt at more distant sites that are innervated at approximately the same spinal level as the disordered structure

Skin prick test Allergen extract is introduced superficially into the skin

Tympanometry (impedance audiometry) Useful in diagnosis of middle ear disease and some types of sensorineural hearing loss. The compliance of the eardrum is measured by varying the pressure in the ear canal. It is very useful for screening for effusions and assessing eustachian tube function

Valsalva manoeuvre A technique used to examine eustachian tube function, and thus middle ear pressure. Keeping nostrils tightly pinched, an attempt is made to blow out; air enters the eustachian tube, the tympanic membrane is seen to move, and a click is often heard

Vertigo Symptoms of imbalance with hallucination of movement and rotational sensation. Not to be confused with light-headedness.

Books for patients

The NHS Home Healthcare Guide 1998 NHS Executive/ Health Education Authority

The NHS Direct Healthcare Guide 1999 and online at www.nhsdirect.nhs.uk NHS Direct/DPP 2000 Ltd

Both provide useful self-help advice and advise when medical attention should be sought

References

British Society for Allergy and Clinical Immunology 1998 Rhinitis management guidelines.

Butler C, Rollnick S, Kinnersley P, Jones A, Stott N 1998 Reducing antibiotics for respiratory tract symptoms in primary care: consolidating 'why' and considering 'how'. Br J Gen Pract 48(437):1865–1870
Summarises recent evidence for poor benefit of antibiotic and explores means to better management including better consultation skills and patient information.

Dagnelie C F, van der Graaf Y, de Melker R A, Touw-Otten F W 1996 Do patients with sore throat benefit from penicillin? A randomized double-blind placebo-controlled clinical trial with penicillin V in general practice. Br J Gen Practice 46:589–593.

Del Mar C, Glasziou P, Hayem M 1997 Are antibiotics indicated as initial treatment for children with acute otitis media? A meta-analysis. Br Med J 314:1526–1529.

Diamond L, Dockhorn R J, Grossman J et al 1995 A dose–response study of the efficacy and safety of ipratropium bromide nasal spray in the treatment of the common cold. J Allergy Clin Immunol 95:1139–1146

Dobbs F 1996 A scoring system for predicting group A streptococcal throat infection Br J Gen Practice 46:461–464.

Drugs and Therapeutics Bulletin 1999 Any place for depot triamcinolone in hay fever. Drugs and Therapeutics Bulletin 37:3 March.

Eisenthal S, Lazare A 1976 Evaluation of the initial interview in a walk-in clinic. J Nerv Mental Dis 162:169–176
Explains how patients whose expectations were discovered and addressed are more likely to accept treatment plan even if their initial expectations were not fulfilled. Could be useful to help behaviour change in reducing antibiotic prescribing.

Evans K 1994 The diagnosis and management of sinusitis. Br Med J 305:684–687.

Gonce Morton 1990 Health assessment, Nurse's clinical guide. Springhouse Corporation, Springhouse, Pennsylvania

Howard J C, Kantner T R, Lilienfield L S et al 1979 Effectiveness of antihistamines in the symptomatic management of common cold. JAMA 242:2414–2417.

Jones A, Macfarlane J, Pugh S 1991 Antibiotic therapy, clinical features and outcome of 36 adults presenting to hospital with proven influenza: do we follow guidelines? Postgrad Med J 67:988–989.

Little P, Williamson I, Warner G, Gould C, Gantley M, Kinmouth A L 1997 Open randomised trial of prescribing strategies in managing sore throats. Br Med J 314(7082):722–727.

Lund V J, Aaronson D et al 1994 International consensus report on the diagnosis and management of rhinitis. Allergy 49 (suppl 19):1–34.

Mossad S B 1998 Fortnightly review: treatment of the common cold. Br Med J 317:33–36.

National Institute for Clinical Excellence (NICE) 1999 Zanamivir (Relenza) in the management and treatment of influenza, October.

Paradise J L 1995 Treatment guidelines for otitis media: the need for breadth and flexibility. Pediatr Infect Dis J 14:429–435.

Raza S A, Denholm S W, Wong J C 1995 An audit of the management of acute otitis externa in an ENT casualty clinic. J Laryngol Otol 109:130–133.

Ruddy J, Bickerton R C 1992 Optimum management of the discharging ear (Review). Drugs 43:219–235.

Scadding G, Martin J A, Alles R, Hawk L, Darby Y 1993 Glue ear guidelines (letter; comment). Lancet 341(8836):57; January 2.

Seller R H 1996 Differential diagnosis of common complaints, 3rd edn. W B Saunders, Philadelphia

Smith A P, Thomas M, Brockman P, Kent J, Nicholson K G 1993 Effect of influenza B virus on human performance. Br Med J 306:760–761.

Stalman W, van Essen G A, van der Graff Y, de Melker R A 1997 The end of antibiotic treatment in adults with acute sinusitis-like complaints in general practice? A placebo double-blind randomised doxycycline trial. Br J Gen Practice 47:794–799.

Standing Medical Advisory Committee 1998 The path of least resistance. Department of Health, London
An important paper which examines antibiotic prescribing patterns, the issue of resistance, and makes recommendations for changing practice.

Tyrell D, Barrow I, Arthur J 1989 Local hyperthermia benefits natural and experimental colds. Br Med J 289(6683):1280–1283

Wiselka M 1994 Influenza: diagnosis, management, and prophylaxis. Br Med J 308:1341–1345.

Further reading

Baloh R W, Baringer J R 1998 Dizzy patients: the varieties of vertigo. Hospital Practice (office edition). 33(6):55–58, 61–63, 76–77; June 15.

Coley Kay 1998 ENT practice for primary care. Churchill Livingstone, Edinburgh. *A useful book written by GPs with clear advice on referral.*

Fry J, Sandler G 1993 Common diseases. Their nature, presentation and care, 5th edn. Kluwer Academic Publishers, London.

Mainous A G, Hueston W J, Clark J R 1996 Antibiotics and upper respiratory infections: do some folk think there is a cure for the common cold? J Family Practice 42:357–361.

Scully C (ed.) 2000 The ABC of oral health. BMJ Books, London.

Souhami R L, Moxham J (eds) 1990 Textbook of medicine. Churchill Livingstone, Edinburgh, pp. 883–884.

RESPIRATORY SYSTEM

Linda Pearce

- Respiratory disease is one of the most common reasons for people to attend their general practice and accounts for a large number of consultations in primary and secondary care. In any year approximately 30% of the population will consult their GP at least once with a respiratory problem

- Respiratory conditions account for the single largest cause of certified absence from work, with infections being the most common reason

- For children, 1 in 3 consultations will be as a result of respiratory problems

- Asthma is the most common chronic disease amongst children and young adults (Russell & Helms 1997)

- Studies also suggest that chronic obstructive pulmonary disease is underdiagnosed in general practice, and that the incidences of occupational lung disease are likely to be underestimated. In the last decade there has been a significant increase in the number of people consulting their GP with respiratory problems (The Lung Report II 2000)

- General principles of care include comprehensive history taking and accurate assessment to ensure accurate diagnosis and appropriate referral for further investigation

Introduction

The assessment of the respiratory system constitutes a critical aspect of any health assessment.

The function of the respiratory system is primarily to maintain the exchange of oxygen and carbon dioxide in the lungs and tissues and regulate the acid–base balance. Therefore any change in this system will affect and may present in other systems in the body.

This chapter outlines the normal physiological processes in the respiratory system, describes in detail the history taking and examination of the system, and then describes the presentation and clinical findings specific to respiratory disorders.

Ventilation and perfusion in the lungs

The normal lung

In the normal lung, ventilation and perfusion are perfectly matched. During activities such as exercise, ventilation may increase up to 20-fold and perfusion in the lungs by up to 6-fold. Exercise capacity is not limited by the healthy lung, but rather by the rate at which oxygen can be delivered to the tissues. Cardiac output may increase to accelerate delivery of oxygen to the tissues.

The abnormal lung

Where ventilation, perfusion or both are compromised, the supply of oxygen to the tissues may be reduced. Ventilation/perfusion mismatches may result in blood from the pulmonary circulation passing, without being oxygenated, into the systemic circulation. As a result, a reduced level of oxygen will reach the tissues. Where the level of oxygen reaching the tissues is inadequate to cope with the demand, systemic signs of oxygen insufficiency may develop.

Abnormalities of ventilation

Diseases causing obstruction of the airways may cause a fall in the ventilation side of the ventilation/perfusion equation. For example, the narrowing of the small airways through bronchoconstriction and inflammation in uncontrolled asthma, even when partially compensated for by an increased rate of ventilation, may result in a reduced volume of air reaching the alveoli.

Other diseases causing obstruction of the airways may also reduce ventilation. These include chronic obstructive bronchitis and bronchiectasis, where damage to the airways themselves causes obstruction. Such damage leading to obstruction is, in general, irreversible.

Abnormalities of perfusion

Obstructive disorders may also cause abnormalities of perfusion. For example, emphysema, a major feature in many patients with chronic obstructive pulmonary disease (COPD) involves the destruction of the normal alveolar architecture. This destruction reduces the area available for gas exchange. Such damage is irreversible and often progressive.

The mechanics of respiration

Expansion and contraction of the muscles of respiration produce pressure differences between the outside environment and the lungs, allowing the movement of air in and out of the respiratory system.

During inspiration, the diaphragm contracts and descends, and the intercostal muscles contract causing the development of intrapulmonary negative pressure. Because of the adherence of the pleural surfaces, the negative pressure is transferred to the alveoli and air is drawn into the lungs.

During expiration, the diaphragm and the intercostal muscles relax. The volume of the chest cavity falls and a positive intrapulmonary pressure is created, forcing air out of the lungs.

Where respiration demands greater effort than can be produced by the diaphragm and intercostal muscles, the accessory muscles of respiration may be brought into use.

Assessment of the patient

Subjective assessment

Assessment of the patient consists of history taking followed by examination.

History taking

A careful, detailed history is essential for establishing the correct diagnosis. It is often said, with justification, that if you listen to the patient they will tell you the diagnosis.

Before commencing, it is necessary to assess quickly the person for any signs of respiratory distress, such as inability to talk, restlessness or laboured breathing, which may require immediate attention.

General history should include details of:
- past medical history – especially respiratory or cardiac disease
- drug history – this must include prescribed and over-the-counter (OTC) medicines as well as complimentary medicines and self-administered drugs
- smoking history – past and present including passive exposure
- family history
- social history – including hobbies, pets and home environment
- psychosocial factors
- occupation – present and past.

Symptoms

Specific respiratory symptoms can be categorised as:
- breathlessness (including wheeze)
- cough (including sputum and haemoptysis)
- chest pain
- other symptoms of lung disease.

Each of this group of symptoms should be the subject of detailed enquiry. It should be remembered that respiratory symptoms may be indicative of disease of that system or may be markers of diseases of other systems. Presenting symptoms will vary according to the pathophysiology.

Breathlessness

It is necessary to establish what the patient means by breathlessness. Patients must then be asked about the details of their breathlessness. The questions need to be specific to the lifestyle of the individual patient. The responses should be compared with those that would be expected from a healthy person of the same age and sex.

Duration. When were they last completely well? When did the breathlessness start? How rapidly did it develop: for example, in minutes, hours, days, weeks, months or years? Is it still progressing?

Severity. Does it limit their ability to carry out normal day-to-day activities or exercise? If so, to what degree? Can they climb stairs? Can they go shopping? Can they carry their shopping home? Does it affect their sleep? How do they sleep, propped up with pillows or in a chair?

Variability. Is the breathlessness a constant feature of their lives both day and night? Is it worse at certain times or in certain seasons? Is it worse at work or soon afterwards? Does it occur at rest? Are they aware of any precipitating factors, such as specific environments, eating certain foods or exposure to specific trigger factors? Are they aware of precipitating events such as stress or exercise? Is it affected by eating or posture? Are they aware of anything that improves their breathlessness, such as temperature changes or medication?

Associated symptoms. Are they aware of any symptoms that are associated with their breathlessness, such as tingling of the fingers, noisy breathing, wheezing, faintness, fatigue, general muscle pain or headache?

Cough

Patients must be asked about their awareness of a cough. It may be thought that cough is regarded as a normal part of their lifestyle: for example, with smokers or with certain industrial environments.

Duration. When did the cough develop? How has it progressed?

Severity. What impact does the cough have on their lifestyle? Does it wake them at night or stop them sleeping? Does it hurt to cough?

Type of cough. Is it a tickly cough? Does it feel as though the cough comes from the back of the throat or deep in the chest?

Variability. Is the cough persistent through the day and/or the night? Does it occur in the early morning? Is it nocturnal? Do specific factors, positions or events trigger it?

Sputum. Is the cough productive? When is sputum produced? What colour is it and is the colour constant? Has there ever been black or bloody sputum? Have they ever coughed up fresh or altered blood? How much sputum is produced over a 24-hour period (useful descriptive terms are teaspoon/tablespoon/egg cup/teacup)? Has it increased in volume or purulence recently? How often does it do this? (i.e. number of times a year). Does it usually require a course of antibiotics to clear? Does the patient feel unwell when this occurs?

Chest pain

Chest pain may be associated with respiratory and cardiac disease as well as other disorders. The lungs themselves do not have pain receptors, so many serious respiratory diseases may not present with pain. Chest pain may be associated with pleural disease, musculoskeletal disease, pressure on other organs or infiltration of lung disease into other areas. It may also be a cardinal sign of cardiac disease. The patient must be asked to describe the pain as carefully and completely as possible.

Duration. When did the pain start? How sudden was the onset? Is it getting worse or better?

Severity. How bad is the pain? What does it stop them doing? Does it affect their daytime activities or sleep? Does the severity vary? Is it associated with any other symptoms, i.e. breathlessness, palpitations?

Variability. Is the pain constant? Does anything cause the pain? What makes the pain worse: for example, moving, breathing or coughing? Is it affected by posture? What makes the pain better or eases it?

Site of pain. Is the pain localised to one part of the chest or is it generalised? Where is it worse? Does it radiate to other parts of the chest or body?

Type of pain. What is the pain like? Is it sharp? Is it heavy or crushing? Is it burning or sore? Is it stabbing? Is there any area of tenderness over the chest wall?

Other symptoms of lung disease

Enquiry may elicit general symptoms or symptoms localised to other parts of the body that may be indications of disease in the respiratory system. Examples of these are:

- fevers – these may be associated with infections such as community-acquired pneumonia, pulmonary embolism, tuberculosis or sarcoidosis
- hoarseness – this may indicate either local disease, psychological disease, side effects of medication or secondary effects of lung disease

- neurological symptoms – these may indicate the presence of secondary effects of respiratory disease such as lung cancer, local neurological pressure with referred symptoms or may be secondary to hypoxia
- muscle pain and weakness – this may be secondary to respiratory insufficiency, such as is found in COPD, or may be because of debility due to malignant or other chronic disease
- bone pain – this may be due to an associated neuromuscular disorder or associated with secondary spread of malignant disease
- weight loss with or without anorexia – these may be associated with many respiratory diseases
- psychological disorders – conditions such as depression and anxiety may impact upon respiratory disease and affect response to treatment.

General approach and techniques of examination

Objective assessment

Examination should at all times be respectful and gentle. To gain experience in examination, it will be necessary to practice techniques in the normal chest.

An appropriate format for the examination is:
- inspection
- palpation
- percussion
- auscultation.

These should be carried out separately for the anterior and posterior chest.

Examination of the chest

The anterior thorax and lungs are best examined in a supine position. This position has an added advantage in women, as the breasts are less likely to be in the way. The posterior thorax and lungs may be examined with the patient in the sitting position. The patient's arms should be folded across her chest with her hands resting on the opposite shoulders. This helps to ensure the scapulae are moved partly out of the way, increasing access to the lung fields.

If appropriate and more comfortable for the patient, both the posterior and the anterior chest may be examined in the sitting or standing position.

If the person is unable to sit up, even with aid, to examine the posterior thorax it will be necessary to roll her to one side and then to the other, carrying out all parts of the examination of each part of the chest in each position.

Inspection

General observation

The following should be observed and noted:
- scars, especially those which may relate to operations carried out on the respiratory system

- other lesions of the chest wall, such as swellings and tumours
- the condition and colour of the skin
- the presence of venous congestion.

Shape

The general shape of the chest should be noted. In a normal adult, the ratio of anteroposterior to lateral diameter is 1:2. This ratio is 1:1 in children and the elderly. The presence of structural deformities or abnormalities should be noted. The presence of a barrel-shaped chest may indicate chronic hyperinflation; this may be as a result of reversible or irreversible obstructive disease. The chest may be funnel-shaped, keel-shaped or Harrison's sulcus (a horizontal indrawing of the lower ribs) may be present. These may signify obstructive disease which was present during the development of the chest in infancy and childhood.

Other abnormalities of the shape of the chest may be congenital features, or may be associated with abnormalities of the spine such as kyphosis and scoliosis.

Movement on respiration

- The patient should be discretely observed from the front while breathing quietly.
- The rate, pattern and distribution of movement of the chest wall should be observed carefully as important diagnostic indicators may be noted.
- Did undressing cause the patient to become breathless?
- Is breathing deep or shallow?
- Do both sides of the chest move evenly?
- Is respiration obviously restricted by pain?
- Is the rate pattern and ease of respiration affected by changes in position?
- Is the patient using accessory muscles of respiration (sternocleidomastoid, scalenus, trapezius and alae nasae muscles), or using the arms to support the chest while breathing?
- Intercostal recession may also be noted.

The posterior chest is examined in the same way.

Palpation

Palpation of the thorax may reveal abnormalities of the skin and underlying structures, asymmetry and also areas of localised or generalised tenderness. It may also be used to further assess respiratory excursion.

Trachea

The trachea should lie in the midline. To assess its position, place the tips of the index and middle fingers at the suprasternal notch, gently move them upwards and separate them until they lie on each side of the trachea where it emerges from the thorax. They should be equidistant from the midline.

Chest

The palpation should, as with all examinations, take place in a structured way to avoid omitting any part of the thorax. It may be carried out with the fingers or with the palmar areas as appropriate for the particular part.

For the anterior chest the palpation should commerce in the supraclavicular region, progressing to the infra-clavicular, sternal, rib and axillary areas. The posterior chest is then examined in a similar way, commencing in the supraclavicular region, progressing to the supras-capular and infrascapular regions, then to the lateral wall of the thorax.

The depth and symmetry of respiratory movements may be noted by spreading the hands over the posterior chest wall so that the thumbs touch in the midline over the spine and the fingers spread towards the lateral walls of the thorax. As the patient breathes in and out, any inequalities in movement of the two sides of the chest wall will be apparent by the relative movement of the thumbs away from and towards the midline. Asking the patient to take deep breaths may highlight differences.

Structural abnormalities or asymmetries may be further noted, as should the presence and location of swellings, which may not always be apparent on observation. If there are any areas of tenderness, their location and extent, as well as their association with respiration or movement, should be noted.

The sensation of crackling under the fingers on palpating the chest wall (surgical emphysema) should be noted.

Tactile vocal fremitus can help assess the various conditions of the underlying lung and pleura. The flat of the hand is placed on the part of the chest to be assessed and the patient is asked to make a noise (usually the words 'ninety-nine' or 'one hundred and one'). A vibration (fremitus) may be felt through the chest wall. If the vibration if difficult to feel, the patient may be asked to speak more loudly. Where there is obstruction to the passage of vibrations, the fremitus is reduced.

Percussion

The purpose of percussion is to set up a vibration which is audible. It is used to help assess areas of varying density within the lungs. The presence of fluids, solids and air will produce different resonances.

The middle finger of the non-dominant hand is placed on the chest wall, with the distal interphalangeal joint firmly pressed against the chest; the finger should be extended at this joint. The tip of the middle finger of the dominant hand is then brought sharply down on the distal interphalangeal joint. The movement of the percussing hand should be from the wrist, and the percussing finger should be in contact with the distal interphalangeal joint for as short a time as possible to avoid damping the vibration.

The clavicles are percussed directly with the percussing finger. The percussion should then proceed down the anterior, posterior and lateral chest (Figs 7.1 and 7.2).

Normal areas of dullness over the liver and heart should be noted.

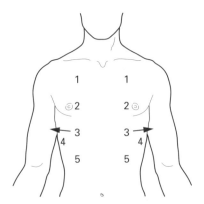

Figure 7.1 *Sites for routine percussion and auscultation (anterior).*

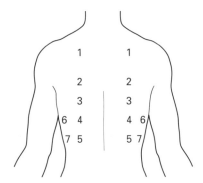

Figure 7.2 *Approximate sites for routine percussion (posterior).*

When percussing, it is especially important to compare one side with the other. Each percussion note should be evaluated for resonance and be noted as resonant, hyper-resonant, dull or stony dull. The presence of morbid obesity makes percussion more difficult.

Auscultation

Auscultation is the evaluation of breath sounds with or without the aid of a device such as a stethoscope. The stethoscope amplifies breath sounds; these may be listened to through the bell (better for low-frequency sounds) or diaphragm (better for high-frequency sounds). The bell may produce better results in the very thin or those with hairy chests. The two sides of the chest should be directly compared, at each position of auscultation.

The patient should be asked to breathe in and out through the open mouth to reduce added sounds from the oral cavity.

The patient's breathing should be evaluated. In the healthy person, breath sounds should not be audible to the naked ear. If there is an element of obstruction, breath sounds may be audible.

The examination should begin on the anterior chest at the upper lobes and move down over the chest wall. The examination should be at least 1 inch from the midline to exclude the sounds transmitted from the central airways. One full inspiration and expiration should be evaluated in each position. The examination should proceed from the anterior to the posterior chest, again progressing from the upper to the lower lobes.

The presence and timing of normal and added sounds should be noted. Normal sounds increase throughout inspiration, fading away quickly during expiration. Turbulent airflow in the central airways produces the tracheal and bronchial sounds and the vesicular breath sounds occur somewhere between the trachea and the alveoli. Tracheal and bronchial breath sounds are not transmitted well through air-filled lungs; therefore, vesicular breath sounds predominate in the normal lung.

The different sounds may be described as:
1. Crepitations – fine crackles that are produced by small airways popping open during inspiration or the passage of air through areas of secretion. They may be caused by inflammation or small amounts of fluid in the airways and, depending on the cause, may be heard at any time during respiration.

   Early inspiratory crackles are often fewer in number and much coarser: causes include asthma and chronic bronchitis.

   Late inspiratory crackles may begin in the early phase of inspiration and continue into late inspiration. Usually they first appear at the base of the lungs and spread as the condition worsens. Causes include fibrosis, pneumonia and left ventricular failure.
2. Rales – coarse crackles that are caused by fluid in the airways and, depending on the cause, may be heard at any time during respiration.
3. Rhonchi – wheezing that are caused by narrowing of the airways; they may be of varying intensity and volume and, depending on the cause, may be heard at any time during respiration.

   Generalised continuous sounds are associated with asthma, chronic bronchitis and congestive cardiac failure. In chronic bronchitis, the wheeze often clears after coughing. In asthma, the wheeze is more commonly heard on inspiration but may occur in both phases of the respiratory cycle.

   A persistent localised wheeze would suggest partial obstruction of the bronchus, caused either by a foreign body or a tumour.
4. Pleural rub – normal pleura move soundlessly; creaking or grating noises throughout the respiratory cycle (occasionally only during inspiration) may indicate pleural inflammation or infection.
5. Stridor – a wheeze that occurs predominately or completely during the inspiratory cycle; it tends to be louder in the neck than over the chest wall. Stridor is significant of major obstruction of the trachea or large airways.

The absence of breath sounds either locally or generally may be important markers of chest disease.

Cyanosis

Central cyanosis is recognised if the tongue, lips and nails are a blue discoloration. Common causes include acute severe asthma, severe pneumonia, pulmonary embolus, left ventricular failure, chronic airflow obstruction and pulmonary fibrosis.

Peripheral cyanosis may be observed in the nailbeds only or generally in the hands and feet. Common causes include cold weather and peripheral vascular disease. The identification of cyanosis by observation may often be difficult, especially in artificial light.

Expiratory lip pursing

If the patient purses their lips on expiration it may be a sign of severe airflow obstruction, most commonly seen in severe COPD and emphysema.

Nasal flaring (use of the alae nasae muscles)

This may be associated with the use of other accessory muscles of respiration in respiratory distress.

Clubbing

The pathogenesis of finger clubbing is unknown and a large number of conditions are associated with it. Signs of clubbing are a loss of the angle between the nail and the nailbed with an increase in the curvature of the nails. The nailbed becomes spongy and the ends of the finger become bulbous.

Clubbing may be congenital. Respiratory causes of clubbing include bronchial carcinoma, fibrosing alveolitis and chronic pulmonary sepsis.

Superior vena caval obstruction (SVCO)

Signs of SVCO are engorged non-pulsatile jugular veins, dilated veins on the anterior chest wall and, depending on severity, oedema of the face, neck and conjunctiva. The cause is usually bronchial carcinoma, with the collateral circulation bypassing the obstruction using the azygos and intercostal systems to return blood to the heart.

The lymphatic system

This should be examined for enlarged glands, which may be indicators of secondary disease from primary respiratory causes. Enlarged glands in the supraclavicular fossa may be associated with bronchial carcinoma, tuberculosis, sarcoidosis or lymphoma.

Specific disorders of the respiratory system

If there is ever a doubt about the diagnosis, or concern regarding non-responsiveness to appropriate therapy, referral to a consultant respiratory physician should always be considered.

Asthma

Definition. Definitions have changed over the past 50 years. Recently, there has been a broad consensus regarding an appropriate definition, and the British Thoracic Society guidelines published in 1993 gave the following description:

> *Asthma is a common and chronic inflammatory condition of the airways whose cause is not fully understood. As a result of inflammation the airways are hyper-responsive and they narrow easily in response to a wide range of stimuli. Narrowing of the airways is usually reversible, but in some patients with chronic asthma the inflammation may lead to irreversible airflow obstruction.*

The disease may vary either spontaneously or in response to treatment.

The prevalence of asthma is thought to have doubled in the UK over the past 10 years and current estimates are about 10% for adults and 20% for children.

Subjective findings

Although asthma most commonly presents for the first time in childhood it may start at any age. Frequently, there is a family history of asthma or other atopic disease. In late-onset asthma there is less of an association with atopy.

Frequently, there is a history of reaction to specific triggers, such as pets (cat dander being the most common), house dust mite, grasses and pollens. In childhood the disease is often triggered by upper respiratory tract infections. Other trigger factors may include drugs (such as beta-blockers, aspirin or nonsteroidal anti-inflammatory drugs (NSAIDs), cigarette smoke, exercise and food. This list is not exclusive and careful enquiry should be for specific trigger factors. Careful enquiry should be made into the possibility of occupational asthma.

Asthma is frequently worse at night or when exposed to specific triggers; therefore, presenting signs may be absent when the patient is seen in the clinic. Accordingly, a comprehensive history will help the health professional make a diagnosis.

Symptoms

Symptoms are usually intermittent, and may consist of episodic breathlessness, wheeze, recurrent or paroxysmal cough. This breathlessness, cough and/or wheezing may be clearly identified by the patient as being triggered by a particular event or factor. The patient may complain of chest tightness, and commonly there is a strong element of anxiety in the patient and her carers.

Objective findings

Because of the intermittent nature of the disease, there may be no clinical signs when the patient is reviewed in clinic or the patient may present with breathlessness, coughing and/or wheezing. When wheezing is present it is generalised; in children crackles may also be heard.

Severe asthma presents with the following signs: tachycardia, tachypneoa, wheeze, chest tightness and pain; the patient may be too breathless to complete whole sentences. In some cases wheezing may be heard without the aid of a stethoscope. In the most severe attacks extreme breathlessness, drowsiness, cyanosis and silent chest may be present.

Where the disease has been present from childhood, chest deformities associated with asthma, such as Harrison's sulcus, may be present.

Plan and investigations

Every step should be taken to identify likely triggers.

As airflow obstruction is variable, serial peak flow readings can be charted to give a clear picture of peak flow variability. It is usual to record morning and evening peak flows for a minimum of 2 weeks. Classically, patients with untreated asthma show diurnal variation, with a fall in peak flow in the morning. Falls in peak flow may also be seen following exercise.

Reversibility testing

The diagnosis may be supported by reversibility testing to either bronchodilators or corticosteroids.

β_2-agonist reversibility. A record is made of the best of three peak flow manoeuvres and the patient is given 200–400 g of β_2-agonist. Repeat peak flow 15 min later and record variability. Increase in peak flow of 15% or more is supportive of a diagnosis of asthma.

Corticosteroid reversibility. A short course (2 weeks) of 30–40 mg of prednisolone is given to the patient. Serial peak flow is measured and the response assessed. This test may also be carried out with high-dose inhaled steroids (800 μg/day) given for a period of 6 weeks.

Exercise tolerance test. The patient is asked to exercise for 6 minutes either by free running or treadmill test, and peak flow before and 10 minutes afterwards is measured. A fall in peak flow of 15% or greater is supportive of a diagnosis of exercise-induced asthma.

In the hospital environment bronchial provocation or challenge tests may also be carried out with inhaled histamine or methacholine.

The chest X-ray is usually normal between acute attacks and is of little diagnostic value unless the asthma is prolonged or severe. However, it may be performed to exclude other causes of wheezing or coughing, such as pneumonia, an inhaled foreign body, malignancy or alveolitis. In long-standing disease, signs of hyper-inflation may be present.

If there is doubt in the differential diagnosis, full lung function testing, including gas transfer factor and flow volume loop, may be helpful.

Management of chronic asthma

The avoidance of specific trigger factors should be advised. Skin prick testing may be carried out as a guide to allergen avoidance, and may also provide supportive evidence to convince the patient of the importance of removing certain triggers from their environment.

Tobacco smoke is a potent trigger of asthma, and active and passive exposure should be strongly discouraged.

Associated conditions which are known to have an influence on asthma, for example allergic rhinitis, should be appropriately managed (see Chapter 6).

For many patients whose asthma is stable, daily monitoring of peak flow is generally unnecessary. However, for those whose disease is more variable or brittle, a regular record of their lung function may provide a useful guide both to the patient and the health professional as to the appropriate management of their condition.

In many patients monitoring of symptoms may be a more useful way of monitoring their asthma, although the relationship between symptoms and lung function is not well established.

Therapeutic intervention

■ Treatment should follow the British guidelines on asthma management (British Thoracic Society 1993).

■ Occasional or intermittent symptoms may be managed with an inhaled β_2-agonist prescribed for use as required.

■ However, for all but the patients with very mild asthma, routine prophylactic therapy should be prescribed, usually in the form of inhaled corticosteroids, although NSAIDs such as sodium cromoglicate or nedocromil may be used.

■ Patients who remain symptomatic may be managed with an increased dose of inhaled steroid, or a long-acting β_2-agonist may be added to their low-dose inhaled steroid.

■ Other therapies that may be sequentially added include leukotriene antagonists, oral β_1-agonists, theophyllines and, for the most severe and unresponsive cases, oral steroids.

❶ Management of acute severe asthma

Immediate management should include careful assessment of the severity of the attack, administration of oral or injectable steroids, high-dose β_2-agonists and anti-cholinergic agent delivered via a metered dose inhaler (MDI) and large-volume spacer or by nebuliser, and oxygen. Administration of oxygen is important and may be life-saving, as many patients will be hypoxic. The choice between oral or injectable steroids should depend upon the ability of the patient to take the treatment, as there is no difference in time taken for the drug to have an effect.

The patient should be monitored until recovery is observed. Where peak flow is below 50% predicted, or remains below 60% predicted after treatment, the patient should be admitted to hospital. It is generally advisable for a course of oral steroids to be given for 10 days after such an attack.

Following the acute episode, asthma management should be reviewed.

Patients who are high risk or who have had a previous admission should be placed on a register in order that they can be more rapidly identified in future emergencies. This register may include those with brittle asthma, history of acute severe attacks, history of oral steroid courses and patients who are at risk for other reasons, e.g. pregnancy.

Inhaler devices

There are a variety of inhaler devices available with a variety of drugs. It is important that an appropriate device is selected for the individual patient (Pearce 1998). Most inhaler devices deliver between 10 and 30% of the drug into the lungs; the rest is deposited in the oral cavity and swallowed.

In the UK the MDI is the most commonly prescribed device; however, there is good evidence that many patients are unable to use an unadapted MDI effectively.

For infants and small children, inhaled medication should be delivered via an MDI, spacer device and mask. Children of about 3–6 years should use an MDI and large-volume spacer device. Over this age, medication may be delivered via an MDI and large-volume spacer device, breath-actuated MDI or a dry powder inhaler.

Spacer devices reduce the amount of drug that is swallowed and will reduce the potential for systemic absorption. They may also increase the amount deposited in the lungs by removing the need for coordinating actuation and inspiration, and give the patient time to inhale the dose, which may be taken from the device by tidal breathing.

Breath-actuated MDIs are triggered by the negative pressure of the patient's inspiration and then deliver a dose of medication. They remove the need for the coordination of inspiration and device actuation, which is frequently a cause for the failure to deliver effective doses of medication with MDIs.

Dry powder inhalers are breath-operated. As the patient inhales, the drug is drawn out of the device. As the drug is drawn out of the device, it is disaggregated, producing a respirable fraction.

The choice of a particular device should be made according to the ability and willingness of the patient to use the device, and the medication available in that device. With dry powder inhalers, the ability of a patient to use a particular device may be assessed by using a variable resistance inspiratory flow meter (Pearce 1999).

In the adolescent it may be important that the selected device has 'street cred' among the patient's peers.

Nebulisers should be reserved for those few patients who are unable to use another form of inhaler device.

Patient education

Education, while important, will not alone improve compliance. Where appropriate, patients should be educated in allergy and trigger factor avoidance, and encouraged to avoid both active and passive tobacco smoke.

The patient must be taught how to recognise when their asthma is deteriorating, and what steps should be taken to manage these events. They should be encouraged to lead normal lives uninhibited by their asthma. They may be encouraged by examples of the many people with asthma who have excelled in their chosen sporting activities, even to international level.

The patient's general environment and social circumstances must be evaluated, as psychosocial factors are implicated in many cases of poorly controlled or even fatal asthma.

Referral

Referral is indicated where there is doubt about the diagnosis, where there is suspected occupational asthma or where asthma is interfering with the patient's lifestyle despite treatment changes.

Other indications for referral include brittle asthma, pregnant women whose asthma is poorly controlled, patients with uncontrolled asthma in spite of high-dose inhaled steroids and patients who are being considered for long-term nebulised bronchodilators or oral steroids.

Complications

Uncontrolled asthma will lead to exacerbations, with a corresponding effect on the health and lifestyle of the patient.

The main complication, apart from death, which is uncommon, is the development of COPD. This follows airway remodelling from poorly controlled asthma.

In children, chest deformities may develop as a result of inadequate or inappropriate treatment.

Prognosis

The prognosis for the majority of patients with asthma is excellent providing that there is appropriate and adequate treatment.

Where psychosocial factors play a major part in poorly controlled asthma, the prognosis may be unfavourable.

Chronic obstructive pulmonary disease

Definition: COPD is defined as a chronic slowly progressive disorder characterised by airways obstruction (FEV_1 < 80% predicted and FEV_1/FVC ratio < 70%) that does not change markedly over several months. The impairment of lung function is largely fixed but is partially reversible by bronchodilator or other therapy (British Thoracic Society 1997b).

COPD encompasses several previously used disease labels: in particular, chronic obstructive bronchitis and emphysema, which both have chronic airflow obstruction with little or no reversibility. Usually the two conditions coexist within COPD, but may occasionally be seen separately.

Chronic obstructive bronchitis is defined as a chronic, product cough present for at least 3 consecutive months of the year for at least the last 2 years, associated with airflow obstruction.

Emphysema is characterised by destruction of the alveolar wall, causing enlargement of the air spaces in the lungs.

Subjective findings

History

Cigarette smoking is the single most important factor in the causation of COPD. Certain occupations such as coal mining, which may be related to parenchymal lung disease, are also associated with COPD.

Enquiries should be made into family history of respiratory disease – there has been some suggestion that a family history of asthma may predispose towards the development of COPD, and a deficiency of α_1-antitrypsin increases the risk of developing emphysema.

Symptoms

Patients with mild COPD may have few or no symptoms. As the disease progresses, there is usually a history of chronic cough with mucoid sputum, usually in the early morning. The mucus may become discoloured (yellow/green) during infective exacerbations. The patient may complain of a gradual increase in breathlessness on exertion (usually developing over years). There may be recurrent exacerbations of acute bronchitis during the winter months.

In the most severe cases the breathlessness is such as to be completely disabling, restricting the patient to a bed or chair, and even requiring oxygen at rest and during sleep.

Objective assessment

In mild and even moderate cases there may be few clinical signs. In some moderate cases rhonchi may be heard on auscultation. Hyperinflation may also be apparent.

In patients with severe COPD, chronic hyperinflation will be obvious. Rhonchi will be heard except in cases where air entry is so poor that the breath sounds are reduced. Signs of pulmonary hypertension (raised jugular venous pressure (JVP), right ventricular heave, peripheral oedema) may also be present. In the most severe cases cyanosis may be present.

❶ During exacerbations, rales as well as rhonchi may be heard throughout the lung fields, and signs of high arterial CO_2 levels may be seen.

Table 7.1 *Diagnosis of COPD (From British Thoracic Society 1997b)*

COPD staging	FEV_1 % predicted
Mild	60–80%
Moderate	40–60%
Severe	<40%

Investigations and plan

Investigations should be carried out to establish and confirm the diagnosis, and to exclude cardiac or other respiratory diseases.

Spirometry

The diagnosis of COPD follows spirometric tests. The FEV_1 is used to grade the disease (British Thoracic Society 1997b; Table 7.1). The FEV_1/FVC ratio is reduced and is generally below 70%.

Gas transfer studies will help evaluate lung function. The carbon monoxide gas transfer factor will be reduced with severe emphysema. Total lung capacity is increased for emphysema and the residual volume will be increased both in chronic obstructive bronchitis and emphysema.

Peak flow measurements provide a poor diagnostic aid for COPD.

Chest X-ray

- Mild COPD – chest X-ray may be normal
- Moderate and severe COPD – hyperinflation may be apparent; emphysematous bullae may be seen.

The chest X-ray is of importance in helping to exclude lung cancer, which is more common in patients with COPD.

Bronchodilator reversibility

Although a degree of FEV_1 reversibility may be found on testing (as for asthma), this should be less than a 200 ml or 15% improvement on the pre-test value. Reversibility testing may be carried out with both β_2-agonists and anticholinergic agents. A degree of bronchodilator reversibility may be seen, but this will be less than with asthma.

Corticosteroid reversibility

Reversibility may be carried out as for asthma, with the same criteria for FEV_1 improvement as with bronchodilators. A response may support the use of regular inhaled steroids in the management of the individual.

Blood tests

Anaemia should be excluded. There may be a degree of polycythaemia. Where there is a family history of chronic lung disease or investigations confirm the presence of emphysema under the age of 40 years, α_1-antitrypsin should be measured.

Blood gas analysis may be useful in exacerbations and late-stage disease to assess for short- or long-term oxygen use.

Computed tomography (CT) scan

This may be useful to assess the extent of emphysema, especially if the presence of bullae are suspected, or the patient is being considered for lung transplantation or lung reduction surgery.

Sputum

Sputum culture during exacerbations may be of help in identifying pathogens.

Management

- Stop smoking: this is the single most important intervention.
- Pulmonary rehabilitation covers a number of activities designed to help the patient manage their disease and prevent deconditioning. It involves an educational as well as an exercise programme and may be tailored to the individual need or circumstance.
- The patient should be encouraged to maintain daily activity and exercise capacity; pulmonary rehabilitation programmes will include exercise modules that may help improve the patient's quality of life.
- Weight reduction if necessary should be encouraged, as it will help improve the patient's ability to exercise.
- Annual influenza immunisation and 10-yearly pneumococcal vaccination should be encouraged.

Management of perception of breathlessness

There is often an increase in anxiety or depression with such a chronic deteriorating, usually self-inflicted condition, and therefore psychological support may be of benefit. Arrangements for social support may be required – also a link in with appropriate services, e.g. occupation therapy and physiotherapy.

Therapeutic intervention

Maintenance

Bronchodilators. Bronchodilator therapy may be prescribed on an 'as required' or regular basis. Even if bronchodilator reversibility testing has been negative, individuals may experience some benefit.

Anticholinergics and β_2-agonists are generally thought to be equally effective in the management of COPD, and may have an additive effect. Long-acting β_2-agonists may also be of benefit; again, individual assessment is advised.

Theophyllines have a variable effect on symptoms, and some patients experience side effects even within the therapeutic range. A trial of therapy is advised after other therapeutic options.

Corticosteroids. There is a theoretical rationale for the use of corticosteroids to help control the inflammatory process in COPD; however, many trials of this group of drugs have been disappointing. More recently, it has been suggested that an adequate dose of corticosteroids, although only producing a modest reduction in the decline of FEV_1, may reduce exacerbations and improve quality of life.

A response to corticosteroids should be confirmed prior to commencing or increasing the strength of inhaled corticosteroids.

Oxygen. Breathlessness in severe COPD may make even the simplest of activities impossible. If the patient is hypoxic, oxygen may be helpful. A decision on this should be supported by blood gases: for portable oxygen, a demonstration of improved exercise tolerance with oxygen. The oxygen may be recommended to be used for short periods, or if the $Po_2 < 7.3$ kPa it may need to be used for more than 16 hours a day to reduce long-term mortality. Long-term oxygen therapy (LTOT) has been shown to improve survival by up to 60%.

Surgery. In patients with giant emphysematous bullae, surgical removal of the bullae may improve FEV_1 significantly.

Lung reduction surgery, where areas of severe emphysema are removed from one or both lungs, has been shown to improve FEV_1.

Exacerbations

Presenting features of an acute exacerbation (not all may be present):

- worsening of previous stable condition
- increased dysponea
- increased sputum volume
- increased sputum purulence
- chest tightness
- fluid retention.

Management in community

- Prescribe appropriate antibiotics.
- No clear benefit has been shown with courses of oral steroids, but in individual cases they may be helpful.
- Admission to hospital so that oxygen and/or ventilatory support can be given may be necessary.

However, increasingly, hospitals are looking to manage more patients with exacerbations at home.

Patient education

Advice regarding smoking cessation and the avoidance of passive exposure is crucial to any education plan. It is most important that the results of continued smoking are explained to the patient (the Fletcher/Peto (Fletcher & Peto 1977) chart is a useful aid).

Advice regarding maintenance or increase in exercise capacity, weight control and healthy diet should be given. If a patient has severe COPD they may be less able to prepare and even eat appropriate food.

Referral

Referral may be necessary to confirm the diagnosis if spirometry is not available in the primary care setting. Patients with severe COPD should be referred for full assessment.

Complications

The most common complications are exacerbations, precipitated by bacterial or viral respiratory tract infections. Where the exacerbation is severe and, especially when caused by a virus, there may be a high mortality as in influenza epidemics.

Prognosis

The prognosis of COPD depends on the stage at which the diagnosis is made. In mid or early moderate disease, smoking cessation may return the lung function to the normal rate of decline before a significant degree of disability is present.

In severe COPD, the prognosis is poor, with disability, frequent hospital admissions and death following a short number of years.

INFECTIONS OF THE LOWER RESPIRATORY TRACT

Acute bronchitis

Definition: Acute bronchitis may be an isolated event. It is usually viral in origin but can be bacterial, and causes inflammation of the bronchial tree. Acute bronchitis is a term which is often used liberally.

Subjective findings

History

It is most prevalent in the winter months and cold climates. It is more common in cigarette smokers, those exposed to passive smoking and people with chronic respiratory conditions. It is often concurrent with upper respiratory tract infections or where there has been exposure to respiratory irritants.

Symptoms

- Cough with production of coloured sputum
- Fever may be present.

Objective findings

- Erythema of nasal mucosa and pharynx
- Enlarged and tender anterior cervical nodes
- There may be widespread crackles and wheezing on auscultation.

Investigations

Usually no investigations are carried out, but if the infection is severe, sputum culture to identify the causative organism may be arranged.

Management and therapeutic intervention

Hydration of the patient must be maintained. Therapy is not usually required, except in cases of acute on chronic bronchitis when bronchodilator usage may be increased and antibiotics prescribed. Analgesia may be required, especially in infants, to control pyrexia.

Patient education

As for management and therapy.

Referral

Improvement should be expected in a few days; otherwise, review is appropriate.

Complications

Usually none, but a misdiagnosis of other respiratory infection, e.g. rhinovirus, pneumonia or influenza, may lead to inappropriate management.

Prognosis

For isolated instances with no concurrent respiratory conditions, the prognosis is good. For acute or chronic bronchitis, recovery may take longer.

Croup

Definition: Croup is a non-specific term used to describe a set of symptoms consisting of a barking cough, hoarseness and inspiratory stridor. It is usually caused by viruses such as influenza, and parainfluenza when these are circulating during the winter months. The respiratory syncytial virus (RSV) is another cause and can occur at any time of year.

Subjective findings

History

Usually a mild viral infection with hoarseness and cough which lasts for about 7 days.

Symptoms

Distinct cough – often referred to as old man cough.

Objective findings

- Increased respiratory effort with inspiratory wheeze and inspiratory stridor
- Increase in nasal mucus production
- Pyrexia
- Exhaustion
- Laryngeal swelling
- ❶ Indications of increasing severity include progressive dyspnoea and stridor, hyperpyrexia, restlessness, pallor or cyanosis.

Investigations

The diagnosis of croup is usually made by the history.

Management and therapeutic intervention

Children with mild clinical symptoms can be managed at home with symptomatic treatment, e.g. relief of pyrexia and maintaining fluid intake. Maintain a clear airway and use humidified air to relieve the cough.

Patient education

Croup is a relatively common respiratory infection in the under 3s, and the carer should be taught how to identify deteriorating symptoms.

Referral

Hospitalisation is indicated for those with severe features.

Complications

- Laryngeal obstruction can occur, leading to death.
- Common complications are otitis media, bronchiolitis and pneumonia.

Prognosis

Although croup is a distressing group of symptoms, the prognosis is good.

Bronchiolitis

Definition: Bronchiolitis is predominantly a disease of infancy that occurs most commonly in the first 6 months of life. Acute bronchiolitis is an acute lower respiratory tract condition characterised by mechanical and inflammatory changes in the bronchioles. It is usually due to RSV infection. Although the infection is of short duration, usually 7–10 days hospitalisation may be necessary (1–2% of all infants require hospitalisation).

Subjective findings

History

The onset is gradual, usually beginning with a simple upper respiratory tract infection.

Symptoms

- Cough is the main symptom
- Serous nasal discharge
- Low-grade pyrexia, becoming more pronounced.

Objective findings

- Auscultation will reveal widespread inspiratory crackles rather than rhonchi
- ❶ 48–72 hours after onset, respiratory distress may be shown by dyspnoea, tachypnoea, flaring nares and intercostal and subcostal recession.

Investigations

Chest X-ray will show hyperinflation.

Management and therapeutic intervention

Management is usually conservative, consisting of rehydration and oxygen to relieve hypoxia. Antibiotics, bronchodilators or corticosteroids are not usually indicated.

Patient education

Passive smoking should be avoided, as this will further compromise the wheezy infant. Modification of the feeding regime may be required for the wheezy infant.

Referral

Frequent cause of infant hospitalisation during the winter.

Complications

- Difficulty feeding due to dyspnoea
- Severe respiratory failure.

Prognosis

Up to 90% of infants will suffer recurrent episodic viral wheeze during early childhood.

Influenza

Definition: Influenza is an acute respiratory tract illness caused by the influenza virus. There are three types of influenza virus: A, B and C. Of these, types A and B cause significant illness, whereas type C is associated with mild upper respiratory symptoms mostly in children. Influenza C will not be further discussed. Influenza A and B are associated with substantial morbidity and mortality. The prime site of replication of the influenza virus is the respiratory tract, and the virus has not, to date, been found to replicate elsewhere.

Subjective findings

Symptoms

The symptoms of influenza can be categorised as systemic and local (respiratory). The symptoms are of sudden onset and usually begin to reduce within 7 days of onset, though they may continue for longer, and it is quite common for affected individuals to feel unwell, listless and depressed for several weeks afterwards.

The systemic symptoms are caused by circulating cytokines and reflect the immune response to infection: they do not indicate systemic infection with influenza virus. They typically include fever (38–40°C), headache, chills, myalgia, anorexia and malaise, and tend to resolve (apart from malaise) before the local symptoms.

The respiratory symptoms caused by local infection typically include dry cough, sore throat, nasal congestion and conjunctivitis.

The diagnosis is usually based on clinical signs and symptoms – abrupt onset, high fever, severe malaise, cough and headache. Diagnostic rates based on clinical symptoms are probably in the region of 60–70% during epidemics. In clinical trials, using the common symptoms as diagnostic criteria, the rate is reported as being between 70 and 80%.

Objective findings

In the absence of primary viral pneumonia or secondary infection, fever is the most reliable sign. There may also be evidence of pharyngitis and conjunctivitis.

Investigations

The diagnosis may be confirmed using laboratory methods. The virus may be identified from nasopharyngeal or throat swabs. Currently work is in progress to establish effective near-patient testing, although at present the diagnostic rates of these tests are lower than with clinical diagnosis.

Management and therapeutic intervention

Vaccination

The mainstay of management is an effective programme of vaccination. Current guidelines suggest that individuals considered at risk because of age (> 65) or concomitant disease should be offered prophylactic vaccination prior to the commencement of the influenza season. Vaccination is effective in reducing the infection rate by 80–90% in young fit adults. It is less effective in the elderly (20–30%) and in children (Nicholson 1999).

Immunity to vaccination usually takes 1–2 months and there may be a risk of influenza infection during this time.

Disease management

Historically, the mainstay of clinical management has consisted of relieving the symptoms with analgesia, encouraging fluid intake and bed-rest, and treating secondary infection as and when it appears

Antiviral agents

Amantadine is an antiviral agent available for the prevention and treatment of influenza A.

Neuraminidase inhibitors are a new therapeutic approach to influenza treatment. Zanamivir is the first member of this class. It prevents the release of progeny virus from the infected host cells, preventing viral spread to other cells in the respiratory tract. It is effective against influenza A and B viruses. Zanamivir is delivered topically to the respiratory tract, by a dry powder inhaler.

Patient education

Education programmes, both in primary care and through the media, can improve the management of influenza by alerting patients to the benefits of vaccination, helping them diagnose influenza from other viral infections such as the common cold and advising them as to when to seek medical advise and treatment.

Complications

Lungs: primary viral pneumonia, secondary bacterial pneumonia, mixed pneumonia, croup, exacerbations of chronic lung conditions.

❶ Primary viral pneumonia caused by the influenza virus is a devastating illness with a rapid onset and high mortality.

Secondary bacterial pneumonia is more common among patients with diseases of the respiratory tract such as (COPD). It should be treated aggressively with appropriate antibiotics.
Heart: myocarditis, pericarditis.
Nervous system: meningitis, encephalitis, transverse myelitis, Guillain–Barré syndrome (paralysis).
Other: otitis media, sudden infant death syndrome, myositis, Reye's syndrome, febrile convulsions, renal failure, toxic shock syndrome.

Referral

Patients who are considered 'at risk' should be referred if it appears that they may be severely affected by influenza. If primary viral pneumonia is suspected, immediate referral to a centre with life-support facilities is indicated.

Prognosis

The prognosis of most influenza infections is good. Spontaneous recovery takes place in the majority of cases over the course of 7–10 days. Post-viral debility may persist and delay return to normal activities. Symptomatic support during the course of the infection and avoidance of spread of infection are important.

Pneumonia

Definition: Pneumonia is an inflammatory infection of the pulmonary parenchyma caused by microorganisms. It is usually caused by either a highly virulent organism infecting a healthy person or a less virulent organism infecting a person with compromised defences.

Pneumonia is classified as community-acquired or hospital-acquired; the causative organisms may be different. Knowledge of current epidemics is helpful.

History

Community-acquired pneumonia

A ratio of 1:100 of the population suffer an episode of pneumonia per year: it is twice as common in the winter months and the highest rates are seen in the elderly and the young. About 10% of cases are viral, although viral infection is more common in infants. The most common organisms are pneumococcus, *Mycoplasma pneumoniae* and *Haemophilus influenzae*. *M. pneumoniae* usually occurs in epidemics every few years and staphylococcal pneumonia during influenza epidemics. Legionella infections are most commonly linked with droplet infection through air-conditioning systems.

Hospital-acquired pneumonia

This can develop in up to 50% of patients. The causes include debility, prior chronic chest disease, impaired mucociliary clearance and the use of broad-spectrum antibiotics and high-dose corticosteroids. General health-related issues, such as age, diabetes, obesity, malnutrition, alcoholism and serious chronic disease, may also play a part. There is a high mortality rate (20–25%) for hospital-acquired pneumonia. Organisms most commonly identified are staphylococcus and pneumococcus and Gram-negative bacteria (*Pseudomonas*, *Klebsiella*, *Proteus*).

Subjective findings

- Fever, including hot/cold sensation and shivering
- Cough is often minimal, with or without sputum, but the cough will be out of proportion to the amount of sputum produced unless there is coexisting bronchitis
- Tachypnoea and pleuritic pain, which itself may cause breathlessness.

Objective findings

- Localised crepitations, crackles and rales especially on inspiration.
- In fully developed pneumonia there will be bronchial breathing and dullness on percussion over the affected lobe.
- Transient hypoxaemia is common.
- ❶ Patients may be considered to be at high risk if the following are present:
  central cyanosis
  rapid shallow breathing > 30/min
  hypotension, with a diastolic reading of < 60 mmHg
  confusion
  serum urea > 7 mmol/litre.

Investigations

- Chest X-ray, both posteroanterior (PA) and lateral, to detect any area of consolidation or collapse.
- Blood cultures are usually a more certain way of identifying the organisms than sputum culture. White blood cells (WBC), urea and electrolytes (U&E), lung function tests (LFTs) and, in cases of suspected *Legionella*, serological tests. In severe cases, where hypoxia is suspected, arterial blood gases should be measured.
- In mild cases, especially where the patient is otherwise healthy, full investigation is not usually required. However 'at risk' patients, those with recurrent or severe disease or hospitalised patients should always be fully investigated.

Management and therapeutic intervention

- Pain relief
- Hydration
- Oral and general hygiene

- Antibiotics – sputum culture and local knowledge of sensitivities should be used for guidance
- If analgesia is required, NSAIDs, which do not suppress the cough or respiration, should be used
- Oxygen should be administered for severe cases.

Patient education

Avoid cough suppressants and comply with the above management.

Referral

Patients should be advised to return if no improvement. Patients should be admitted to hospital if they develop severe pneumonia, if they fail to respond to therapy or if they are immunocompromised.

Complications

- Pleurisy
- Pleural effusion
- Empyema – usually secondary to pneumococcal pneumonia
- Lung abscess
- Bronchiectasis may occasionally develop following pneumonia
- Severe pneumonia can be fatal.

Prognosis

Good for uncomplicated pneumonia in a healthy person.

Tuberculosis (TB)

Definition: Tuberculosis is an infection caused by *Mycobacterium tuberculosis*. Tuberculosis most commonly affects the lungs but may affect many other parts of the body. *Mycobacterium tuberculosis* is spread by droplet infection and the primary complex takes approximately 4 weeks to form. Natural defences will heal the lesion in 90% of cases. Clinical disease develops in 5% and relapse of the primary disease at a later stage occurs in 5%.

Subjective findings

History

Contact with known cases is a risk category: this may include family members, friends and health workers. Tuberculosis is linked to poverty and is often found in the immigrant population from Third World countries, especially from Asia and Eastern Europe. Immunocompromised individuals are at particular risk.

❶ Symptoms

- Fever with night sweats
- Persistent cough, with sputum, that does not respond to antibiotics
- Malaise, anorexia and weight loss
- Haemoptysis.

Objective findings

Clinical signs

There may be no abnormalities detected on clinical examination unless pleural effusion is present.

Investigations

- Chest X-ray to identify localisation (a normal chest X-ray usually excludes pulmonary TB).
- Smear test for acid-fast bacilli (AFB). Bacteriological confirmation and drug susceptibilities essential because of rising incidence of drug-resistant tuberculosis.
- Liver function test pretreatment and if the patient becomes symptomatic.
- If risk assessment indicates a risk of AIDS, seek informed consent for HIV (human immunodeficiency virus) testing.

Management

- Referral to a respiratory physician if TB is suspected.
- Notification of the disease is a statutory requirement.
- Contact tracing should be initiated.
- Patients may initially be treated in hospital isolation (respiratory TB only) and then continue therapy at home. They are usually not infectious 14 days after commencing therapy.
- Multidrug-resistant TB patients should be nursed in a negative pressure or lamina airflow room.

Therapeutic intervention

For both adults and children:
- Two months – rifampicin, isoniazid, pyrazinamide. Ethambutol may be added.
- Four months – isoniazid and rifampicin.
- If pyrazinamide cannot be tolerated, treatment should be extended for 9 months. Where possible, combined therapy should be used to encourage compliance.

Patient education

- Allay fears and anxieties
- The patient must be helped to understand the importance of compliance – directly observed therapy may be required.

Referral

All cases of suspected tuberculosis should be referred to a respiratory physician.

Complications

- If there is good compliance with treatment, relapse is uncommon (0–3%)
- Pleurisy
- Empyema
- Pneumothorax
- Bronchiectasis secondary to residual fibrosis or middle lobe as a result of lymph node compression

- Other structures, e.g. kidneys may be infected with TB.

Prognosis

The prognosis is good with appropriate therapy. There is a risk of reactivation if modern therapies have not been used and in patients who are immuno-compromised. Multidrug resistance is increasingly seen and presents serious management problems.

Bronchiectasis

Definition: Bronchiectasis is persistent dilatation of the bronchi. It is caused either by weakening of the walls of the bronchi by infection or retraction of the airways due to interstitial disease or other forces.

Subjective findings

History

There is frequently a history of recurrent childhood chest infection, e.g. bronchiolitis, whooping cough, measles, pneumonia. Other causes include TB, bronchial obstruction, cystic fibrosis, or certain systemic diseases such as ulcerative colitis or Crohn's disease, rheumatoid disease or immunological disease. Acute infective exacerbations usually follow a viral infection.

Symptoms

- Persistent cough with or without purulent sputum. Symptoms do not always correlate with radiological extent of disease.
- Haemoptysis.
- Pleuritic pain, usually in the same site.
- Recurrent pneumonia.

Objective findings

- Auscultation may be unremarkable in the early stages or if there are few secretions.
- Inspiratory crackles may be heard in more severe or extensive disease.
- Finger clubbing, central cyanosis and right heart failure may develop with long-standing widespread disease.

Investigations

- Chest X-ray – may be normal in early stages unless there is active infection.
- High-resolution CT scan is now standard for the diagnosis.
- Lung function to determine degree of airway obstruction.
- Sputum specimen to identify organisms.

Management

Physiotherapy to aid drainage of secretions.

Therapeutic intervention

- Treat infections with antibiotics
- Annual influenza vaccination
- Pneumococcal vaccination
- Inhaled bronchodilator for breathlessness and to aid sputum expectoration
- Regular bronchodilators and low-dose inhaled steroids to treat chronic airflow obstruction.

Patient education

Maintain a healthy lifestyle, including non smoking, regular physiotherapy and exercise. Infections should be treated promptly and with more prolonged course of antibiotics.

Referral

- If reinfection becomes a problem or to determine the extent or cause of the condition
- Most patients will be under long-term hospital follow-up.

Complications

- Frequently misdiagnosed as asthma
- Progressive loss of lung function.

Prognosis

Is variable depending on severity, coexisting lung disease and active management.

Diffuse parenchymal disease

Definition: The term parenchyma covers the epithelium of the alveoli as well as the endothelium of the small blood vessels and the septal tissues between these structures. The alveolar spaces may also be involved as they become affected by fluid or damaged cells. There is a large group of over 200 lung disorders that affect these tissues and the term 'diffuse parenchymal lung disease' is used as a generic term for these disorders (British Thoracic Society 1999), which include asbestosis, extrinsic allergic alveolitis (e.g. farmer's lung, bird fancier's lung), sarcoidosis and cryptogenic fibrosing alveolitis.

This group of disorders have varying presentations, pathology and prognoses, and there is no general agreement as to the management of many of the conditions within this grouping.

This section deals with the more common of these disorders within the classification suggested by the British Thoracic Society:

- acute: bacterial (e.g. tuberculosis), toxins (e.g. amiodarone), vasculitis (e.g. Churg–Strauss syndrome, Wegener's granulomatosis), adult respiratory distress syndrome (ARDS) (trauma, septicaemia)
- episodic: extrinsic allergic alveolitis, Churg–Strauss syndrome
- chronic secondary to occupational or environmental agents: asbestosis, silicosis, coal-miner's lung, farmer's lung, bird fancier's lung, illicit drugs, amiodarone, radiation

- chronic with evidence of systemic disease: rheumatoid arthritis, lymphoma, Wegener's granulomatosis, sarcoidosis, HIV-associated, inflammatory bowel disease, post-transplantation
- chronic with evidence of no systemic disease: cryptogenic fibrosing alveolitis (CFA), sarcoidosis, cryptogenic organising pneumonia, bronchoalveolar carcinoma.

Subjective findings

History

The history may give important clues as to the origin of the lung disease.

Although industry has taken many steps over recent years to reduce the risk of workers being exposed to occupational danger in the form of inhaled agents, the legacy of previous practice is still presenting, e.g. in the form of asbestosis in shipyard workers and pneumoconiosis in coal miners.

The history may reveal long-term exposure to industrial agents or more short-term or recent exposure to drugs (although reaction to some drugs may take years to develop). Risk factors for immunosuppression, HIV or drug exposure should be sought.

Exposure may also occur through pets (birds).

Sarcoidosis and CFA may on rare occasions be familial.

Symptoms

- Breathlessness, but cough may also be a prominent feature
- Haemoptysis may occur with vasculitis
- Other symptoms such as pleurisy, pneumothorax or chest pain may more rarely occur
- Erythema nodosum/joint pains due to sarcoidosis.

Objective findings

- Fine crepitations (crackles) heard at the end of inspiration in CFA and asbestosis. They are less commonly heard in extrinsic allergic alveolitis and sarcoidosis. Inspiratory 'squeaks' are often heard in extrinsic allergic alveolitis.
- Finger clubbing is common in disease due to CFA and rheumatoid arthritis. In severe disease, breathlessness is apparent even at rest and cyanosis may be observed.
- Weight loss and fatigue are non-specific, but if weight loss is a major factor in the presentation malignancy should be suspected.
- Presence of pyrexia may suggest infective causes.
- General malaise and systemic symptoms such as diarrhoea, lymphadenopathy and oral candidiasis may be suggestive of HIV infection.

Investigations

1. In most cases the chest X-ray will be abnormal. With CFA, asbestosis and collagen-related diseases diffuse

shadowing in the lower lung zones may be seen. With TB, sarcoidosis and pneumoconiosis the upper zones are more likely to be affected. Hilar lymphadenopathy may be present in sarcoidosis and lymphoma and carcinoma. Pleural thickening may be present in asbestosis, silicosis and TB.

2. Lung function tests should be carried out. In moderate disease FEV_1 and FVC will be reduced, with a normal FEV_1, FVC ratio. Lung volume and gas transfer factor will be reduced.

3. Chest X-ray and lung function tests will help differentiate this group of disorders from COPD.

4. Full blood count (FBC), eosinophil count, U&E, antinuclear factor and rheumatoid factor should be taken. If a vasculitis is suspected, antineutrophil cytoplasmic and antibasement antibodies should be measured. Serum angiotensin-converting (ACE) enzyme levels may be raised in sarcoidosis but the test is non-specific. Serum calcium levels may be raised in about 10% of cases.

5. With extrinsic allergic alveolitis, specific precipitins (e.g. avian precipitins) may be raised but the test is non-specific as raised levels are found in many asymptomatic subjects.

6. High-resolution CT scanning may be pathognomonic in some cases of sarcoidosis, CFA and some occupational lung diseases.

7. Often transbronchial biopsy (sarcoidosis, extrinsic allergic alveolitis (EAA)), or in other cases, open-lung biopsy or video-assisted thoracoscopic biopsy may be needed to confirm the diagnosis.

Management and therapeutic intervention

Many of this group of disorders have little evidence for successful management regimes.

Sarcoidosis

Although sarcoidosis responds well to corticosteroids, many patients do not need treatment. Treatment should be reserved for patients with symptoms and pulmonary shadowing. These should be delivered in the form of oral prednisolone, as there is no good evidence of the effectiveness of inhaled steroids in this disease. In resistant cases, other anti-inflammatory agents such as azathioprine or methotrexate may be used.

CFA

Oral corticosteroids are generally first-line choice in CFA and are given together with immunosuppressive therapy such as azathioprine or cyclophosphamide.

Extrinsic allergic alveolitis

First-line management is avoidance of further exposure to the precipitating agent. This may lead to complete resolution. The recovery may be speeded by the use of oral corticosteroids, but these are unlikely to change the end-stage lung function deficit. If the underlying cause of the parenchymal lung disorder is infective, this must be dealt with by appropriate therapy.

Churg–Strauss syndrome

This is thought to be related in some cases to the withdrawal of treatment with oral (or high-dose inhaled) steroids. In these cases, the vasculitis may regress with the administration of systemic steroids.

Other parenchymal lung diseases

With vasculitis such as Wegener's granulomatosis, regression may be achieved with oral steroids or immunosuppressive drugs, but the condition often recurs in spite of continued therapy. Many disorders within this grouping will have transplantation as the only management option with a chance of improving survival rates.

The therapeutic options for this group of disorders have significant side effects, and patients must be monitored carefully for the development of osteoporosis (due to oral steroids) and blood cell and liver function abnormalities (due to immunosuppressives).

Patient education

With extrinsic allergic alveolitis, the patient must be helped to understand the cause of his disease and the importance of avoiding further exposure.

The possible side effects of therapy, where it is used, must be explained and the patient must be advised as to the necessity of following the recommended regime and of regular monitoring of appropriate blood levels.

In many cases the progression of the condition is relentless and education of the patient and his carers as to the prognosis is essential.

Referral

Where any of this group of diseases is suspected, referral to a specialist respiratory unit is mandatory.

Complications

The complications are varied and generally result from uncontrolled disease. They include pneumothorax, chest pain and haemoptysis.

Prognosis

- Extrinsic allergic alveolitis may respond well to avoidance and, in bird fancier's lung, may stabilise even in the presence of continued exposure to allergen
- Most cases of sarcoidosis respond well to corticosteroid therapy
- CFA has a variable and often disappointing response to therapy
- However, the prognosis of many diseases within this grouping is poor, with progression towards increasingly restrictive lung disease and death.

Malignant disease of the lung

Definition: The term is used to describe any malignant disease affecting the lungs, whether the disease has arisen in the lungs or has invaded or metastasised into the lungs. There are four main groups within this description:

- bronchial
- mediastinal
- parenchymal
- pleural.

Subjective findings

History

❶ Eighty to ninety percent of bronchial carcinomas occur in people who smoke. Those exposed to high levels of passive smoking have an incidence above that of non-exposed nonsmokers.

Certain industrial exposures, such as asbestos, nickel and arsenic, increase the risk of lung cancer; for example, asbestos workers have an increased risk of mesothelioma (a malignant disease affecting the pleura).

The incidence of lung cancer is falling in younger males but is rising among women.

Symptoms

- The disease may be asymptomatic and be diagnosed as an incidental finding on chest X-ray
- Haemoptysis
- Weight loss
- Anorexia
- Unremitting cough, which may be worsening
- Stridor, where the large airways are affected
- Extensive disease may cause breathlessness, wheeze or chest pain
- General respiratory symptoms
- Nerve involvement or infiltrative disease may cause hoarseness
- Pressure from the tumour or associated lymphadenopathy may cause dysphagia
- An associated infection may result in the presentation of pneumonia
- Parenchymal disease may present with signs of large airway obstruction
- Pleural lesions may present with pleuritic pain, persistent chest wall or shoulder pain, as well as coughing and haemoptysis.

There should be a suspicion of lung cancer in a patient over the age of 30 who smokes and who presents with any of the above symptoms.

Objective findings

- There may be no obvious signs of disease on clinical examination.
- Occasionally, localised signs of airflow obstruction (rhonchi and rales) may be heard. Where there is a pleural effusion, this may be detectable on auscultation and percussion.
- Finger clubbing may be early and can occur in patients with stage I – II tumours.
- Finger clubbing, cachexia and weight loss may be apparent in advanced disease.
- Metastatic lymphadenopathy may be apparent, especially in the supraclavicular region.
- Occasionally, the disease may present with metastases such as brain secondaries.

Investigations

- Chest X-ray
- Sputum cytology, FBC, U&E, calcitonin and LFTs
- Bronchoscopy or needle biopsy
- Staging CT scan
- Electrocardiogram (ECG).

Management and therapeutic intervention

1. The management will depend upon the location, nature and the extent of the tumour, as well as on the general condition of the patient.
2. The majority of lung cancers are inoperable, either due to the extent of the lesion, the presence of multiple metastases or the location of the lesion in relation to other organs. Mediastinal and pleural lesions are generally inoperable.
3. For some patients with non-small cell cancer, early diagnosis and localised disease may allow operative removal of the tumour. This may be combined with radiotherapy or chemotherapy.
4. Small cell cancer is generally treated with radiotherapy or chemotherapy, but the prognosis is significantly worse than other forms of bronchial carcinoma.
5. Haemoptysis or symptoms associated with local obstruction may sometimes be relieved by radiotherapy. Occasionally, laser treatment, cryotherapy or the application of stents is used to relieve local obstruction.
6. Large pleural effusions may be treated by aspiration and drainage with subsequent chemical or talc pleurodesis, which can give rise to good long-term palliation.
7. In many cases the only treatment available or appropriate will be palliative. In the later stages of the disease, analgesia is the main form of treatment, and continuous subcutaneous analgesia is often effective in providing 24-hour pain relief.

Patient education

The patient and their carers will need education and information concerning the type of cancer and the management. Involvement of the palliative care team is necessary from a very early stage.

The disease is generally rapidly progressive and there is a high level of awareness among patients of the significance of the diagnosis. Careful counselling is necessary to deal with the hopes, fears and expectations of the patient and their carers.

Referral

Where malignant disease of the lung is suspected, immediate referral to a chest physician is necessary, and an urgent appointment received within 1–2 weeks of referral.

Complications

- Complications include secondary infections and pneumonia, local pressure on other organs from the disease or metastases and metastatic involvement of other organs.
- Haemoptysis may become frequent.
- Pleural effusion may occur, especially where there is secondary disease. It may cause severe dyspnoea.

Prognosis

The mean survival time is less than 1 year and over 90% of patients die within 5 years.

Pulmonary embolus (PE)

Definition: Pulmonary embolus (pulmonary thromboembolism) is a term used to describe an embolus or clot that has originated in the venous system, which lodges, because of its size, in the arteries within the lung. Depending on their location and size, emboli may cause a significant obstruction to arterial blood flow through the lungs. Air or fat embolism may occur less commonly. If PE is suspected, urgent referral to hospital is required.

❶ Subjective findings

History

Risk factors include:
- immobility (due to major surgery, injury, stroke, infirmity or other causes)
- malignant disease
- pregnancy
- history of thromboembolic disease
- familial thrombotic disorders
- oral contraception (oestrogens) is a minor risk factor.

Symptoms

The patient will present with some or all of the following symptoms:
- dyspnoea
- pleuritic pain
- tachypneoa and tachycardia
- cough
- haemoptysis
- leg pain (if a lower leg, deep vein thrombosis is present)
- the patient is generally anxious.

Objective findings

- The patient is often anxious and sweating
- Tachypnoea and tachycardia may be present
- There are generally no abnormal signs on auscultation
- PE is easily missed in the elderly or in patients with severe cardiac or respiratory disease.

Investigations

1. X-ray of the chest is often non-specific, but is often valuable in excluding other causes of dyspnoea, pleuritic pain, tachypnoea and tachycardia, such as pneumothorax, pneumonia or cardiac failure.
2. With PE, a segmental collapse, pleural effusion and a raised hemidiaphragm may be seen.
3. An ECG is important in excluding myocardial infarction. With PE, although it may be abnormal, the changes, usually in the ST segment, are generally non-specific.
4. Blood gases, except in severe cases, are generally normal.
5. In low probability cases, a nasal D-dimer level excludes the diagnosis. The initial investigation is most usually ventilation/perfusion (V/Q) isotope scanning. This test should be performed as soon as possible as the V/Q ratio may return to normal quite quickly. The test has a high level of accuracy in confirming or excluding PE, when the scan is either normal (misses 4% of cases) or graded as high probability. However, in many patients the scan is indeterminate and other tests such as leg ultrasound or CT angiogram are required to confirm the diagnosis.
6. Ultrasound or other imaging of the lower leg is often used to determine the source of the suspected PE.

Management and therapeutic findings

1. Anticoagulation is the first-line treatment for PE. Heparin should be started immediately the diagnosis is suspected, and continued for at least 6 days and after warfarin has been established as anticoagulation therapy. Increasingly, single dose low molecular weight heparin is being substituted for continuous infusions of unfractionated heparin.
2. Thrombolytic therapy may be used in massive PE.
3. The risk/benefit ratio of anticoagulant or thrombolytic therapy must be carefully assessed, especially in postoperative patients.
4. High-risk patients may need permanent anticoagulation; they may also be advised to wear anti-embolus stockings.

Patient education

High-risk patients must be advised as to methods of risk reduction. Anticoagulation may be advisable for high-risk patients where surgery or pregnancy is planned. Where the risk may be short term (as during a long journey by air) short-term prophylactic anticoagulation may be advised. These patients should also be advised on the importance of avoiding immobility of their lower limbs.

For all patients who have suffered a PE, advice regarding extended periods of immobility and dehydration as occur in air travel, should be given.

Referral

Where PE is suspected, refer to a hospital with facilities to make appropriate investigations should be made as soon as possible.

Complications

- Large emboli may cause right heart failure, hypotension, cyanosis and death
- The risk of further emboli from the primary site must be considered
- Haemorrhage is a major complication of anticoagulation treatment of PE.

Prognosis

The prognosis depends upon the risk level of the individual. For those with an established high risk, the risk of further emboli may be high unless appropriate avoidance measures are taken.

Where there is no apparent risk factor for PE, the presence of an underlying cause such as malignancy should be suspected and investigated.

OTHER LUNG DISORDERS

Pneumothorax

Definition: A pneumothorax occurs when air enters the cavity between the parietal and visceral pleura allowing the underlying lung to collapse partially or completely.

Subjective findings

History

Pneumothorax most commonly occurs spontaneously in healthy young males or it can be secondary to trauma, including penetrating injury; to infection, e.g. tuberculosis, staphylococcal pneumonia; to airway obstruction, e.g. COPD, malignancy; or to congenital disorders, such as Marfan's syndrome. Rarely, bilateral pneumothorax is seen.

Symptoms

❶ Sudden onset of chest pain followed by breathlessness.

Objective findings

- Deviated trachea may be seen with large pneumothoraces
- Hyperinflated chest, limited respiratory excursion

- No audible breath sounds over the affected area
- Hyperresonance on percussion
- Hypotension.

Investigations

On chest X-rays, it is important to assess severity and differentiate between pneumothorax, pulmonary embolus and emphysematous bullae.

Management

- With small-to-moderate pneumothoraces with no dyspnoea and no chronic lung disease, no treatment may be required, as the lung may reinflate spontaneously.
- Chest X-ray should be repeated the following day, or sooner if dyspnoea develops.
- If symptomatic, the pneumothorax should be aspirated. Intercostal tube drainage with an underwater seal will be required for more severe cases.
- If recurrent, pleurodesis may be considered.

Therapeutic intervention

Nil.

Patient education

Advise against air travel for 3 months.

Referral

Referral is generally indicated to establish the extent of the pneumothorax and to determine the appropriate treatment, as well as to identify possible precipitating factors.

Complications

- If pressure builds up in the pleural cavity as a result of tension, there is a risk of compression of the heart and major vessels.
- Haemothorax, if the cause is a penetrating injury.
- Surgical emphysema can occur with a penetrating injury or if the chest drain is not correctly sited.

Prognosis

In uncomplicated cases, the prognosis is good. With recurrent pneumothorax, careful assessment of the underlying causes must be made.

Empyema

Definition: Empyema is a collection of pus in a cavity. This may occur in the lungs following a generalised or localised lung infection.

The empyema may be a single locus or may be multilocular. Treatment with appropriate antibiotics should be initiated and the fluid drained with a fine-bore catheter. Intrapleural streptokinase appears to reduce the need for subsequent surgical intervention. Most empyemas will resolve with treatment, but there may be residual damage to the structures in the lung.

Pleural effusion

Definition: Pleural effusion is a collection of fluid between the layers of the pleura; the fluid may be infective or non-infective. Pleural effusion may occur following pleurisy, and may be secondary to an infection or secondary to the presence of malignant or non-malignant local disease.

If the effusion is large, it may cause respiratory embarrassment, and may need drainage. Tapping or drainage may also be needed for diagnostic purposes in association with biopsy of the pleura. Where the cause is malignant, the effusion may re-accumulate quickly after drainage.

Smoking cessation

The effects of smoking-related disease are frequently evident in respiratory disease. Lung function naturally declines with ageing, but for some smokers the decline is ever greater. It has been shown that irrespective of age the rate of decline can be slowed down with smoking cessation.

Several factors are involved in the process of cigarette smoking. These include nicotine dependency, habit and often a psychological dependency. The addiction to nicotine is said to be equivalent to heroin addiction. Nicotine is suspended in tar droplets and drawn into the lungs; about 90% of the nicotine is absorbed into the bloodstream and it is a powerful stimulant which causes vasoconstriction. A large number of chemicals (creating a tar) are found in cigarette smoke, many of which are known carcinogens. This tar also irritates the airways, causing cough and an increase in mucus production, which damages the cilia.

Carbon monoxide gas is inhaled with cigarette smoke and irreversibly forms carboxyhaemoglobin, thereby reducing the number of red cells able to form oxyhaemoglobin.

Cigarette smoking has the potential to affect many body systems:

- cardiovascular system, including stroke, heart disease and peripheral vascular disease
- respiratory system, causing COPD, exacerbations of asthma and throat and lung cancer
- gastrointestinal system, causing cancer of the mouth, oesophagus and stomach
- genitourinary system, causing cancer of the kidneys and bladder
- reproductive system, increasing the risk of cervical cancer and causing low infant birth weight.

Smoking cessation is a difficult process and requires determination on the part of the patient. Guidelines advise health professionals of their role in assisting smokers to quit. These should include the following:

- ask – about present and past smoking and passive smoking
- assess – interest in stopping smoking

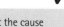

Top Tips
1 Always take a careful history; it may highlight the cause and nature of the disease and give pointers to management options
2 Persistent cough or wheezing in a child with an atopic history make asthma a likely diagnosis
3 Avoidance of precipitating factors may reduce or remove the need for treatment for asthma and other respiratory diseases
4 Inhaled corticosteroids are the cornerstone of asthma treatment
5 Smoking is the prime cause of COPD and smoking cessation the cornerstone of management
6 Malignant disease must be suspected in a current or ex-smoker with haemoptysis
7 Appropriate use of antibiotics in bacterial lung infections may be lifesaving
8 Compliance with treatment is key to the successful management of TB
9 Overuse and inappropriate use of antibiotics in respiratory disease may lead to the development of resistance
10 The use of oxygen in patients with respiratory distress may be lifesaving

- advise – discuss the value of stopping smoking, ensuring it is personalised
- assist – at all stages, if a person is showing an interest in quitting
- arrange – follow-up visits; recommendations are at 1, 2, 4, 8 and 12 weeks. Relapse is not unusual and most people take 3–4 attempts before being successful.

Both the physical and psychological aspects of smoking cessation need to be addressed by preparing for a quit day, which is appropriate for the person. Quit with the aid of nicotine replacement (NRT), which is a temporary nicotine replacement that is gradually reduced over a period of time. NRT is available in the form of patches, gum, nasal spray, vaporisers and sublingual tablets. This should be used in conjunction with behavioural changes compatible with breaking the habit of smoking. Oral anti-smoking therapy (bupropion) has been shown to be effective in the management of smoking cessation.

Glossary

α₁-Antitrypsin   A glycoprotein in the serum which can inactivate protein splitting enzymes such as trypsin, elastase and collagenase. An hereditary deficiency can lead to liver disease in childhood and emphysema in adults

Atopy   A hypersensitivity reaction associated with an immunoglobulin E (IgE) response to the presence of allergen. There is an hereditary tendency

Cachexia   Severe muscle wasting and weakness occurring in the late stage of serious illness

CT scanning   Computed tomography internal X-ray scanning built up by computer from thousands of separate low-intensity readings. Images can be reconstructed from stored readings in any plane or orientation

Emphysematous bullae   Acute overinflation of the lungs, with breakdown of the alveoli to form large air sacs

FEV$_1$ Forced expiratory volume in 1 is the volume of air expelled in the first second of a forced expiration starting from full inspiration

FEV$_1$/FVC ratio   Often known as forced expiratory ratio (FER). Normally the FEV$_1$ is 75–85% of the FVC, decreasing with age

FVC   Forced vital capacity is total volume of air expelled and is used as an indication of lung size

Hyperinflation   Overinflation of the air spaces in the lungs

Hypoxic   Deficiency of oxygen, due to relative failure of the passage of oxygen

Marfan's syndrome   A genetic disorder involving weakness of the structural protein fibrillin, characterised by arachnodactyly, tall stature, lens dislocation and aortic aneurysm

Pathognomonic   Symptom or physical sign that is uniquely characteristic of a particular disease as to establish the diagnosis

Pleural effusion   An excessive accumulation of fluid between the layers of the pleura that may compress the underlying lung

Pleurisy   Inflammation of the pleura

Polycythaemia   An abnormal increase in the number of red blood cells

Sarcoidosis   Disease of unknown cause featuring granulomas in many parts of the body, especially the lymph nodes, liver, lungs, skin and eyes. It mainly affects young adults

References

British Thoracic Society, British Paediatric Association, Royal College of Physicians et al 1993 Guidelines for the management of asthma. Thorax 48:S1–24.

British Thoracic Society, the National Asthma Campaign, Royal College of Physicians of London et al 1997a The British Guidelines on Asthma Management 1995 review and position statement. Thorax 52:S1–21.

British Thoracic Society Guidelines for the Management of Chronic Obstructive Pulmonary Disease 1997b The COPD Guidelines Group of the Standards of Care Committee of the BTS. Thorax 52(suppl 5):S1–S28.

British Thoracic Society 1999 The diagnosis, assessment and treatment of diffuse parenchymal lung disease in adults. Thorax 54(suppl. 1):S1–S30.

Fletcher C, Peto R 1977 The natural history of chronic airflow obstruction. British Medical Journal 1:1645–1648.

Nicholson K G 1999 Managing influenza in primary care. Blackwell Science, London.

Pearce L 1998 Know how: a guide to asthma inhalers. Nursing Times 94 (9) (Suppl.):72.

Pearce L 1999 The development of a device to help in the assessment of inhaler technique. Airways 9:6–8.

Russell G, Helms P J 1997 Trends in occurrence of asthma among children and young adults. Br Med J 315:1014–1015

The Lung Report II 2000 Lung disease: a shadow over the nation's health. British Lung Foundation, London.

Further reading

Holgate S T, Boushey H A, Fabbri L M (eds) 1999 Difficult asthma. Martin Dunitz, London.

Levy M, Hilton S 1999 Asthma in practice, 4th edn. Royal College of General Practitioners, London.

National Asthma & Respiratory Training Centre 1998 Simply COPD. A practical pocket book on chronic obstructive pulmonary disease. Direct Publishing Solutions, Berkshire.

National Asthma & Respiratory Training Centre 2000 Simply stop smoking. A practical handbook. Direct Publishing Solutions, Berkshire.

Silverman M (ed.) 1996 Childhood asthma and other wheezing disorders. Chapman and Hall Medical, London.

8

THE CARDIOVASCULAR SYSTEM

Morag White

Key Issues

- The publication of the governments consultative paper 'Our Healthier Nation' (DHSS 1998), highlights coronary heart disease (CHD) and stroke prevention as priority health areas in the United Kingdom. Latest figures show that CHD accounts for one-third of deaths in men and one-fifth of deaths in women under the age of 65

- The volume of evidence in support of both primary and secondary interventions to prevent CHD and other atheroslerotic disease necessitates careful appraisal of the scientific evidence in order to implement changes in the clinical context

- The long-term consequences of hypertension are well understood. Elevated blood pressure is a major risk factor for the development of stroke and an important risk factor for the development of CHD. Reduction in blood pressure have been shown to reduce stroke, myocardial infarction (MI), heart failure and other cardiovascular events, and should have a major public health impact

- The British Hypertension Society (BHS) Guidelines (Ramsey et al 1999) have added impetus to reduce blood pressures further. BHS Guidelines target diabetics (L 135/85 mmHg) and non-diabetics (L 140/90 mmHg).

- Evidence from randomised control trials and meta-analysis has strengthened our understanding of the effectiveness of lifestyle and therapeutic interventions in reducing coronary artery disease. Recommendations to reduce lipid levels in high-risk individuals have come from studies such as the Scandinavian Simvastatin Survival Study (1993) and the West of Scotland Coronary Prevention Study (1996)

- In 1998 the European societies of Cardiology, Atherosclerosis, and Hypertension joined forces to publish recommendations on the prevention of CHD in clinical practice

Introduction

Cardiovascular disease can be congenital or acquired and encompasses a wide range of conditions. Common cardiological conditions which are seen by Nurse Practitioners include angina, hypertension, post-myocardial infarction, pericarditis and vascular disease. Less commonly, practitioners are faced with cardiological emergencies such as acute MI, acute heart failure or even cardiac arrhythmias

There is increasing awareness amongst the general population of the possible significance of chest pain; however, it is important to remember that any structure in the chest can give rise to pain and that careful history and examination are the cornerstones of good management. Hypertension, ischaemic heart disease and peripheral vascular disease are all more common in the elderly and give rise to particular problems. Infants and children presenting with cardiological problems are also discussed in this section.

The heart as a pump

The core functions of the cardiovascular system are to ensure an adequate circulation of blood, the transport of nutritional substances, the removal of carbon dioxide and metabolic end products and the dissipation of heat away from the active tissues, helping to establish normal body temperature. The heart functions as a pump that, together with the vascular system, assists in the transport of these nutrients and waste products.

The walls of the heart consist mainly of muscle called the myocardium, which is responsible for pumping the blood into the circulation. The myocardium is divided into two layers of epithelium: the endocardium, which lines the internal surface of the heart; and the valves and the outer surface of the myocardium, which is known as the epicardium. Inflammation of these layers can give rise to conditions known as myocarditis, endocarditis and epicarditis.

In the adult heart there are two pumps working together. The right side of the heart has a low-pressure system, which receives blood from the systemic system, and pumps it to the lungs. It consists of the right atrium, tricuspid valve, right ventricle, pulmonary valve and pulmonary artery. The left side of the heart acts as a high-pressure pump and is responsible for receiving blood from the lungs and pumping it round the body. The main structures of the left heart are the left atrium, mitral valve, left ventricle, aortic valve and aorta (Fig. 8.1).

Oxygenated blood is carried to the cardiac muscle by the right and left coronary arteries and their branches. The pressure in the aorta is responsible for maintaining blood flow to the cardiac muscle. In normal circumstances a equilibrium in pressure is maintained by a baroreceptor mechanism. However, changes in the resistance of coronary artery vessels will lead to changes in coronary artery flow. A major factor affecting the resistance of the coronary vessels is the demand for oxygen. At rest, oxygen extraction from the coronary circulation is almost three times greater than the normal circulation. Angina results from an imbalance between myocardial oxygen supply and demand, and in most cases is due to fixed atheromatous obstructions in the larger epicardial coronary arteries.

The conduction system

For the heart to pump effectively the atria and the ventricles must be coordinated, and this is dependent on the electrical activity of the heart. Coordination is achieved through precise timing and the routing of the impulse conduction. The signal for contraction of each heart muscle cell is the electrical depolarisation of its membrane. The electrical signal is transmitted from cell to cell, which allows cardiac muscle to function as a whole. In the healthy heart, impulses originate in the sinoatrial (SA) node and spread rapidly through the atria. These cells normally undergo cyclical depolarisation and repolarisation at a faster rate than other parts of the heart. The impulses pass slowly through the atrioventricular (AV) node with a delay of 0.12–0.20 s. The impulses then spread rapidly through the ventricles. The SA node, located in the roof of the right atrium near the entrance of the superior vena cava, and the AV node, located at the base of the right atrium, possess a spontaneous intrinsic rhythm (Fig. 8.2).

Note. The electrical activity of the heart is important to the understanding of the electrocardiograph (ECG).

The vascular system

The vascular system is divided into the arterial system and the venous system and is made up of arteries, arterioles and veins. The structure of these vessels in different parts of the vascular system varies according to their

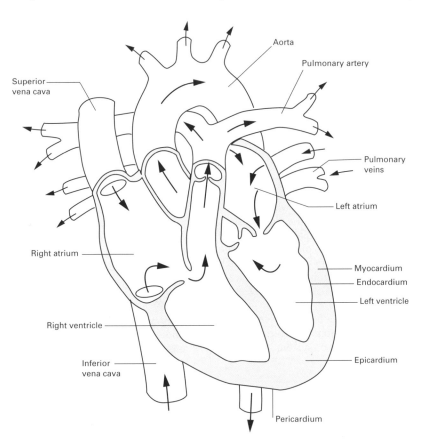

Figure 8.1 *Flow of blood around the body.*

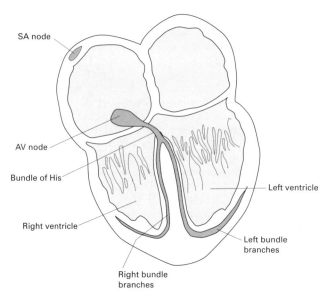

Figure 8.2 *The conduction system.*

specific function; for example, the aorta and most of the large arteries have a wider diameter and a lower resistance, allowing blood to flow freely through them. The smaller arteries or arterioles have a smaller diameter with a thicker muscle wall; here the resistance to blood flow is very much increased due to a narrower radius. The narrower the radius of the vessels therefore determines the amount of peripheral resistance. The smallest of the vessels in the arterial system are the capillaries. There are estimated to be 40 000–50 000 million capillaries, which have an important role in the exchange of nutrients, gases and fluids and in the elimination of metabolic waste products. Consequently, they are sometimes known as the exchange vessels.

The venous system functions differently by returning blood from the capillary system to the heart. This occurs through a pressure gradient, which in the venules must always be greater than the right atrium. The vessels have a relatively large diameter and, like the arteries, offer a low resistance to blood flow. A large volume of blood is contained within the system, which merges to form venules. Venous return to the heart is determined by even small variations in the vessels radius and resistance.

Peripheral vascular disease can be considered under two headings: disease of the peripheral arterial system and disease of the peripheral venous system.

Assessment

Subjective assessment

History taking is a fundamental prerequisite to the efficiency of the subsequent physical examination of the cardiovascular system.

The principal symptoms of heart disease can be of dyspnoea, pain, oedema, palpitation or claudication. Some heart disease is asymptomatic, and is only detected during routine examination, or when a complication develops. Heart disease may be one of many non-specific symptoms, such as tiredness.

Questions to ask if the presenting symptom is chest pain

Onset. Ask whether onset was gradual, sudden, recurrent or new.

Provocation. The patient may present with symptoms of chest pain that are characteristically triggered by exercise. This may also occur at rest, but is usually during stress or sometimes after a meal. Symptoms are often atypical in the elderly; shortness of breath may be the only symptom. Ask about the consistency with which the symptoms are reproduced by exercise and other stressors.

Palliation. Ask if resting, taking medication, i.e. nitroglycerin or antacids to relieve chest pain, changing position or applying heat.

Quantity and quality. Quality, site and radiation of pain is important, but duration of pain is equally significant, as angina usually lasts less than 5 min and is relieved by short-acting nitrates. Ask if pain is sharp, dull, stabbing, burning or feels like pressure. Elicit whether the pain is mild, moderate, severe or disabling on a scale from 1 to 10.

Region and radiation. Is the pain retrosternal, precordial, epigastric, localised or diffuse. Does it radiate into the neck, jaw, arms, abdomen or back.

Associated symptoms. Ask the patient if there have been any symptoms of nausea, vomiting, shortness of breath, headache, fever, cough or syncope.

Underlying disorders. Any previously diagnosed diseases? Risk factors for potential causes of chest pain? Ask about family history of ischaemic heart disease: normally, it is the patient's immediate family that is most significant. Patients often cannot differentiate between sudden death from other causes and ischaemic heart disease, so carefully phrase your questions. A vague history, which cannot be substantiated, should be discounted. Equally, a history of a relative who dies from heart disease over the age of 70 years is less significant than a parent or sibling who has had a significant event leading to hospitalisation or death under the age of 70. Ask about other risk factors for atheromatous disease, such as smoking, hypertension, high cholesterol and diabetes mellitus. Smoking is by far the most important. Ask about alcohol intake and exercise.

Patients with heart disease that causes breathlessness characteristically experience it during physical exertion (*exertional dyspnoea*) or sometimes when they lie flat in bed (*orthopnoea*). The patient who suffers from *paroxysmal nocturnal dyspnoea* may wake from their sleep gasping for breath; this may be accompanied by a cough and white frothy sputum.

If the presenting symptom is dyspnoea, then ask:

- Do you feel short of breath?
- What makes you short of breath?
- Do you have a cough or are you bringing up any sputum?
- Do you get short of breath climbing one flight of stairs or walking on the flat for a few metres?
- How far can you walk before becoming short of breath?
- What do you do when you get short of breath?
- Do you feel short of breath when you lie down?
- Do you ever wake up gasping for breath?
- What do you do then?

❶ It can sometimes be difficult to determine whether a patient's breathlessness is caused by heart or lung disease. Paroxysmal nocturnal dyspnoea or orthopnoea would point towards heart disease, whereas wheezing is more symptomatic of lung disease. It is more appropriate to make this distinction with the addition of a physical examination.

Palpitation

Palpitation is an abnormal awareness of the heart beat and can be due to:
- extrasystoles
- paroxysmal atrial fibrillation
- paroxysmal supraventricular tachycardia
- anxiety
- thyrotoxicosis
- anaemia.

It is important to determine the exact nature of the palpitation by asking a series of questions:
- What do you mean by palpitation?
- How is the heart beating when you have an attack?
- Is it regular or irregular?
- How fast does it go?
- Does anything set off an attack?
- How long does an attack last?
- Do you get other symptoms with an attack?
- Do you get chest pain with an attack?
- Are you able to tap out on the table how your heart sounds?
- Is it regular or irregular?
- Do you ever feel dizzy or blackout with an attack?

It is often helpful to ask the patient to tap out the heart rhythm on the table. Ask about the circumstances when the patient feels the palpitation. Paroxysmal tachycardia is often precipitated by exercise or particular movements (bending or reaching), whereas ectopic beats, or extrasystoles, may be experienced when the patient has a very forceful beat. Patients may be anxious about this as they feel the heart is about to stop.

In some patients, palpitation is precipitated by the ingestion of certain foods such as tea, coffee, wine or certain medications that contain sympathomimetic compounds such as decongestants. Careful questioning may be useful to determine the exact cause.

❶ It is important to remember that the sort of questions asked are determined by the severity of the condition.

❶ Any patient presenting with acute symptoms of chest pain, shortness of breath or a rapid pulse should be assessed very quickly to determine the exact nature of the presenting problem.

Objective assessment

The physical exam starts as soon as the nurse practitioner meets the patient and includes an assessment of general appearance, dress, demeanour, and personal hygiene. Risk factors such as obesity or increased arterial neck pulsation that occurs in aortic incompetence may be observed. Physical signs can easily be missed during a routine examination unless the practitioner is specifically looking for them.

General approach

- Signs of nervousness, dyspnoea, tachycardia and tremor should be noted at the time of the initial examination.
- Examine the patient's hands to assess warmth, sweating and peripheral cyanosis. Examine the nails for clubbing or splinter haemorrhages.
- Palpate brachial pulse: assess quality and measure the blood pressure.
- Palpate carotid pulse. Listen for bruits.
- With the patient lying supine at 45°, assess the jugular venous pressure and the jugular venous pulse form.

- Examine the face further, looking for cyanosis, e.g. tongue, lips. Look for features of hypercholesterolaemia.
- With the patient's chest exposed, inspect the precordium and assess the breathing pattern and the presence of any abnormal pulsation.
- Palpate the precordium, locate the apex best and assess the character. Assess the feel of the rest of the precordium and the presence of any abnormal vibrations or thrills.
- Auscultate the heart with the stethoscope and assess heart sounds and murmurs.
- Percuss and auscultate the chest from both front and back. Listen for crepitations. Look for sacral oedema.
- Examine the abdomen. Palpate the liver and look for only dilation of the abdominal aorta. Listen for renal bruits.
- Assess the femoral pulses and the popliteal and foot pulses. Look for ankle and sacral oedema.
- Examine the optic fundi.
- Test the urine.

Physical assessment

Inspect the hands

A patient's hands can provide important signs to suggest cardiac disease and give a guide to peripheral vasodilatation and sweating. Heart failure can cause vasoconstriction. Hands can feel cold and sometimes sweaty from increased adrenaline secretion. Finger clubbing can indicate subacute bacterial endocarditis or cyanotic congenital heart disease. Splinter haemorrhages can occur in subacute infective endocarditis or cyanotic congenital heart disease. Xanthoma (palmar or tendon) may be observed, which are a feature of hyperlipidaemia but can also be observed on the elbows, knuckles, buttock or Achilles tendon.

Inspect the face

There are important clues to the possible existence of ischaemic heart disease, which can be seen when examining the face. The colour of the skin is of great importance in assessment.

Corneal arcus. This is due to precipitation of cholesterol crystals at the periphery of the cornea. In young people, it is strongly associated with hypercholesterolaemia (non-specific in the over 50s).

Xanthelasma. This is a yellowish exception at the corner side of the eyelids. This is also associated with hypercholesterolaemia (non-specific in the over 50s.)

Inspect the pallor. The degree of pallor or redness of the skin depends largely on the blood flow through the surface vessels; hence, the person who has collapsed peripheral blood vessels, which can occur in shock, i.e. – with the severe pain experienced after myocardial infarction or in cold conditions – may appear very pale.

Adrenaline (epinephrine) also causes vasoconstriction, so the frightened or anxious patient may also appear pale.

Inspect for cyanosis

This occurs when more than 5 g Hb/dl is in the reduced state. Thus cyanosis, a blue coloration, occurs relatively early in patients who are polycythaemic but is rarely seen in those who are anaemic. Cyanosis may be *central*, e.g. over the face and lips, or peripheral, where the extremities are effected. Cyanosis is difficult to assess in non-caucasian patients, whose skin pigments may obscure the condition. The inside of the lips, palms and soles may, however, give some indication of the problem (Hinchliffe & Montague 1988).

Peripheral pulses

The cardiovascular system should be examined for the presence of all major arterial pulses. Absent or delayed femoral pulses may indicate coarctation of the aorta. Collaterals may be palpated on the posterior surface of the scapula. Thickening of the wall of the radial artery is often felt in hypertensive elderly subjects.

Look for evidence of peripheral vascular disease. Peripheral arterial disease is mainly due to acute or chronic impairment of blood supply to a limb and may result from atheromatous narrowing of the artery or from thrombus formation. Acute arterial obstruction presents with a cold, pulseless limb. Chronic arterial insufficiency is much more common in the lower limb and usually presents as intermittent claudication. Examination of the leg reveals weak or absent foot, knee or sometimes femoral pulses.

The patient may be aware of pain in the leg, thigh or buttock on walking, which can become progressively worse until the patient even experiences pain at rest. Diabetes mellitus affects both large and small blood vessels and therefore predisposes some patients to develop arterial disease. Complications of diabetic neuropathy complicate the situation, as the patient may sustain injury to the lower limb without any discomfort.

Look for varicose veins, varicose ulcers or oedema. Oedema means swelling of the tissues due to an increase in interstitial fluid. Generalised oedema may be due to a disorder of the heart, kidneys, liver or gut. Clinically, oedema is detected in peripheral tissue, usually in the legs, back of the thighs and the lumbosacral area in the semirecumbent patient and can be displaced by firm finger pressure, which leaves a pit when the finger is removed. Cardiac oedema differs from stasis oedema, which occurs in the elderly or immobile patients. Looking for other signs of heart failure makes the distinction. In a patient who has normal jugular venous pressure, peripheral oedema is rarely the result of heart failure.

Brachial pulse

Assessment of the brachial pulse is best undertaken by using the thumb of the right hand, applied to the front of the elbow first medial to the biceps tendon with the fingers cupped round the back of the elbow. A large volume pulse occurs in patients with vasodilatation or aortic reflux, a small volume pulse where the peripheral arteries are constricted, or the cardiac output is low. A pulse with two *bumps*, called a bisferious pulse, is occasionally felt at the elbow in patients with aortic stenosis/incompetence.

The carotid pulse

The carotid pulse is more accurate for assessing pulse character than the brachial pulse and is a better reflection of left ventricular function:

- The best way to take the carotid pulse is to have the patient lying on a bed or couch. Carotid artery pressure can cause bradycardia and hypotension (carotid sinus syncope).
- Bilateral massage of the carotid sinus should never be attempted.
- Use the left thumb for the carotid, and vice versa.
- Press the thumb gently *backwards* to feel the pulse against the front of the cervical vertebrae.

The radial pulse

The radial pulse is readily felt just laterally to the tendon of the flexor carpi radialis muscle. It is used to assess heart rate and rhythm. As the radial pulse is a relatively long way from the heart, it is not a good pulse from which to assess the pulse character. In patients with suspected coarctation of the aorta, it is helpful simultaneously to feel the radial and the femoral pulse. Where coarctation exists, there is a diminished volume of the femoral pulse but it is also appreciably delayed compared with the radial pulse.

The popliteal pulse

The popliteal pulse lies deep within the popliteal fossa. To examine this pulse it is important to compress it against the posterior surface of the distal end of the femur. With the patient lying flat and knee slightly bent, press the tips of the finger of one hand into the popliteal fossa. With both hands around the knee, use the fingers of the other hand to apply pressure. The popliteal pulse is a useful pulse to locate in patients with peripheral vascular disease where there is absence of foot pulses.

Evaluation of jugular venous pressure

1. Assessment of the jugular venous pressure (JVP) is an important evaluation of the 'input' side of the heart.
2. There are no valves between the right atrium and the internal jugular vein. This lies deep to the sternal and clavicular heads of the sternomastoid. This muscle needs to be relaxed to examine the internal jugular.
3. The internal jugular vein is in direct communication, with the superior vena cava and the right atrium.
4. The normal pressure in the right atrium is equivalent to that exerted by a column of blood 10–12 cm tall. Therefore, when the patient is standing or sitting upright, the internal jugular vein is collapsed and when the patient is lying flat, it is completely filled. If the patient lies supine at approximately 45°, the point at which jugular venous pulsation becomes visible is usually just above the clavicle. This is the position actually chosen for examination of the JVP. Measurement of the JVP is usually undertaken with the neck slightly flexed and looking straight ahead.
5. Once the JVP has been identified, the examiner must try to assess first, the mean height of pulsation above the right atrial level and secondly, the wave form of jugular venous pulsation above the manubriosternal angle. The height of the manubriosternal angle above the mid-right atrium is approximately constant, irrespective of whether the patient is lying, sitting or standing. A normal JVP is less than it was above the manubriosternal angle. If jugular venous pulsation can be seen with the patient sitting upright, then the JVP is raised (Fig. 8.3).

Causes of a raised jugular venous pressure

- Hypervolaemia (fluid overload)
- Cardiac failure
- Pulmonary embolism
- Pericardial constriction or tamponade
- Pericarditis.

Distinction of the JVP from the carotid pulse involves the following five features

- timing
- the ability to compress and obliterate the JVP
- the demonstration of hepatojugular reflux
- the alteration of the JVP with position
- the site of the pulsation itself.

Examination of precordium

Inspection. With the patient's chest exposed, examine the precordium and assess the breathing pattern. An active heart may indicate ventricular dilatation from aortic or mitral regurgitation.

Palpation. Palpate the precordium by laying the flat of the hand and the outstretch fingers on the chest wall to the left of the sternum.

Check for thrills, apex beat, abnormal pulsation and palpable sounds. The normal adult apex beat with the patient lying supine at 45° is in the fifth and sixth intercostal space, in the midclavicular line. To assess the quality of the impulses the patient should be rolled on his left side. This is particularly important in obese patients or those suffering from emphysema.

Abnormalities of the apex beat:

- Diffuse or dyskinetic apex beat can appear post-MI where there has been damage to the myocardium.
- Sustained or 'heaving' in the presence of left ventricular hypertrophy.
- In mitral stenosis, the cardiac apex is described as tapping. The loud first heart sound is palpable as well as audible.
- Right ventricular hypertrophy is felt as a heave close to the left sternal border.

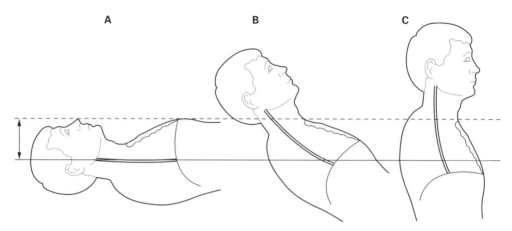

Figure 8.3 *Measuring jugular venous pressure:* **A** *the jugular vein is completely filled when the patient is lying flat;* **B** *jugular vein pulsation just becomes visible above the clavicle when the patient is positioned at 45 degrees;* **C** *the internal jugular vein is collapsed when patient is standing.*

During palpation, feel for vibration or thrills: these present as palpable murmurs, which accompany the murmurs of aortic stenosis, ventricular septal defect and pulmonary stenosis.

Standard methods for auscultation of the heart

- Before trying to decipher what may be the underlying cause of a murmur, it is important to first understand what the normal heart sounds are, and what normal variations of these sounds may occur.
- A good stethoscope is essential. The diaphragm of the stethoscope filters out low-pitched sounds and helps to identify high-pitched ones, such as the second heart sound.
- The bell is essential for listening to the low-pitched sounds, such as the murmur of mitral stenosis.

Cardiac auscultation

The most obvious of the heart sounds are the first and second sounds of S_1 and S_2, which demarcate systole from diastole. S_1 is the sound that marks the approximate beginning of systole, and is created when the increases in intraventricular pressure during contraction exceed the pressure within the atria, causing a hidden closing of the tricuspid and mitral valves. The ventricles continue to contract throughout systole, forcing blood through the aortic and pulmonary, or semilunar valves. At the end of systole, the ventricles begin to relax, the pressures within the heart become less than that in the aorta and pulmonary artery. A brief back flow of blood causes the semilunar valves to snap shut, producing S_2.

Although S_1 and S_2 are considered to be discrete sounds, you will notice that each is created by the near-instantaneous closing of two separate valves. For the most part, it is enough to consider that these sounds are single and instantaneous. However, it is worth remembering the actual order of the closures, because certain conditions can split these sounds into separate valve components. During S_1, the closing of the mitral valve slightly precedes the closing of the tricuspid valve, while in S_2 the aortic valve closes just before the pulmonary valve. Rather than memorise this order, if you remember that the pressure during systole in the left ventricle is much greater than in the right, you can predict that the mitral valve closes before the tricuspid in S_1. Similarly, because the pressure at the start of diastole in the aorta is much higher than in the pulmonary artery, the aorta valve closes first in S_2. Knowing the order of valve closure makes understanding of the different reasons for splitting of heart sounds easier. When listening to a patient's heart, the cadence of the beat will usually distinguish S_1 from S_2. However, certain conditions can shorten diastole to the point where it is difficult to discern which is S_1 and which is S_2. For this reason, it is important to *always* palpate the carotid or radial pulse when auscultating. The heart sound you hear when you first feel the pulse is S_1 and when the pulse disappears it is S_2.

When a valve is stenotic or damaged, the abnormal turbulent flow of blood produces a murmur which can be heard during the normally quiet times of systole or diastole. This murmur may not be audible over all areas of the chest, and it is important to note where it is heard best and where it radiates to (Fig. 8.4).

Third and fourth heart sounds

These are abnormal heart sounds that are heard in addition to the normal sounds in patients with certain specific conditions. The third heart sound is a low-pitched thudding sound that occurs in diastole and coincides with the end of the rapid phase of ventricular filling. It occurs in two distinct sets of circumstances: one is physiological, the other pathological. A physiological heart sound occurs in young fit athletes, in the presence of fever or during pregnancy. It is of no pathological significance. A pathological third heart sound is usually a marker for severe impairment of left ventricular function. It can be heard in dilated cardiomyopathy, after acute myocardial infarction (specifically the right ventricle) or in acute massive pulmonary embolism. In patients with a pathological third heart sound, there is nearly always a tachycardia. The name gallop rhythm has been given to describe the first, second and third heart sound, which can be heard as 'da-da-boom'. A fourth heart sound is an extra heart sound that coincides with atrial contraction. It is usually best heard in patients whose left atrium is hypertrophied (e.g. as a consequence of systemic hypertension or hypertrophic cardiomyopathy. It is not, however, heard in mitral stenosis. A fourth heart sound sounds like 'da-lub-dub, de-lub.'

Added sounds

Ejection Click. This is a high-pitched ringing sound that very quickly follows after the first heart sound and is associated with aortic or pulmonary valve stenosis.

The murmur of aortic stenosis is typically a mid-systolic ejection murmur best heard over the aortic area or right second intercostal space, with radiation into the right neck.

Opening Snap. There is a loud S_1, as the mitral valve opens throughout diastole and is suddenly slammed shut by ventricular systole.

Innocent cardiac murmurs in the paediatric patient

One of the more common cardiac-related problems in primary health care is the child who has a heart murmur. Between 50% to 90% of children will have a detectable heart murmur during some point in their lives. The advanced practitioner needs to be able to detect and evaluate these murmurs, differentiating between the functional and non-functional presentation. Guidelines for identifying innocent cardiac murmurs will be presented here. Further readings for more in depth cardiac assessments are provided at the end of the chapter.

Definition: An innocent cardiac murmur is a murmur that is not associated with any structural or physiological abnormality. This is in contrast to a pathological or non-functional heart murmur which is caused by cardiovascular structural abnormalities or a physiological murmur resulting from a physiological change in the body such as anaemia.

Subjective findings

The child that has a functional murmur will present with a history that is normal in relation to:
■ Age-appropriate growth rate and developmental levels.

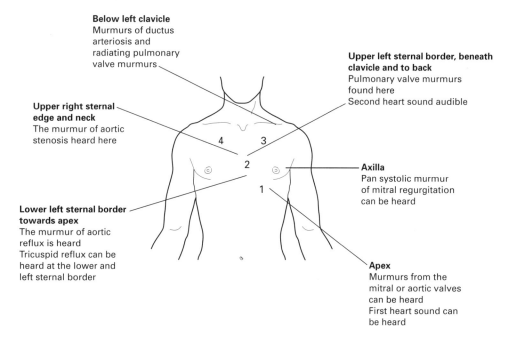

1. Mitral regurgitation: apex, axilla
2. Aortic regurgitation: lower left sternal border
3. Pulmonary stenoses: upper left sternal border/clavicle
4. Aortic stenoses: apex, upper right sternal border, neck

Figure 8.4 *Cardiac auscultation.*

Table 8.1 *Paediatric cardiac murmurs*

Characteristics of murmur	Age of child when most commonly detected	Type of murmur
Short, midsystolic blowing murmur. Grade 1/6–2/6. May be heard in front, back and axillae. Noted in right chest as well as the left. Disappears by about 3 months of age	Infant	Peripheral pulmonic stenosis (PPS)
Low-pitched systolic ejection murmur with a musical or vibratory quality. Best heard halfway between the lower left sternal border and the apex. Intensifies in supine position. Sounds louder with fever or exercise	Toddler–middle childhood. May be present as late as adolescence	Still's murmur
Heard continuously throughout systole and diastole. Noted best on the right side of the chest at the level of the clavicles. Turning the child's head away from the murmur or compressing the internal jugular vein on the side of the murmur may modify or obliterate it. Disappears in supine position	Toddler–middle childhood	Venous hum
High-pitched systolic ejection murmur ranging from 1/6–3/6. Best heard in supraclavicular area and may radiate to lower neck. Accentuates with light pressure on subclavian artery, but disappears with firmer pressure	Middle childhood and adolescents	Supraclavicular bruit
Systolic ejection murmur that is loudest at the upper left sternal border, particularly in the recumbent child. It may disappear when the child sits up. High-pitched, it may be soft or harsh. The intensity is 1/6–3/6	Middle childhood and adolescents (most common innocent murmur noted in the adolescent)	Pulmonary flow murmur
A usually continuous murmur that may be related to systolic ejection. Best heard in 2nd or 3rd interspace in the mid-clavicular line, either right or left haemothorax. Light pressure with the stethoscope may accentuate it, firm pressure abolishes it.	Adolescents	Mammary-souffle.

- Activities of daily living, particularly feeding in the infant and activity levels in the toddler and child.
- Negative complaints for signs and symptoms that may be indicative of heart disease. This would include such symptoms as circumoral cyanosis in the infant while feeding, poor exercise tolerance in the toddler and older child, and respiratory distress.

Objective findings

Vital signs. Vital signs will be within normal limits for the child's age.

Physical exam. Findings will be normal. Innocent cardiac murmurs, with the exception of a venous hum and mammary souffle, are never heard in diastole and never associated with other adventitious cardiac sounds or signs of cardiac disease. They are characteristically soft,

not louder than a grade 3/6, vary in intensity with change in position and are associated with normal S_1 and S_2 sounds. Table 8.1 lists the paediatric cardiac murmurs that may be auscultated by the practitioner on cardiac examination.

Assessment: Refer to Table 8.1. R/O pathological or physiological murmur.

Plan

Consult with other members of the team regarding follow-up and further evaluation.

Diagnostics: Consider ECG, if functional murmur status is questionable.

Management: Parental education is paramount. Reassure parents that the murmur is innocent and commonly noted. It is likely to come and go throughout childhood and the child does not have a heart condition. No limitations should be placed on the child's activity. Written material to further reinforce information discussed during the consultation is often helpful.

Indications for referral

Immediate. Any child that is unstable or acutely ill with suspected heart disease should be referred on an emergency basis. Children with suspected heart disease and whose conditions are stable should also be referred but on a less immediate basis. Always consult with your GP.

Follow-up. Children should return for further monitoring if signs and symptoms of heart disease are noted. Periodic checks of normal growth and development should be carried out per practice protocol.

Complications

No complications should be noted with a functional heart murmur.

Diagnostic tests

Blood tests

Full blood count

- Anaemia can cause heart failure, angina or shortness of breath on exertion.
- Raised mean cell volume can occur with excess alcohol.
- A raised erythrocyte sedimentation rate (ESR) could indicate vasculitis.

Electrolytes (potassium, K)

- Normal value: 3.5–5.0 mmol/l
- low K < 3.0 mmol/l: low U-wave amplitude on ECG.
- low K < 2.7 mmol/l: low T-wave amplitude on ECG.
- *Note.* with elderly patients, consider diuretic use.
- High K 5.5–6.5 mmol/l: peaked T waves on ECG.
- High K 7.0–8.0 mmol/l: low P waves on ECG.
- High K 9.0–11.0 mmol/l: widening QRS on ECG.
- *Note.* If potassium is high, there is a likelihood of arrhythmias, especially sinus bradycardia, AV block and ventricular fibrillation. NB Consider angiotensin converting enzyme (ACE) inhibitor use and renal failure as contributory causes.

High and low values of calcium (Ca) and magnesium (Mg) also affect the normal ECG pattern.

Thyroid function test

- Thyroid-stimulating hormone (THS): 0.3–5.0 U/l.
- Tri-iodothyronine (T_3): 1.1–2.8 nmol/l (under 65); 0.5–2.2 nmol/l (over 65).
- Thyroxine (T_4): 9–23 pmol/l.
- *Note.* Hyperthyroidism can cause tachycardia/heart failure/atrial fibrillation. Myxoedema may cause bradycardia.

Cardiac enzymes

These are released by necrotic cellular tissue. The first assay is often normal if taken < 12 hours after the onset of pain, with at least three-fold increases seen in subsequent analyses. Administration of a thrombolytic drug can stop the enzyme rise.

Creatinine kinase (CK). This enzyme peaks within 24 hours of an MI, usually returning to normal after 48 hours. The brain and skeletal muscle also produce CK; the myocardial-bound (MB) isoenzyme fraction (CK-MB) is specific for heart muscle damage. Large infarcts usually produce high serum levels of CK (upper limit of normal (ULN)=1201 U/l).

Aspartate aminotransferase (AST). This enzyme, is a less specific indicator of MI as it is also released following injury to red blood cells, kidney, liver and lungs. In MI, AST peaks at 24–48 hours and may fall to normal by 72 hours. The normal level is <40 IU/l.

Lactate dehydrogenase (LDH). After MI the level of LDH peaks at 4–5 days and can take 2 weeks to return to normal. The typical range of normal is 200–560 U/l. LDH is also released following damage to the liver, skeletal muscle and red blood cells.

Troponin T or I. Some laboratories use the cardiac muscle enzymes for acute MI and for risk stratification in unstable angina. The levels begin to rise 4 hours post MI; 12–24 hours gives the highest reading, but elevation can persist up to 7 days after MI. The test is around eight times more expensive than the CK-MB. ULN is 0.2 µg/l (MIMS 2000).

The electrocardiogram

The electrocardiogram (ECG) is an invaluable aid to studying heart rhythm. It works by picking up and amplifying the very small electrical potential changes between different points on the surface of the body caused by the cyclical depolarisation and repolarisation of the heart cells. The electrocardiograph (also abbreviated ECG) is a record of the electrical activity of the heart recorded at the skin surface. Three bipolar leads (1.11.111) and nine unipolar leads (AVR-V6) are usually displayed (Fig. 8.5A). The potential differences coming from the heart are represented by the **vector v** whose origin is at the centre of the Einthoven triangle and whose projection on each of the three sides of the triangle produces the corresponding standard leads 1 11 111. One can imagine the three standard leads as the sides of a triangle with the heart in the centre (Fig. 8.5B).

The sinus rhythm

The sinus node is the pacemaker of the normal heart. It depolarises spontaneously at regular intervals, which determines the heart rate. The sinus node is influenced by a variety of neurohumoral factors, particularly vagal and sympathetic activity. Atrial depolarisation (P wave)

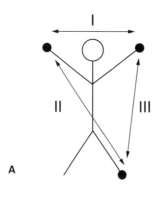

Figure 8.5 *Electrocardiogram (ECG) record of the electrical activity of the heart recorded at the skin surface.*
A Three bipolar leads (I–III) and nine unipolar leads (aVR–V$_6$) are usually displayed. B The paper speed is 25 mm per second, such that each small square (1 mm) represents 0.04 seconds and each large square (5 mm) represents 0.20 seconds. The square wave is a calibration signal: 1 cm vertical deflection = 1 mV. A calibration signal should be included with every 12 lead ECG recording.

is followed by ventricular depolarisation (QRS) complex and ventricular repolarization (T wave). The sequence of ECG deflections occurring at regular intervals is the hallmark of sinus rhythm.

Abnormalities of the heart rhythm can be divided into those in which the heart goes too slowly (bradycardia) and those in which the rate is abnormally rapid (tachycardia). Physiologically, heart rate can vary in a normal young adult from 40 beats/min during sleep to 180 beats/min or more during vigorous exercise.

Note. Vagal tone (slows the heart); sympathetic force (speeds up the heart).

Supraventricular dysrythmias

Supraventricular dysrythmias are arrhythmias that arise in areas of the heart above the ventricles. Supraventricular dysrhythmias per se are not especially harmful. This is because dysrhythmic activity within the atria does not significantly reduce cardiac output (except in patients with valvular disorders and heart failure). Supraventricular tachy dysrhythmias *can* be dangerous, however, in the AV node, resulting in excitation of the ventricles. If the atria drive the ventricles at an excessive rate, diastolic filling will be incomplete and cardiac output will decline. Hence when treating supraventricular dysrythmias, the objective is frequently one of (blocking impulse conduction through the AV node and *not* elimination of the dysrhythmia itself.

Common supraventricular dysrythmias

Atrial flutter and fibrillation

Atrial flutter and fibrillation are two disorders of rhythm characterised by an atrial tachycardia in which the activation of the atria is ectopic and proceeds at a rate which is higher than normal:

- Between 200 and 400 beats/min for flutter and between 400 and 700 beats/min for fibrillation.
- In flutter, each atrial (F) ends at the AV node which rarely responds to each stimulus (producing a 1:1 block at 300/min). More often to one out of two or three (flutter called 2:1, 3:1) causing a functionally incomplete AV block.
- In atrial fibrillation, the atrial stimuli are numerous (400–700/min) and this results in grossly disorganised activity of the atrial myocardium, which shows itself by fibrillation waves clearly seen in V$_1$. The ventricles respond irregularly to these multiple disorganised auricular stimuli. The AV node is blocked to a proportion of these; hence, the irregular ventricular rate produces a complete arrhythmia. Generally, the ventricular rate is rapid, producing a complete tachyarrhythmia.

Supraventricular tachycardia

Supraventricular tachycardia (SVT) is caused by a rapidly firing ectopic focus located in the atria or in the

AV node. Heart rate is increased to 150–250 beats/min. In the case of atrial tachycardia, the P waves are equal in number to the ventricular responses. Ventricular rate is rapid and regular, usually equal or faster than 160 beats/min with normal ventricular complexes.

❶ The need to treat the arrhythmia is determined by the haemodynamic effect it is having: for example, a rapid atrial arrhythmia can precipitate heart failure and a drop in blood pressure. Further investigations are required in the hospital-setting where DC conversion (cardioversion) may be carried out followed by commencement on antiarrhythmic medication and an anticoagulant such as warfarin.

A 24-hour ambulatory ECG is a useful diagnostic technique for arrhythmias. The patient wears the chest electrodes attached to a tape recorder worn around the waist. Recordings over a period of time are analysed via a computer. These are available for use by the GP; however, they are commonly given to patients when they are under investigation by the hospital consultant.

Ventricular dysrythmias

Ventricular premature beats are beats that occur before they should in the cardiac cycle. These beats are caused by ectopic ventricular foci. The ventricular ectopics can arise from a single ectopic focus or from several foci. In the absence of additional signs of heart disease, ventricular ectopies are benign and not usually treated. However, in the presence of acute MI, ventricular ectopics may predispose the patient to ventricular fibrillation.

Ventricular fibrillation

Ventricular fibrillation is a life-threatening emergency and requires immediate treatment. This dysrythmia results from the asynchronous discharge of multiple ventricular ectopic foci. Because many different foci are firing, and because each focus indicates contraction on its immediate vicinity, localised twitching takes place all over the ventricles, making coordinated ventricular contraction impossible. As a result, the pumping action of the heart stops. In the absence of blood flow, the patient becomes unconscious and cyanotic. If heart beat is not restored rapidly, death soon follows.

- ❶ There are legal issues surrounding the area of cardiopulmonary resuscitation.
- Make sure you are properly trained and that the area in which you work has the right equipment to undertake this.
- There are many good courses available through local hospitals. Find out what the local policy is and discuss it with the primary care team.
- Appointing appropriate persons to maintain and check emergency equipment, oxygen and drugs is essential to the management of the emergency situation.
- If you are in an area that is covered by a cardiac ambulance be familiar with the telephone number and how to request this. Speedy action could save the

patient's life as the cardiac team or ambulance personnel will carry the appropriate equipment to treat the patient appropriately.

The following tests are common diagnostic tests, which are available by referral to hospital.

Exercise (stress) ECG

Exercise tests while time consuming, are particularly useful in symptomatic (anginal patients). They are also used to evaluate cardiac function, post-MI recovery and exercise induced arrhythmias.

The stress test is a graduated treadmill exercise usually with 3-min segments at an increasing gradient up to 12 min, followed by a recovery phase of about 10 min. Blood pressure is measured simultaneously. Tests must be carried out under medical supervision, with full resuscitation provision available.

Note. Contraindications to stress ECG

Contraindications comprise aortic stenosis; myopericarditis; fever; unstable angina; and heart failure.

In fit post-MI patients who can climb a flight of stairs, a stress ECG at 7–10 days post-infarct is acceptable. Termination usually occurs at 85% of maximal predicted heart rate. Other reasons for stopping the test are worsening angina, progressive ST segment depression (> 2 mm), falling blood pressure, arrhythmias and heart block.

Where possible, digoxin should be stopped for 1 week prior to the test, to avoid spurious ST changes. Beta-blockers can be continued, but may reduce the sensitivity of the test for diagnosing angina (MIMS 2000).

Angiography

The advent of echocardiography has reduced the need for cardiac catheterisation in both congenital and adult heart disease and more modern techniques such as digital subtraction angiography and the use of radionuclides have reduced this need further.

Coronary angiography (catheterisation) is often combined with balloon angioplasty and stent insertion for coronary artery stenoses.

Useful hints

- As well as all invasive procedures, full informed consent is mandatory.
- All medication, except for morning diuretics can be continued, but warfarin should be stopped at least 4 hours before the test.
- Nil by mouth for 24 hours is advised.
- Most operators prefer the femoral artery entry site. The brachial route can also be used.

Echocardiography

Echocardiography is now a standard non-invasive investigation. It will confirm the diagnosis of heart failure, assess the degree of heart failure and determine the aetiology. Indications for open access echocardiography are:

- suspected heart failure
- murmur
- borderline hypertension
- atrial fibrillation
- screening relatives of patients with hypertrophic cardiomyopathy.

M-mode and two-dimensional screening

An M-mode or (motion mode) recording is constructed by transmitting and receiving ultrasound along only one scan line, thus giving substantially greater sensitivity than two-dimensional echocardiography for recording moving structures. The returning echoes are displayed as a graph against time. M-mode is used for timing events within the heart and measurement of cardiac dimensions (Chambers 1996). In two-dimensional echocardiography, a fan-shaped wavefront is produced. The anatomical views usually studied are parasternal long and short axis, four-chamber view and subcostal view.

Differential diagnosis

The aetiology of chest pain can be divided into cardiac and non-cardiac pain (Fig. 8.6):
- gastro-oesophageal disease
- ischaemic heart disease
- chest wall syndromes

- pericarditis
- pleurisy/pneumonia
- pulmonary embolism
- lung cancer
- aortic aneurysm
- herpes zoster.

Acute MI can be differentiated from angina pectoris in that pain caused by MI lasts longer (20–30 min) and is not relieved by nitroglycerine. Some patients confuse the pain of MI with indigestion. An organised history and physical assessment will provide the basis of a differential diagnosis. The information solicited during the chest pain history includes the character of the chest pain, associated symptoms, risk factors for common aetiologies and past medical history.

Angina

Angina can be defined as chest tightness occurring on exertion or at rest and is caused by myocardial ischaemia. Angina results as an imbalance between myocardial oxygen supply and demand, and in most cases is due to atheroma of the larger epicardial coronary arteries. Coronary artery spasm also causes angina but is unusual in the absence of at least some evidence of atheromatous plaque disease. Other conditions that more rarely cause angina include aortic valve

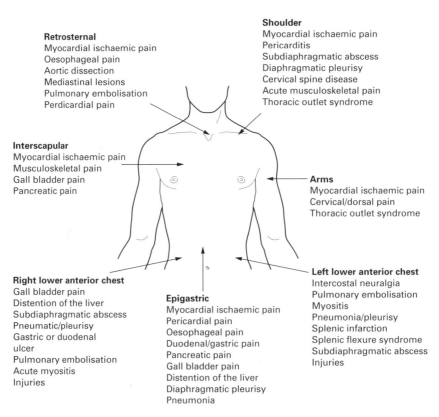

Shoulder
Myocardial ischaemic pain
Pericarditis
Subdiaphragmatic abscess
Diaphragmatic pleurisy
Cervical spine disease
Acute musculoskeletal pain
Thoracic outlet syndrome

Retrosternal
Myocardial ischaemic pain
Oesophageal pain
Aortic dissection
Mediastinal lesions
Pulmonary embolisation
Perdicardial pain

Interscapular
Myocardial ischaemic pain
Musculoskeletal pain
Gall bladder pain
Pancreatic pain

Arms
Myocardial ischaemic pain
Cervical/dorsal pain
Thoracic outlet syndrome

Right lower anterior chest
Gall bladder pain
Distention of the liver
Subdiaphragmatic abscess
Pneumatic/pleurisy
Gastric or duodenal ulcer
Pulmonary embolisation
Acute myositis
Injuries

Epigastric
Myocardial ischaemic pain
Pericardial pain
Oesophageal pain
Duodenal/gastric pain
Pancreatic pain
Gall bladder pain
Distention of the liver
Diaphragmatic pleurisy
Pneumonia

Left lower anterior chest
Intercostal neuralgia
Pulmonary embolisation
Myositis
Pneumonia/pleurisy
Splenic infarction
Splenic flexure syndrome
Subdiaphragmatic abscess
Injuries

Figure 8.6 *Sites of pain.*

disease, left ventricular hypertrophy, anaemia and a variety of metabolic disorders.

Variant angina

This is also known as Prinzmetal's angina and is caused by spasm of the coronary artery. It usually occurs at rest and in response to cold. Often it occurs at a consistent time of the day, usually at night or early morning. It is distinguished from other forms of angina by the presence of ST segment elevation on the ECG during periods of ischaemia (in contrast to more usual ST segment depression seen in other forms of angina).

Oesophageal pain versus cardiac ischaemia

Chronic or intermittent oesophageal pain is central and, like angina, may radiate to the arms and back. It does not, however, radiate to the jaw or teeth. It may apparently be induced by exercise (which can cause oesophageal reflux) but then it lasts longer than angina. It is not induced by emotional stress and is not affected by cold or windy weather. There is usually a relationship between the pain and eating. This can also be true of angina (typically exercising after a meal). Antacids relieve oesophageal pain unlike angina, and a trial for a period of 1 month can be a good diagnostic test.

Subjective findings

- *Onset*. Usually > 1–2 min.
- *Provocation*. Physical exertion, emotional stress, or cold.
- *Palliation*. Rest, nitroglycerin, beta-blockades, calcium channel antagonists.
- *Quality*. Pressure/squeezing, also dull or sharp.
- *Quantity*. Variable, with greater demand on the heart.
- *Radiation*. Retrosternal or precordial. It can radiate to left shoulder, ulnar aspect of arm, interscapular or epigastric region.
- *Associated symptoms*. Dyspnoea, palpitations; nausea or weakness.
- *Underlying conditions*. Hypertension, diabetes mellitus, hyperlipidaemia, smoking, family history, obesity and sedentary lifestyle.

Objective findings

- If physical findings are present, they are often subtle. The baseline function in patients presenting with angina is limitation of physical activity. An important aspect of the onset of exertional angina is the lag period. A certain amount of physical activity must be sustained before the pain occurs. The pain will usually subside after a period of rest. Absence of a lag period suggests a non-ischaemic aetiology.
- A careful examination should detect signs of significant aortic valve disease, which may be the cause of angina, or simply a compounding factor.
- Signs of heart failure should also be looked for, since these will require specific therapy and carry an adverse prognosis.

- Angina patients often have vascular disease elsewhere and evidence for this should be sought during physical examination.
- The carotid and peripheral pulses should be examined carefully.
- A hypertensive tendency might be due to coexistent renovascular disease.

Diagnosis and investigations

- Physical examination and resting ECG are usually normal. An abnormal resting ECG is associated with a worse prognosis and left ventricular dysfunction.
- Full blood count, renal function, cholesterol and possibly T_4 should be considered.
- Treadmill exercise ECG does not necessarily exclude a diagnosis of angina; however, a negative treadmill is associated with a good prognosis.

Therapeutic intervention

1. Patients with mild symptoms are usually started on a trial of glyceryl trinitrate (nitroglycerin). If no response, consider re-diagnosis. Aspirin has been shown to reduce the incidence of infarction and many patients are now commenced on 75 mg per day (Hanssom et al 1998).
2. Moderate to severe symptoms are relieved by the addition of prophylactic oral therapy. Beta-blockade is commonly prescribed as first-line anti-anginal agents.
3. Angina shows a marked circadian variation, with characteristic early morning ischaemic episodes. It is important to initiate medication that gives 24 hour cover.
4. In the majority of cases, intervention will be on symptomatic grounds after failure of optimal medical therapy.
5. Coronary angiography is often reserved for cases where intervention is contemplated.

Patient education

- Patients should be given lifestyle advice, such as stopping smoking, reduction in alcohol and advice on lipid management.
- Patients can present with anxiety and a fear of the impending diagnosis. This is important to remember in your management plan.
- The patient may be unsure of his limitation regarding exercise or sexual activity. Some patients may find it difficult to discuss these issues. There are some useful leaflets produced, which can help reduce anxiety. Try the British Heart Foundation or your local coronary care unit.
- Patients may ask about fitness to drive. Group I licence can be issued for patients with controlled symptoms. Group II licences are obtained from Vehicle Licensing (Medical Advisory branch) – see Useful Addresses.

Referral

- All patients presenting for the first time with symptoms of angina should be referred for investigation after initial assessment.
- *Unstable angina.* The term unstable angina describes either the onset of typical angina (within the last 2–4 weeks); that occurring at rest or a changing pattern with increasing frequency and/or severity for no obvious reason. Each of these suggests an unstable atheromatous plaque in the coronary arteries. *Urgent referral is recommended.*

Acute myocardial infarction

Note. If you suspect an acute myocardial infarction do not hesitate in seeking medical help. The chest pain of acute MI is typically crushing, central and often associated with breathlessness. Pain can radiate anywhere around the chest, arms and neck. This is a cardiological emergency and necessitates a quick diagnosis. Patients undergoing acute MI typically experience severe substernal pressure that they characterise as unbearable crushing or constructing pain. The World Health Organisation defines cardiac pain as:

> *In the front of the chest, mid or upper sternum radiating to the left arm or both arms, round the chest or into the jaw. Rarely of more than 30 minutes duration unless a coronary thrombosis has occurred. The words used to describe it are tight, heavy, constricting, numbing or burning.*

The important points in the history are the site of the pain, its quality and intensity, the time sequence and duration and the factors affecting it, e.g. eating, exercise, breathing or movement. Secondary features such as sweating, vomiting, other symptoms, and his approach to his condition are also important. Past history of similar events and a drug history, whether he is working, and his smoking habits, are all most relevant (Mead & Patterson 1992).

Remember *site, radiation, character, severity and duration, aggravating factors and relieving factors.*

General points

1. Do not waste time.
2. An ECG is an urgent priority to back up clinical findings.
3. Intravenous access makes easier access of drugs, such as diamorphine, for pain relief and an antiemetic.
4. Oxygen and oral aspirin 300 mg should be given.
5. If there is ST elevation of 1 mm in a limb lead or 2 mm in a chest lead, or if there is bundle branch block with a clinical infarct, then thrombolysis should be started as soon as possible if there are no contraindications. Each centre varies in the management of thrombolysis. Some GPs are happy to instigate treatment and others to await the arrival of an appropriate ambulance.
6. Provide gentle reassurance until the patient is transported to hospital by ambulance.
7. Be up to date with recussitation procedures and equipment use.
8. Biochemical markers play no role in the initial assessment, but are important later in confirming diagnosis.
9. There is controversy over which thrombolytic is best used in practice. Tissue plasminogen activator (t-PA) is safer in the hypotensive patient and is used in many hospitals where there is evidence of large anterior infarcts. Streptokinase, however, is much cheaper (MIMS 2000).

❶ Acute myocardial infarction is a condition that occasionally presents in general practice and therefore professionals need to keep abreast of current trends in its management in practice.

Post–MI, therapeutic intervention

Post-MI patients should be targeted for secondary prevention:

1. In clinical practice the top priority for prevention should be patients with CHD or other major atherosclerotic disease, with the object of reducing the risk of a further major ischaemic event.
2. In patients with CHD, rigorous control of blood pressure, lipids and glucose is recommended with the following treatment targets:
   - blood pressure less than 140 mmHg systolic and less than 85 mmHg diastolic
   - total cholesterol less than 5.0 mmol/l (low-density lipoprotein (LDL) cholesterol less than 3.0 mmol/l).
3. Diabetes mellitus should be optimally controlled with insulin during and immediately following acute MI, and blood pressure reduced to <130 mmHg systolic and < 80 mmHg diastolic.
4. Cardioprotective drug therapy should be considered and prescribed in selective patients: i.e. aspirin for all patients; beta-blockers particularly in high-risk patients (where there is no contraindication); cholesterol lowering therapy; ACE inhibitors for those patients with symptoms or signs of heart failure at the time of MI; anticoagulants for patients at risk of systemic embolisation with large anterior infarctions, severe heart failure, left ventricular aneurysm or paroxysmal tachycardia (Wood et al 1998).

Patient education

- The aims of rehabilitation are to restore normal social and economic living and to prevent further progression of the disease. This requires a multidisciplinary approach to education from the specialist nurse and other health professionals to deliver a mix of education counselling and physical exercise.
- Lifestyle intervention, to discontinue smoking, make healthier food choices, increase aerobic exercise and moderate alcohol consumption.
- Involvement of the whole family is important if changes are to be implemented.

Hypertension

Hypertension affects approximately 23% of the adult population. Prevalence is approximately equal in men and women, although men tend to be affected at a younger age. Elevated blood pressure is associated with increased cardiovascular morbidity and mortality.

Additionally, abnormalities of lipid and glucose metabolism are found more commonly in hypertensive patients than in the general population. In recent years evidence from randomised control trials and meta-analysis has strengthened our understanding of the effectiveness of lifestyle and therapeutic interventions in reducing coronary and other atherosclerotic risk.

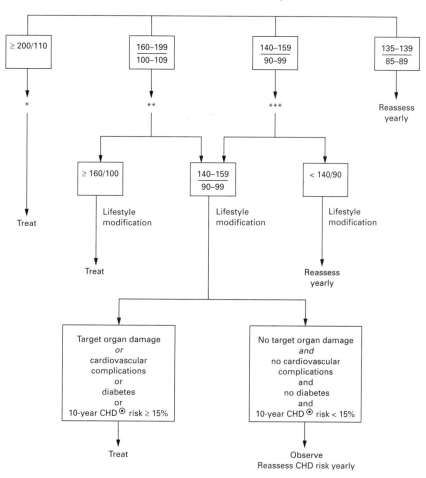

* Unless malignant phase, or hypertensive emergency, monitor for a short period of time then treat

** If cardiovascular complications, target organ damage, or diabetes is present, confirm over 3–4 weeks, then treat; if absent, remeasure weekly and treat if blood pressure persists at these levels over 4–12 weeks

*** If cardiovascular complications, target organ damage, or diabetes is present, confirm over 12 weeks, then treat; if absent, remeasure monthly and treat if these levels are maintained and if estimated 10-year CHD risk is ≥ 15%

⊙ Assessed with Cardiac Risk Assessor computer program or coronary heart disease risk chart

Figure 8.7 *Diagnosis and management of hypertension. Initial blood pressure are in millimetres of mercury (mmHg).*

All adults should have their blood pressure measured at least every 5 years. Those with high normal values (135–139/85–89) and those that have had high readings recorded at any time previously should have their blood pressure measured annually. The British Hypertension Guidelines (BHG) for measurement should be followed (Fig. 8.7).

Unfortunately, recent studies in both the UK and in the USA have shown that blood pressure is often poorly controlled. The BHG advocate reducing blood pressure below 140/85 mmHg; however, in practice, only a small proportion of hypertensive patients actually attain good blood pressure control. The Hypertension Optimal Treatment (HOT) Study showed that about 80% of subjects aged > 50 years with mild/moderate hypertension need at least two antihypertensive agents to achieve target blood pressure and about 30% need three or more drugs.

Note. There has been much debate on the relative importance of systolic blood pressure (SBP) and diastolic blood pressure (DBP), but in practice SBP should be regarded as the most important. SBP and DBP correlate closely. Outcome trials of antihypertension treatment based on thresholds of SBP and DBP have shown similar reductions in cardiovascular events. This has implications for thresholds for treatment and targets during treatment. Thus, when treatment is recommended at a blood pressure threshold of 140/90 mmHg, this means 140 mmHg systolic or 90 mmHg diastolic. A target of <140/85 mmHg means <140 mmHg systolic and < 85 mmHg diastolic (Passmore 2000).

Subjective assessment

- Ask about family history of ischaemic heart disease or stroke
- What age were parents or siblings when event occurred?
- Ask alcohol, smoking, salt intake, and diet
- Ask about physical exercise
- Note any previous documentation regarding lifestyle or blood pressure
- History of diabetes
- Record any medication currently in use.

Objective assessment

1. Assessment of the severity of hypertension should include a search for target organ damage, i.e. kidneys, arteries and heart.
2. Use of a standardised measurement is invaluable in clinical practice.
3. British Hypertension Guidelines on measurement are advocated.
4. Blood pressure should be measured in the sitting position from the right arm, after a resting period of 5 min, using a conventional sphygmomanometer with an appropriate cuff size.
5. The reading of the diastolic BP should be taken at the disappearance of the second sound (phase 5) and should be read to the nearest 2 mmHg.

6. At least two measurements are to be made at each visit. Three different readings are necessary to a diagnosis of hypertension.
7. In elderly patients and in patients with diabetes mellitus, standing blood pressure should be taken due to the problem of orthostatic hypotension.
8. 24-hour ambulatory blood pressure measurement (ABTM) may now be considered as indispensable to the diagnosis and management of hypertension. This should be incorporated into the total risk profile of patients with hypertension.

Indications for ambulatory blood pressure monitoring

- When clinical blood pressure shows unusual variability
- Hypertension is resistant to drug treatment
- When symptoms suggest the possibility of hypotension
- To diagnose 'white coat hypertension'.

Remember. Most patients with hypertension are asymptomatic and the condition is usually discovered by screening or casual blood pressure reading. The onset of symptoms may signal the onset of major complications (angina, heart failure or stroke).

Note. Personal estimations of cardiovascular risk are very inaccurate but improve when all major risk factors are weighted and counted using risk functions such as the Framington function. The formal estimation of CHD risk has been proposed as an aid to treatment decisions in hypertension and it is recommended that this is performed using the cardiac risk computer program or the CHD risk chart issued by the Joint British Societies. Cardiovascular risk can be estimated by multiplying the coronary risk by 4/3 (Passmore 2000).

Investigations

1. ECG and chest X-ray may demonstrate the presence of left ventricular hypertrophy or heart failure, although ECG is much more informative.
2. Measuring serum levels of urea and creatinine, as well as urinary blood and protein, can assess renal function.
3. Serum total: high-density lipoprotein (HDL) cholesterol ratio if one other risk factor for coronary heart disease, e.g. smoking, diabetes, obesity and family history of premature *secondary hypertension*.

Treatment for secondary hypertension depends on the underlying cause: surgery may be needed for renal artery stenosis, coarctation of the aorta, phaeochromocytoma or Conn's syndrome.

Therapeutic intervention

- Drug therapy for hypertension is usually lifelong. It is therefore better to try non-medical approaches first
- Drug treatment should be tailored to the individual to maximise compliance
- The most commonly used antihypertensives include diuretics, beta-blockers, calcium antagonists, alpha-

blockers, ACE inhibitors and angiotensin II antagonists..

Education

- For patients without clinical atherosclerotic disease the absolute risk of developing CHD (non-fatal MI or coronary death), or other athersclerotic disease, during the next 10 years should influence the intensity of the lifestyle and therapeutic intervention.
- As the absolute CHD risk increases, so should the intensity of the intervention: thus, maximising the potential benefit from risk factor reduction.
- Lifestyle intervention to discontinue smoking, making healthier food choices, increasing aerobic exercise and moderating alcohol consumption in all coronary and other atherosclerotic disease prevention programmes, both primary and secondary (Wood et al 1998).

Referral

Occasionally a patient with either essential or secondary hypertension may develop malignant hypertension, i.e. a hypertensive crisis. This is characterised by markedly elevated blood pressure, often with severe headache, vomiting, papilloedema or haemorrhages and exudates, cardiac and renal dysfunction, and convulsions or even coma. Treatment involves bed rest and reduction of blood pressure *gradually* over 24 hours to a DBP of between 90 and 100 mmHg (MIMS 2000).

Heart failure (chronic)

Direct myocardial impairment is usually the result of coronary artery disease and myocardial ischaemia, viral myocarditis, drugs and toxins. In the failing heart, increasing end-diastolic volume does not result in a proportionate increase in the volume of ejected blood, as occurs in healthy hearts, and therefore left ventricular end-diastolic pressure rises. This results in pulmonary congestion and oedema. In addition to excessive fluid overload, valvular regurgitation (aortic or mitral), atrial septal defects and post-infarction ventricular septal defect all contribute to an increase in preload. Afterload refers to the force the heart must generate to overcome peripheral vascular resistance. Hypertension is the commonest cause of increased afterload, but aortic stenosis, subvalvular stenosis and coarctation of the aorta must be considered. Other causes of heart failure are amyloid and sarcoid disease, iatrogenic causes, i.e. beta-blockers, antiarryhthmics, calcium antagonists, steroids and non-steroidal anti-inflammatory drugs (NSAIDs), and arrhythmias such as atrial fibrillation.

Subjective assessment

- Ask about fatigue, exhaustion. Patient may get fatigued on minimal exertion.
- Dyspnoea, orthopnoea, paroxysmal nocturnal dyspnoea or nocturnal dry cough may be a presenting feature, so ask about breathlessness.

- Is the breathlessness recent or has it been present for some time?
- Is it constant or does it come and go?
- What can't you do because of the breathlessness?
- What makes your breathing worse?
- Does anything make it better?
- Does the patient suffer from nocturia (reverse of diurnal rhythm).
- Does the patient cough up any sputum? What colour and consistency is it? Is it pink or frothy?
- Have they noticed any ankle swelling? Oedema may present at later stages in the thigh and sacral area.
- Ask about recent and past medical history.
- Current medication.

Left ventricular failure can lead to all of the above symptoms, but cold peripheries, palpitation, loss of appetite, weight loss, muscle wasting and cachexia can also be presenting symptoms. Right heart failure may also present with symptoms of nausea and anorexia.

Objective assessment

Carry out a full cardiovascular assessment. Observe in particular for:
- cold peripheries
- tachycardia
- low pulse volume
- pulsus alternans
- atrial fibrillation
- low blood pressure
- examine the carotid pulse for raised JVP
- listen for third and fourth heart sounds (gallop rhythm)
- listen for chest signs such as wheezes, fine basal crepitations and pleural effusion
- examine the abdomen for hepatomegaly and ascites
- observe any peripheral oedema.

Any valvular lesion, either obstruction (stenosis) or incompetence (regurgitation) can impair the circulation, resulting in heart failure.

Investigations

1. The initial investigations should include full blood count, renal and thyroid biochemistry, serum albumin.
2. A resting ECG.
3. A good quality chest X-ray. The chest X-ray is probably the single most important investigation as it has both prognostic and diagnostic importance. It can be repeated to monitor the clearing of pulmonary oedema and heart size.
4. Referral for ECG to distinguish between heart muscle abnormalities and valvular disease.
5. Referral for coronary angiography is important in patients with ongoing myocardial ischaemia who may be considered for revascularisation either by percutaneous coronary artery angioplasty or coronary artery bypass surgery.

Therapeutic intervention

- Diuretics reduce preload by causing diuresis and reducing breathlessness.
- ACE inhibitors are used widely in the management of heart failure. ACE inhibitors improve dyspnoea, exercise tolerance, reduce hospital admissions and prolong life expectancy.
- Angiotensin II antagonists have similar effects on symptoms as ACE inhibitors, but their effect on mortality is still under study (MIMS 2000).
- The use of inotropic agents such as digoxin are well established in patients with atrial fibrillation.
- Evidence is available that beta-blocking drugs can improve morbidity. However, patients with heart failure should be stabilised on a diuretic and ACE inhibitor before a beta-blocker is commenced and the starting dose must be very low.

Patient education

- Heart failure is often confined to the elderly, and the use of many different drugs (polypharmacy) can be confusing.
- Careful attention to the needs of the elderly includes a multidisciplinary approach in primary care: particularly, how and where they are able to obtain their prescriptions and how and when they take their medication.
- Take time to explain the purpose of the medication patients are taking, particularly in patients with hearing difficulties.
   ❶ Remember, elderly patients often have multiple pathology and may be taking a variety of medications, some of which can cause cardiovascular problems. For example, NSAIDs can cause fluid retention and raise blood pressure.

Acute heart failure

Clinical features of acute heart failure include (Ebstein et al 1997):
- acute dyspnoea (pulmonary oedema)
- hypotension (may be marked general vaso-constriction)
- cold clammy skin (peripheral vasoconstriction)
- anxiety
- confusion (impaired cerebral blood flow, hypoxaemia)
- oliguria.
   Acute heart failures (left ventricular failure or cardiogenic shock) are cardiological emergencies that are rarely seen in general practice and necessitate prompt medical intervention. Treatment with diamorphine 2.5–5 mg and furosemide 40 mg intravenously, sublingual GTN (glyceryl trinitrate) and oxygen. Sitting the patient upright reduces pulmonary oedema. Consider admission.

Pericarditic pain

Pericarditis is inflammation of the pericardium, the serous sac that surrounds the heart. It may be a complication of MI or occur as a result of viral or bacterial infection. Another important cause is uraemia.

Pericarditis causes pain that is retrosternal and may radiate to the shoulders or upper arm. It is accentuated by, or may only be present in, inspiration and also varies with posture. Unlike the pain of angina or MI, pericardic pain is related to movement (e.g. turning in bed) but not to physical exertion. It sometimes radiates to the tip of the shoulder.

Subjective findings

- *Onset.* Subacute, i.e. hours or days.
- *Provocation.* Pleuritic and/or positional. It is worsened by deep inspiration, coughing, lying supine or on the left side.
- *Palliation.* Position change or leaning forward.
- *Quality/quantity.* The pain of pericarditis is moderate but tends to be oppressive in nature.
- *Radiation.* Precordial. Posterior neck or trapezius region.
- *Associated symptoms.* Fever dyspnoea or orthopnoea.
- *Underlying conditions.* Viral, vascular, or post-MI.

Objective findings

- On physical examination the heart sounds are normal or soft.
- Pericardial friction rub (a specific sound) may be heard at the left sternal edge. These sounds are best heard if the patient is made to sit up, lean forward and breathe out fully.
- Patients with acute pericarditis are often pyrexic and may feel systemically unwell.
- There may be reduced blood pressure.
- Pulsus paradoxus with pericardial effusion.

Investigations

- Chest X-ray.
- ECG.
- Referral for electrocardiography. This is most valuable in detecting an effusion.
- Referral for cardiac catheterisation only in chronic cases.

Therapeutic intervention

- This depends on the underlying cause.
- In acute pericarditis, pain relief is of value. Aspirin or nonsteroidal drugs are useful.

Referral

1. Pericardial effusion can develop in cases of viral or bacterial pericarditis.
2. Referral to hospital is necessary for aspiration of pericardial effusion if indicated for the relief of symptoms and tamponade. Fluid specimens can be sent for pathology.

3. If pericardial effusion develops then there will be an inevitable pericardial tamponade with limited cardiac filling and reduced cardiac stroke volume. An increase in heart rate, increased dyspnoea and fall in blood pressure are the inevitable outcomes. Signs of tamponade include increasing dyspnoea, facial engorgement, peripheral oedema and raised JVP.

❶ This is a medical emergency. The patient is often very ill, hypotensive and peripherally constricted. There may be a pulses paradoxus (a variation in pulse volume with respiration) and the JVP is very high.

Musculoskeletal chest pain

Musculoskeletal disease is a common cause of chest pain. Costochondritis and hypertrophic osteoarthritis of the cervical spine are the most common causes. Pain arising in the chest wall or thoracic spine is often mistaken for cardiac pain. Characteristically, it tends to be an aching pain, the onset of which may relate to a particular twist or movement; the pain persists at rest. There is often localised tenderness, particularly over the costal regions.

Costochondritis

The costochondral and chondosternal articulations are common sites of inflammation causing anterior chest pains. The onset, which may be gradual or sudden, is exacerbated by coughing, breathing, laughing and sneezing or with shoulder movement and is typically described as dull. The sole physical finding is tenderness at the costochondral articulations. The key distinguishing feature is intensification of the pain with respiratory movement and point tenderness that produces pain.

Hypertrophic osteoarthritis of the cervical spine

Pain is caused by initiation of sensory nerve roots due to the degenerative changes in the vertebral ostia. There is usually a gradual onset of pain – changes in body position such as bending, lifting, lying down, or prolonged sitting will elicit pain that is exacerbated by coughing, deep breathing and exertion. It is not relieved by rest or nitroglycerin and is described as having the angina qualities of pressure, heaviness or vice-like constriction.

Tsetse's syndrome

Tsetse's syndrome is chest pain caused by inflammation of one or more of the costal cartilages, usually at the costochondral junction. The cartilage becomes swollen and protuberant, and is tender on palpation. The cause is unknown; inflammation persists for months or years but is usually self-limiting. It can be treated by NSAIDs

Top Tips

1 The approach to physical examination will depend upon the condition of the patient

2 When measuring blood pressure it is important to access the patient for cuff size before measurement

3 Pulsile elevation of the internal JVP is a reliable sign of right heart failure or fluid overload

4 The single most characteristic feature of angina is that it is brought on by exertion and relieved by rest

5 Crescendo, or unstable angina, may culminate in MI and is an indication of urgent assessment

6 The severity of cardiac symptoms depends upon normal daily activity. The occupational history may exert a major influence on management

7 Patients with severe coronary artery disease may have a normal resting ECG

8 Echocardiography is a valuable technique for assessing abnormalities of heart valves, cardiac hypertrophy, the size and arrangement of the cardiac chambers and the presence of pericardial effusion

9 Doppler cardiography is a sensitive method of detecting and measuring abnormal blood flow

10 Never palpate both carotids simultaneously

or by local injection of drugs. In its classical form, Tsetse's syndrome is rare, but minor degrees have been recorded.

Shingles

After an attack of chickenpox, the varicella-zoster virus lies dormant in a dorsal root or cranial nerve ganglion. Reactivation of the virus causes a localised eruption called shingles.

Subjective assessment

- Patient experiences tingling, paraesthesia, or a burning pain in the distribution of a single dermatome.
- Patient notices a rash 24 hours later.

Objective assessment

- Erythema, then macular papular and vesicular lesions, progressing to pustules, crusts and finally scars.
- Shingles is always unilateral. It is most likely to appear on the trunk, but the face is often affected.
- Secondary bacterial infection of the vesicles is common, indicated by yellow slough or crusts.
- If the rash is in the trigeminal nerve root distribution, look for spread to eye or nose.

- Postherpetic neuralgia, i.e. continued pain after the rash has gone, may complicate shingles, especially in the elderly.

Therapeutic intervention

- Pain relief is often necessary, e.g. co-proxamol, 2 tablets, 4-hourly.
- Secondary bacterial infection can be treated with fusidic acid ointment three times a day or oral flucloxacillin 250 mg every day.
- Postherpetic neuralgia can be treated with amitriptyline 25 mg at night, increasing to 25 mg three times a day in younger patients.
- There is some evidence that zoster-associated pain can be lessened by the use of valaciclovir in patients over 50 years of age presenting within 72 hours of the rash.

Referral

- Arrange for the patient to be seen by an ophthalmologist if the rash involves the eye.
- Admit the patient under the medical or infectious diseases team if the rash becomes extensive (Cartwright & Godlee 1998).

Glossary

Arterial pulse and pressure   Rate, rhythm, wave form and volume of radial pulse and blood pressure

Auscultation   First and second heart sounds; added sounds; murmurs

Bruits   Abnormal turbulent sound heard from auscultation of the arteries and represents vessel disease

Cardiomyopathy   A general term meaning 'heart muscle disease'. Clinically, cardiomyopathy can be classified into hypertrophic, dilated and restricted (HOCM) types

Dextrocardia   Position of the heart in the opposite side of the chest, i.e. right instead of left

Dyspnoea   Pulmonary congestion leading to shortness of breath. In left heart failure the rise in left arterial pressure also produces a sharp rise in pulmonary capillary pressure, predisposing to pulmonary congestion and shortness of breath. The symptoms are worse on exertion or on lying flat

Ebstein anomaly   Abnormality of the tricuspid valve

Haemoptysis   Coughing up blood from the lower respiratory tract. Frank haemoptysis may be fatal due to pulmonary infarction. Recurrent episodes over many years and associated with purulent sputum is often a feature of bronchiectasis

Hyperlipidaemia   Elevation of plasma lipid levels. Elevations of total or low-density cholesterol without triglyceride elevation are termed hypercholesterolaemia, whereas triglyceride elevations are termed hypertriglyceridaemia. Concomitant hypercholesterolaemia and hypertriglyceridaemia is termed hyperlipidaemia

Jugular venous pressure (JVP)   Note form of the jugular pulse wave and height of the JVP

Orthopnoea   Gravitational pooling of blood in the upright posture ensures a relatively low PAWP (pulmonary artery wedge pressure), but lying flat causes it to rise sharply, particularly in patients with heart failure. This produces orthopnoea, which may disturb normal sleep. In advanced cases, pulmonary oedema in the supine position can cause very severe dyspnoea – *paroxysmal nocturnal dyspnoea*

Palpation   Position of the apex beat, character of the apical impulse and other pulsations; thrills

Pectus excavatum: 'funnel chest'   A condition where the sternum is depressed. This is a benign condition and needs treatment. It can produce unusual chest radiographic appearances

Pulmonary hypertension   Pulmonary or systemic hypertension results from ventricular hypertrophy due to ventricular outflow obstruction by stenosed aortic or pulmonary values or because the resistance in the pulmonary or systemic circulation is high

Scoliosis   Lateral curvature of the spine

Xanthoma   Clinical feature of familial hypercholesterolaemia (autosomal dominant). Can be present as yellowish eruptions at the inner side of the eyelids or may present as skin, palmar or tendon xanthomas.

Useful addresses

Vehicle Licensing (Medical Advisory Branch), Olway Centre, Orchard Street, Swansea SA99 ITU.

References

Cartwright, Godlee 1998 Churchill's pocket book of general practice. Churchill Livingstone, Edinburgh.

Chambers J 1996 Echocardiography in primary care. Parthenon Publishing Group, London.

DHSS 1998 Our healthier nation. A contract for health. DHSS, London.

Ebstein O, Perkin D, de Bono D, Cookson J 1997 Clinical examination, 2nd edn. Mosby, London.

Hanssom L, Zanchetti A, Carruthers S G et al 1998 Effects of intensive blood pressure lowering and low dose aspirin in patients with hypertension: principle results of the hypertension optimal treatment (HOT) randomised control trial. Lancet 351:1755–1762.

Hinchliff S, Montague S 1998 Physiology for nursing practice; 1st edn. Baillière Tindall, London.

MIMS 2000 Handbook of cardiology, MAPP Pharmaceuticals.

Mead M, Patterson H 1992 Tutorials in general practice, 2nd edn. Churchill Livingstone, Edinburgh.

Passmore P 2000 Hypertension beyond 2000. Northern Ireland Medicine Today March:18–21.

Ramsay L E, Williams B, Johnson G D et al 1999 for the British Hypertension Society Guidelines for Management of Hypertension: Report of the Third Working Party of the British Hypertension Society. J. Hum. Hypertension 13:559–592.

Wood D, Durrington P, Poulter N, McInnes G, Rees A, Wray R 1998 Joint recommendations on prevention of coronary heart disease in clinical practice. Heart 80(Suppl 2).

Further reading

Moody L, Yakowich 1997 Pediatric cardiovascular assessment and referral in the primary care setting. Nurse Pract. 22(1):120–134.
This is an easy-to-read article written by a nurse practitioner. It not only reviews the basic assessment of the innocent paediatric cardiac murmur but focuses on paediatric assessment techniques, specific key findings, management and referral parameters.

9

THE GASTROINTESTINAL SYSTEM

Jane Bayliss

Key Issues

- Comprehensive history taking and accurate assessment are the key to accurate diagnosis

- Signs and symptoms that appear to be gastrointestinal in origin may be from other sources. This is especially relevant when assessing women

- Symptoms that may appear relatively innocent may be masking a more serious underlying condition. This is particularly true in the elderly population

- Children with abdominal disease may present differently from adults with the same condition and can deteriorate rapidly

Introduction

Full assessment of the gastrointestinal (GI) system is one of the most complex situations faced by the nurse practitioner in primary care. The presenting signs and symptoms can be misleading because of the variety of internal organs that are situated in the thorax and abdomen. The physical proximity and closely allied innervation of these structures can make for a difficult diagnosis.

The five main functions of the GI tract are ingestion, digestion, absorption and metabolism of nutrients and the removal of indigestible and secretory waste. This is achieved by the coordinated functioning of a long muscular tube comprising the mouth, oropharynx, oesophagus, stomach, small intestine, large intestine, rectum and anal sphincter and a number of accessory organs – the salivary glands, liver and gall bladder and the pancreas.

Digestion commences in the mouth, with the secretion of saliva containing the enzymes amylase and ptyalin; this continues in the stomach by the production of a variety of compounds, including gastrin and pepsinogen (which aid in the digestion of protein).

Very little absorption occurs in the stomach; the small intestine is the site at which the majority of nutrients are absorbed into the system. Bile, from the liver and gall bladder, and pancreatic juices are secreted into the upper portion of the small intestine, the jejunum. These aid in the breakdown of fats and carbohydrates, and absorption of these and other products of digestion, e.g. simple sugars and amino acids, occurs throughout the remaining length of the small intestine. The large intestine, which extends from the ileum to the anus, is responsible for the absorption of water and ions. It commences at the caecum, a blind-ended sac to which is attached the worm-like appendix (which in humans plays very little part in digestion), and ends at the anal sphincter.

The accessory organs have crucial functions in the process of digestion. The liver secretes bile, which is stored and concentrated in the gall bladder. This stimulates peristalsis and has an emulsifying action, aiding the breakdown and absorption of fats. The liver absorbs glucose from the hepatic portal circulation and converts it into glycogen. The pancreas has both an exocrine and endocrine function. The exocrine function is the secretion of pancreatic juice, which aids in the digestion of all classes of food; the endocrine function includes the secretion of the two hormones insulin and glucagon that are crucial in carbohydrate metabolism.

Presenting signs and symptoms of GI disturbance will be directly dependent on the underlying pathophysiology, but there tends to be a common theme running throughout. Common problems associated with GI disease include pain or discomfort, anorexia, nausea, vomiting, heartburn (pyrosis) or 'indigestion', reflux or regurgitation of gastric contents, excessive gas either in terms of eructation or flatulence and changes in normal bowel habit, which may be a combination of diarrhoea and/or constipation.

Important symptoms to note are mucus in the stools, any fresh bleeding seen in either vomit or stools or a black 'tarry' stool, which might indicate bleeding higher up in the GI tract; slow onset, progressive dysphagia and excessive weight changes may also be significant.

Gastrointestinal problems are some of the most common encountered in primary care and the key to ensuring an accurate diagnosis is a comprehensive history and assessment.

Assessment

Subjective assessment

The physical assessment of the GI system will be based on what the patient tells you, so it is extremely important that you take an accurate history first. This history is your most effective diagnostic and management tool. Based on the variety of symptoms that patients can present with, it is vital that you adopt a systematic approach to the history.

The questions you should ask should be initially open ended and, then, if necessary, focus the patient to provide as accurate a description of their symptoms as possible.

Types of question to ask

1. Can you describe the problem for me?
2. When did it start?
3. What have you eaten and drunk in the last 24 hours?
4. Is there any pain or discomfort?
5. Where exactly is the pain/discomfort? Point to where it hurts the most.
6. How long does it last?
7. Does the pain/discomfort go anywhere else? Show me where.
8. What makes the pain better, or worse?
9. Can you describe the pain/discomfort? Is it sharp and stabbing or more like a dull ache?
10. When you have the pain, are there any other associated symptoms (e.g. nausea, diarrhoea, vomiting, reflux, a feeling of fullness/emptiness)?
11. Apart from the symptoms you have already described, are there any other changes you would like to tell me about? These might include:
    - a change in frequency and/or consistency of the stools
    - the presence of blood, pus or mucus in the stools
    - a change in appetite
    - any difficulty swallowing
    - any heartburn or regurgitation
    - any unusual or rapid weight changes.

It is also important that you ask about urinary symptoms and, for women, the presence of any possible gynaecological problem, for example:

12. Are you having any problems when you pass water?
13. How often do you have to empty your bladder?
14. Is that more frequently than usual?
15. Is there any discomfort or pain when you pass water?
16. Can you describe it for me?
17. When you pass water is the stream as good as usual?
18. Do you have any problems starting or stopping the flow of urine?
19. Have you noticed any unusual vaginal discharge?
20. Please describe it for me, i.e. the colour, odour and appearance.
21. When was your last menstrual period?
22. Was your period of normal flow and duration?
23. Are you having any unusual bleeding?
24. Do you experience any pain or discomfort on intercourse?

It may also be relevant to obtain an obstetric history if any gynaecological problems are highlighted.

The answers to these questions form the basis for the focus of your objective assessment of the patient.

Objective assessment

Obviously, the GI system will form the basis of your objective assessment but, as can be seen from the above questions, it may be necessary to assess other systems dependent on what the history and appearance of the patient reveal. The order of the assessment is important, as it is different from all other systems. When examining the abdomen it is essential to inspect *then* auscultate before percussion and lastly palpation.

General approach

- Observe patient for general appearance and nutritional status. Colour or pallor of skin and any signs of dehydration should be noted.
- Check vital signs as appropriate: temperature, if fever is suspected, pulse and blood pressure.

Physical assessment

1. Depending on the history, it may be necessary to examine the patient's mouth and throat. If they are having difficulty eating or swallowing, check mouth for dental caries or ill-fitting dentures, signs of soreness or infection, any abnormal lesions or dryness. The tongue should also be inspected.
2. You need to carry out the abdominal assessment in a good light and with the patient undressed and supine. Their arms should be at their sides or crossed loosely over their chest. For the purpose of examination, the abdomen is divided into four sections or quadrants. This ensures that symptoms can be located more accurately. The subdivisions commonly used are right upper and lower and left upper and lower quadrants. These are formed by imaginary vertical and horizontal lines that cross at the umbilicus.
3. *Inspect* the abdomen for shape, symmetry and any pulsations. Observe any lesions, scars or unusual blood vessel formation (the presence of spider naevi on the abdomen may indicate liver disease).
4. *Auscultate* for bowel sounds using the diaphragm of a stethoscope and for bruits and friction rubs using the bell of a stethoscope. The abdomen should be auscultated for up to 5 min in each quadrant. Normal bowel sounds are high-pitched, irregular gurgles and occur 5–35 times per minute. Note the absence or any hyperactivity (borborygmus) of sounds. There should be no bruits, venous sounds or friction rubs heard in the abdomen. If a bruit is heard, then the abdomen should not be palpated, as it may be indicative of a narrowed vessel or aneurysm (Weber 1988).
5. *Percuss* the abdomen to assess the underlying structures for consistency and size. The percussion notes will range from dull to tympanic (drum-like). Tympany will be heard over the hollow organs such as the stomach, intestines, aorta, bladder and gall bladder. Dull notes will be heard over the solid internal organs, i.e. the liver, spleen, pancreas, kidneys and uterus. Percussion can also be used to assess the size of the internal structures by percussing from

dull to hollow to establish where the border of the internal organ lies. Percussion may also highlight any tender or painful areas.

6. *Palpation* should be carried out in two ways – lightly then deeply – and all four quadrants should be palpated systematically, ensuring you do not omit any areas. You should palpate lightly at first, noting any tender or painful areas, and then palpate more deeply, leaving the painful areas until last. This ensures the patient's abdomen remains soft until you have finished the examination.

7. Signs to look out for when palpating the abdomen are tenderness or severe pain, guarding or rigidity of the abdominal muscles and rebound tenderness. You should observe the patient's face during the examination for signs of pain or distress.

Special manoeuvres

These manoeuvres are used to palpate the liver, kidneys and spleen for size, tenderness and masses.

The liver

1. Stand on the patient's right side.
2. Place your left hand under their ribs at the position of ribs 11 and 12.
3. Place your right hand with the fingers parallel to their right costal margin.
4. Ask them to breathe in and out deeply.
5. Press upwards with each inhalation.
6. The lower border of the liver may be just palpable. If felt, it should be smooth, firm and with a clearly defined edge. The edge of the liver does not usually extend beyond the costal margin. It is normal in some individuals for the liver to be unpalpable. The lower liver border is more easily palpated in the elderly and in infants and young children.

The kidneys

1. Place one hand on the patient's back between the lowest rib and the iliac crest.
2. Place your other hand on the corresponding anterior surface.
3. Ask the patient to take a deep breath in.
4. Pull upwards with lower hand while at the same time pushing inwards with upper hand while the patient breathes out, i.e. bring hands towards each other and palpate with palmar surfaces of fingers. *This should be done gently.*
5. Repeat on the opposite side.

The kidneys are rarely palpable, and this manoeuvre can be uncomfortable for the patient.

The spleen

1. Stand on the right of the patient
2. Lean over patient and place your right hand under patient's right lower ribs and push upwards
3. Place your left hand below the anterior costal margin
4. Ask patient to breathe in deeply

5. Move hands towards each other during inspiration to try and palpate spleen
6. The spleen is not normally palpable and there should be no tenderness.

Depending on the history, it may also be necessary for you to carry out a pelvic examination on a female patient to determine whether the symptoms are of GI tract or gynaecological origin. All findings should be documented and any deviations from normal, noted.

Diagnostic tests

The tests you consider will be totally dependent on your subjective and objective assessments. They may range from nothing through to a whole range of investigations, including X-rays, a variety of endoscopic examinations, ultrasound and/or a range of microbiological and biochemical tests. The most common or most frequently helpful include:

- Full blood count and white cell differential: these will indicate anaemia, chronic inflammation, infection or leukocytosis of another cause.
- Erythrocyte sedimentation rate or plasma viscosity: these provide an indication of generalised inflammation; your choice will depend on local policy.
- Urinalysis and/or urine culture.
- Pregnancy test (urinary human chorionic gonadotrophin (HcG) levels).
- Vaginal/cervical swabs to detect gynaecological infection.
- Stool smear on a *fresh* stool sample for direct microscopy.
- Stool culture to detect bacterial or viral infection.
- Faecal occult blood to detect GI haemorrhage. Three consecutive stool samples should be collected and sent to the laboratory together.
- Stool sample for microscopy, to detect ova or parasites.
- Liver function tests, if liver disease is suspected.
- Serum amylase, if pancreatic disease is suspected.
- Urea and electrolytes to observe renal function.

These tests can all be carried out in the primary care setting; it may be necessary, however, to refer to secondary care for other investigations. The most common would be:

- X-ray, either plain film or using contrast medium, e.g. barium. Contrast radiography may be used to establish a possible diagnosis of inflammatory bowel disease or malignancy prior to endoscopic examination and biopsy. In some units it may be deemed inappropriate to request plain abdominal films to investigate certain conditions, e.g. constipation, if there is an absence of other clinical signs.
- Ultrasound, e.g. abdominal scan. This is used to detect abnormalities such as masses, and is often the initial investigation of choice in this case (Hope et al 1996). The Pelvic scan is now a routine assessment in the management of normal pregnancy but is also used to detect ovarian, uterine and testicular masses.

Ultrasound would be the first investigation of choice if a malignancy were suspected, e.g. in the liver or in the GI tract, or to assess for gall bladder disease or renal abnormalities.

- A range of endoscopic examinations: oesophago-gastroduodenoscopy (Hope et al 1996) (commonly called an endoscopy), colonoscopy, sigmoidoscopy and proctoscopy are the most common. These are the investigations of choice if malignancy or peptic ulceration is suspected or if there is a GI bleed of unknown origin. There are age limitations in some areas, however, e.g. in a patient under 50 years of age some units will only carry out barium X-ray as the first line of investigation. You need to be familiar with local policy.

Differential diagnoses

There are a huge variety of conditions of the GI tract that can present in primary care. The most common will be discussed in the following section but it is important to consider other possible diagnoses. These might include:

- partial or total obstruction of the bowel
- inflammatory bowel disease, e.g. Crohn's disease, ulcerative colitis
- malabsorption syndromes, e.g. coeliac disease, chronic pancreatitis
- liver disease, e.g. cirrhosis, chronic hepatitis
- malignancy
- chronic diarrhoea.

For some of these conditions initial investigations may be implemented by the primary care nurse practitioner. This would depend on the presenting condition of the patient. Subsequent management, however, would require specialised care.

SPECIFIC DISORDERS

Gastroenteritis

Gastroenteritis is an inflammation of the stomach, small intestine and the colon. It can be divided into bacterial and non-bacterial, dependent on the causative agent. Non-bacterial gastroenteritis is usually caused by a viral agent; the most common are a group of small round structured viruses (SRSV) collectively called rotavirus. Gastroenteritis caused by this group tends to be acute, short lived and with projectile vomiting and tends to occur more frequently in the very young and the very old (Winter 1998). There are a number of bacterial agents that can cause bacterial gastroenteritis. These tend to be less common than viral gastroenteritis, but the more common species are *Salmonella*, *Shigella*, *Campylobacter*, *Escherichia coli* and *Clostridium difficile*. The initial assessment of both types of gastroenteritis is very similar.

Subjective findings

- The patient complains of sudden onset diarrhoea, which may or may not be accompanied by nausea and/or vomiting.
- They may give a history of eating something different (for them), e.g. shellfish.
- Assess whether they have recently travelled abroad and where their destination was.
- Check whether they know of anyone else with similar symptoms.
- They may complain of abdominal cramping pains and in some cases rectal urgency and tenesmus.
- They may feel feverish or have a normal temperature.
- There may be a feeling of malaise and there may be headache.
- Establish how long they have had the symptoms and whether they have experienced the condition before.
- Assess whether the symptoms are associated with eating and/or drinking and what the time interval is before symptoms reappear.
- Ask whether the symptoms are exacerbated by any particular type of food, e.g. dairy products.
- Assess their use of any medication, either prescribed or bought over the counter (OTC), especially laxatives.
- Assess patient's definition of diarrhoea. There are a number of definitions of diarrhoea, ranging from the frequent passage of stool to the passage of unformed stool (Shaw 1996). Probably the most useful definition is the passage of more than 300 ml of liquid faeces in 24 hours (Hope et al 1996).

Objective findings

1. Vital signs: the temperature may range from normal to 39°C or above. If the temperature is acutely raised, i.e. 39°C or above, and is accompanied by blood-stained diarrhoea and dehydration, then consider admission to hospital.
2. Observe for signs of dehydration, specifically assessing skin turgor, moistness of mucous membranes and presence of oliguria. You should also check for signs of postural hypotension, as this is significant of more severe dehydration. Dehydration is more significant in children and in the older adult, as homeostatic mechanisms are less efficient and deterioration can occur more rapidly. Special precautions should also be taken in pregnant women, as the pregnancy can be at risk if dehydration occurs.
3. Examine the abdomen. There will be hyperactive bowel sounds and probably a diffuse tenderness. It is unlikely there will be any guarding or rebound tenderness.
4. Assess abdominal lymph nodes for tenderness and enlargement.
5. Where possible, assess stool for consistency, colour, odour and the presence of blood or mucus.
6. In the older adult, carry out a rectal examination to exclude constipation with overflow.

Plan

Most episodes of gastroenteritis are self-limiting; therefore, management is primarily concerned with relief of symptoms and the prevention of deterioration:
- provide advice regarding a self-management regime
- discuss any necessary therapeutic interventions
- negotiate a time for review with the patient
- refer for further investigation or stabilisation as appropriate.

Advice

1. Bed rest.
2. Restrict oral intake to fluids only for 24 hours while vomiting.
3. Avoid milk or milky drinks for at least 24 hours: longer if an intake of dairy products causes a return of diarrhoea.
4. In children and the older adult, every episode of diarrhoea and/or vomiting should be followed by an attempt at fluid replacement (see below). Fluid replacement is important for the younger adult population but is less crucial than in the above two groups.
5. Women who are pregnant are especially at risk from dehydration and vitamin depletion. They should be monitored carefully and if symptoms persist should be referred for management.

Investigations

- Symptoms should resolve quickly, i.e. within 24–48 hours, although diarrhoea can persist for up to 2 weeks.
- If patient remains unwell and there is no improvement in symptoms after 48 hours, then a stool sample for culture and sensitivity and microscopy is indicated.
- If diarrhoea persists beyond 2 weeks, refer for further investigation.

Therapeutic intervention

1. Replace fluid and electrolyte loss with a proprietary rehydration product (e.g. Rehidrat, Diocalm Junior or Dioralyte) (BNF 36 1998).
2. Alternatively, a home-made fluid replacement mixture can be made using a pinch of salt and a teaspoon of sugar to a pint of water. This can be added to fruit juice to make it more palatable.
3. If stool culture is required and a bacterial pathogen is isolated, then an appropriate antibiotic may be necessary (Table 9.1). Often, however, bacterial gastroenteritis will resolve spontaneously and antibiotics should be avoided except in the more severe infections. This avoids the possibility of enhancing the carrier state of salmonellosis (Shaw 1996), and triggering antibiotic-induced diarrhoea. There is always a risk of inducing pseudomembranous colitis following

Table 9.1 *Antibiotic therapy for bacterial gastroenteritis*

Infection	Antibiotic therapy	Dosage
Campylobacter enteritis	Ciprofloxacin	500–750 mg twice per day (not suitable for children) for 5 days
	Erythromycin	Adults and children over 8: 250–500 mg, 6 hourly Child 2–8 years: 250 mg, 6 hourly Child under 2: 125 mg, 6 hourly, for 5 days
Salmonella infection	Ciprofloxacin	500–750 mg twice per day (not suitable for children) for 5 days

	Trimethoprim	200 mg every 12 hours for 7 days
		Children: doses to be given 12 hourly:
		  2–5 months: 25 mg
		  6 months–5 years: 50 mg
		  6–12 years: 100 mg

Shigella infection	Ciprofloxacin (drug of choice for trimethoprim-resistant strains)	500–750 mg twice per day (not suitable for children) for 5 days

	Trimethoprim	200 mg every 12 hours for 7 days
		Children: doses to be given 12 hourly:
		  2–5 months: 25 mg
		  6 months–5 years: 50 mg
		  6–12 years: 100 mg

Pseudomembranous colitis	Oral vancomycin	125 mg, 6 hourly for 7–10 days
	Oral metronidazole	400 mg three times per day for 7 days

antibiotic therapy. This is caused by an overgrowth of *C. difficile* and should be suspected if diarrhoea presents after treatment for another infection.

4. It is rarely appropriate to administer an adsorbent, e.g. kaolin, or a drug to reduce gut motility, e.g. an opiate such as codeine phosphate or the anti-diarrhoeal drugs loperamide hydrochloride (Imodium) and co-phenotrope (Lomotil) (BNF 36 1998), as they merely prolong the course of the disease by delaying the expulsion of the pathogen.

Patient education

- The maintenance of hydration is the key to managing gastroenteritis effectively.
- Good hygiene practices are essential to avoid the spread of infection, i.e. hand washing, washing of soiled linen, disinfection of surfaces.
- Check patient's employment and advise that they should refrain from working until 48 hours after the symptoms have ceased. This is of particular importance if they are employed in the food industry, with children or in a caring environment (hospital, residential or nursing home).
- Discuss food preparation practices, e.g. keeping cooked and raw meat separate, ensuring poultry is completely defrosted and thoroughly cooked before consumption and ensuring refrigerators are at the correct temperature.

Referral

- Reassess patient after 48 hours, 24 hours if an infant or older adult; and if no improvement, consider referral to hospital.
- If satisfactory rehydration is not being achieved, consider admission to hospital for intravenous (IV) fluids. This is particularly important in children and the older adult.
- Some bacterial causes of gastroenteritis are 'notifiable diseases'. They tend to cause 'dysentery' with bloody diarrhoea, i.e. *Salmonella*, *Shigella*, *Campylobacter* and *E. coli*. In these cases, you should inform the Consultant for Communicable Disease Control (CCDC) or the Director of Public Health.
- If diarrhoea becomes a chronic problem, i.e. persists longer than 2 weeks, then further investigation and referral to a specialist may be necessary, e.g. proctoscopy, sigmoidoscopy, colonoscopy or possibly barium enema, to exclude the possibility of inflammatory bowel disease.

Complications

- The main risk from gastroenteritis is dehydration, i.e. fluid and electrolyte depletion. The very old and the very young are more susceptible to this and should, therefore, be monitored very closely, possibly even warranting early admission to hospital.
- Severe dehydration can result in hypovolaemic shock and organ failure.

Danger signs

- ❶ Sudden onset bloody diarrhoea of less than 2 weeks' duration. This may have an infectious cause. Check whether patient has recently been abroad and either refer or take prompt direct faecal smear and then sample for culture. Notify the CCDC or the Director of Public Health.
- ❶ Slow-onset bloody diarrhoea may be indicative of inflammatory bowel disease, especially if it lasts more than 7 days. It may also be a sign of amoebic dysentery; check whether patient has travelled abroad (it can occur years after original infection). Refer if suspicious.
- ❶ Signs of dehydration, especially in children, the older adult and pregnant women. Refer for IV fluid replacement if not resolving within 24 hours.
- ❶ Persistent diarrhoea without vomiting may be caused by non-GI conditions, e.g. autonomic neuropathy caused by diabetes mellitus, thyrotoxicosis, anxiety or medication. This may be prescribed, e.g. antacids, cimetidine, antibiotics or OTC, e.g. antacids, laxatives. Manage underlying condition where possible.
- ❶ Vomiting accompanied by weight loss and dysphagia may be indicative of oesophageal stricture, malignancy or possibly be psychological in origin. Refer for investigation.
- ❶ A bloody and/or purulent anal discharge may be an indication of an acute or chronic infection of the rectal mucosa caused by, for example, gonorrhoea, *Chlamydia*, herpes and syphilis.

Constipation

There is no universally accepted definition of constipation; the term can have a variety of meanings. It is vital, therefore, that you assess what a patient means when they inform you they are constipated. For some people, constipation means a hard stool that may be difficult to evacuate; for others it means having their bowels open infrequently or the stools are bulky (Winney 1998); it may even mean they have diarrhoea! A useful assessment is that the frequency of defaecation has decreased significantly for the patient and/or the stools are dry, hard and difficult to pass. Another guide is that straining to pass stools has occurred more than 25% of the time (Norton 1996). The problem of constipation can cause distress and discomfort to many, which is highlighted by the number of consultations it results in: almost half a million per year in general practice (Norton 1996). Table 9.2 shows some possible causes of constipation.

Subjective indications

- Patients may complain that they have not had their bowels open for a period of time.
- It is important to establish what their normal bowel pattern is and how long they have had the current problem.

Table 9.2 *Factors that may contribute to constipation (Adapted from Winney 1998, Norton 1996.)*

Contributory factor	Rationale
Diet	Inadequate fibre and/or fluid Inadequate intake of food
Ignoring the desire to defaecate	'Too busy' Inconvenient Embarrassment/inadequate toilet facilities Immobility Confusion or intellectual impairment
Underlying condition	Hormonal, e.g. hypothyroidism Neuropathy, e.g. diabetes or local problem, e.g. damage to myenteric plexus in gut wall Bowel disorders, e.g. irritable bowel syndrome, diverticular disease, carcinoma of bowel or pelvic organs Psychiatric disorder, e.g. depression, anorexia nervosa Megacolon or megarectum
Decreased abdominal pressure	Pelvic floor problems, e.g. rectocoele Paradoxical pelvic floor contractions (anismus) Hirschsprung's disease Prolapse of rectal mucosa Position during defaecation General debility leading to reduced abdominal effort
Anorectal pain	Hard stools Haemorrhoids Anal fissure Perianal Crohn's disease Solitary rectal ulcer syndrome Postpartum perianal pain
Medication	Opiate analgesics Oral iron Anticholinergic drugs Some antacids Antihistamines Antidepressants
Other	Hormonal, e.g. pregnancy, premenstrual syndrome

- Ask the patient to describe the stool, paying particular attention to the presence of fresh blood or a black, tarry stool.
- Patients may be complaining of a variety of other symptoms, such as tenesmus, abdominal pain or cramps. Some may complain of feeling bloated and they may experience a general feeling of malaise or tiredness.
- In very severe cases, there may also be nausea, headache and halitosis (Norton 1996).
- Establish dietary intake of both food and fluid, including type and volume.
- Ask about weight changes and any alteration in appetite.
- Enquire whether this is an isolated event or a recurrent problem.
- If recurrent, how have they managed it before? Have they used proprietary laxatives?
- Establish the use of any current medication, especially opioid analgesics and oral iron. Iron may cause constipation in some individuals and can result in a black tarry stool.
- Ask about any previous GI problems or surgery.
- Constipation in children often presents at around 5 months and 2 years of age, i.e. when weaning and potty training commence. In the older child, it is often accompanied by soiling, and foul-smelling wind. This can cause considerable embarrassment to the child and his family.

Objective findings

- Assess the patient's general demeanour, skin colour and texture, observing for any signs of dehydration.
- Assess mouth and tongue: there may be dryness and a coating on the tongue and their breath may be fetid.
- Vital signs should be normal.

- Inspect and auscultate the abdomen: there may be visible abdominal distension. Bowel sounds may be normal, decreased, increased or absent. If increased with a tinkling quality, this may be an early sign of intestinal obstruction; if decreased, then absent, it may indicate a paralytic ileus or peritonitis. These conditions, however, would be accompanied by other physical signs and an ill patient!
- Percuss the abdomen. There should be tympany; this may be exaggerated if there is excessive gas in the gut. If the colon is full of faecal matter, there may be dullness to the percussion note. Assess the extent of the dullness.
- Palpate the abdomen in all four quadrants. There may be mild tenderness over the xiphoid area, the caecum and the sigmoid colon, which is normal. You may be able to palpate a full descending colon. It should feel soft and pliable without nodules.
- Perform a rectal digital examination and assess for hard dry faeces, haemorrhoids, any fissures or masses. Observe the gloved finger on removal, for faeces or fresh blood.
- If available, it may also be useful to directly view the rectum using a proctoscope. It may be possible to visualise internal haemorrhoids or rectal polyps.
- You may need to carry out a vaginal examination in some women to detect any gynaecological problems that could be causing the problem.

Plan

The management of the constipation will depend on the cause and duration of the problem. Simple transient constipation will often resolve spontaneously and, therefore, advice may be all that is necessary.

- Discuss dietary practices with patient, i.e. alter the diet to increase fibre and fluids. This should include a variety of fibre and not just an increase in wheat bran. Fluid should be increased to approximately 2 litres per day.
- Discuss exercise and encourage an increase in the patient's level of activity, where possible.
- Decide if any therapeutic intervention is indicated.
- Refer for further investigations as appropriate.
- Review the patient regularly. The length of time will depend on the age of the patient, the use of any medication and the severity of the condition. It may range from 2 days to 1 week.

Investigations

- The history is most important in revealing the likely cause.
- Faecal occult blood and full blood count may be necessary to assess any occult blood loss.
- Plain abdominal film if there is any doubt about faecal loading (Norton 1996). This may not be acceptable in

some centres for the investigation of constipation; it is therefore important to be aware of local policy.

- Transit studies, which examine colonic transit time, to detect whether the problem lies in the colon or whether there is rectal stasis.
- Barium enema, which would reveal obstruction, malignancy or megacolon.

Despite numerous investigations, there is often no cause found and there are often complex reasons for the problem that are psychological, behavioural and cultural in origin (Norton 1996).

Therapeutic intervention

1. If lifestyle changes alone do not resolve the problem and a full assessment has resulted in no obvious underlying cause, then it may be appropriate to prescribe a laxative and/or an enema.
2. There are a variety of different types of laxative; these are summarised in Tables 9.3. Table 9.4 summarises the different types of enema preparation.
3. The choice of product will depend on the patient's circumstances and duration of the problem.
4. If the constipation is severe, with faecal impaction, it may be necessary to prescribe an enema prior to the introduction of laxatives.
5. A sudden increase in fibre can exacerbate the problem by causing bloating and discomfort. This can be a particular problem for immobile elderly people and may result in faecal incontinence (Barrett 1993).
6. The prolonged use of stimulant laxatives is thought to cause damage to the myenteric plexus, although there is currently no conclusive evidence (Christensen 1994). This might explain, in part, the reliance that some older adults have on the use of stimulant laxatives.
7. The use of laxatives should be monitored and a programme established to gradually wean the patient off. This should not be hurried, however, as the constipation will return.
8. It is common practice to maintain the older adult on long-term laxative therapy, especially if they are in long-term care. Little research has been done on the management of constipation in the older adult in primary care.
9. Constipation in children may also be managed by the use of laxatives but a multidisciplinary approach can also be useful, involving the nurse practitioner, health visitor, paediatric community nurse and GP (Lewis & Muir 1996).
10. Abdominal massage may also be helpful in relieving constipation. A self-massage technique using a tennis ball can be particularly effective and is useful in children. The routine employed is up the ascending colon, across the transverse colon and down the descending colon. The aim is to ease gut spasm and assist peristalsis (Richards 1998).

Table 9.3 *Common laxatives and their mode of action (Adapted from BNF 36 1998.)*

Mode of action	Generic	Brand name	Dosage
Bulking agent (fibre)	Ispaghula husk	Fybogel	1 sachet in water twice daily
		Isogel	2 × 5 ml spoons twice daily
		Regulan	1 sachet in water 1–3 times/day (children always have a smaller dose)
	Sterculia	Normacol	1–2 5 ml spoons washed down with water twice daily (children-half adult dose)
	Methylcellulose	Celevac	3–6 tablets twice daily with 300 ml water
	Natural bran	Trifyba	1 sachet 2–3 times daily added to food (children half-1 sachet 1–2 times daily added to food)

Osmotic	Lactitol	Generic	20 g daily in single dose with food
			Child:
			  1–6 years 2.5–5 g
			  6–12 years 5–10 g
			  12–16 years 10–20 g
			In all cases adjust dose to produce 1 soft stool/day

	Lactulose	Generic	15 ml twice daily adjusted as required
			Child:
			  under 1 year 2.5 ml
			  1–5 years 5 ml
			  5–10 years 10 ml twice daily

	Magnesium salts	Magnesium hydroxide	25–50 ml when required
		Magnesium hydroxide and liquid paraffin (Milpar)	5–20 ml when required
		Magnesium sulphate (Epsom salts)	5–10 g in water (rapid action)
Stimulant	Senna	Generic	2–4 tablets at night Child: over 6 years half adult dose Start with low dose and increase (all ages)
	Bisacodyl	Generic	5–10 mg at night Child under 10 years 5 mg
	Danthron (only for use in older adult and terminally ill)	Co-danthramer (generic) Co-danthrusate (generic)	1–2 capsules at bedtime 1–3 capsules at night
Combination	Senna and ispaghula husk	Manevac	1–2 × 5 ml spoons/sachets at night with liquid Child: 5–12 years 1 × 5 ml spoon

Patient education

- Maintain adequate fluid (approximately 2 litres per day) and fibre intake (30 g per day – five portions of fruit and/or vegetables and wholegrain cereal and bread) with appropriate exercise where possible.
- Discuss the use of laxatives and explain their use as a last resort, not as first-line treatment. If the patient has used laxatives regularly, then this may be the most difficult part of management.
- Discuss openly the possible reasons for constipation and address environmental factors, e.g. lack of privacy, lack of physical height; the provision of a footstool may be useful for children and the older adult, allowing correct use of abdominal muscle contraction.
- Monitor the use of any laxative and advise the patient accordingly.
- Teach the use of abdominal massage to the patient and/or his carer.

Table 9.4 *Rectal preparations (Adapted from BNF 36 1998.)*

Mode of action	Generic	Brand name	Dosage
Faecal softener	Arachis oil	Fletchers' Arachis Oil Retention Enema	130 ml single dose pack
Stimulant	Docusate sodium	Fletchers' Enemette	5 ml unit
		Norgalax Micro-enema	10 g unit
	Glycerol	Glycerol Suppositories (generic)	1 suppository when required
Osmotic	Phosphates	Fleet Ready-to-use enema	Single dose pack
		Fletchers' Phosphate Enema	Single dose pack
	Sodium citrate (rectal)	Fleet Micro-enema	Single dose pack
		Micolette Micro-enema	Single dose pack
		Micralax Micro-enema	Single dose pack
		Relaxit Micro-enema	Single dose pack

- Encourage the patient to 'retrain' his bowel, allowing sufficient time to have their bowels open, not ignoring the sensation and trying to establish a routine.
- Be patient and explain that it may take weeks (or longer) to establish a more regular bowel pattern.

Referral

Indications for referral are:
- passage of dark tarry stools implies a potential underlying pathology, such as peptic ulceration (see below), diverticulosis or neoplasm
- constipation accompanied by sudden weight loss, serious abdominal pain, and nausea or vomiting with general malaise
- any fresh bleeding per rectum without a previous diagnosis of haemorrhoids
- any sudden onset change in bowel habit in adults over 50 should be investigated, even if there are no other symptoms.

Complications

- Bowel obstruction can be precipitated by the inappropriate management of constipation, especially in the elderly, by a sudden increase in dietary fibre without adequate fluid intake
- Avoid the use of stimulant laxatives if faecal impaction is suspected, and in those patients with diverticular disease there is a possibility of bowel rupture
- Atonic bowel, as a result of overuse of stimulant laxatives.

Danger signs

- ❶ Passage of a black tarry stool may indicate a GI bleed or neoplasm, but it may also indicate oral iron therapy
- ❶ Passage of fresh blood with a hard dry stool may indicate anal fissure or haemorrhoids. It can also be a sign of malignancy or polyposis syndromes

- ❶ Passage of blood and mucus with a formed stool may indicate ulcerative colitis (confined to the rectum) or diverticulitis
- ❶ Any sudden onset change in bowel habit in an individual over the age of 50 should be investigated.

Irritable bowel syndrome (IBS)

(IBS) is a syndrome usually diagnosed by exclusion. It is a chronic irritation of the bowel characterised by a variety of symptoms, including abdominal pain, which may be mild or extremely severe, and an altered bowel pattern, ranging from constipation to diarrhoea, which is often a combination of the two. Other symptoms experienced are bloating, flatulence, abdominal distension, tiredness, lethargy and sometimes nausea. It is a syndrome more often experienced by women than men in the ratio 2:1 (Ness 1997) and, consequently, it has been labelled as psychogenic in origin. There is currently no known cause, however, and unfortunately no known cure. It often first appears in late adolescence but can affect anyone at any age (Ness 1997) and the main principle of management is to alleviate the symptoms. There is some recent evidence to suggest that patients with IBS may also have an irritable bladder (Monga et al 1997).

Subjective findings

Symptoms may be of a wide variety linked to the problem of impaired gut motility.
- The patient may complain of constipation or diarrhoea or a combination of both.
- Many patients complain of several small volume loose stools occurring in the morning (Shaw 1996).
- There may be associated anorectal problems, e.g. anal fissure or haemorrhoids.
- Symptoms can be intermittent or prolonged.
- Lower abdominal pain is usually present and has a cramp-like quality. It may be mild through to severe.

- The pain may be eased by defaecation. It is usually associated with a change in bowel frequency or stool consistency.
- Excessive gas and bloating may be a problem and there may be abdominal distension.
- There may be a wide variety of other symptoms such as urinary frequency, dyspareunia, backache, heartburn and nausea.
- Patients may also complain of urgency to have their bowels open, tenesmus, passing mucus and a need to strain to pass soft stools.
- A careful history is needed to eliminate other conditions.
- A patient presenting with weight loss, nocturnal diarrhoea, faecal incontinence and the presence of blood in or on the stools should have further investigations (Shaw 1996).
- Assess the patient's diet and lifestyle.
- Explore the possibility of laxative abuse.
- Assess stress and/or anxiety levels in the patient's life or any recent major life events.
- Is this an isolated problem or has the patient experienced it before?
- Is the problem associated with the menstrual cycle?
- Has the patient recently travelled abroad?

Objective findings

- Vital signs should be normal.
- Assess colour, body mass index and general demeanour.
- Inspect and auscultate the abdomen. Bowel sounds should be normal to mildly hyperactive.
- Percuss and palpate the abdomen. There should be nothing remarkable. Percussion should reveal appropriate sounds, and palpation might show mild tenderness over the colon in the left or both lower quadrants.
- Tenderness associated with spasm tends to disappear or move under constant pressure, whereas pain associated with inflammation becomes worse under constant pressure.
- Digital rectal examination may not be necessary but, if performed, should reveal nothing of note.

Plan

The main aim of the management of IBS is the control of symptoms, which may be achieved through lifestyle changes, use of antispasmodics and/or antidiarrhoeal drugs:

- Establish the cause of symptoms, where possible, through investigations appropriate for the age of the patient.
- Initiate dietary and lifestyle changes as appropriate.
- Enable the patient to cope with stress/anxiety if appropriate.
- Review the symptoms regularly, i.e. at 2–4 weekly intervals initially.

- If lifestyle changes seem ineffective, initiate a trial of antispasmodic/antidiarrhoea therapy and review after 2 weeks.
- If still no improvement, consider referral for specialist intervention.

Investigations

The extent of the investigations will depend on the history and age of the patient. Because of the wide range of symptoms that may present, however, it is possible to initiate a whole battery of tests and procedures that reveal nothing:

1. If there is no history of excessive weight loss or passage of blood in the stools and the patient is under 40 years old with no relevant family history (e.g. familial adenomatous polyposis), it may be appropriate to manage the situation conservatively with minimal investigation
2. If over 40 years old and the problem has never appeared before then it may be appropriate to investigate further, i.e. request plain abdominal film, barium enema and/or possibly refer for colonoscopy
3. Possibly take stool samples for faecal occult blood
4. It may be appropriate to take blood for a full blood count and thyroid function if clinically indicated.
5. If diarrhoea predominates, it might be useful to carry out a random blood glucose test to elicit any underlying diabetes.
6. If history indicates, then take a stool sample to assess for ova or parasites.

Therapeutic intervention

The management of IBS is highly individual for each patient because of the wide variety of symptoms that present. The cornerstone of good management, however, is a good supportive relationship between the patient and nurse practitioner.

- A gradual increase in dietary fibre is usually helpful if constipation is a problem. If there is alternating diarrhoea and constipation, then a bulking agent such as ispaghula husk may be helpful. It is essential to advise an appropriate increase in fluid intake if fibre is increased, however.
- If chronic diarrhoea is a problem and is causing a major disruption to a patient's lifestyle, then it may be appropriate to use an antidiarrhoeal drug, e.g. Lomotil or Imodium. Advise against overuse, as there is a danger of paralytic ileus.
- Antispasmodic therapy may be useful to alleviate the pain, e.g. Colofac (mebeverine hydrochloride). This should be taken three times per day, approximately half an hour before a meal, but should not be used continuously as they can lose effectiveness.
- An alternative to Colofac is peppermint oil capsules. The dosage is 1–2 capsules three times per day 30–60 min before food. Treatment should be continued for up to 3 months.

Patient education

- Advise on diet and lifestyle, e.g. an increase in a variety of dietary fibre (not just wheat fibre, as this can exacerbate the problem in some individuals).
- General advice to avoid those foods that seem to aggravate the problem, providing the diet remains well balanced.
- If appropriate, reduce alcohol intake.
- Allay their fears with adequate explanation and education on the condition. People who suffer from IBS are often extremely anxious that they have a serious underlying pathology.
- If patients experience levels of stress they find difficult to cope with it may be appropriate to teach or refer for relaxation therapy and stress management.
- Some patients find complementary therapies such as aromatherapy and reflexology helpful.
- Help patients to control their symptoms rather than their symptoms controlling them.

Referral

Patient should be referred to a gastroenterologist if:
- symptoms that were previously well controlled on the above measures suddenly worsen
- a patient presenting over 40 years old with a sudden onset disturbance of bowel function, especially if there is blood in the stools
- any episode of bloody diarrhoea
- any worsening of constipation accompanied by weight loss
- any doubt or inconsistency in the diagnosis.

Complications

There are few direct complications of IBS alone. Complications are more likely to arise by an initial misdiagnosis. It is therefore vital that an accurate and comprehensive history forms the basis of your initial diagnosis of the condition.

Danger signs

- ❶ Refer if there is a sudden and/or dramatic change in symptoms with no apparent cause. This is especially important in a patient over 40 years old.
- ❶ Onset of symptoms of alternating constipation and diarrhoea in patients over 40 years old, especially if accompanied by weight loss and no previous history.
- ❶ If previous management loses its effectiveness and symptoms deteriorate – refer.

Appendicitis

Appendicitis is an acute inflammation of the appendix caused by bacterial infection. It often occurs after obstruction of the lumen by a foreign body, adhesions or lymphoid tissue. The bacteria invade the mucosal wall of the appendix, causing ischaemia, gangrene and eventual perforation. It is most common in young adults and approximately 1 in 20 of the population will experience this condition at some time during their lives (Mead 1996).

Subjective findings

Appendicitis, although a common GI complaint, can be difficult to evaluate as it can present in a variety of ways:
- Initially the patient might complain of epigastric discomfort.
- There may be constipation at first, which may change to diarrhoea as the condition progresses.
- Nausea and/or vomiting may be present. The patient may complain of a slight fever and have anorexia.
- The discomfort progresses to pain and becomes more localised over the right iliac fossa.
- Sometimes there is pain on the left too.
- The patient, especially if a child, finds it more comfortable to lie down with their knees drawn up.

Objective findings

1. Vital signs: mild fever, less than 39°C, tachycardia, shallow respirations.
2. Inspect and auscultate abdomen. Bowel sounds may be reduced or absent.
3. Percussion and palpation will reveal pain and possibly guarding in the right lower quadrant.
4. There are three classical abdominal signs indicative of appendicitis:
   - *McBurney's point* occurs where the inflamed appendix or bowel touches the abdominal wall. It is situated one-third of the distance from the anterior iliac crest to the umbilicus and rebound tenderness at this point is a classical sign.
   - *Rovsing's sign* occurs when palpation of the left lower quadrant induces pain in the right lower quadrant. This is caused by peritoneal inflammation (Wright 1997).
   - *Psoas sign*. Place your hand on the patient's right thigh, just above the knee and ask him to raise his leg against your hand (flexion of the hip). Alternatively, ask him to lie on his left side and you extend his right leg at the hip. If either of these manoeuvres causes pain, that constitutes a positive psoas sign. It is caused by irritation of the psoas muscle by an inflamed appendix (Bates 1991).
5. Digital rectal examination results in tenderness on the right (but this may also be due to pelvic inflammatory disease, especially in young women).
6. Sometimes the appendix is displaced, which can lead to a different presentation. There may be pain on micturition and left-sided pain. In a pregnant woman, the appendix is situated much higher in the abdomen.
7. Children and older adults can also present very differently. Children can be more systemically ill with vomiting, rather than abdominal pain and tenderness.

In older adults, the perception of pain from internal organs is altered and they may present with only relatively mild discomfort, even on perforation.

Plan

- If unsure of diagnosis, review patient in 2–3 hours (often useful for children and the older adult who do not present initially with classical symptoms).
- If diagnosis is confirmed or seems likely, refer.

Referral

As the condition can be difficult to diagnose, any suspicion of appendicitis should be referred to the surgical team for further assessment, without delay.

Patient education

- In this instance, the main area of education would be management of the healing wound.
- Discuss healing and its relationship to wound integrity.
- Many appendicectomies are now carried out using a laparoscopic technique and therefore there may only be a very small wound.
- Discuss lifestyle to ensure adequate fibre, fluids and exercise to maintain a regular bowel action.

Complications

The main complication of appendicitis is peritonitis following perforation of the inflamed appendix. Other complications are an appendix mass and an appendix abscess. Differential diagnosis is important and can be difficult, particularly in young women, children and the elderly. Conditions that might be confused with appendicitis include diverticulitis, pelvic inflammatory disease, ovarian pathology, ectopic pregnancy, Crohn's disease and mesenteric adenitis (Hirsh & McKenna 1996, Mead 1996).

Danger signs

- ❶ If appendicitis is suspected in a child, do not delay requesting a surgical opinion.
- ❶ Take care in the older adult, as an altered perception of abdominal pain can mask the severity of the condition and perforation can occur if left untreated. Refer if in doubt.
- ❶ In women of child-bearing age exclude the possibility of ectopic pregnancy as a cause for right lower quadrant pain and guarding. It is also possible that acute pelvic inflammation can cause similar pain to appendicitis.
- ❶ Appendicitis in the pregnant woman is more difficult to diagnose because of the upward displacement of the appendix by the uterus. Pain tends to be in the right lateral region and prompt effective diagnosis is important. If surgical intervention is initiated prior to perforation, then the outcome is usually favourable. However, there is a 30% fetal mortality if perforation occurs (Hope et al 1996).

Cholecystitis

Gall bladder disease can be acute or chronic. The cause is usually cystic duct obstruction or irritation by a stone in, or inflammation of, the gall bladder. The five 'Fs' were used to describe the classic patient with cholecystitis – 'fair, fat, fertile, female and forty' and, although it is more common in older, overweight women, it can also occur in other groups. Patients with diabetes are more likely to develop gallstones (Shaw 1996).

Gallbladder disease is asymptomatic in many individuals who have gallstones, but it may result in recurrent bouts of abdominal discomfort accompanied by nausea, flatulence and fat intolerance. These symptoms, however, can also be caused by other conditions such as IBS, gastro-oesophageal reflux disease, peptic ulcers, chronic relapsing pancreatitis and malignancy (Hope et al 1996). The acute form of the disease usually occurs following impaction of a stone in the cystic duct.

Acute cholecystitis

Subjective findings .

- The patient complains of acute upper right quadrant pain. This is often accompanied by nausea and/or vomiting and fever.
- The patient may complain that the pain radiates to their back.
- It may be sudden onset, but the pain classically builds in intensity over 2–4 hours.
- Pain may radiate to the right or left upper scapula.
- Patients may say it is difficult to take a deep breath.

Objective findings

- Vital signs should be normal. There may be a slight tachycardia if the patient has severe pain but there should be no fever.
- Observe the colour of the patient; there may be jaundice present or the patient's colour may be normal. Jaundice occurs if a stone becomes lodged in the common bile duct.
- Inspection and auscultation of the abdomen should reveal nothing abnormal.
- Percussion may be too painful for the patient but reveals normal sounds.
- Palpation again will be painful, but observe for *Murphy's sign*. Place two fingers of your right hand under the right costal margin and ask the patient to take a deep breath. Sudden inspiratory arrest due to pain is a positive sign. It is only positive, however, if the same manoeuvre in the left upper quadrant produces no pain (Hope et al 1996).
- There may be localised peritonism.

Plan

- Following assessment decide on probable diagnosis
- Refer if appropriate.

Referral

- For a patient with evidence of acute cholecystitis the most appropriate action is referral to the surgical team.
- Often the patient requires an intravenous (IV) infusion with IV antibiotics and should be nil by mouth.
- Cholecystectomy may be performed within 48 hours, or once the acute episode has settled patients may be brought back for surgery within 3 months (Hope et al 1996).

Chronic cholecystitis

Subjective findings

- The patient may complain of vague intermittent abdominal discomfort in the right upper quadrant. This may radiate to the back.
- The condition may be exacerbated by an intake of fatty food.
- Patients may also experience some nausea, flatulence and abdominal distension (remember these can have other causes).

Objective findings

- Vital signs will be normal
- Observe the patient's colour for any signs of jaundice
- The patient may be overweight and female (see above), but this is not inevitably so
- Abdominal examination is usually unremarkable unless there is an acute episode (see above)
- The gallbladder is rarely palpable (Shaw 1996).

Plan

- Carry out appropriate investigations
- Provide the patient with appropriate advice
- Refer if appropriate.

Investigations

- Take blood for white cell count (WCC), liver enzymes and serum amylase to eliminate other causes.
- Request abdominal ultrasound. This is the preferred diagnostic test for the detection of gall bladder disease; oral cholecystogram and IV cholangiogram are less reliable (Hope et al 1996).

Therapeutic intervention

There is no appropriate medication for the treatment of chronic cholecystitis other than relief of symptoms. If patient discomfort is mild and the diagnosis of gall bladder disease has been confirmed, then advice on diet and lifestyle together with reassurance may be all that is needed. It may also be appropriate to reduce or change preparation for some drugs that may trigger stone formation, e.g. oestrogen and thiazides (Shaw 1996).

Referral

- As symptomatic gallbladder disease tends to recur, then referral to the surgical team for possible cholecystectomy may be appropriate.
- Cholecystectomy is often carried out using a laparoscopic technique, which tends to reduce postoperative morbidity.
- There are other techniques that can be used to disintegrate gallstones. The administration of oral agents to dissolve stones is only of use for small to medium-sized radiolucent stones and is used under close radiological supervision.

Patient education

- Reduce fat and calorie intake to ensure appropriate body mass index (BMI).
- There is some evidence that a moderate daily intake of alcohol protects against the incidence of symptomatic gallbladder disease (Shaw 1996).
- If there is no acute distress, then reassurance about the benign nature of the disease should be given.

Complications

There are generally few complications of chronic cholecystitis, but untreated acute disease can result in jaundice, cholangitis, empyema or pancreatitis owing to the obstructive nature of the disease. Another possible complication of gallstones is gallstone ileus. This is caused by a gallstone perforating the gall bladder, eroding through the duodenum and possibly eventually lodging and causing an obstruction in the terminal ileum (Hope et al 1996).

Danger signs

- ❶ Possibly the most important danger sign for acute and chronic cholecystitis is an accurate differential diagnosis.
- ❶ The pain of acute cholecystitis may also be indicative of pancreatitis, peptic ulcer, diverticulitis, hepatitis, possible pelvic inflammatory disease or myocardial infarction (MI). Refer for investigation.
- ❶ Chronic cholecystitis may also be confused with other conditions, e.g. reflux, peptic ulcers, IBS, chronic pancreatitis or malignancy. Refer for further investigation.

Gastrointestinal bleeding

A GI bleed can be an acute or chronic haemorrhagic event and can occur anywhere in the GI tract. The most common sites for haemorrhage are the oesophagus, stomach and duodenum at the proximal end and the colon, anus and rectum at the distal end of the GI tract. In the primary care setting the most common causes of GI bleed encountered are peptic ulcer disease (PUD) (see separate section below), diverticulitis, colitis, malignancy and anorectal problems such as haemorrhoids or anal fissure. Other less common causes are oesophageal varices and a Mallory–Weiss tear (Hope et al 1996, Selfridge-Thomas 1998).

Acute gastrointestinal haemorrhage

Subjective findings

- The patient may complain of blood-stained vomitus or stools.
- Patients may feel weak and faint.
- There may be abdominal pain or discomfort.
- There may be a history of melaena with visible clots in the stool.
- If possible establish any history of excessive alcohol consumption (a clue to the possibility of oesophageal varices).
- Discover what medication may have been used, including OTC products. Drugs such as aspirin and other nonsteroidal anti-inflammatory drugs (NSAIDs) may be of significance.

Objective findings

- Vital signs may show evidence of shock: tachycardia with 'thready pulse', hypotension.
- The patient may be pale and restless with an altered state of consciousness. Look for evidence of jaundice.
- Inspection and auscultation of the abdomen may reveal normal, hyporeactive or hyperactive bowel sounds (Selfridge-Thomas 1998). There may be spider naevi and ascites present.
- Percussion and palpation may show abdominal tenderness. Check for an enlarged spleen or liver.

Plan

- Following assessment, decide on probable diagnosis.
- Refer urgently, if appropriate.

Referral

This tends to be an acute situation that needs urgent referral to hospital for stablisation.

Chronic gastrointestinal bleeding

Subjective findings

Many of the symptoms described will overlap with those for PUD (see below).

- Other symptoms may include feelings of weakness, dizziness, palpitations and shortness of breath (owing to anaemia)
- Patients may complain of intermittent black, tarry stools or fresh blood in their stools
- There may be weight loss and changes in bowel habit
- Assess any changes in appetite and establish whether this is associated with early satiety or difficulty in swallowing
- Are patients passing any mucus with their stool as well as blood?

- Patients may complain of abdominal pain and urgent diarrhoea
- Establish diet and alcohol intake and enquire about oral medication, including OTC preparations
- Assess any previous history of GI disturbance or treatment.

Objective findings

- Assess the patient's colour and appearance. Observe mucous membranes and nail beds for pallor or jaundice
- Vital signs may indicate mild tachycardia or normal pulse; blood pressure may be normal, hypotensive or hypertensive, depending on the severity of the bleeding and any other underlying condition
- Inspection and auscultation of the abdomen may reveal nothing unusual.
- Percussion and palpation may highlight areas of tenderness, e.g. in the epigastrium (see PUD) or anywhere over the colon
- There may be localised peritonism if there is a severe diverticulitis (this can be confused with appendicitis and/or PID)
- Digital rectal examination and proctoscopy may reveal rectal haemorrhoids, polyps or even malignancy.

Plan

- Establish presence of anaemia, if any
- Investigate possible cause of GI bleed
- Provide appropriate information and health promotion advice for the patient
- Refer on as necessary for further investigations or treatment.

Investigations

1. Take blood for a full blood count, to assess the extent of any anaemia.
2. Request endoscopy if an upper GI bleed is suspected (i.e. patient is passing melaena stools).
3. Alternatively, a barium meal X-ray could be requested. The choice will depend on local policy and the age of the patient.
4. Send a faecal sample for culture and sensitivity. Some bacterial infections can cause bleeding (Davies et al 1998).
5. Obtain faecal samples for faecal occult blood to detect subacute GI bleeding.
6. It may be necessary to order a repeat proctoscopy where samples of rectal mucosa can be taken.
7. Request sigmoidoscopy or colonoscopy. Sigmoidoscopy allows inspection and possible sampling of the sigmoid colon up to the splenic flexure, approximately 60 cm. A colonoscopy enables the whole of the lower bowel to be visualised and/or sampled, i.e. from the anus to the start of the ascending colon, a distance of 165–185 cm. A sigmoidoscopy would be used to exclude ulcerative

colitis or Crohn's disease, either of which would be suspected with bleeding from the colon with or without diarrhoea and pain.

8. A barium enema is an alternative to colonoscopy but should not be performed if an obstructing annular carcinoma is suspected or within 48 hours of a rectal biopsy (Davies et al 1998).

Therapeutic intervention

- Any intervention will depend on the outcome of the investigations and the cause of the GI bleed. This may range from oral iron through transfusion, ulcer eradication therapy (see below) to radical surgery, depending on the cause.
- If ulcerative colitis or Crohn's disease are diagnosed, the initial management is usually conservative. Oral therapy is prescribed to reduce the activity of the disease and induce remission. Neither disease is curable but they are treatable. The drugs of choice are initially corticosteroids (topical by suppository or enema, oral or IV in severe cases) to suppress the disease process. Maintenance of remission is then achieved by the use of aminosalicylates: sulfasalazine and mesalazine are the most common. Care of patients with inflammatory bowel disease is usually shared between primary care and a gastro-enterology specialist. Surgical treatment is some-times required.
- All intervention should be carried out in a supportive and educative way, providing the patient with adequate explanation and information.

Patient education

- General education regarding diet and other lifestyle advice should be given, explaining the importance of adequate fibre in the diet and the beneficial effects of eating five portions of fruit and vegetables every day
- Explain the need to stop smoking and reduce alcohol consumption, if appropriate
- Diet is particularly important if the cause of the GI bleed was haemorrhoids or anal fissure, both of which can be caused by constipation
- Clear advice about the early reporting of any rectal bleeding should be given
- If the patient needs to self-treat, e.g. for some ano-rectal disorder, then provide clear instruction on how the condition should be managed
- For patients with inflammatory bowel disease, pastoral care – i.e. providing advice, information and support for the patient within his environment – may be particularly important (Finlay 1999).

Referral

- Any case of unexplained GI bleeding should be referred for further investigation
- Depending on the outcome of the investigations you initiate, you may need to refer the patient to a gastroenterologist or the surgical team.

Complications

- The sequelae of a GI bleed again depend on the cause.
- The obvious most serious complication is haemor-rhagic shock and subsequent death. A GI bleed is a serious complication of oesophageal varices, which can remain undetected until they rupture, causing a massive haematemesis.
- Inflammatory bowel disease can lead to bowel obstruction, perforation and fistula formation.
- Diverticulitis can also result in perforation of the bowel and subsequent peritonitis.
- Malignancy can develop from Crohn's disease in either the large or small bowel.

Danger signs

- **!** All episodes of GI bleed require further investiga-tion.
- **!** Special vigilance is required when caring for older adults, especially if they are taking NSAIDs for musculoskeletal disorders. They are very susceptible to the slow, 'silent' GI bleed as a result of gastric irri-tation and may not display overt symptoms. Alternatively, they may assume that symptoms of tiredness, lethargy and breathlessness, due to anaemia, may be a consequence of ageing.
- **!** Patients often do not seek help for episodes of rectal bleeding. Opportunistic health education is vital.
- **!** If a young adult or child presents with hae-matemesis, assess the possibility of swallowed blood from a nosebleed first.
- **!** In teenagers and adults exclude the possibility of excessive use of alcohol when presenting with hae-matemesis.

Peptic ulcer disease (PUD)

PUD is a chronic inflammatory disorder of the lower oesophagus, stomach and/or duodenum. It is a common disorder, although incidence has been declining in the UK since the 1950s (Cottrill 1996). It tends to affect men more than women (in the ratio 2:1), reaching a plateau during middle age (Hope et al 1996, Shaw 1996). Peptic ulceration occurs in the sites that come into contact with pepsin and gastric acid – the distal end of the oesopha-gus, the stomach and the duodenum – but in over 95% of cases of duodenal ulcer and over 85% of gastric ulcer the bacterium *Helicobacter pylori* is also present (Shaw 1996). This microorganism was discovered and linked with PUD in the early 1980s but it was only acknowl-edged as one of the main causes of the disease in the mid-1990s (Aronson 1998). *H. pylori* bacteria are S-shaped or curved rod-shaped organisms with flagella at one end. The bacteria burrow into the wall of the stomach, causing a local inflammatory reaction and a systemic immune response. They also decrease the production of the gastroduodenal hormone somatostatin. This hormone suppresses the production of gastric acid when gastrin is released, so the end result of the infection is over production of gastric acid, gastritis and ulcer formation (Cottrill 1996, MacConnachie 1997). PUD is a common cause of upper GI bleed (see above) but non-bleeding ulcers can also occur.

Subjective findings

1. The most common symptom is epigastric pain, which can radiate through to the back.
2. The pain is classically relieved by antacids and occurs in episodes of a few weeks, interspersed with several pain-free months (Shaw 1996).
3. The pain of a duodenal ulcer tends to be relieved by food, whereas in a gastric ulcer food makes it worse.
4. As a result of the above, there may be weight fluctuations – a patient with a duodenal ulcer may tend to put weight on, whereas a patient with a gastric ulcer may lose weight. However, this is by no means an inevitable rule.
5. Often a patient with a duodenal ulcer will complain of intermittent pain that wakens them at night but does not usually occur before breakfast. This is not always the case for everyone, however.
6. Gastric ulcer pain tends to radiate from the epigastric area behind the sternum and into the back.
7. Patients may also describe other symptoms, such as pyrosis (heart burn), excessive gas, belching, nausea and dysphagia.
8. If there is a bleeding peptic ulcer, patients may describe a black melaena stool as in other causes of upper GI bleed (see above).
9. The pain may be described as dull, aching, gnawing or burning.
10. It is important to establish lifestyle factors, especially smoking and drinking alcohol. Although these are now believed not to cause PUD, they are still considered to be exacerbating factors.
11. Establish the use of any OTC medication, such as aspirin or other NSAIDs and any antacids.

Objective findings

- Assess the patient's colour and mucous membranes, particularly for signs of anaemia.
- Vital signs will probably be normal.
- Inspection and auscultation should be unremarkable. Bowel sounds should be normal.
- Palpation and percussion will probably reveal a tender epigastrium but little else.

Plan

- Establish the presence of anaemia, if suspected
- Request appropriate investigations to establish cause of symptoms
- Once cause is established, commence appropriate therapy or refer for further investigation and/or treatment

- Provide appropriate information and advice for the patient in relation to the outcome of the above.

Investigations

1. Take blood for a full blood count and possibly an *H. pylori* antibody titre. This will depend on local policy and facilities at the laboratory. The presence of antibodies in a symptomatic individual may be used as the only initial investigation prior to treatment, but there are risks with adopting this method in isolation (see below).
2. Abdominal ultrasound may be requested first to rule out gall bladder disease (see above).
3. If the patient is under 40–45 years of age, it will probably be more appropriate to request subsequent barium meal X-ray studies.
4. If the patient is 40–45 years old or over, then refer for endoscopy. This is the 'gold standard' diagnostic procedure for peptic ulcer, but the age of the patient and the availability of local resources will determine its use. Patients in this age group should automatically have endoscopy to exclude gastric malignancy.
5. Endoscopy allows for biopsy and histological identification of the bacterium and a direct measure of urease, a product of metabolism of the bacterium.
6. Once the ulcer has been treated (see below), a repeat test may be needed. This is usually a 'breath test'. Urease is detected in the breath of an individual with *H. pylori* infection, and following treatment it should be undetectable. If symptoms are removed, it may not be necessary to do this, but if a patient has persistent problems or a history of previous complications, such as perforation or GI bleed, then eradication should be verified.

Therapeutic intervention

- The prime objective of any intervention is to alleviate symptoms, encourage healing and prevent recurrence.
- The first line of treatment will be to remove or reduce exacerbating factors such as smoking and alcohol intake.
- Special diets or excluding certain foods are no longer recognised to be necessary, but patients may still discuss this with you. If they feel more comfortable avoiding certain foods, then so long as they are not overly restrictive it will do no harm.
- The main drug therapy options for the treatment of PUD are shown in Table 9.5.
- Once a diagnosis of PUD is confirmed, then the treatment of choice is 'ulcer eradication therapy'. This consists of a combination of two antibiotics and a proton pump inhibitor, which together destroy the bacteria and reduce the gastric acid secretion to allow healing of the ulcer. Table 9.6 shows the different combinations of drugs in common use for eradication therapy.
- During the time of investigation, it is appropriate to use antacid therapy to alleviate symptoms.

Table 9.5 *Main drug therapy options for PUD* *(Adapted from BNF 36 1998.)*

Type of product	Generic	Brand	Dose
Antacids: aluminium and magnesium salts	Aluminium hydroxide/ magnesium hydroxide	Maalox (suspension)	10–20 ml when required
		Maalox TC (tablets)	1–2 tablets when required
	Magnesium carbonate	Generic only	10 ml three times a day in water
	Magnesium trisilicate	Generic only:	
		tablets	1–2 tablets when required
		mixture	10 ml three times a day in water
		oral powder	1–5 g in liquid when required
Compounds of aluminium hydroxide, magnesium trisilicate, sodium bicarbonate and alginic acid	Compound alginic acid preparations	Gastrocote tablets	1–2 tablets four times a day
		Gastrocote liquid	5–15 ml four times a day
		Gaviscon liquid	10–20 ml after meals and at night
		Gaviscon tablets	1–2 tablets to be chewed and followed by water
H_2-receptor antagonists	Cimetidine	Tagamet	400 mg twice per day (with breakfast and at night) or 800 mg at night for 4–8 weeks maintenance 400 mg daily
	Ranitidine	Zantac	150 mg twice daily or 300 mg at night as above; maintenance 150 mg at night
	Famotidine	Pepcid	40 mg at night as above; maintenance 20 mg at night
	Nizatidine	Axid	As for ranitidine
Proton pump inhibitors	Omeprazole	Losec	20–40 mg for 4–8 weeks; maintenance 20 mg daily
	Lansoprazole	Zoton	30 mg daily for 4–8 weeks; maintenance 15 mg daily
	Pantoprazole	Protium	40 mg daily for 2–8 weeks

- In the younger symptomatic adult, i.e. under 40–45 years of age, it is possible that some clinicians may treat with an H_2-receptor antagonist alone for 4–8 weeks, allowing the ulcer to heal. The problem with this therapy alone if *H. pylori* is present is that the symptoms, i.e. the ulcer, are extremely likely to recur.
- Once eradication is established, some individuals may need to continue indefinitely with a maintenance dose of proton pump inhibitor or H_2-receptor antagonist and antacid if they have a persistent problem with pain. These individuals may have concurrent non-ulcer dyspepsia.

Patient education

1. Perhaps the most important part of patient education is a clear understanding of the need to take antibiotic therapy for 'indigestion' or 'acid stomach'.
2. Secondly, the importance of compliance with the eradication therapy regimen. Without completion of the course there is a strong possibility that the bacterium will develop resistance to the antibiotics and obviously the ulcer will not heal.
3. Related to this is a clear explanation of the possibility of side effects of the combination therapy. These tend to be minor, but if not expected they may preclude compliance.
4. Generally, the regimens are well tolerated but minor GI upsets may be associated with any or all

of the drugs (see Table 9.6 for regimens). Inform patients that if abdominal pain with bloody diarrhoea presents they should stop the medication and consult promptly for further investigations. This may be an indication of pseudomembranous colitis.
5. You also need to inform patients receiving metronidazole as part of their treatment to avoid alcohol while taking the medication. There is an interaction between the two compounds, which can result in 'flu-like' illness or a prolonged 'hangover' effect.
6. If patients smoke and are taking H_2-receptor antagonists, then they should be warned that smoking reduces the effect of the drug. Advise them that if they are unable to stop smoking entirely, then they should not smoke before the bedtime dose of the drug.
7. Advise patients taking proton pump inhibitors that they should take them once per day on an empty stomach. This may be before breakfast or at bedtime.
8. It is important to discuss with patients their use of antacids, especially if they use OTC preparations. Some of these can contain high levels of sodium, calcium and/or magnesium, which can cause potential problems, particularly in elderly patients and in those with impaired renal function (Aronson 1998).

Table 9.6 *Ulcer eradication therapy regimens (Adapted from BNF 36 1998.)*

Therapy regime	Drug combinations
Triple therapy: 1-week regimens	Amoxicillin 500 mg three times daily + Metronidazole 400 mg three times daily + Omeprazole 20 mg twice daily or 40 mg once daily for 7 days
	Clarithromycin 250 mg twice daily + metronidazole 400 mg (or tinidazole 500 mg) twice daily + omeprazole 20 mg twice daily or 40 mg once daily for 7 days
	Amoxicillin 1 g twice daily + clarithromycin 500 mg twice daily + omeprazole 20 mg twice daily or 40 mg once daily for 7 days
	Lansoprazole 30 mg twice daily + *two* of the following: amoxicillin 1 g twice daily, clarithromycin 250 mg twice daily or metronidazole 400 mg twice daily
Triple therapy: 2-week regimens	Tetracycline 500 mg four times daily + metronidazole 400 mg three times daily + tripotassium dicitratobismuthate (bismuth chelate) 120 mg four times daily
	Amoxicillin 750 mg three times daily + metronidazole 500 mg three times daily + ranitidine 300 mg at night (or 150 mg twice daily) for 14 days
Dual therapy: 2-week regimens	Ranitidine bismuth citrate 400 mg twice daily + either: amoxicillin 500 mg four times daily or clarithromycin 250 mg four times daily (or 500 mg three times daily) for 14 days

9. Antacid products containing aluminium and magnesium can cause constipation and diarrhoea, respectively, so advise patients to keep their consumption to a minimum.
10. Antacids can also interact with other drugs, including proton pump inhibitors, so it is important to separate these drugs by at least 1–2 hours.
11. Interestingly, although many patients take milk as an antacid, it can exacerbate the problem. The high calcium content of milk over a prolonged period can cause an increase in gastric acid production (Brozenec 1996).
12. Although stress is no longer believed to cause ulcers, it does cause an increase in gastric acid production, so it might exacerbate an existing condition. Encourage patients to review their coping mechanisms and stress management techniques (Brozenec 1996).
13. It is essential that patients are encouraged to report any return or exacerbation of symptoms immediately. They should also be advised that taking antacids indefinitely might be masking a more serious underlying condition.

Referral

- Currently, apart from referral for investigations, PUD may be managed in the primary care setting
- If symptoms persist or return following apparent eradication, then refer the patient to a gastroenterologist for further investigation and treatment.

Complications

- The main complication of PUD is bleeding and perforation.

- There is a strong association with gastric cancer in some countries, e.g. Japan (Cottrill 1996). This seems to be linked with some strains of *H. pylori*, which may lead to the development of chronic atrophic gastritis, a precursor for gastric cancer (Seifrit 1997).

Danger signs

- ❶ The pain of what appears to be peptic ulcer disease may be an undetected MI.

Glossary

Aneurysm A ballooning of an artery wall. This puts the artery at risk of rupture. It may have a congenital cause, but often is due to a weakening effect caused by chronic hypertension and arteriosclerosis

Bruit An abnormal sound heard over a blood vessel. It may be caused by narrowing of the vessel or by an aneurysm

Cholangitis Infection in the bile duct that causes a high temperature with rigors, jaundice and right upper quadrant pain

Chronic atrophic gastritis Chronic inflammation of the gastric mucosa that seems to be associated with *H. pylori* infection. It occurs over a number of years and results in a wasting of the gastric mucosa and a decline in acid production, which in turn seems to be a precursor for gastric cancer

Empyema A collection of pus in an internal organ or potential body space, e.g. an infected gall bladder filled with pus or a collection of pus between the pleural membranes

Familial adenomatous polyposis (Gardner's syndrome) A genetic disorder that is dominantly inherited. It results in multiple pre-malignant polyps in the colon together with bone and soft tissue tumours. Symptoms include bloody diarrhoea

Guarding A reflex contraction of the abdominal muscles during palpation that is caused by local or general peritoneal inflammation

Top Tips ✓

1 A comprehensive and accurate history is the key to effective management, because of the variety of symptoms that can occur in gastrointestinal (GI) disease

2 Symptoms in women that may appear to be of GI origin may be caused by gynaecological problems and vice versa

3 Older adults and young children may not present with 'classical symptoms' in GI disease

4 Dehydration in gastroenteritis is of particular significance in the very young, the very old and in pregnant women. Fluid replacement is essential

5 Confirmed bacterial gastroenteritis will often resolve spontaneously and antibiotics should be avoided unless the infection is very severe

6 Vomiting with dysphagia and weight loss may be indicative of malignancy and should be referred for further investigation

7 Abdominal massage may be a useful non-pharmacological intervention in mild constipation, particularly in children

8 Any sudden onset change in bowel habit over the age of 50 years should be referred for investigation

9 Exclude pelvic inflammatory disease or ectopic pregnancy in women of child-bearing age who present with right lower quadrant pain and guarding

10 All episodes of GI bleeding require further investigation.

H₂-receptor antagonists H_2-receptors are a group of histamine receptors found in the parietal cells of the stomach mucosa. They respond to histamine and stimulate the production of hydrochloric acid necessary for digestion

HcG (human chorionic gonadotrophin)   A hormone produced by a newly fertilized embryo that stimulates the corpus luteum to continue secreting oestrogen and progesterone. This overrides the pituitary/ovarian control mechanism and allows continuation of the endometrial layer ready for implantation of the embryo

IV cholangiogram   An IV injection of a radio-opaque contrast medium, which shows up the outline of the gall bladder on X-ray

Mallory–Weiss tear   A tear in the oesophagus caused by prolonged vomiting of any cause, which results in haematemesis

Mesenteric adenitis   This occurs in young children and is pain in the abdomen following an upper respiratory tract infection. It is extremely difficult to differentiate from appendicitis

Myenteric plexus   An autonomic nerve plexus, i.e. a network of converging and diverging nerve fibres. It is found between the two smooth muscle layers of the gut and controls gut motility

Non-ulcer dyspepsia   This can be described as a burning epigastric pain that occurs approximately 1 hour after meals. It is easy to confuse with a peptic ulcer but *H. pylori* eradication therapy makes little difference to the symptoms as the organism tends not to be present

Oesophageal varices   Hypertension in the hepatic portal venous system, which may be due to alcohol-induced cirrhosis, leads to a bypassing of some of the circulation into veins at the base of the oesophagus. If the pressure continues to rise, then these vessels become distended resulting in varicose veins at the base of the oesophagus. Once this happens, rupture is common and can be catastrophic

Oral cholecystogram   A radio-opaque contrast medium is given orally. This is concentrated by the gall bladder, which then shows up on X-ray

Peritonism   A sign that can be observed in the abdomen following rupture of an organ or perforation of an inflamed appendix or peptic ulcer. It consists of tenderness guarding and rebound tenderness

Proton-pump inhibitors   Also known as gastric acid pump inhibitors, proton pump inhibitors are powerful drugs that stop gastric acid secretion by up to 95%. They act on the parietal cell of the gastric mucosa at the chemical level, blocking the chemical reaction that results in the secretion of gastric acid

Rebound tenderness   On abdominal examination, if an increase in pain is felt briefly following removal of the examiner's hand, then rebound tenderness is present. This is due to an inflamed peritoneum rebounding into place after being moved by the pressure of the fingers

Spider naevi   Distended arterioles visible on the abdomen that are often associated with liver disease and consist of a central arteriole 'body' with spider-like 'legs' branching out from the centre. They blanch when pressure is applied and usually, though not always, are on areas drained by the superior vena cava

Tenesmus   The sensation that the rectum has not been emptied fully even after having the bowels open. It is common in irritable bowel syndrome but can also be caused by a tumour

References

Aronson B 1998 Update on peptic ulcer drugs. American Journal of Nursing 98(1):41–46.

Barrett J A 1993 Faecal incontinence and related problems in the older adult. Edward Arnold, London.

Bates B 1991 A guide to physical examination and history taking, 5th edn. Lippincott, Philadelphia.

British National Formulary (BNF) 36 1998 British Medical Association, London.

Brozenec S 1996 Ulcer update therapy. RN 59(9):48–50, 52–54.

Christensen J 1994 Possible effects of laxatives on the nerve plexuses of the colon. In: Kamm M A, Lennard-Jones, J E (eds) Constipation. Wrighton Biomedical Publishing, Petersfield: 321–326.

Cottrill M R B 1996 *Helicobacter pylori*. Professional Nurse 12(1):46–48.

Davies P, Button C, Foster M 1998 Rectal bleeding. Nursing Times 94(16):46–49.

Finlay T 1999 Inflammatory bowel disease. Nursing Times 95(8):50–53.

Hirsh M P, McKenna C J 1996 Abdominal pain in children: surgical consideration. Topics in Emergency Medicine 18(3):49–61.

Hope R A, Longmore J M, Hodgetts T J, Ramrakha P S 1996 Oxford handbook of clinical medicine, 3rd edn. Oxford University Press, Oxford.

Lewis C, Muir J 1996 A collaborative approach in the management of childhood constipation. Health Visitor 69(10):424–426.

MacConnachie A M 1997 Eradication therapy in peptic ulcer disease. Intensive and Critical Care Nursing 13:121–122.

Mead M 1996 Detecting appendicitis. Practice Nurse 11(7):486–487.

Monga A K, Marrerro J M, Stanton S L et al 1997 Is there an irritable bladder in the irritable bowel syndrome. British Journal of Obstetrics and Gynaecology 104(12):1409–1412.

Ness W 1997 Irritable bowel syndrome. Primary Health Care 7(10):18–20.

Norton C 1996 The causes and nursing management of constipation. British Journal of Nursing 5(20):1252–1258.

Richards A 1998 Hands on help. Nursing Times 94(32):69–75.

Seifrit B 1997 *Helicobacter pylori*. AORN Journal 65(3):614–616, 619–620.

Selfridge-Thomas J 1998 Gastrointestinal bleeding. American Journal of Nursing 98(1):16BB.

Shaw B 1996 Primary care for women. Management and treatment of gastrointestinal disorders. Journal of Nurse-Midwifery 41(2):155–172.

Weber J 1988 Nurses' handbook of health assessment. Lippincott, Philadelphia.

Winney J 1998 Constipation. Nursing Standard 13(1):46–56.

Winter G 1998 A gut feeling. Nursing Times 94(37):41.

Wright J A 1997 Seven abdominal assessment signs every emergency nurse should know. Journal Emergency Nursing 23(5):446–450.

Further reading

Primary health care clinical update 1997 Bowel disease 7(10):17–19.

Shaw B 1995 Primary care for women. Comprehensive assessment of gastrointestinal disorders. Journal of Nurse-Midwifery 40(2):216–230.

Shaw B 1996 Primary care for women. Management and treatment of gastrointestinal disorders. Journal of Nurse-Midwifery 41(2):155–172.

Weber J 1988 Nurses' handbook of health assessment. Lippincott, Philadelphia.

ENDOCRINE DISORDERS

Rosie Walsh

- Diabetes is the commonest endocrine disorder, costing the NHS over £2 billion a year and accounting for 9% of hospital costs (Audit Commission 2000)

- Diabetes affects 3% of the population (Audit Commission 2000) and may be undetected in approximately 50% of people (Griffith et al 1996)

- One in four Asian people over 60 have diabetes (Audit Commission 2000)

- Type 1 diabetes is more common in people of European extraction in the second and third decades of life (Griffith et al 1996)

- Type 2 diabetes is more common after middle age but can present in the fourth decade of life or earlier and particularly occurs in populations characterised by modern rather than traditional lifestyles and diets (Griffith et al 1996)

- Graves' disease (hyperthyroidism) usually presents between 30 and 60 years of age and 90% of cases are in women (Conway & Betteridge 1996)

- Toxic multinodular goitre usually develops in late middle age (Conway & Betteridge 1996)

- The annual incidence of hypothyroidism in women is 2/1000 and 90% of patients are female (Conway & Betteridge 1996)

- Hypothyroidism may occur at any age but is most common from middle age onwards (Conway & Betteridge 1996)

- Hyperthyroidism is more common in iodine-replete areas and hypothyroidism is more common in iodine-deficient areas (Conway & Betteridge 1996)

Introduction

Presenting signs and symptoms of endocrine disorders vary according to the underlying pathophysiology. The common symptoms of endocrine disorders are fatigue, weight change or altered mental function (Conway & Betteridge 1996). Although these general symptoms are common to a number of other diseases, if present, the more specific features of an endocrine disorder in each hormone system should be explored. For example, weakness, lethargy and depression may be features of Cushing's syndrome, hypothyroidism, sex hormone deficiency or hypopituitarism. Hypothyroidism may also be accompanied by dry skin and alopecia, while Cushing's syndrome may feature thin skin, bruising, purple striae and hirsutism. Weight gain may be generalised in hypothyroidism or truncal in Cushing's syndrome (Conway & Betteridge 1996). The symptoms may often be subtle and insidious and may go unnoticed by the patient.

Subjective assessment

As endocrine disorders may affect any body function, the detailed history taken should be broad and include details of any family history of autoimmune endocrinopathies or endocrine neoplasia. A full history of developmental milestones will be required, particularly if an endocrine disorder is suspected in a child. Key components that you will need to investigate in the history of a patient presenting with a suspected endocrine disorder (Conway & Betteridge 1996) are:

- General well-being – explore when the patient was last completely well, his energy levels, mood, sleeping pattern, appetite and weight, changes in skin and hair.
- Pattern of disease onset and progression – explore how symptoms have developed (most endocrine disorders are gradually progressive rather than relapsing).
- Impact on lifestyle – explore whether there is anything that the patient now has difficulty in doing (physical, social or psychological). Check for history of stressful life events or difficulties.
- Enquire about alcohol intake.
- Drug history – some endocrine disorders may be iatrogenic, e.g., corticosteroid-induced Cushing's syndrome.
- Past medical history – previous head injury may cause hypopituitarism; previous partial thyroidec-

tomy may cause hypothyroidism; and previous radiation or cytotoxic therapy may be related to gonadal failure. Enquire about any previous mental health problems (may have a history of anxiety or depressive disorders).

- Family history – may be important indicators of thyroid disease and diabetes.
- In children, endocrine disorders may manifest as failure to thrive. The three common metabolic diseases in children are diabetes mellitus, phenylketonuria (PKU) and galactosaemia (Burns et al 1996).

Objective assessment

Assessment of the patient with a suspected endocrine disorder will include a general physical examination. In some disorders, e.g. suspected pituitary tumours, examination of the central and peripheral nervous system will also be necessary and, unless you are competent in these assessments, you may need to refer the patient to a medical practitioner. It may be necessary to examine the genitalia if a gonadal disorder is suspected.

1. Measure height and weight. Growth rate is particularly important in children with suspected endocrine disease and it is helpful to review serial measurements. A growth rate of more or less than 2 inches a year may need to be investigated (Burns et al 1996). Key areas to note are the height of the child's parents, any medication that may affect growth (e.g. steroids) and diet and exercise history. In a child, check also for proportionate appearance by measuring sitting and standing heights for upper to lower segment ratio (Burns et al 1996).
2. Vital signs – pulse, for rate and character, and blood pressure (hypertension may indicate Cushing's syndrome or phaeochromocytoma).
3. Physical examination – observe overall appearance and note fat distribution (important feature in Cushing's syndrome and hypothyroidism). Key areas to inspect are the hands for tremor or pigmentation, skin (note vitiligo, which is associated with autoimmunity, dryness, hirsutism, bruising), hair (note alopecia and dryness), abdomen (note pigmented striae associated with Cushing's syndrome).
4. Test visual acuity and visual fields (field changes occur with pituitary tumours).
5. Diagnostics – consider these blood tests: full blood count (FBC), urea and electrolytes, biochemistry tests for specific hormone levels, immunology for autoantibodies, diagnostic imaging (may follow referral to a medical practitioner).

Differential diagnosis

The list of conditions that may present in primary care with fatigue (remember, fatigue is one of the most common symptoms of endocrine disorders) as a symptom is long and varied. Some common endocrine disorders will be considered in the next section. However, also be sure to consider (Ford & Nixon 1995):

- psychological/psychiatric disorders – stress, anxiety and depression
- infections – glandular fever-like illnesses
- blood disorders – anaemia, chronic bleeding, marrow disorders
- malignancy
- drugs – iatrogenic or self-administered
- alcohol abuse
- endocrine disease – thyroid, adrenal, pituitary, diabetes
- connective tissue diseases – rheumatoid arthritis, systemic lupus erythematosus, polymyalgia
- cardiac disease – ischaemic heart disease, cardiac failure
- respiratory disease – chronic respiratory failure.

SPECIFIC DISORDERS

Diabetes mellitus

Definition: A raised blood glucose concentration caused either by a lack of insulin or factors present in the body that oppose the action of insulin. Other metabolic abnormalities occur, notably an increase in ketone bodies in the blood when there is a severe lack of insulin (Watkins 1998). A new classification which identifies five types of diabetes, grouped according to pathogenesis, has recently been recommended (Alberti & Zimmet 1998, Watkins 1998):

- Type 1 – immune mediated and idiopathic forms of β-cell dysfunction which leads to absolute insulin deficiency. This type is insulin-dependent diabetes mellitus (IDDM).
- Type 2 – disease of adult onset, which may originate from insulin resistance and relative insulin deficiency or from a secretory defect. Subgroups include those with various genetic defects and diseases of the exocrine pancreas. This type is non–insulin-dependent diabetes (NIDDM).
- Maturity-onset diabetes of youth (MODY) 1, 2 and 3 – families in these groups have dominantly inherited NIDDM with different clinical characteristics. Children in these families are often affected (Watkins 1998).

Subjective findings

For the purposes of this chapter, because of the overlaps, all types of diabetes will be considered together, but the differences in symptoms, signs and treatments will be highlighted.

The patient will often give a history (Makinnon 1998) of

- polydipsia
- hunger
- urinary symptoms of polyuria, nocturia (frequency and dysuria if associated urinary tract infection), bedwetting in children, incontinence in the elderly

- pruritis vulvae or balanitis (usually caused by candidiasis)
- weight loss (especially in patients with IDDM)
- weakness, tiredness and lethargy
- deteriorating or blurred vision
- neuritis, causing exquisite pain in the feet, thighs or trunk
- mood changes (irritability)
- foot ulceration and recurrent sepsis, particularly in the elderly
- non-specific abdominal pain, particularly in children
- positive family history of diabetes.

The patient may well be of non-European origin, now resident in the UK. The prevalence in Indo-Asians is approximately four times higher than that found in the White population (2%) and increases with age to 16% in the 40–65 age range. Afro-Caribbean people also have a slightly higher prevalence of NIDDM associated with weight gain.

Also, explore lifestyle factors – smoking history, eating habits, alcohol intake and exercise levels.

These symptoms will often develop more rapidly in patients with IDDM, either over a few days or over several weeks or months. In patients with NIDDM, symptoms are often insidious in onset and, for that reason, may be denied.

Objective findings

1. Height and weight. Calculate the body mass index (BMI). Patients with NIDDM are frequently overweight, with BMI > 25 (those with android obesity, apple-shaped, waist–hip ratio > 0.9, are more prone to NIDDM). Data from the Framingham study (2000) have shown that there is a 33% reduction in the risk of developing diabetes in obese individuals (BMI in excess of 27) if there is a modest weight reduction of 1 lb (0.45 kg) a year. Patients with IDDM are usually underweight.
2. Vital signs – pulse and blood pressure. Hypertension may be present (associated with nephropathy or cardiovascular disease). There may be postural hypotension, which is a feature of autonomic neuropathy (Griffith et al 1996).
3. May detect acetone (similar to the smell of sweet apples) on the patient's breath.
4. Urinalysis may demonstrate proteinuria (sign of nephropathy or urinary infection).
5. Test for visual acuity (may be reduced) and perform fundoscopy (there may be evidence of cataracts or retinal degeneration) (see Chapter 5 for details of eye examination).
6. Physical examination – key areas to examine in a patient with suspected diabetes:
   - Inspect the skin and tongue for signs of dehydration.
   - Look for evidence of infection (staphylococcal skin infection is common).
   - Inspect the feet for signs of infection, ulceration or gangrene. Palpate the pedal pulses. Test the ankle reflexes and foot sensation to check for peripheral neuropathy (ankle reflexes may be absent and sensation may be reduced or altered in a sock distribution) (see Chapter 11 for details of examination).
   - Palpate the pulses in the legs to check for evidence of peripheral vascular disease.
   - Cardiac examination – for signs of cardiovascular disease (atrial fibrillation and cardiac failure) (see Chapter 6).

Assessment

- Impaired glucose tolerance
- Diabetes mellitus.

Plan

Diagnostics

Consider urinalysis for glycosuria, ketonuria and proteinuria, random plasma glucose (capillary blood sample can be analysed on presentation) and a fasting plasma glucose if the random level is elevated, after a fast of 10–16 hours (Bennett 1991). An oral glucose tolerance test (OGTT) may also be undertaken as previously recommended by WHO in 1985 (DECODE Study Group 1998).

1. Urinalysis may show glycosuria, but this may be absent in a patient with type 2 diabetes (MacKinnon 1998). Ketonuria is more likely to be present in the patient with type 1 diabetes. Proteinuria may be present if there are renal microvascular changes, one of the complications of diabetes.
2. The revised criteria for diagnosis in the USA are symptoms of diabetes and a casual (random) plasma glucose concentration ≥ 11.1 mmol/l or a fasting plasma glucose ≥ 7.0 mmol/l or a 2-hour plasma glucose ≥ 11.1 mmol/l during a standard 75 g OGTT (Expert Committee 1997). Most experts in the UK continue to support the previous WHO criteria for diagnosis (fasting glucose ≥ 7.8 mmol/l *and* 2-hour glucose ≥ 11.1 mmol/l) (Fig. 10.1) (DECODE Study Group 1998). A decision about whether to accept the revised criteria now used in the USA is expected imminently. It is also recommended that the diagnosis is confirmed by a second test.
3. A plasma glucose of 5.5–6.6 mmol/l indicates an equivocal result and the patient should be re-screened in 6–12 months (McDowell 1996). The OGTT may also be used for asymptomatic patients with equivocal blood glucose results (Bennett 1991).
4. An elevated result just lower than the values above would indicate impaired glucose tolerance (IGT) which carries an increased risk of macrovascular disease such as stroke and coronary artery disease. Patients with IGT should also be screened for hyperlipidaemia (McDowell 1996).

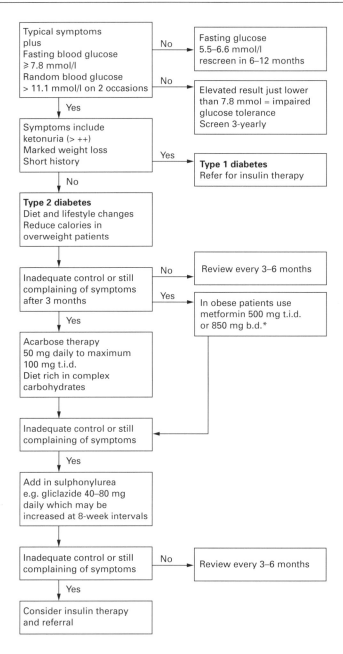

Figure 10.1 *Management flow chart for diabetes.*

5. Patients with IGT are at increased risk of developing diabetes in the future and should be screened every 3 years (Patterson 1993).

Management

Negotiating a management plan with the patient develops a therapeutic partnership that enhances patient empowerment (Jones 1998, Lee 1999). Empowerment ensures that the person with diabetes has the knowledge, skills and self-awareness necessary for optimum self-care, makes early and effective responses to everyday problems and has the confidence to obtain the best input from the health care team (European Diabetes Policy Group 1999). Shillitoe (1994) identifies the potential benefits of empowerment as a positive self-concept; increased personal satisfaction; self-efficacy, a sense of mastery and control, justice, in that patient choices have been respected, and improved quality of life. The management plan should be designed to incorporate aspects of the patient's culture and lifestyle: 'For people with the disease, diabetes is not an academic subject; it is a lived experience' (Feste 1992).

1. Psychological care – the patient's reaction, when diabetes is first diagnosed, can vary from total disbelief and shock to relief at finally having an explanation for their symptoms (Lee 1999). A varying amount of support will be required while the patient comes to terms with having a chronic illness and the lifestyle changes which may inevitably form part of the treatment.

2. Good blood glucose control reduces the risk of developing diabetic complications or their progression (DCCT Research Group 1993, Groeneveld et al 1999). The UK Prospective Diabetes Study Group (UKPDS 1998a) has also shown that good control decreases the risk of myocardial infarction (MI) by 16% and microvascular incidents by 25% (Simpson 1999). For type 2 diabetics, the primary focus is on healthy eating. The principles involved are

   - low sucrose intake (25 g per day is recommended by the BDA (1992a) now known as Diabetes UK)
   - low fat intake (< 10% saturated fat; additional 10% fat either monounsaturated or polyunsaturated)
   - carbohydrate foods should form 50–55% of daily energy requirements (use complex carbohydrate foods naturally high in soluble fibre, e.g. bread, rice, cereals, potatoes and fruit)
   - high fibre (30 g daily)
   - protein should form no more than 10–15% of daily energy requirements
   - low salt of < 6 g per day (McDowell 1996, BDA 1997)
   - obese patients will also need to reduce daily calorie intake in order to reduce weight (and risk of macrovascular complications)
   - over-restricting the fat content of the diet of the elderly diabetic is not recommended, as this could seriously affect the nutritional quality of the diet (Phillips 1994)
   - diabetic foods are not recommended due to their high fat content and addition of sorbitol or another sweetener that has a laxative effect (BDA 1992b).

Diet is often cited as the most traumatic aspect of diabetic treatment (Aitken 1997). The patient should be encouraged to have more frequent smaller meals or snacks each day to optimise glycaemic control. Early referral of all newly diagnosed diabetics to a dietician is recommended. Patients should also be taught the principles of either urine or blood glucose monitoring according to their preference.

Pharmacotherapeutics. Type 1 diabetics require insulin. Consider oral hypoglycaemics in type 2 diabetics if dietary modifications are not achieving optimal glycaemic control after 3 months. This can be assessed by monitoring glycated haemoglobin levels, $HbA1_c$ (if necessary 2–4 monthly until stable). Results are reported as the percentage of total haemoglobin:

- A level of 6.2–7.5 is adequate.
- A level > 7.5 is inadequate (European Diabetes Policy Group 1999). Acarbose (an α-glucosidase inhibitor) should be the first-line medication (Beckwith 1998). The dose should be titrated upwards from 50 mg daily to a maximum 100 mg three times a day over a few weeks to limit flatulence. A diet rich in complex carbohydrates will also help. Metformin (a biguanide) 500 mg three times a day or 850 mg twice a day may be used in the obese patient. A sulphonylurea, such as gliclazide may also be used: 40–80 mg initially (glibenclamide is not recommended for patients over 65 years of age).

Screen for risk factors for the complications of diabetes. The UKPDS 38 (1998a) has shown that tight control of blood pressure (mean 144/82 mmHg over 9 years compared with 154/87 mmHg in controls) resulted in a 24% reduction in any diabetic complications (macrovascular and microvascular) and a 32% reduction in death related to diabetes, mostly from MI and strokes.

It appears from a second study that an angiotensin-converting enzyme (ACE) inhibitor (captopril) and a β-blocker (atenolol) were equally effective in reducing hypertension, the risk of clinical end points and of progression of retinopathy (UKPDS 39 1998b). Nine years after the trials commenced, one-quarter of the patients required three or more hypotensive agents and the results show that lowering the blood pressure may be important in reducing the complications of type 2 diabetes rather than the treatments used. Tight blood pressure control has been found to be cost effective and comparable with other widely supported preventive strategies (UKPDS 40 1998c). Current recommendations are that for patients with normal albumin excretion rate, the blood pressure should be controlled at < 135/85 mmHg; but in patients with abnormal albumin excretion rates, the target is < 130/80 mmHg or lower if easily attained (European Diabetic Policy Group 1998).

In 1989, the St Vincent Declaration Action Programme set a target of reducing cardiovascular disease among diabetics through vigorous programmes of risk factor reduction (Krans et al 1992). In 1997, all medical practitioners were circulated with guidelines on the use of lipid-lowering therapy (statins) by the Standing Medical Advisory Committee (SMAC) of the Department of Health. Criticism of these guidelines, which recommend that the Sheffield risk tables are used as a simple calculation of coronary heart disease (CHD) risk, is that the tables make no provision for the lower high-density lipoprotein (HDL) cholesterol which occurs in type 2 diabetes mellitus (UKPDS 1984, Jones 1997, Colhoun et al 1999). Yudkin & Chaturvedi (1999) have developed revised risk charts which include the impact of micro albuminuria and lipid fractions by including the total cholesterol: HDL cholesterol ratio.

Current advice is that diabetics with risk factors for hyperlipidaemia (family history, smoker, higher than recommended alcohol intake, obesity, sedentary lifestyle, previous coronary event) should be screened yearly. Treatment targets for plasma lipid levels are:

- total cholesterol < 6.5 mmol/l and triglycerides < 4.5 mmol/l (McDowell 1996)
- for those with known vascular disease, a total cholesterol < 4.8 mmol/l, low-density lipoprotein (LDL) cholesterol < 3.0 mmol/l, HDL cholesterol > 1.2 mmol/l and triglycerides < 1.7 mmol/l are recommended (European Diabetes Policy Group 1999)
- the normal LDL:HDL ratio should be < 3.

Patient education. The patient will need information about foot health, lifestyle factors (exercise levels, alcohol intake, diet, risks of smoking, stress management and the positive benefits of relaxation, contraception and pregnancy, driving), employment issues, illness and infections, vaccination (e.g. annual flu), travel, dental treatment and hypoglycaemic attacks if treated with insulin or sulphonylureas. The patient may well feel overwhelmed if all these subjects are discussed on the first visit. The information should therefore be prioritised and staged to suit the individual and supported by audiovisual material, such as patient information leaflets. It is important to explore patient education in terms of needs and achievements in future consultations.

Regular review. Time of review will vary according to the needs of individual patients. For those with stable disease, review should occur annually and include:

- Urinalysis.
- Microalbuminuria screen.
- Blood tests – HbA1$_c$, cholesterol and lipid profile, serum creatinine, urea and electrolytes. Honess (1999) also suggests that all diabetics should be routinely screened for thyroid disease.
- Blood pressure.
- Weight and BMI.
- Visual acuity and fundoscopy (may involve retinal photography).
- Foot health.
- Review of medication.
- Lifestyle factors – dietary behaviours, smoking habits, physical activity and patient self-management skills.
- The review should include negotiated agreement on targets for future months, interval to next consultation and explanation and agreement on changes in therapy.

Indications for referral

- *Immediate* – a child with suspected diabetes needs to be referred to the diabetologist.

- *Immediate* – a patient with type 1 diabetes, usually under 40 years of age, presenting with a short history of dramatic weight loss, polydipsia and polyuria. The patient may demonstrate heavy ketonuria on urinalysis and signs of ketoacidosis.
- *Immediate* – foot ulceration in the elderly or signs of ischaemia of the lower limbs.
- *Immediate* – a patient with proteinuria > 1 g per 24 hours not related to urinary infection and plasma creatinine 300–350 μmol/l. This indicates a glomerular filtration rate of 20–30 ml/min, where the residual renal tissue is progressively damaged, leading to chronic renal failure. Dialysis will be required when plasma creatinine > 600 μmol/l and urea > 40 mmol/l (Kingswood & Packham 1996, Griffith et al 1996).
- A diabetic patient contemplating pregnancy (a type 2 diabetic will need to change to insulin therapy during pregnancy).

Complications

1. Macrovascular – diabetes mellitus is a risk factor for the development of atherosclerosis (Griffith et al 1996). Atheroma may lead to MI, peripheral vascular disease and cerebrovascular accidents.
2. Microvascular – may occur throughout the body but clinically important changes give rise to nephropathy, diabetic eye disease (retinopathy, cataract formation and, occasionally, glaucoma caused by new blood vessel formation in the iris) and neuropathy.
3. Reduced libido and impotence – erectile dysfunction (see Chapter 13) in a diabetic patient is caused by vascular disease and autonomic neuropathy. It has been estimated that between one-third and one-half of all male diabetic patients are affected by impotence (Fairburn et al 1982). Erectile impotence is age related (McDowell 1996) but occurs at much younger ages in diabetic men than in the general population. Once it develops, it is progressive and permanent. It also appears to be the most underdiagnosed complication of diabetes (McDowell 1996). It is often a hugely embarrassing subject for the patient (and possibly also for the health worker) and usually causes immense distress to the patient and his partner. Exploration of any sexual problems may therefore need to be initiated by the health professional. This will require sensitive handling, particularly if the health worker is female and youthful. An explanation that this is a common complication of diabetes will often give reassurance. It is important to establish whether there are any treatable causes or any underlying psychological or personal relationship problems that may have precipitated the difficulty. Erectile dysfunction may lead to psychological problems and it is sometimes difficult to identify which came first. Some medications may also cause impotence, e.g. beta-blockers, bendroflumethiazide (bendrofluazide and tricyclic antidepressants. In the absence of organic causes, psychological or

relationship problems, the patient may be offered a number of differing forms of treatment:

- Vacuum tumescence devices may be offered in primary care. These create a vacuum in a solid condom apparatus around the penis and induce an erection which is maintained by an elastic band. It may be an unpopular choice as the penis is filled with venous blood and feels cold and the band prevents ejaculation but it may be a useful alternative in older men (Dinsmore 1999).
- Intracorporeal injection of vasoactive agents, such as papaverine or prostagladin E_1, is normally provided by a diabetologist or urologist with a special interest in this treatment. There may be a number of unpleasant side effects: penile pain, haematoma, fibrosis, erythema, testicular or perineal pain, penile deviations, haemosiderin deposits in the penis or priapism (Dinsmore 1999).
- MUSE (medicated urethral system for erection), which is a transurethral delivery of alprostadil, is generally considered to be less effective than intercavernosal injection but may be more acceptable to some men (Dinsmore 1999).
- Penile prosthetics which are either inflatable or semi-rigid and malleable: the semi-rigid options may be difficult to conceal and the inflatable options have a 2% infection and erosion risk, which may be best avoided in the diabetic male (Dinsmore 1999).
- Sildenafil (Viagra) is the only oral treatment available and may now be prescribed for diabetic erectile dysfunction (Department of Health 1999). It has been suggested from studies that the normal frequency of sexual intercourse in the 40–60 age range is once a week (Johnston et al 1994) and the guidance suggests that, although each case should be considered individually, the prescribing pattern perhaps should follow this rate (Department of Health 1999). It is worth noting that sildenafil is ineffective in the absence of arousal and is completely contraindicated in patients on nitrates, where it may cause fatal hypotension (Boulton 1999). The usual treatment dose is 50 mg taken 1 hour before intercourse on an empty stomach. The dose may be titrated up to 100 mg or down to 25 mg according to response. It is important to warn the couple that this drug will not induce an automatic erection and that the person treated will still need stimulation (Dinsmore 1999). Studies have shown that improved erections were obtained in 50–56% of diabetic men (Price et al 1998, Langtry & Markham 1999, Rendell et al 1999, Spollett 1999).

In all cases it is important that the patient and his partner take plenty of time to select the device that is most suitable to them in privacy.

A National Service Framework identifying national standards for diabetic care is expected in 2001.

Hypoglycaemia

Definition: Hypoglycaemia is a low blood glucose level below 3 mmol/1 (Hall 1998). Diabetes UK recommends that the blood glucose level should be maintained at 4 mmol/l or above. The signs and symptoms of hypoglycaemia are particularly unpleasant and distressing for patient and carers, particularly if the patient is a child. Hypoglycaemia can be caused by:

- delayed or missed meals (or low food intake in the elderly)
- increased exercise (hypoglycaemia may be delayed by many hours)
- stress
- alcohol (causes reduced hypoglycaemia awareness, impaired normal response to fall in blood glucose and prolonged onset of hypoglycaemia some hours after intake)
- very tight diabetic control
- an increase in medication or overdose.

Patients treated with insulin or sulphonylureas, particularly glibenclamide (due to its long duration of action), are at risk. It is more likely to occur in hot weather in insulin-dependent diabetics as insulin is absorbed more rapidly (MacKinnon 1998). Occasionally, it may also occur with the change of injection site where one site has been used repeatedly before changing it. A decrease in weight in elderly patients or renal failure may also increase the risk of hypoglycaemia.

Subjective findings

The patient will give a history of (Hall 1998):
- sweating
- dizziness and faintness
- hunger
- trembling, shakiness
- anxiety
- palpitations
- unusual behaviour (especially elderly patients treated with long-acting sulphonylureas)
- epilepsy in diabetic children (as the result of severe hypoglycaemia – if this occurs nocturnally the child may fail to wake before the fit occurs)
- poor concentration
- visual disturbance
- poor coordination
- tingling around mouth
- confusion
- weakness
- nausea
- dry mouth
- headache
- severe hypoglycaemia may present with symptoms resembling a transitory stroke (limb weakness and/or paralysis may be evident)
- impaired consciousness or coma in severe cases.

It is important to note that recurrent hypoglycaemia may lead to reduced awareness of impending attacks. In patients with prolonged periods of hyperglycaemia, e.g. at diagnosis, the symptoms of hypoglycaemia may occur at blood glucose levels > 4 mmol/l (MacKinnon 1998). The symptoms may also be mistaken for excessive alcohol intake.

Objective findings

- Vital signs – tachycardia may be present.
- Physical examination – as this is often an emergency situation, examination will need to be limited. However, examination should include general observation of the patient for signs of trembling, shakiness, anxiety, confusion and impaired consciousness, and inspection of the skin for signs of pallor and sweating.

Assessment

- Hypoglycaemia.

Plan

Diagnostics

If the patient is diabetic, medication with sulphonylureas or insulin treatment will need to be given quickly to prevent the patient lapsing into a coma. If there is any doubt about the diagnosis, particularly if the patient has reduced awareness of impending attacks, a random blood sugar may quickly be performed and analysed using a glucometer. A glycated haemoglobin, which is normal or close to normal, may also indicate hypoglycaemia.

Management

The aim of the management plan is to prevent or significantly reduce hypoglycaemic attacks. Remember that recurrent attacks lead to impaired awareness. The BDA Working Party Report (1996) accepted that, although there is no conclusive evidence, recurrent severe hypoglycaemic attacks may be implicated in the development of altered cognitive function. Hypoglycaemia occurring in children who have developed diabetes before the age of 5 or 6 is likely to impair intelligence (McDowell 1996). For this reason, tight metabolic control should not be the aim of treatment in young children.

Pharmacotherapeutics. In mild or moderate hypoglycaemia, an oral rapidly absorbed carbohydrate snack or drink is generally the first choice (Box 10.1). This should be followed by a more substantial snack or meal containing complex carbohydrate, particularly if a meal has been delayed or the patient has taken increased exercise.

Moderate hypoglycaemia with no loss of consciousness can be treated with Hypostop, a glucose gel (either bought OTC or available on prescription), which is massaged into the gums. Treacle or jam can be used in the same way in an emergency. Patients taking acarbose should treat hypoglycaemia with dextrose tablets (as acarbose acts by inhibiting the absorption of carbohydrate from the gut).

Severe hypoglycaemia is treated with subcutaneous, intramuscular (IM) or intravenous (IV) glucagon (a hormone produced by the α cells in the islets of Langerhans of the pancreas which increases plasma glucose by mobilising glycogen stored in the liver). Two presentations of this emergency kit exist: a syringe pre-filled with diluent and one vial or two vials that must be mixed. Patients or their carers may be taught how to give glucagon in an emergency. However, a study by Yanai et al (1997) has found that, although patients were educated about the use of glucagon, only a small number used it when required. It is important to note that glucagon may cause nausea and vomiting.

Whatever treatment is used, it is important to check that the blood glucose level has returned to normal after a hypoglycaemic attack.

Behavioural. In the IDDM patient who is unaware of hypoglycaemic episodes, blood glucose monitoring should occur four or more times a day (European Diabetes Policy Group 1999). Results (date, time, insulin dose, hypoglycaemia) need to be recorded to form a cumulative record on which to base daily changes in therapy. Regular bedtime tests are recommended in patients prone to nocturnal hypoglycaemia. A 3 a.m. test may be required if the Somogyi effect is suspected (glucose released by the liver to combat a nocturnal hypoglycaemic attack leads to an elevated blood glucose in the morning, which may often be treated with extra insulin by the patient, thus increasing hypoglycaemia).

Some patients may not wish to monitor their blood glucose for a variety of reasons. It is important that any fears or concerns are adequately explored. If the positive benefits of this method in the control of hypoglycaemia are highlighted, then it may be possible to

Box 10.1	*Management of hypoglycaemia*
Mild or moderate hypoglycaemia	Oral rapidly absorbed carbohydrate snack or drink followed by substantial snack/ meal containing complex carbohydrate
Patients taking acarbose	Dextrose tablets
Moderate hypoglycaemia with no loss of consciousness	Hypostop (glucose gel) massaged into gums or treacle/jam in an emergency
Severe hypoglycemia	Subcutaneous, IM or IV glucagon

Note Always check that the patient's blood glucose has returned to normal after an attack

negotiate a short trial period with the patient, with offers of support when needed. Patients may find in practice that this method is not as bad as they feared. Overall, however, it is important that the patient's wishes are respected. In type 2 diabetics, blood glucose monitoring is not so important and it is just as satisfactory to use urine testing and glycated haemoglobin results. This is helpful with the elderly, in whom blood glucose monitoring may be particularly difficult (and most elderly patients have type 2 diabetes).

Patient education. It is important that patients know the warning signs, understand the likely causes and are aware of the risks of operating machinery or driving if prone to attacks. Current laws prevent new diabetics treated with insulin from driving C1 vehicles (3.5–7.5 tonnes) and D1 vehicles (9–16 seat minibuses). The DVLA criteria state that for those who have previously driven C1 vehicles, they may continue within the UK provided annual review by a diabetologist is satisfactory (Hall 1998). Treatment choices should be negotiated with the patient, although carrying rapidly absorbed carbohydrate (or dextrose if treated with acarbose) may be all the treatment needed for mild attacks.

Indications for referral

- Immediate – if the patient does not regain consciousness after glucagon (takes approximately 15–20 min)
- Immediate – a child with suspected nocturnal hypoglycaemia
- Immediate – a type 1 diabetic with frequent hypoglycaemic episodes
- Follow-up – should occur as often as warranted until the condition has been controlled.

Complications

These may include altered cognitive function, coma and, if untreated, death.

Hyperthyroidism

Definition: Hyperthyrodism, which is sometimes known as thyrotoxicosis, is overactivity of the thyroid gland and is characterised by excessive secretion of the thyroid hormones, T_3 and T_4. It may be caused by Graves' disease, toxic multinodular goitre which may develop in a long-standing goitre, toxic adenoma, thyroid-stimulating hormone TSH-secreting tumour or may be iodine induced (Conway & Betteridge 1996).

Subjective findings

The patient may give a history of
- Anxiety.
- Nervousness and tremors.
- Increased sweating.
- Heat intolerance.
- Tachycardia and palpitations. It is important to check the patient's meaning of palpitations in terms of the

nature (regular/irregular), rate and duration. This may be helped by getting the patient to tap out the rhythm of the heart beat during an attack for you. Explore the nature of the palpitations by checking for associated symptoms (shortness of breath, faintness, chest pain), precipitants (none, exercise or emotion) and whether the patient takes stimulant drugs or caffeine-containing drinks (coffee, fizzy drinks). Also check on family history.
- Fatigue.
- Weakness.
- Weight loss.
- Increased appetite.
- Frequent bowel action, possibly diarrhoea.
- Eye symptoms – the patient will often complain of a 'gritty' feeling in their eyes and blink less frequently.
- Swelling of the neck (goitre).
- Difficulty in swallowing or eating (if goitre is present).
- Psychosis (rare).
- Oligomenorrhoea.
- 25–40% of older people may also present with absent or atypical thyroid symptoms (Bailes 1999). Often, because the elderly have several other chronic diseases, hyperthyrodism may be hidden. The atypical presentation (apathetic thyrotoxicosis) may include anorexia and weight loss, apathy and lassitude, depression, confusion and constipation. Hyperthyroidism may exacerbate underlying chronic disease and, in people with known coronary artery disease, there may be increased angina, dyspnoea and congestive cardiac failure. Peripheral signs may include claudication and poor tissue healing.

Objective findings

1. Vital signs – resting tachycardia, but this may be absent in the elderly. Pulse may be irregularly irregular if atrial fibrillation is present. Temperature may be slightly elevated.
2. Physical examination – observe the patient for any difficulty in breathing or stridor which may be present with severe goitre. The key areas to inspect are the hands, the neck for swelling, the eyes for lid lag (this may be absent in the elderly patient) or exophthalmos and the upper arms and thighs for myopathy. On inspection, the hands will be warm and moist with a fine tremor of the outstretched fingers. Tendon reflexes are brisk. In severe cases, proximal myopathy may be evident (Conway & Betteridge 1996). Atrial fibrillation may be confirmed from inspection of the jugular venous pulse (JVP). If the patient is in sinus rhythm, two waves are present ('a' corresponding to atrial systole and 'c' transmitted pulsation of carotid artery at onset of ventricular systole) but, in atrial fibrillation, the 'a' wave is absent.
   - Palpation of the thyroid gland – this should first be inspected from the front for swelling. On swallow-

ing, thyroid swellings move upwards because the gland is encased within the pretracheal fascia. The thyroid is then gently palpated from behind, while the patient holds the head slightly flexed. Check whether the gland is uniformly enlarged or nodular, whether hard or soft and whether it is tender or not on palpation. It may also be helpful to palpate while the patient swallows to feel the lower border of the gland, which will identify any retrosternal extension (Conway & Betteridge 1996). Also palpate the cervical lymph glands for enlargement (this may indicate a thyroid cancer).

■ Cardiac examination – this will be necessary if any pulse abnormalities are detected (see Chapter 8 for details). You need to exclude other common causes of atrial fibrillation, such as mitral valve disease, ischaemic heart disease, alcohol-related heart disease, atrial septal defect and impaired ventricular function (de Bono & Macpherson 1996) and also congestive heart failure in the elderly (Bailes 1999). Some of these abnormalities will be easier to detect on electrocardiogram (ECG).

■ In elderly patients, assess for signs of congestive cardiac failure – raised JVP, pitting oedema of the lower extremities, inability to lie flat without shortness of breath. Auscultation of the chest may demonstrate the presence of crackles (crepitations), especially in the bases of both lungs.

It is worth noting that presentation in primary care may be far more subtle than described and, where there is no conclusive physical findings just the patient's subjective description of symptoms, basic investigations such as thyroid function tests may be carried out as screening tests rather than to confirm the results of physical examination.

Assessment

■ Hyperthyroidism
■ Graves' disease (see later).

Plan

Diagnostics

Consider ECG, full blood count (FBC), which should precede antithyroid therapy (which can result in agranulocytosis), and thyroid function tests (TFTs). In most cases of hyperthyroidism, T_4 and T_3 are elevated (Fig. 10.2) but, in some cases, only T_3 levels are raised (this occurs in cases of toxic adenoma). In all cases, the TSH level is abnormally low. The new immunoradiometric assay test for TSH is very sensitive and in future it may be the only screening test necessary to detect hyperthyroidism (Fry & Sandler 1993, Conway & Betteridge 1996, Ramachandran et al 1998)

Management

The patient, who is often very anxious and irritable as a result of the disease, can feel immensely relieved to know that there is a pathophysiological reason for how they are feeling and that it is curable. The three main options for treatment of hyperthyroidism are antithyroid drugs, radioactive iodine therapy and thyroid surgery.

Pharmacotherapeutics. Antithyroid drugs are the first line of treatment. Even when the preferred treatment is radioactive iodine or surgery, it is important to render the patient euthyroid with drugs first to prevent thyroid crisis. The most commonly used drug in the UK is carbimazole. Initial doses vary from 20–60 mg daily, reducing to 5–15 mg daily once the patient becomes euthyroid. It will be necessary to review the patient's FBC and TFTs regularly, according to previous results, because two of the side effects of carbimazole are agranulocytosis (rare) and hypothyroidism. The antithyroid drug propylthiouracil may be used as an alternative in pregnancy or if carbimazole is not tolerated. Treatment invariably continues for 1 year then stops. In over 50% of cases, hyperthyroidism will recur (Fry & Sandler 1993).

Patient education. It is important to advise the patient of the complications of antithyroid therapy; in particular, to

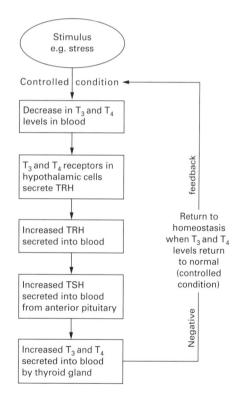

Key
TRH Thyrotropin releasing hormone
TSH Thyroid stimulating hormone or thyrotropin

Figure 10.2 *Negative feedback system for regulation of T_3 and T_4 concentration in the blood.*

stop the drug if a rash or sore throat develops and seek medical attention. Patients should also be made aware of the possibility of relapse and to look for recurrence of the symptoms of thyrotoxicosis. The importance of regular review and blood tests should be stressed.

Indications for referral

- Immediate – thyrotoxic crisis. This is an emergency situation. The patient will have marked anxiety and agitation (occasionally psychosis), pronounced tachycardia, marked tremor, fever, dehydration and cardiac failure.
- Immediate – failed antithyroid therapy. The patient will need thyroid surgery (once euthyroid) or radioactive iodine therapy. Some physicians restrict the use of radioactive iodine in women to those over 40 years of age.
- All patients with thyroid nodules and goitre will need to be referred for assessment. Thyroid imaging, involving iodine or technetium uptake, and thyroid ultrasound can help determine the nature of thyroid cysts or nodules. Fine needle aspiration of suspicious nodules for cytology may be performed.

Complications

- Thyrotoxic crisis (see under referral above)
- Hypothyroidism as a result of antithyroid treatment.

Graves' disease

Definition: Graves' disease is autoimmune thyroid disease characterised by the presence of immunoglobulin, IgG (thyroid-stimulating antibodies which bind to the TSH receptors of the thyroid and produce a similar effect to TSH). Other systems may be affected, notably the eyes. Graves' disease is the most common cause of hyperthyroidism. It usually presents between the ages of 30 and 40 years old and 90% of patients are women (Conway & Betteridge 1996). It is more common in areas with high iodine levels. There is also a familial tendency.

Subjective findings

The patient may present with some or all of the symptoms of hyperthyroidism and also:

- hyperactivity – the patient is often unable to sit still.
- wide-eyed expression (forward protrusion of the eyeball caused by autoimmune inflammatory reaction within the orbit).
- diplopia, and the patient is also unable to gaze upwards and outwards (ophthalmoplegia). In severe cases blindness may occur.
- nausea and vomiting.

Objective findings

- Physical examination – the findings are similar to those found in a patient with hyperthyroidism plus:
- Skin inspection may reveal vitiligo.

- Inspection of the neck reveals a symmetrical goitre, with a smooth outline, which moves on swallowing.
- A thyroid bruit is present on auscultation of the goitre caused by the increased vascularity.
- Examination of the eyes – inspection may reveal corneal damage (keratitis) in severe cases of exophthalmos. Proptosis (where the white sclera is visible between the cornea and the lower eyelid) may be visible when the patient looks straight ahead. Assessment of the visual fields may show ophthalmoplegia (with inability to gaze upwards and outwards). Visual acuity may be affected. Fundoscopy may reveal papilloedema in severe cases. It is worth noting that ophthalmic Graves' disease may be present without any of the signs and symptoms of hyperthyroidism.

Assessment

- Graves' disease
- ? Thyroid adenoma.

Plan

Diagnostics

All the tests identified for hyperthyroidism plus an immunology test for thyroid receptor antibodies. Ultrasound and technetium scanning may help differentiate Graves' disease from adenoma.

Management

Management is the same as for any patient with hyperthyroidism.

Patient education. Patient education is the same as for any patient with hyperthyroidism. However, many patients find the exophthalmos and ophthalmoplegia very distressing and need opportunities to express their feelings. The treatment options in severe cases should be discussed.

Indications for referral

As for hyperthyroidism and:

- For treatment of Graves' ophthalmopathy. This severe progressive eye damage may lead to blindness. Treatment available includes high-dose steroid therapy, tarsorrhaphy, orbital irradiation and surgical decompression of the orbit (Fry & Sandler 1993).

Hypothyroidism

Definition: Hypothyroidism results from decreased secretion of thyroid hormones. It tends to occur more frequently in women (90% of cases) from the middle years onwards. It is associated with a familial tendency to autoimmunity (Conway & Betteridge 1996). It is more common in iodine-deficient areas. Hypothyroidism can lead to secondary hypercholesterolaemia with accelerated ischaemic heart disease and atherosclerosis.

Subjective findings

- The patient may have had previous treatment for hyperthyroidism.
- Family history of thyroid disease.
- Weight gain and obesity.
- Cold intolerance.
- Tiredness and lethargy.
- Constipation.
- Poor memory.
- Mental slowness.
- Generalised aches and pains.
- In later stages, puffiness around the eyes and thickening of the lips and tongue (myxoedema). In some cases puffiness may extend to the entire face.
- Skin which is dry, flaky and sometimes has a yellow tinge.
- Hair thinning and alopecia.
- Hoarse voice.
- Goitre.
- Angina (if there is associated ischaemic heart disease).
- Other autoimmune disease (for example, pernicious anaemia or rheumatoid arthritis).

Symptoms may be non-specific at first and are therefore sometimes attributed to ageing. Severe cases may present with dementia.

- In neonates, congenital hypothyroidism occurs in 1:4000–5000 births (Conway & Betteridge 1996). Screening now takes place 5–7 days postnatally.
- Children born to iodine-deficient mothers may exhibit severe neurological defects (cretinism) associated with hypothyroidism. Diagnosis is difficult and delay may lead to permanent mental retardation.
- Autoimmune thyroiditis may occur in childhood. It is more common in girls. Hypothyroidism in childhood is associated with retarded growth and sexual development. The long bones and facial bones fail to develop and there is delayed epiphyseal healing. Usually, puberty is delayed but, rarely, precocious puberty may occur. In a girl, delayed puberty is defined as absence of breast budding by 13.2 years of age (Castiglia 1991) and precocious puberty as the appearance of secondary sexual characteristics before the age of 7.5 years or the onset of menses before 9.5 years (Rosenfield 1990 cited in Castiglia 1991). Hypothyroidism in childhood does not cause permanent mental retardation.

Objective findings

1. Vital signs – bradycardia is present and sometimes hypothermia. Dyspnoea may be observed (if there is associated heart failure) and the patient may be unable to lie in a recumbent position.
2. Physical examination – you may find that the patient is very slow to comprehend instructions during the examination. Sometimes these will need to be repeated a number of times. Observe overall demeanour (depression is common) and inspect the skin for dryness, flakiness and a yellow tinge and the hair for thinning and alopecia. Inspect the face for the typical facies of myxoedema.

   - Inspect the neck for goitre. This should be palpated gently (see section about examination in a patient with suspected thyrotoxicosis). Note, however, that even when goitre is present, the thyroid gland may not be palpable. Ease of swallowing and breathing should also be checked.
   - Chest examination may show pleural effusions. This is demonstrated by dullness on percussion and diminished vesicular breath sounds (rustling) on auscultation over the site of the effusion (see Chapter 7 for examination details).
   - Cardiac examination. The patient may show signs of cardiac failure. Inspect the lips and fingernails for cyanosis. The patient may also be pale and sweaty. Check for pitting oedema of the extremities. The JVP will tend to be high. There may be a mild tachycardia, but this may not be evident, as a feature of hypothyroidism is bradycardia. On auscultation, the first and second heart sounds tend to be quiet and there may be a third sound (gallop rhythm, i.e. sounds like a galloping horse). Pericardial effusion may also be present which causes retrosternal chest pain at rest (see Chapter 8 for further details).
   - Abdominal examination may reveal ascites. In tense ascites the dipping technique for palpation, where the examining hand is placed flat on the abdomen and moved around with quick dipping movements may help to detect hepatic or splenic enlargement. In ascites, there is dullness in the flanks (lumbar regions), with central abdominal resonance on percussion.
   - The patient will have slowly relaxing reflexes on testing, e.g. ankle jerks.

In primary care, the presentation of symptoms may be much more subtle than described with no conclusive physical findings, so that thyroid function tests may be carried out as a screening procedure rather than to confirm physical findings.

Assessment

- Hypothyroidism
- ? Concomitant cardiac failure
- ? Concomitant ischaemic heart disease and hypercholesterolaemia.

Plan

Diagnostics

Consider FBC (may reveal a mild macrocytic anaemia), TFTs (low circulating T_4 and raised TSH confirm primary hypothyroidism; if TSH is not raised, hypothyroidism may be secondary to pituitary or hypothalamic disease), immunology for autoantibodies (e.g.

microsomal: – both microsomal and thyroglobulin autoantibodies are present in Hashimoto's thyroiditis), lipid profile (secondary hypercholesterolaemia is often present) and chest radiography (CXR) if there is suspicion of pleural or pericardial effusions; and ECG if ischaemic changes or heart failure are suspected. Patients with hypothyroidism may also have low serum sodium levels and abnormal liver function (Fry & Sandler 1993).

Management

The mainstay of treatment is drug therapy.

Pharmacotherapeutics. Lifelong treatment with thyroxine, usually up to 200 μg daily. If there is associated angina or heart failure, which is more likely to occur in the elderly, the initial dose should be small (25 μg instead of 50 μg daily). Subsequent increase in doses should be determined by well-being and monitoring the TSH levels (normal reference range 0.15–3.50 mIU/l) and increments made every 2–4 weeks (Fry & Sandler 1993). Once the patient is euthyroid, annual checks of TSH levels should continue throughout life.

Patient education. It is important that the patient understands the importance of continuing the therapy for life and also the rationale for regular blood tests. The principles of a low saturated fat diet and healthy eating should also be discussed with the patient (particularly if there is associated ischaemic heart disease and hypercholesterolaemia).

Indications for referral

- Immediate – a child with suspected hypothyroidism.
- Immediate – myxoedema coma, a rare medical emergency more common in the elderly, in poor socioeconomic groups and in cold climates (Conway & Betteridge 1996). It is characterised by hypothermia and coma as well as the features of hypothyroidism.
- Hypothyroidism secondary to pituitary or hypothalamic disease.

Complications

- Myxoedema coma
- Accelerated ischemic heart disease
- Cretinism in children.

Glossary

Diplopia Double vision: in Graves' disease this is caused by weakness and tethering of the inferior rectus muscles
Euthyroid Normal thyroid functioning
Galactosaemia A disorder of galactose metabolism in which there is a deficiency of galactose-1-phosphate uridyltransferase. Without this enzyme, galactose metabolites accumulate in the tissues, which may cause vomiting, weight loss, diarrhoea and lethargy
Goitre Enlargement of the thyroid gland which may be associated with hypothyroidism, hyperthyroidism or normal thyroid functioning

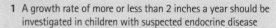

Top Tips ✓

1 A growth rate of more or less than 2 inches a year should be investigated in children with suspected endocrine disease

2 Always test for glucosuria in the elderly, as sepsis and incontinence may be related to diabetes

3 Similarly, bed-wetting in children may be associated with diabetes

4 Tight blood glucose control increases the risk of hypoglycaemia, and it is important to educate the diabetic person about this

5 Tight blood pressure control (<135/85 mmHg for patients with normal albumin excretion rates and <130/80 mmHg for patients with abnormal albumin excretion rates) is important to reduce macrovascular and microvascular complications in diabetics significantly

6 The first line of treatment in type 2 diabetics is a healthy diet and lifestyle changes, which may include increased exercise

7 Remember that all diabetics with risk factors for hyperlipidaemia (family history, smoker, high alcohol intake, obesity, sedentary lifestyle, previous coronary event) should have lipid screening yearly

8 Erectile dysfunction is a common problem in diabetic men, and it is important to ask sensitive questions about this subject

9 The secret to successful diabetic management is patient empowerment, where a therapeutic partnership develops that ensures that the patient has the knowledge, skills and self-awareness necessary for optimum self-care

10 All elderly people with atrial fibrillation should have thyroid function tests for hyperthyroidism

Hashimoto's disease A lymphocytic thyroiditis which produces the clinical features of hypothyroidism
Lid lag Retraction of the upper eyelid which produces the staring appearance of a person with thyrotoxicosis. In severe cases the sclera is visible above the cornea. It is caused by spasm of the levator palpebrae superioris muscle in the presence of excess thyroid hormones
Phaeochromocytoma A rare malignant tumor of the adrenal medulla
Phenylketonuria (PKU) A disorder of amino acid metabolism in which phenylalanine cannot be converted to tyrosine because of a deficiency of the enzyme phenylalanine hydroxylase. If undetected, phenylalanine causes mental retardation
Toxic adenoma An autonomous hyperfunctioning thyroid nodule. As the nodule enlarges, additional amounts of thyroid hormones are produced. The thyrotoxicosis produced in this way is often mild
Vitiligo A patchy skin depigmentation that may be found in a patient with Graves' disease

References

Aitken G 1997 Nutrition and diabetes: putting guidelines into practice. British Journal of Nursing 6(18):1035–1040.

Alberti K G M M, Zimmett P Z 1998 Definition, diagnosis and classification of diabetes mellitus and its complications. Part 1. Provisional report of a World Health Organisation consultation. Diabetic Medicine 15:539–553.

Audit Commission 2000 Testing times: a review of diabetes services in England and Wales (National Report). Audit Commission Publications, Abingdon.

Bailes B K 1999 Hyperthyroidism in elderly patients. AORN Journal 69(1):254–256.

Beckwith S 1998 Focus on diabetes. British Journal of Community Nursing 3:3:135–136.

Bennett P H 1991 Classification and diagnosis of diabetes mellitus and impaired glucose tolerance. In: Pickup J C, Williams G (eds) Textbook of diabetes. Blackwell Scientific, Oxford.

Boulton A J M 1999 Sildenafil: what is it? International Diabetes Federation Bulletin 43:20–22.

British Diabetic Association (BDA) 1992a Dietary recommendations for people with diabetes: an update for the 1990s. Diabetic Medicine 9(2):189–202.

British Diabetic Association (BDA) 1992b Discussion paper on the role of diabetic foods. Diabetic Medicine 9:413–416.

British Diabetic Association (BDA) 1996 Working Party Report: diabetes and cognitive function: the evidence so far. BDA, London.

British Diabetic Association (BDA) 1997 Balance for beginners: starting out with non-insulin dependent diabetes. BDA, London.

Burns C E, Barber N, Brady M A, Dunn A M 1996 Pediatric primary care: a handbook for nurse practitioners. W B Saunders, Philadelphia.

Castiglia P T 1991 Delayed sexual development. Journal of Pediatric Health Care 5(4):213–214.

Colhoun H M, Dong W, Barakat M T, Mather H M, Poulter N R 1999 The scope for cardiovascular disease risk factor intervention among people with diabetes mellitus in England: a population-based analysis from the Health Surveys for England 1991–1994. Diabetic Medicine 16:35–40.

Conway G S, Betteridge D J 1996 Endocrine disease. In: Axford J (ed) Medicine. Blackwell Science, Oxford, ch 12.

De Bono D P, Macpherson D S 1996 The cardiovascular system. In: Munro J, Edwards C R W (eds) Macleod's clinical examination, 9th edn. Churchill Livingstone, Edinburgh.

DECODE Study Group 1998 Will new diagnostic criteria for diabetes mellitus change phenotype of patients with diabetes? Reanalysis of European epidemiological data. British Medical Journal 317:371–375.

Department of Health (DoH) 1999 Treatment for impotence: HSC 1999/148 DH, London.

Diabetic Control and Complications Trial (DCCT) Research Group 1993 The effect of intensive treatment of diabetes on the development and progression of long-term complications in insulin-dependent diabetes mellitus. New England Journal of Medicine 329(14):977–986.

Dinsmore W 1999 Top 100 erectile dysfunction, parts 1 and 2. GP Medicine July 16 and 23 1999.

European Diabetes Policy Group (International Diabetes Federation 1998) 1999 A desktop guide to type 1 (insulin dependent) diabetes mellitus. Diabetic Medicine 16:253–266.

Expert Committee 1997 Report on the diagnosis and classification of diabetes mellitus. Diabetes Care 20:1183–1197.

Fairburn C G, McCullooch D K, Wu F C 1982 The effects of diabetes on male sexual function. Journal of Clinical Endocrine Endocrinology and Metabolism 11:749–767.

Feste C 1992 A practical look at patient empowerment. Diabetes Care 15(7):922–925.

Ford M J, Nixon S 1995 The analysis of symptoms. In: Munro J, Edwards C R W (ed) Macleod's clinical examination, 9th edn. Churchill Livingstone, Edinburgh.

Framingham Study 2000 Epidemiology 11:269–272.

Fry J, Sandler G 1993 Common diseases: their nature, presentation and care, 5th edn. Kluwer Academic Publishers, Dordrecht.

Griffith D N W, Betteridge D J, Axford J S 1996 Diabetes mellitus, lipoprotein disorders and other metabolic diseases. In: Axford J (ed) Medicine. Blackwell Science, Oxford, ch 13.

Groeneveld Y, Petri H, Hermans J, Springer M P 1999 Relationship between blood glucose level and mortality in type 2 diabetes mellitus: a systematic review. Diabetic Medicine 16:2–13.

Hall G 1998 Living with hypoglycaemic attacks. Practice Nurse 16(7):432–434.

Honess T M 1999 Should we routinely screen for thyroid disease in diabetes? Diabetic Nursing 30:16–18.

Johnston M, Maes S, Leventhal H 1994 International review of health psychology: volume 3. John Wiley, Chichester.

Jones A F 1997 Statins and hypercholesterolaemia: UK Standing Medical Advisory Committee guidelines. Lancet 350:1174–1175.

Jones K 1998 Keeping diabetic patients informed of their treatment options (report of the Primary Care Diabetes UK meeting). Practice Nurse 16(4):232.

Kingswood J C, Packham D K 1996 Renal disease. In: Axford J (ed) Medicine. Blackwell Science, Oxford, ch 13.

Krans H M J, Porta M, Keen H (eds) 1992 Diabetes care and research in Europe: the St Vincent Declaration Action Programme: International Diabetes Federation. WHO Regional Office for Europe, Copenhagen.

Langtry H D, Markham A 1999 Sildenafil: a review of its use in erectile dysfunction. Drugs 57(6):967–989.

Lee M 1999 Compliance or empowerment? Diabetic Nursing 30:5–7.

McDowell J R S 1996 Diagnosis and screening for diabetes. In: McDowell J R S, Gordon D (eds) Diabetes: caring for patients in the community. Churchill Livingstone, New York.

MacKinnon M 1998 Providing diabetic care in general practice, 3rd edn. Class Publishing, London.

Patterson K R 1993 Population screening for diabetes mellitus. Diabetic Medicine 10:77–81.

Phillips P A 1994 Dietary assessment and therapy. In: Kesson C M, Knight P V (eds) Diabetes in elderly people: a guide for the health care team. Chapman and Hall, London.

Price D E, Gingell J C, Gepi-Attee S et al 1998 Sildenafil: a study of a novel treatment for erectile dysfunction in diabetic men. Diabetic Medicine 15(10):821–825.

Ramachandran S, Milles J J, Wells M B, Hall R A 1998 Development of a thyroid strategy for general practice. British Journal of General Practice 48:1683–1684.

Rendell M S, Rajfer J, Wicker P A et al 1999 Sildenafil for treatment of erectile dysfunction in men with diabetes: a randomised controlled trial. Sildenafil Diabetes Study Group. Journal of the American Medical Association 3:281:5:421–426.

Rosenfield R L 1990 The ovary and female sexual maturation. In: Kaplan S A (ed) Clinical pediatric endocrinology. W B Saunders, Philadelphia. Cited in Castiglia P T 1991 Precocious puberty. Journal of Pediatric Health Care 5(5):267–268.

Shillitoe R 1994 Counselling people with diabetes. British Psychological Society, Leicester, pp 44–46.

Simpson H 1999 Management of type 2 diabetes: Where are we now? Diabetic Nursing 30:9.

Spollett G R 1999 Assessment and management of erectile dysfunction in men with diabetes. Diabetic Education 25(1):65–73.

Standing Medical Advisory Committee 1997 The use of statins. Department of Health, London.

UK Prospective Diabetes Study Group 1998a Tight blood pressure control and risk of macrovascular complications in type 2 diabetes: UKPDS 38. British Medical Journal 317:703–713.

UK Prospective Diabetes Study Group 1998b Efficacy of atenolol and captopril in reducing risk of macrovascular and microvascular complications in type 2 diabetes: UKPDS 39. British Medical Journal 317:713–720.

UK Prospective Diabetes Study Group 1998c Cost effectiveness analysis of improved blood pressure control in hypertensive patients with type 2 diabetes: UKPDS 40. British Medical Journal 317:720–726.

UK Prospective Diabetes Study Group 1984 Biochemical risk factors in type 2 diabetic patients at diagnosis compared with age-matched normal subjects: UKPDS 11. Diabetic Medicine 11:534–544.

Wareham N J, O'Rahilly S 1998 The changing classification and diagnosis of diabetes. British Medical Journal 317:359–360.

Watkins P J 1998 ABC of diabetes, 4th edn. BMJ Publishing Group, London.

World Health Organisation 1985 Technical Report Series No 72: diabetes mellitus. World Health Organisation, Geneva.

Yanai O, Pilpel D, Harman I, Elitzur-Lieberman E, Philip M 1997 IDDM patients' opinions on the use of Glucagon Emergency Kit in severe episodes of hypoglycemia. Practical Diabetes International 14:2.

Yudkin J S, Alberti K G M M, McLarty D G, Swai A B M 1990 Impaired glucose tolerance. British Medical Journal 301:397–402.

Yudkin J S, Chaturvedi N 1999 Developing risk stratification charts for non-diabetic and diabetic subjects. Diabetic Medicine 16:219–227.

Further reading

Axford J (ed.) 1996 Medicine. Blackwell Science, Oxford.

This is an excellent, comprehensive medical text. It is easily readable with numerous 'at a glance' summaries of common diseases and boxes in the text showing the causes, clinical features and management of specific conditions. It is also illustrated throughout with colour photographs. There is a helpful summary of contents at the beginning of each chapter and a section in each chapter identifying important questions to ask the patient and the principles of examination.

McKinnon M 1998 Providing diabetes care in general practice. 3rd edn. Class Publishing, London.

This book is written as a practical guide for all members of the primary care team and inspires confidence when dealing with diabetic issues. It is filled with useful checklists and sample protocols. It would be useful as a quick reference guide in clinical practice.

Munro J, Edwards C R W 1996 Macleod's clinical examination. 9th edn. Churchill Livingstone, Edinburgh.

This book is an excellent resource for accurate history taking and physical examination techniques and contains helpful details of the relevant symptoms and examination appropriate to the clinical problem presented.

Watkins P J 1998 ABC of Diabetes. 4th edn. BMJ Publishing Group, London.

This easily readable book is an excellent introduction to the practical management of diabetes. It includes useful up-to-date material on the aetiology and genetics of NIDDM. It is filled with charts, tables and colour photographs.

11

NERVOUS SYSTEM

Daphne Miller

Key Issues

- The nervous system is a complex, rapid, fantastic work of art. It is the master control and communication centre of the body

- Comprehensive history and assessment in relation to neurological symptoms are critical to accurate diagnosis and appropriate referral

- Common neurological symptoms which may appear relatively innocent may mask more serious pathology

- A sound knowledge of cranial nerves and dermatomes is essential

Introduction

The presenting signs and symptoms of neurological disorders vary according to the underlying pathology. The common symptoms of neurological disorders include pain, headache, visual disturbance, deafness, dizziness, behavioural changes, dysphasia, dysphagia, seizures, syncope, muscle hypertrophy or weakness, unsteady gait, paralysis, numbness, tingling or increased sensation and sphincter disturbance (Bates 1995, Epstein et al 1997).

The nervous system is so complex that nurse practitioners (NPs) often approach neurological examination with some trepidation. This chapter hopes to alleviate those anxieties by providing the NP with the skills necessary to elicit abnormal physical signs. Remember, as neurology is a highly specialised subject, when an abnormal physical sign has been detected by the NP it is commonly referred to the neurological experts in the secondary care team. Therefore, in primary care our aim is to accurately recognise abnormalities and to understand their physiological relevance.

Subjective assessment

Assessing neurological symptoms is not only heavily influenced by the patient's history but is also affected by patient cooperation, conscious state and degree of fatigue. Taking a detailed, accurate history is crucial to the assessment of any presenting complaint. Throughout the history further symptoms may be elicited, for each of which a detailed description is essential:

1. How long has the patient been experiencing the symptom?
2. Onset – sudden or gradual?
3. What has happened since:
   - Constant or periodic?
   - Getting worse or better?
   - Frequency?
4. Precipitating or relieving factors.
5. Affect or restriction on lifestyle.
6. Associated symptoms.
7. Previous episodes.
   Where pain is a symptom, also determine:
- site
- radiation
- character or type
- severity on a scale of 1–10.

The usual structure of a systematic, comprehensive health history applies.

Past history

- Previous illness, childhood and adult
- Immunisation and recent contact with infectious diseases
- Previous emotional or nervous problems
- Previous operations, accidents, hospitalisation
- Allergies.

Family history

Family history identifies predisposition to illness:
- Ask about parents, siblings and children. Note diseases, cause of death and age at time of death.
- History of familial disease, heart disease, diabetes, hypertension? This line of questioning can be varied to take into account the presenting complaint.

Social history

The aim of the social history is to gather some idea of what type of person the patient is, their home circumstances and how their illness affects themselves and their family:
1. Who lives at home?
2. Family problems or worries.

3. Who is the key carer?
4. Accommodation.
5. Job.
6. Hobbies.
7. Alcohol – estimate weekly consumption.
8. Exercise.
9. Diet.
10. Smoking.
11. Recreational drugs.

Drug history

- Prescribed
- Those bought 'over the counter' (OTC)
- Herbal or alternative therapies
- Specific drug allergies

Neurological systems enquiry

- Pain
- Headache
- Visual disturbance
- Deafness
- Dizziness – may be cardiac in origin, so ask about palpitations
- Behavioural changes
- Dysphasia
- Dysphagia
- Syncope
- Seizures
- Muscle wasting
- Muscle weakness
- Paralysis
- Numbness
- Increased sensation
- Unsteady gait
- Sphincter disturbance – difficulty in holding urine or motions.

Objective assessment

Assessment of a patient with a suspected neurological disorder will require motor neurological examination, sensory neurological examination, or examination techniques specific to individual cranial nerves.

Motor neurological assessment

Gait

A practitioner generally examines a patient's gait on entering the consultation room; however, the following tests are specific to elicit possible neurological disorders. Be prepared to support the ataxic patient when you ask them to walk or perform tests independently. With the patient barefoot, observe the following:

- have the patient walk away from and towards the examiner
- have the patient perform a tandem walk (heel to toe)
- have the patient walk on the heels then on tiptoes.

Unless there is substantial disorder of midline cerebellar structures, patients do not demonstrate any insta-

bility of the trunk when sitting. On standing, however, oscillations of the body may materialise even before gait is initiated.

When walking, the patient will often use a wide-based gait and may show caution when turning. Any attempt to turn quickly will result in imbalance. If a patient has a lesion of one cerebellar hemisphere, deviation to that side will occur on walking. The tandem walk test is performed to detect a more subtle disturbance of cerebellar function. The practitioner must appreciate how variably normal individuals perform this test.

Romberg test

The Romberg test is a test of position sense or proprioception. When performing this manoeuvre the practitioner must be positioned behind the patient to give support if necessary:

- Have patient stand with feet together, eyes open, then close eyes for 20–30 seconds without support.
- Note the patient's ability to maintain an upright posture. Normally only minimal swaying occurs and the patient can self-correct this: however, where there is loss of proprioception, the patient immediately loses stability. This loss of stability is noted as a positive Romberg test.

Coordination

Coordination of both upper and lower limbs must be tested:

- have the patient hop on one leg at a time
- while still standing have the patient perform shallow knee bends
- rapid alternating movements of hands – have the patient rapidly pat knees alternately with palm and back of hand
- rapid alternating movement of feet – have the patient rapidly pat the examiner's hands with soles of feet.

The performance of rapid alternating movements of hands and feet is variable in normal individuals and is commonly less smooth in the non-dominant limb.

- Point-to-point test. Ask the patient to touch his nose with his index finger, then to touch your finger, held approximately 0.5 m in front of him.
- Continue the point-to-point test but move your target finger randomly.

In cerebellar ataxia, a tremor emerges that becomes more obvious as the target is approached. The random point-to-point test may make a mild ataxia become more evident.

To assess lower limb coordination, perform the 'heel to knee to shin' test:

- Have the patient slide the heel of one foot in a straight line down the shin of the other leg. In the presence of cerebellar ataxia the heel wavers around the intended pathway.
- When the heel has reached the bottom of the shin, ask the patient to flex the leg and bring the heel back down to the shin just below the knee. If there is

cerebellar incoordination, the heel may fall short of its target or thump into the shin rather than landing gently.

Dermatomes (Figs 11.1 and 11.2)

Key terms

Dermatome – an area of skin innervated by the cutaneous branches of a single spinal nerve
Myotome – an area of muscle innervated by a spinal nerve
Sclerotome – other deep structures, such as bones or joints, innervated by a spinal nerve.

At each segmental level, the dorsal root (sensory) and the ventral root (motor) join to form a mixed spinal nerve that produces two branches: the posterior primary ramus and the anterior primary ramus. The areas of skin supplied by the branches of the dorsal roots are the dermatomes (Epstein et al 1997). Dermatome regions are not as clearly separate as a dermatome map might indicate: the regions of the trunk may overlap up to 50%, therefore destruction of a single spinal nerve will not result in complete numbness anywhere on the trunk. In the limbs the dermatomes overlap much less, and in some areas are innervated by only one spinal nerve.

Sensory neurological assessment

Sensory neurological examination is difficult, with assessment dependent on the patient's subjective responses. The practitioner need not test all sensory areas in all parts of the body; the focus should be on

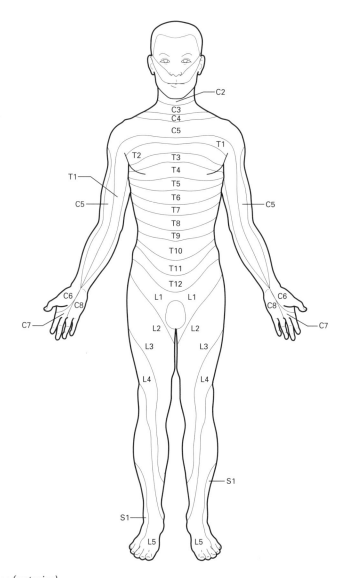

Figure 11.1 *Dermatomes (anterior).*

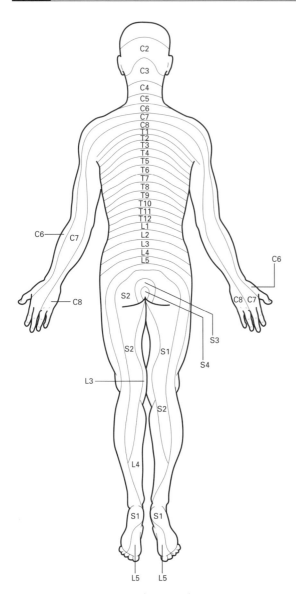

Figure 11.2 *Dermatomes (posterior).*

those areas indicated by the type of sensory disturbance suggested by the patient's history.

Always begin testing from an area of reduced skin sensation, moving out gradually to determine the area of change to normal sensation. Some of the following tests will not be carried out in primary care, but are included as a matter of interest as to what tests may be performed in a secondary setting.

Light touch

Note that distal areas of a limb are more sensitive than proximal areas, and skin containing hair is more sensitive than smooth skin. If the patient indicates unilateral

sensory change, the practitioner should compare equivalent parts on the opposite side of the body:

- do not drag the cotton wool along the surface of the skin, just apply it at a single point
- ask the patient to close his eyes and to respond when contact is made.

Pain

Pain is best assessed using a sharp pin. Venepuncture needles tend to puncture the skin, and are unsuitable. Purpose-made sharps for assessing pain sensation are available. Bear in mind that you are testing the painful aspect of the stimulus rather than the appreciation of contact. In some pathological conditions diffuse pain radiates out from the contact site:

- ask the patient to close his eyes and to identify if the contact is painful
- present sharp and blunt ends of the pin randomly and ask the patient to distinguish one stimulus from another.

Temperature

Using temperature as a sensory neurological test is not usually performed in a primary care setting, although it is useful to have a knowledge as to how it is performed:

- use two metal tubes, one holding hot water the other ice chips
- test the tubes on yourself before applying to the patient's skin
- ask the patient to discern hot from cold on comparable areas on two sides of the body.

Proprioception

Proprioception as a sensory neurological test assesses the patient's ability to recognise the position of joints. It is rare to find loss of proximal joint position sense – it is more usual that the problem is confined to the digits:

1. perform all tests with the patient's eyes closed
2. test the patient's ability to discern passive movement of the joints
3. hold the digit between your right finger and thumb at the sides of the distal joint and use your left hand to stabilise the proximal joint
4. the movement should be barely perceptible
5. indicate findings in the notes as joint position sense (JPS) – intact to the movement of distal interphalangeal (DIP) joint of 10°, or whatever range you have chosen
6. active proprioception testing is performed by asking the patient, with eyes closed, to locate a digit on one hand with the index finger of the other hand
7. mimicking as a test of proprioception is performed by moving the limb with intact sensation into a certain posture, and asking the patient to mimic that posture with the affected limb
8. the final test is to ask the patient to hold the hands outstretched with eyes closed – with severe loss of proprioception, the fingers move in an irregular fashion

9. to test proprioception of the lower limbs, assess by Romberg's test.

Vibration

■ Use a 128 Hz tuning fork with a flat base.
■ To test the finger, apply the gently vibrating tuning fork base to the pad of the finger at the DIP joint. If the vibration sense is absent, test gradually more proximally and note the area where the vibration sense is felt.
■ To test the foot, apply the base of the fork to the pad of the big toe or the dorsum of the interphalangeal (IP) joint. As with the fingers, if the vibration sense is absent, test gradually more proximally until it is felt.

Discrimination

Discrimination is assessed using stereognosis, which is the ability to identify a small object placed in one hand at a time. Patients may also be asked to discriminate weight or texture:
■ with eyes closed, place a small object such as a safety pin, penny or hairclip in the palm of the patient's hand; get them to feel it and ask them to identify the object
■ perform the same test on the other palm using a different object.

Reflexes

Reflexes are remarkably variable in normal individuals. They are assessed using a reflex hammer, and the practitioner must note the grade (Box 11.1). Reinforcement may be necessary to elicit a reflex response; this is done by asking the patient to close their eyes, grit their teeth or clench hands. The latter is known as the 'Jendrassik manoeuvre'.

Brachial (supinator). Brachioradialis is found approximately 5 cm above the wrist on the side of the arm in line with the thumb.

Biceps. Expose the whole arm, place your thumb on the antecubital space on the biceps tendon and strike your thumb with the reflex hammer. This is known as the indirect technique.

Triceps. This can be tested either with the arm fully supported by the examiner with the lower arm dangling, or by bringing the patient's arm well across his body, with

the elbow flexed at 90° so that the triceps tendon is adequately exposed and strike with the reflex hammer.

Patellar. With the patient on the couch, insert your left arm under the patient's knees and flex them to approximately 60°. If the patient is properly relaxed, the legs should sag when you remove your arm. Tap the patellar tendon with the reflex hammer. If one or both of the reflexes is exaggerated, test the knee for clonus. Clonus is where a succession of muscular contractions occurs. To test, fit your thumb and forefinger along the upper border of the patella with the knee extended, exert a sudden downward stretch and hold it. If clonus occurs, even if it is only two or three beats, it is indicative of a pyramidal tract disorder.

Achilles. With the patient kneeling on a chair with ankle flexed, strike the Achilles tendon with a hammer. Alternatively, with the patient on the couch, abduct the leg and externally rotate at the hip with knee and ankle flexed. In the case of limited hip abduction, rest one leg across the other to access and strike the Achilles tendon. If the reflex is exaggerated, test for clonus by holding the limb in the same position, forcibly dorsiflexing the ankle and hold. Three or four beats of clonus is acceptable in normal individuals; however, asymmetric or more sustained clonus is of pathological origin.

Plantar (Babinski's reflex). Using an orange stick or similar tool, apply firm pressure to the lateral aspect of the sole of the foot. Maintaining the pressure, move from the heel to the base of the fifth toe and across the base of the toes. While performing this test, observe the joint of the big toe. In the normal adult the toe plantar flexes, but in the presence of a pyramidal tract disorder the toe dorsiflexes. It is a normal finding if dorsiflexion occurs in an adult when a sharp stimulus is applied to the big toe, and in infants if the stimulus is applied over a wider area.

CRANIAL NERVES

It is of some use to cover each cranial nerve (CN) individually, as it affords a greater understanding of the characteristics and possible presenting symptoms that may arise. Cranial nerves are either sensory or motor nerves:

- CN 1 (sensory), olfactory
- CN 2 (sensory), optic
- CN 3, 4 and 6 (motor), oculomotor, trochlear and abducens
- CN 5 (sensory and motor), trigeminal
- CN 7 (sensory and motor), facial
- CN 8 (sensory), acoustic (vestibulocochlear)
- CN 9 (sensory and motor), glossopharyngeal
- CN 10 (sensory and motor), vagus
- CN 11 (motor), spinal accessory
- CN 12 (motor), hypoglossal.

Box 11.1	*Reflexes*

Grade	Definition
0	Absent
+	Present only with reinforcement
±	Just present
++	Brisk, normal
+++	Exaggerated response

CN 1 olfactory (sensory)

Anatomy and physiology

Molecules from odours are absorbed into the mucosa lining the olfactory epithelium. From here, they diffuse via ciliary processes to the receptor cells and bind reversibly to receptor sites. The olfactory nerve carries impulses from the smell receptors, along the floor of the anterior fossa of the skull to the olfactory area of the cerebral cortex (Marieb 1995; Epstein et al 1997).

Key terms

- *Hyposmia* – partial loss of smell
- *Anosmia* – total loss of smell
- *Hyperosmia* – exaggerated sensitivity to smell
- *Dyosmia* – distorted sense of smell.

Symptoms

Disturbances of smell include:

- post-traumatic anosmia
- post-infective anosmia
- olfactory hallucinations in complex partial seizures (temporal lobe epilepsy).

Examination

For anosmia, the practitioner must determine whether it is bilateral or unilateral. Do not use noxious substances such as ammonia to test smell, as they also stimulate receptors of the trigeminal nerve and give a false positive response. Use test odours such as peppermint, clove, lemon, coffee, vinegar or cinnamon.

- Check nasal patency. Occlude one nostril and ask the patient to sniff.
- Ask patient to identify odour with eyes closed. Occlude each nostril in turn and perform smell test using two different odours.

Clinical relevance

1. Women have a more sensitive sense of smell than men; however, in both sexes sensitivity declines with age
2. Olfaction is diminished in dementia
3. Olfaction is commonly disturbed by upper respiratory tract infection
4. Olfaction may be disturbed with local nasal pathology, e.g. polyp, allergic rhinitis, foreign body, trauma, smoking, cocaine usage
5. Hyposmia may be congenital
6. Hyposmia can persist after viral illness
7. Hyposmia can occur after head injury
8. Olfactory hallucinations occur in temporal lobe epilepsy
9. Unilateral hyposmia may rarely be the presenting symptom of a subfrontal meningioma.

CN 2 optic (sensory)

Anatomy and physiology

I have no wish to cover ground already well known but to look at some specific features which are relevant to examination of the eye.

Key terms

- *Scotoma* – an area of blindness in the field of vision
- *Papilloedema* – swelling of the optic disc.

Nerve pathways for vision

The eyeball is spherical in shape and designed to focus light onto the neurosensory rods and cones of the fundus. The fovea contains only cones, with the rods predominating in the periphery. For an image to be seen, light reflected from it must pass through the pupil and be focused onto the rods and cones in the retina. The image projected there is upside down and reversed right to left. Impulses from these neurosensory receptors travel via fibres in the retina to the optic nerve. From the optic nerve, impulses are conveyed along the optic tract, to where they cross at the optic chiasm, and continue along the optic radiation tract to the visual cortex, situated in the occipital lobe of the brain (Bates 1995, Marieb 1995).

Visual fields

A visual field is the entire area seen by an eye when it looks at a central point. When the patient is using both eyes, the central parts of the two visual fields overlap in an area of binocular vision; laterally in the temporal margins vision is monocular. There are eight fields of vision. Visual fields extend farthest on the temporal sides and are limited by the brows above, the cheeks below and by the nose medially.

Examination

Inspection

Inspect both eyes for position and symmetry. Inspect eyelashes, eyebrows, eyelids, lachrymal apparatus, sclera, conjunctivae, irises, and corneas, for colour and absence of lesions. The white sclera may look pale yellow or cream-coloured in the extreme periphery: this should not be mistaken for jaundice, which is more generalised over the sclera and a deeper yellow colour.

Visual acuity

Visual acuity can be checked by gross reading ability, or more accurately by using the Snellen or Rosenbaum charts.

Near vision. When checking gross reading ability, ensure that the patient who normally wears spectacles or contact lenses has them on. Ask the patient to read the reading test types: if these are not available, ask them to read some small print. Remember that near vision does not necessarily equate well with distance vision.

Distance vision. Visual acuity using the Snellen chart should be checked in conditions of high illumination to produce an amount of cone function. The Snellen chart is used for checking distance vision. Ensure that the patient wears their spectacles for distance correction: if these are not to hand, reading through a pinhole card will partly correct myopia. With the patient 6 m from the chart, ask them to cover each eye in turn and identify the smallest line of print that can be read comfortably. Acuity is expressed as the distance between the patient and the chart (6 m), to the figure on the chart immediately above the smallest line. An acuity of 6/18, shows that at 6 m from the chart the patient is able to read only to the 18 m line.

Colour vision

Usually a congenital defect which is checked by using the Farnsworth–Munsell test, which consists of 84 coloured tiles; however, the Ishihara test plates, which assess red/green deficiency more rapidly, are more commonly used. Ask the patient to read the plates 1–15 at a distance of 75 cm from the eyes. Colour vision is regarded as normal if a patient reads 13 or more plates correctly.

Visual fields

There are several types of scotoma; however, for the NP, the aim is to recognise a scotoma and refer to a doctor or Ophthalmology Department in secondary care. There are eight visual fields (Fig. 11.3).

Assess visual fields by confrontation using finger movements or coloured objects. Remember that you are checking the patient's visual fields by comparing them to your own visual fields. Also note that absence of rods and cones in the optic disc produces a blind spot in the normal field of vision of each eye, 15° temporal to the line of gaze. Sit or stand approximately 1 m from the patient. To test the left eye, ask the patient to cover the right eye while you cover your left eye with your right hand. Ensure that the patient's left eye remains fixed on your right eye throughout the examination. Check eight visual fields and repeat for the right eye.

Fundoscopy

Normally it is not necessary to dilate the pupils in order to examine the central fundus; however, if the patient has small pupils, or the background illumination is high, take the patient into a darkened room for the examination.

For those NPs working in a hospital environment, a mydriatic such as mydrilate (cyclopentolate hydrochloride 0.5%), can be instilled. This should never be administered to the unconscious patient, and should always be recorded in the patient's notes. Do not use mydriatics in a patient with glaucoma. Remember to reverse the effects of the mydriatic by instilling 2% pilocarpine at the end of the examination. If the patient wears spectacles with substantial correction, it may facilitate the examination to perform it with the patient's spectacles in place:

- Ask the patient to fix their gaze on a distant target over your shoulder. Use your right eye and right hand to examine the patient's right eye and vice versa.
- Locate the red reflex with the ophthalmoscope and follow towards the eye.

Now that you are looking at the retina, focus your ophthalmoscope if necessary. You may need a different focus for each eye. Examine:

1. The lens for opacity.
2. The optic disc and cup for colour and size.
3. The retinal blood vessels for crossings, nipping and size. Arteries are narrower than veins and a brighter colour.
4. The retinal background for colour, cotton wool spots (exudates) and haemorrhages.
5. The macular area.
6. The fovea.

Findings can be described using the optic disc as a clock face, e.g. 'one large haemorrhage at 6 o'clock'.

Disorders of the retina and visual pathways

- Anterior ischaemic optic neuropathy
- Optic neuritis
- Optic nerve compression
- Papilloedema
- Hypertensive retinopathy
- Diabetic retinopathy
- Chiasmatic compression due to pituitary tumour
- Optic tract radiation or visual cortex lesions due to vascular disease.

Clinical application

Optic atrophy

Follows any process that damages the ganglion cells or the axons between the retinal nerve fibre layer and the lateral geniculate body. Optic atrophy is associated with loss of bulk from the nerve and pallor of the disc. Detection of optic atrophy requires considerable experience.

Papilloedema

Patients often have no visual complaints; some experience a transient obscuring of vision, either occurring spontaneously or generated by postural change. Papilloedema is usually bilateral and sometimes asymmetrical. As yet we are unsure about the causes of

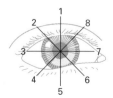 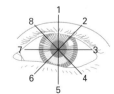

Figure 11.3 *Visual fields.*

papilloedema; however, the term is used for those patients whose papilloedema is secondary to a raised intracranial pressure.

Hypertensive retinopathy

In hypertensive retinopathy the light reflex from the blood vessel walls in the retina is abnormal, appearing like silver or copper wiring. Arteriovenous nipping, which is caused by constriction of the venous wall, is seen at sites of arteriovenous crossing. Both of these symptoms are seen in normal older individuals. A more reliable indication of hypertensive retinopathy is a variation in the diameter of the arterioles. As the disease progresses, cotton wool spots and haemorrhages appear, and in malignant or accelerated hypertension, disc swelling occurs.

Diabetic retinopathy

The main effect of diabetic retinopathy is seen initially in the microcirculation producing the microaneurysm. As the disease progresses small haemorrhages, exudates and cotton wool spots appear. Loss of sight is due either to macular disease such as oedema, infarction or lipid deposition, or to new vessel formation known as proliferative diabetic retinopathy. Proliferative diabetic retinopathy causes traction on the retina from fibrous tissue, which in turn leads to vitreous haemorrhage and retinal detachment.

Glaucoma

Glaucoma is identified by raised intraocular pressure; this occurs either in primary form or secondary to other ocular pathology. Effects on the optic disc involve enlargement of the physiological cup, arcuate field defects, and with advanced disease there is marked undermining of the disc margins and bowing of the blood vessels.

Optic nerve disease

With optic nerve disease, the visual defect is usually monocular, visual acuity is reduced and colour perception, particularly for red/green, is disturbed. The most likely visual field defect is a central scotoma and there is an afferent pupillary defect. Optic atrophy is a late development in optic nerve compression, and proptosis or protrusion is likely if the lesion is within the orbit.

CN 3, 4 and 6 oculomotor, trochlear and abducens (motor)

Anatomy and physiology

Extraocular movements

Six muscles control the movement of each eye: the four rectus and two oblique muscles. Muscle function can be tested by asking the patient to move the eye in the direction controlled by each muscle. There are six cardinal directions of movement (Fig. 11.4).

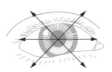 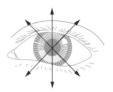

Figure 11.4 *Cardinal directions of movement.*

If your patient is looking up and towards the right, the right eye is moved by the right superior rectus muscle supplied by CN 3; the left eye is moved by the inferior oblique muscle also supplied by CN 3. In the presence of paralysis of the muscles involved, the eye will deviate in the affected muscle from its position in that direction of gaze.

Key terms

- *Strabismus* – squint
- *Anisocoria* – pupil size inequality of less than 0.5 mm
- *Esodeviation* – inverting strabismus
- *Exodeviation* – everting strabismus.

Examination

Inspection

Normal movement of eyebrows and eyelids is innervated by CN 3, 4 and 6: observe movement for symmetry and lack of lag. If there is a ptosis, assess its fatiguability by asking the patient to sustain an upward gaze.

Extraocular movements

Movement of each eye is controlled by the coordinated action of six muscles: four rectus muscles – superior, lateral, inferior and medial – and two oblique muscles – inferior and superior (Fig. 11.5).

To test the function and nerve supply of each muscle, ask the patient to move the eye in the direction controlled by each muscle. As there are six muscles controlling movement in each eye, then there are six cardinal directions. Ask the patient to follow your finger with his eyes: you will be drawing a large 'H' in order to test all the muscles. Start with your finger pointing between the patient's eyes at approximately 20 cm distance. Move your finger smoothly to your right (tests left lateral rectus muscle and CN 6); upwards for approximately 15 cm (tests left superior rectus muscle and CN 3); down to the medial point and further down for the same distance (tests left inferior rectus muscle and CN 3). Move your finger back up to the medial point and across to your left (tests right lateral rectus muscle and CN 6); upwards (tests right superior rectus muscle and CN 3); and downwards (tests right inferior rectus muscle and CN 3). Move the finger back to the starting point and towards the top of the nose to test for convergence. While carrying out this test observe eye movements: note any difficulty or lag in movement. It is considered normal to observe three beats of nystagmus

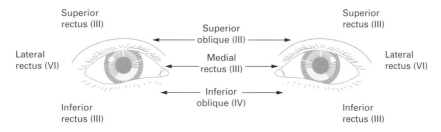

Figure 11.5 *Eye muscles.*

on lateral gaze: however, more than three beats is considered an abnormality. Note that convergence is symmetrical.

Strabismus

A strabismus is an indication that the axes of the eyes are not parallel. If the strabismus is towards the nose (esodeviation), the axes are convergent. If the strabismus is lateral (exodeviation), the axes are divergent. Throughout the range of eye movements the strabismus angle of deviation may remain constant: this is known as a concomitant or nonparalytic strabismus, usually caused by an imbalance in muscular tone. It has many causes, may be hereditary and usually appears in early childhood. Where there is variation of the angle of deviation this is known as incomitant or paralytic strabismus, which is an indication of paresis of one or more of the extraocular muscles (Bates 1995).

The cover test. In nonparalytic strabismus a cover test can be performed. For example, take a patient with a right monocular convergent strabismus; ask the patient to focus on a pen light in front of the eyes. First you will note that corneal reflections are asymmetrical. Cover the normal left eye: the affected eye now moves outward to fix on the light; the covered eye moves inward to the same degree. Remove the cover: the left eye moves outward to fix on the light and the right eye returns to its convergent position.

Pupils

Inspect the pupils for size and shape. Note that pupils are considered large if > 5 mm, and small if < 3 mm. Pupil size inequality of less than 0.5 mm, known as anisocoria, is present in approximately 20% of normal people. If pupillary reactions are normal, anisocoria is considered benign. It is possible to observe variations of shape, e.g. oval or keyhole shaped.

Test the pupillary reaction to light. Ask the patient to fix their gaze in the distance; shine a light obliquely into each eye in turn; the distant gaze and oblique lighting help to avoid a near reaction. Observe the direct reaction, which is pupillary constriction in that eye; and the consensual reaction, which is pupillary constriction in the opposite eye. When a poor reaction is elicited, observe the pupillary reactions in a darkened room.

Accommodation as a pupillary reaction test is performed by the patient fixing the gaze into the distance:

after 30 seconds, ask the patient to focus on an object approximately 20 cm from the eyes. The pupils should constrict to accommodate the shift of gaze. Innervation of the pupils is through CN 3, 4 and 6.

We have often observed in a patient's notes the mnemonic 'PERLA'. This stands for:

P pupils
E equal
R round and reactive to
L light and
A accommodation.

Pupillary reaction

The nerve pathways for pupillary action differ from that of vision. The initial pathways are via retina, optic nerve and optic tract: the pathways then diverge in the midbrain, after which impulses are transmitted through the oculomotor nerve to the constrictor muscles of the iris of each eye (Bates 1995, Epstein et al 1997).

The nerve fibres in the oculomotor nerve resulting in pupillary constriction are part of the parasympathetic nervous system. The iris is also supplied by sympathetic nerve fibres, which when stimulated cause the pupil to dilate and the upper eyelid to rise. The sympathetic pathway originates in the hypothalamus, travels through the brainstem and cervical cord into the neck. From the neck, the pathway follows the carotid artery and its branches into the orbit. A lesion at any site of the sympathetic pathway could result in impairment of sympathetic effects on the pupil (Bates 1995).

The pupil size is altered as a response either to light or to the effort of focusing on a near object. Both light reaction and near reaction are mediated by the oculomotor nerve.

Light reaction. In normal circumstances a light shining onto one retina causes pupillary constriction in both eyes. In the eye into which the light is shining, this pupillary response is known as a direct reaction; in the opposite eye, where there is no direct stimulus, the pupillary response is known as a consensual reaction.

Near reaction. When the gaze is shifted from a far point to a near point, the pupils constrict. Two other factors simultaneously occur in the near reaction: convergence, which is an extraocular movement; and accommodation, which is an increase in the convexity of the lenses caused by constriction of the ciliary muscles. This increased convexity of the lenses brings near objects into focus, but is not visible to the examiner.

Disorders of the pupil and eye movements

Eye movement disorders. Gaze paresis, internuclear ophthalmoplegia, one-and-a-half syndrome, abducens, trochlear and oculomotor nerve palsies.

Pupillary defects. Horner's syndrome, tonic pupil, Argyll Robertson pupil, relative afferent pupillary defect.

Nystagmus. Congenital, vestibular, gaze evoked, downbeat, convergence retractory.

CN 5 trigeminal (sensory and motor)

Anatomy and physiology

The main muscles supplied by the trigeminal nerve are the medial and lateral pterygoids, temporalis and masseter. The smaller muscles supplied are the tensor tympani and tensor palatini. Jaw closure is accomplished by contraction of both the temporalis and masseter muscles. Jaw opening and lateral movements are achieved by the pterygoids. CN 5 innervates the temporomandibular area of the face and jaw, the mucous membranes of the nose and mouth, some sinuses, part of the external auditory meatus and most of the dura (Epstein et al 1997).

Key terms

- *Pterygoid muscles* – the medial pterygoid is a deep, two-headed muscle that runs along the internal surface of the mandible and is largely concealed by that bone. The lateral pterygoid is a deep, two-headed muscle which lies superior to the medial pterygoid muscle.
- *Trismus* – spasm of the masticatory muscles.

Examination

Inspection

Inspect the face for symmetry; look for signs of paralysis or muscle wasting. Look for tremor of the lips, involuntary chewing movements and trismus.

Corneal reflex

It is important to explain this procedure to the patient in advance in order that they know what to expect. To test corneal reflex, ask the patient to look up and away from you. Touch the cornea lightly with a wisp of cotton wool. The normal response is rapid blinking of the eyes. The sensory aspect of this reflex is through the trigeminal nerve, CN 5; the motor response is through CN 7. Please note that use of contact lenses can reduce or eliminate this reflex. Patients who wear contact lenses must remove them for the test: a more dull response can occur which will be symmetrical. In the absent or depressed corneal response, the cotton wool can touch the cornea without provoking a reaction.

Jaw

While performing this test, observe for symmetry of movement, strength and signs of muscle wasting or paralysis. As you palpate the temporomandibular joint, ask the patient to clench their teeth, wriggle the jaw from side to side and to open the mouth – first without, then with resistance. In a unilateral trigeminal lesion, the jaw deviates to the paralysed side.

Jaw jerk. With the patient's mouth slightly open, place your index finger on the apex of the jaw and tap it with the patella hammer. The normal response is contraction of the pterygoid muscles; however, this response varies greatly in normal individuals.

Facial sensation

Areas for testing facial sensation include the forehead, the medial aspect of the cheek and the chin. Test sensations include light touch, pinprick and, occasionally, it is necessary to assess temperature appreciation. With the patient's eyes closed, test light touch using a wisp of cotton wool; do not drag along the skin. It is more common to find a partial loss of sensation, rather than total loss. If this occurs, ask the patient to compare the stimulus with sites on other parts of the trigeminal nerve on the same side, and with comparable areas on the other side of the face. Test pinprick sensation on the same sites. A sensory loss confined to the trigeminal nerve distribution should become normal at the level of the vertex, but well above the angle of the jaw. You can map out any areas of sensation loss by testing around the area and record your findings in diagram form.

Disorders of facial sensation include malignant invasion of the trigeminal nerve, isolated trigeminal neuropathy, involvement in the lateral medullary syndrome, involvement with cerebellopontine tumours and sensory involvement with thalamic, capsular or cortical infarction.

Clinical application

Motor

Involvement of the trigeminal distribution in a unilateral upper motor neurone lesion is not normally clinically detectable. However, the jaw jerk will be exaggerated in a bilateral upper motor neurone lesion.

Sensory

Both sensory and motor loss is evident where there is malignant invasion of the trigeminal nerve or its ganglion. Isolated trigeminal neuropathy results in normal motor function but progressive loss of facial sensation. Spinal lesions above C2 can result in selective loss of facial temperature and pain sense, occasionally with an 'onion ring' type distribution. Loss of facial temperature and pain sense affects the same side of the face in the lateral medullary syndrome. Diminution of light touch eventuates with damage to the main sensory nucleus, although thalamic infarction is liable to affect all facial senses.

Corneal response

As previously mentioned, corneal response can be diminished through use of contact lenses. Loss of response may be an early indication of trigeminal compression. This should be assessed in patients presenting with unilateral facial pain or deafness. Corneal response is diminished in unilateral lower motor neurone facial paresis; the response, however, on the opposite side of the face is normal.

CN 7 facial (sensory and motor)

Anatomy and physiology

The facial nerve leaves the pons along with the acoustic nerve, crosses the cerebellopontine angle and enters the internal auditory meatus. From here it enters the facial nerve canal, runs forwards above the cochlea and bends sharply backwards. At this point the nerve expands to form the geniculate ganglion. From here the CN 7 supplies taste sensation to the anterior two-thirds of the tongue. The nerve then runs through the parotid gland to the muscles of facial expression. The sensory element of the facial nerve innervates the external auditory meatus, the tympanic membrane and a small area of skin behind the ear (Epstein et al 1997).

Key terms

See facial movement disorders.

Examination

Inspection

Facial asymmetry is a common normal finding, as is asymmetry of the lower face during speech. Carefully observe the patient's face while you are taking the history.

Facial examination

Observe the facies at rest. Note any difference in symmetry. Observe the level of the two angles of the mouth. Remember that with a long-standing facial weakness, fibrotic contracture of the mouth can elevate the angle of the mouth, suggesting that the weakness is on the opposite side. Bilateral face weakness is easily overlooked. The face lacks expression and appears to sag.

Observe the facies in movement. The muscles of facial expression are employed in facial movement. The frontalis muscle elevates the eyebrow, the orbicularis oculi closes the eye, the orbicularis oris closes the mouth, and the platysma muscle depresses the angle of the mouth. The buccinator muscle, which assists in mastication, is also supplied by the facial nerve. Again, noting difference in symmetry, ask the patient to smile, frown and wrinkle the forehead. Ask the patient to close the eyes tightly; normally, the eyelashes virtually disappear. A sign of a mild weakness is a marked protrusion of the eyelashes on the affected side.

Clinical application

Causes of peripheral palsies of the facial nerve are usually unknown but occasionally occur in poliomyelitis, tumour, multiple sclerosis, Guillain–Barré syndrome, trauma, Ramsay Hunt syndrome and sarcoid. The most common isolated facial nerve lesion is Bell's palsy.

Facial movement disorders

Fasciculation. Nearly always associated with motor neurone disease.

Myokymia. A fine, almost continuous shimmering contraction of some or all of the muscles supplied by the facial nerve, commonly caused by multiple sclerosis.

Hemifacial spasm. An involuntary contraction of facial muscles. Initially it is often confined to the orbicularis oculi; eventually, a mild facial weakness appears.

Blepharospasm. Uncontrollable blinking due to involuntary contraction of the eyelid muscle.

Tics. An habitual spasmodic muscular contraction.

Orofacial dyskinesia. An involuntary semi-repetitive contraction of muscles around the mouth. This is often accompanied by abnormal movements of the tongue. Orofacial dyskinesia can either occur spontaneously or as a side-effect of phenothiazines.

CN 8 acoustic (sensory)

Anatomy and physiology

A sound stimulus causes vibration of the tympanic membrane, which transmits the stimulus to the three ossicles of the inner ear: the malleus, incus and stapes. The stapes, which is attached to the oval window, vibrates and starts movement in the perilymph within the bony labyrinth, comprising cochlea, vestibule and semicircular canals (Epstein et al 1997).

The semicircular canals each surround a semicircular duct, and at one end of each canal is a receptor organ called the crista ampullaris. The canals open into the vestibule, where the saccule and the utricle contain receptor cells called maculae (Epstein et al 1997).

In the wall of the cochlear duct is the spiral organ of corti, which is innervated by the cochlear component of the auditory nerve. The vestibular component of the auditory nerve innervates the receptors in the utricle and semicircular canals. The saccule and part of the posterior semicircular canal are innervated by fibres from the cochlear division. Within the internal auditory canal, the vestibular and cochlear nerve components join together: this nerve now crosses the subarachnoid space and enters the brainstem at the junction of the pons and the medulla. The semicircular canals are responsible for detection of rotational head movements; the vestibular system gives information on head movement and posture (Epstein et al 1997).

Examination

Damage to CN 8 results in either deafness or vertigo.

Deafness

Almost every form of deafness can be classified under the following headings:

Conductive. Due to wax, perforation, foreign body, otosclerosis, disease of the canal or middle ear such as infection, tumour or abscess.

Sensorineural. Due to Ménière's disease, senile deafness or disturbance of the auditory nerve such as tumour, or occlusion of the internal auditory artery.

Mixed conductive and sensorineural. Where conductive and sensorineural factors are present in the same ear.

Where there is a presenting complaint of deafness, always inspect the ears for an obvious cause, such as wax or foreign body: however, if deafness persists after treatment, a hearing test must be performed.

Hearing tests

Hearing tests include whispered/conversational voice tests, audiogram and Weber and Rinne tests.

Whispered/conversational voice tests. These are simple to perform:

- have the patient stand approximately 2 m away, with his back towards you
- ask the patient to occlude one ear
- whisper a word and ask the patient to identify it
- if the patient is unable to hear at that distance, move approximately 30 cm closer and retest
- note the point where the patient can identify the word and record in notes, e.g. as 'right ear WV at 2 m'
- retest the other ear in the same fashion
- the choice of using whispered voice or conversational voice for the test will depend on the degree of the patient's deafness.

Audiogram. Many surgeries will have their own audiogram equipment: some may refer patients to hospital to have this performed. In any case, audiogram in the surgery is used as a tool for making a decision regarding referral: hospital equipment and environment give a much more accurate assessment:

- learn how to operate the audiogram equipment accurately
- give the patient clear instructions
- perform the test in the quietest room in the surgery
- have the patient sitting with his back to the audiogram before testing.

The Weber and Rinne tests are designed to distinguish if the deafness is conductive, sensorineural or mixed conductive and sensorineural. You will need a 512 Hz tuning fork with a flat base.

Rinne's test. Strike the fork and hold with prongs facing towards the meatus until the patient indicates that the sound can no longer be heard. Apply the base of the fork immediately to the mastoid process. If the patient can hear no sound the result is a normal or positive Rinne, where sound is heard better by air conduction (AC) than bone conduction (BC). This is written as AC > BC. If deafness is present in the ear tested, then the deafness is said to be sensorineural. A negative Rinne is where sound is heard through the mastoid process after the patient has ceased to hear the sound at the meatus. In this case, bone conduction is greater than air conduction, BC > AC, and the deduction is that deafness, if present in that ear, is conductive.

To confuse the issue further, a false negative Rinne in a patient with severe unilateral perceptive deafness means that a patient may appear to hear better by BC than AC in the deaf ear. What is happening is that he is hearing the bone conducted sound transmitted to the good cochlea in the other ear. If a false negative Rinne is suspected, retest, but mask the good ear by some form of noise. The result should then show that either little or nothing will be heard in the affected ear.

Weber's test. Your patient is presenting, for example, with a right ear deafness. Strike the tuning fork and place the base on the vertex; ask the patient in which ear he hears the sound. In conductive deafness, sound is referred to the affected right ear, as the cochlea will pick up the sound through bone conduction. In sensorineural deafness, sound is referred to the good ear. Weber's test is often unreliable.

Vertigo

There are two types of vertigo:

Peripheral vertigo. Disruption of the labyrinthine system. Causes include vestibular neuronitis, benign positional vertigo and Ménière's disease.

Central vertigo. Disruption of the vestibular nerve. Causes include cerebrovascular disease and multiple sclerosis.

If a patient presents with positional vertigo, check the effect of posture during examination:

1. position the patient at the edge of the couch facing away from you
2. tell the patient that vertigo may occur and ask them to keep their eyes open throughout the manoeuvre
3. lower the head and trunk backward so that the head is almost 30° below the horizontal
4. observe the patient's eyes and move the head to one side and then to the other
5. if nystagmus appears, note whether it begins immediately or after an interval of time, whether it persists or disappears, and then if it reappears when the patient returns to the sitting position
6. if the test proves positive, ask the patient if the symptoms resembled those previously experienced.

Clinical application

Vertigo

Vertigo is where a patient experiences a sense of rotation of self or of the environment. The vertigo experienced is rarely persistent, although symptoms such as dizziness may persist. Acute vertigo is often associated with vomiting, ataxia and malaise. Epidemic labyrinthitis and acute vestibular neuronitis are diagnosis applied to patients giving a history of acute vertigo on the suspicion that an acute disturbance of the labyrinth or vestibular nerve has occurred.

Benign postural vertigo. This is sometimes caused by head injury, but is often spontaneous. The patient usually recovers within a few weeks but may be subject to recurrence of the disease in subsequent years. Patients complain of attacks of vertigo that are triggered, for example, by lying down in bed on one particular side. Tests for nystagmus prove positive.

Central vertigo. This tends to persist longer than peripheral vertigo. Cerebrovascular disease and multiple sclerosis are common causes of a central vestibular disturbance. Other symptoms of brainstem disease are usually evident. Ménière's disease is thought to be due to distension of the endolymphatic space. Bouts of vertigo occur together with a persistent unilateral tinnitus and progressive sensorineural deafness.

Tinnitus

Tinnitus is manifested by noise in one or both ears which may be continuous or intermittent and varying in pitch. Tinnitus occurs with cochlear disease or damage, and with compression of the auditory nerve. Some patients with abnormal cranial flow are able to hear the flow and describe it as a type of pulsatile noise. In these patients a bruit may be audible over the skull.

CN 9 glossopharyngeal (sensory and motor)

Anatomy and physiology

CN 9, 10 and 11 use one motor nucleus that innervates the striated muscle of the pharynx, larynx and upper oesophagus. The glossopharyngeal nerve leaves the medulla and exits the skull through the jugular foramen along with the vagus and accessory nerves. The somatic components of the glossopharyngeal nerve supply the tonsillar fossa and sections of the pharynx: however, the general visceral efferent and special visceral efferent fibres are not readily testable. The glossopharyngeal nerve supplies the sensory organs for pain, touch and temperature in the pharynx, fauces and palatine tonsil, and is the nerve of taste for the posterior third of the tongue. CN 9 innervates arterial baroreceptors in the carotid sinus: the vagus innervates those in the aortic arch (Epstein et al 1997).

Examination

Gag reflex

Bear in mind that testing the gag reflex is an uncomfortable experience for the patient:
- explain the procedure to the patient
- using the tip of an orange stick, press first into one tonsillar fossa and then the other
- observe that the soft palate rises in the midline
- check with the patient that the sensation is similar on both sides.

Clinical application

A depressed or absent gag reflex is an indication of a glossopharyngeal lesion. It is extremely rare to find isolated lesions of the glossopharyngeal nerve.

A glossopharyngeal neuralgia is commonly due to distortion of the nerve by vascular anomaly or tumour. Paroxysms of pain in the tongue, tonsil or soft palate are provoked by swallowing, masticating or tongue protrusion. Syncopal attacks occurring at the time of paroxysm or triggered by swallowing are indicative of carotid sinus fibre involvement. In the presence of a nasopharyngeal tumour, the vagus, accessory and glossopharyngeal nerves will all be affected. In cases of Chiari malformation, stretching of CN 9 can lead to unilateral or bilateral depression of gag.

CN 10 vagus (sensory and motor)

Anatomy and physiology

The vagus nerve, the most extensive of the cranial nerves, lies immediately below the glossopharyngeal nerve and leaves the medulla and exits the skull at the jugular foramen (Epstein et al 1997). Like CN 9, the special efferent fibres innervate the striated muscle of the pharynx, larynx and upper oesophagus. The recurrent laryngeal branch supplies all the intrinsic muscles of the larynx except for the cricothyroid, which is innervated by the external branch (Epstein et al 1997).

In the heart, the fibres from the right vagus end chiefly in the sinoatrial (SA) node; the fibres from the left vagus end chiefly around the atrioventricular (AV) node. CN 10 also innervates the baroreceptors in the aortic arch.

Key terms

- *Aphonia* – loss of speech.

Examination

Assessment is made by observing the position of the soft palate and the movements of the uvula and posterior pharyngeal wall:
- observe the soft palate and uvula
- note the position of the uvula, which should be midline at rest
- note the position of the soft palate, which in normal circumstances is symmetrical

- ask the patient to say 'Ah': the soft palate and uvula should move on phonation
- test the gag reflex
- note hoarseness.

Minor deviations of the uvula, particularly those that are inconsistent, should be ignored. A unilateral lesion of the vagus causes paralysis of the soft palate on the same side. At rest, the palate will lie slightly lower on the affected side and deviate to the intact side on phonation or on testing gag reflex. A bilateral vagus palsy will result in severe palatal palsy, nasal regurgitation and aphonia.

Disorders of the vagus nerve

Bilateral supranuclear palsy (pseudobulbar palsy)

- Cerebrovascular accident
- Motor neurone disease.

Bilateral nuclear lesions (bulbar palsy)

- Motor neurone disease.

Unilateral nuclear lesions

- Lateral medullary syndrome.

Recurrent laryngeal palsy

- Aortic aneurysm
- Tumour
- Post-thyroid surgery.

CN 11 spinal accessory (sensory and motor)

Anatomy and physiology

The accessory nerve has both cranial and spinal elements. The cranial element leaves the medulla accompanied by CN 9 and CN 10. The spinal element is formed of rootlets that come from the lateral aspect of the spinal cord down to the fifth segment. The rootlets from a single stem, which ascends alongside the cord, passes through the foramen magnum and unites with the cranial element. The combined cranial and spinal nerve leaves the skull through the jugular foramen (Epstein et al 1997).

The cranial root joins the vagus. The spinal root receives input from the second, third and fourth cervical roots, before innervating the sternomastoid muscle and the upper part of the trapezius muscle. The second and third roots passing to the sternomastoid are probably sensory: the third and fourth roots to the trapezium are entirely motor (Epstein et al 1997).

Examination

The cranial element of the accessory nerve cannot be assessed; however, the spinal element is assessed by examining the trapezius and sternomastoid muscles.

Trapezius

1. Observe the position of the trapezius at rest
2. Ask the patient to shrug the shoulders without resistance and observe for symmetrical movement
3. Ask the patient to shrug the shoulders against resistance and assess the strength for equality.

Sternomastoid (sternocleidomastoid)

1. Inspect the sternomastoid. A patient with a CN 11 lesion presents with a less conspicuous sternomastoid on the affected side.
2. Assess the strength by asking the patient to turn the head to the affected side against resistance. The sternomastoid on the affected side will fail to stand out during rotation.
3. Spasmodic torticollis may also be elicited on rotation.

Disorders of the accessory nerve

1. Involvement of jugular foramen tumours
2. Spasmodic torticollis
3. Accessory palsy of unknown aetiology.

CN 12 hypoglossal (motor)

Anatomy and physiology

The hypoglossal nerve exits the skull through the anterior condylar canal and supplies the intrinsic muscles of the tongue and all its extrinsic muscles, except for the palatoglossus muscle (Epstein et al 1997).

Examination

1. Inspect the tongue in the oral cavity at rest
2. Observe for involuntary movements:
   - fasciculation (a shimmering motion on the surface of the tongue)
   - coarse tremor or unpredictable complex movements
3. Assess the tongue for bulk (as the tongue wastes it becomes thinner and more wrinkled)
4. Ask the patient to protrude the tongue (minor deviations are seen in normal individuals)
5. Assess strength by pushing the tongue on the inside of each cheek or by protruding and pressing to right and left against a tongue depressor
6. Ask the patient to move the tongue rapidly from side to side.

Clinical application

Disturbance of the speed of the tongue on side-to-side movements occurs in extrapyramidal diseases, including Parkinson's disease. Coarse tremor of the tongue is also found in Parkinson's disease, whereas unpredictable complex movements could be associated with Huntington's disease or orofacial dyskinesia.

A unilateral, hypoglossal, lower motor nerve lesion will cause focal atrophy, fasciculation and deviation to the paralysed side. This lesion may occur in isolation or as a result of skull base malignant invasion.

A bilateral involvement of the lower motor neurone projections to the tongue is usually part of a bulbar palsy. There is added involvement of the other lower brainstem motor nerve cells which results in dysphagia and dysarthria. The tongue will appear wasted and immobile.

A unilateral, upper motor neurone lesion will have little effect on the tongue function, although some protrusion may be evident on the side of the hemiparesis.

A bilateral, upper motor neurone lesion is usually the result of cerebrovascular disease, and results in pseudobulbar palsy. Dysphagia, dysarthria and emotional lability will be evident. The tongue is stiff and immobile, there is a weakness of palatal elevation, a brisk jaw jerk and gag reflex.

SPECIFIC DISORDERS

Vertigo

Dizziness and vertigo can be difficult to assess, as in many cases the patient's understanding is different to that of the practitioner. Vertigo may be defined as 'the consciousness of disordered orientation of the body in space' (Bannister 1992, p. 75).

Vertigo may arise as a single episode or in repeated attacks, as in acute vertigo. It is rarely persistent, although symptoms such as dizziness may persist. There are two types of vertigo: peripheral vertigo, a disruption of the labyrinthine system; and central vertigo, which is disruption of the vestibular nerve. Causes include:

- labyrinthitis (infective, traumatic, syphilitic, postoperative)
- neoplasms (acoustic neuroma, glomus tumour, carcinoma)
- vestibular neuronitis
- benign positional vertigo
- Ménière's disease
- cerebrovascular disease (atherosclerosis, hypertension, haemorrhage)
- multiple sclerosis
- ototoxic drugs (streptomycin, quinine, salicylates)
- alcohol abuse
- wax
- head injury.

Subjective assessment

A comprehensive history is essential to elicit symptoms, their duration and frequency and associated symptoms, and to rule out differential diagnoses. From the history you may find:

- The patient experiences a sense of rotation of self or of the environment
- Posture of the limbs, especially the lower limbs, may be felt to be unsteady and ill adjusted

- The patient may experience visceral disturbances such as pallor, sweating, nausea, vomiting and diarrhoea
- Motor disturbances include falling and disorientation of body parts
- Tinnitus may be an associated symptom
- Hearing loss can occur (wax, infection, neuromas, etc.)
- Ask about current and recent medication.

Objective assessment

A neurological examination and auscultation of the carotid for bruits should be checked to rule out other causes. During an attack check the patient for altered pulse and blood pressure. Assess the following:

- vital signs, including blood pressure
- ear examination and, if deafness is a symptom with no obvious cause, audiogram
- positional vertigo test, nystagmus and vertigo may be elicited (brainstem lesions may rarely cause positional vertigo and nystagmus; this nystagmus has no latent interval, persists, does not fatigue and does not reverse direction from sitting to lying and vice versa)
- Romberg's test.

Investigations

Check the following blood tests: full blood picture, erythrocyte sedimentation rate (ESR) and liver function test.

Treatment

Address any underlying cause, e.g. wax, infection or alcoholism. The most common treatment used for vertigo are the phenothiazines, an example of which is prochlorperazine (Stemetil).

- ❶ Any loss of consciousness may be indicative of epilepsy
- ❶ New, persistent nystagmus, or the presence of additional neurological symptoms indicates a neurological problem
- ❶ Consider acoustic neuroma with vertigo in the presence of unilateral sensorineural deafness and tinnitus
- ❶ A patient who suffers chronic otitis media and then develops vertigo should be referred urgently to rule out fistula
- ❶ Consider MS in atypical episodic vertigo in the young or middle-aged, accompanied with transient neurological symptoms.

Headache

Headache is an extremely common presenting complaint in general practice. It has been estimated that 80–90% of the population will suffer a headache in any 1 year (Gambril 1994, Khunti 1997). Although the most common causes for headaches seen in general practice are tension headaches and migraine, it is essential to carefully assess the patient to detect potentially serious causes. Most patients presenting with headache show no abnormal physical signs on examination; therefore, an accurate history, along with familiarity of the differential diagnoses of headache, will aid diagnosis. With this in mind, I will address four types of headache:

- acute
- tension
- migraine
- cluster.

Acute headache

1. Any acute onset occurring in a patient for the first time must be taken seriously and must be referred to the GP
2. Serious causes include subarachnoid haemorrhage, stroke and bacterial or viral meningitis.

Tension headache

1. Bilateral mild or moderate, dull, non-pulsatile headache
2. Feels tight or pressing
3. Often found in the hatband region
4. May radiate down the back of the neck
5. Precipitating factors are variable and may include emotional or psychological stress, or be related to an activity or occupation.

Migraine

1. Commonly unilateral headache but may be bilateral
2. Throbbing pain
3. Associated symptoms include nausea, vomiting, photophobia and phonophobia
4. Neurological symptoms include visual aura, bright spots, shimmering lines, jagged edges, bars, grids and geometric shapes
5. Triggers may include foods, light, exercise, stress and hormonal factors.

Cluster headache

1. Rare: occurs in timed attacks 'clusters', lasting 30–60 min but can last up to 4 hours
2. Usually found in men aged 20–60 years
3. Unilateral deep severe pain
4. Pain can radiate to face, eye, temple
5. Headaches occur on the same side of the head during each attack
6. Cause unknown.

Subjective assessment

- ❶ Abnormal physical signs on examination, e.g. associated meningism, focal neurological symptoms of oculoparesis, palsy, hemiparesis, loss of consciousness, should be investigated.
- ❶ New onset, unilateral headaches, especially >35 years old
- ❶ Suspect subarachnoid haemorrhage with sudden excruciating headache

- ❶ Headaches different from those suffered in the past – more intense, more regular, present on wakening, increased on stooping or accompanied with vomiting and no nausea should be investigated
- ❶ Headache in the third trimester of pregnancy: check ankles for oedema; urine for protein; and blood pressure, may be a symptom of pre-eclampsia.

The subjective assessment is crucial, as there are often no abnormalities to be found on examination. Besides eliciting information to rule out the above types of headache, you will need to know:

- a description of the pain, type, region, radiation, severity
- onset, duration, frequency
- precipitating and relieving factors
- associated symptoms
- presence and type of aura
- history of trauma
- medication
- psychological state, depression, anxiety, life stressors, occupation
- alcohol intake, smoking habit
- sleep disturbances
- fever or malaise
- is pain intensified on coughing or when straining at stools
- past medical history
- family history.

Objective assessment

- Vital signs
- Inspect the scalp and skin for bulges and erythema
- To elicit pain or tenderness, palpate bones of the cranium, temporomandibular joint, face, sinuses
- Palpate carotid and temporal arteries for pulsations and tenderness
- Full examination of the eyes and full neurological examination
- Alternatively, check the '3-minute neuro-examination' of headache:
1. Romberg test
2. heel to toe gait
3. pronator drift
4. light touch-test using the patient's forefinger; ask the patient to – touch their nose with the finger with eyes closed, use both hands
5. tap hands one on top of other, right and left
6. visual fields
7. extraocular movements and convergence
8. facies – screw up eyes, frown, smile, rapid tongue movement
9. tendons, reflexes – elbow, wrist, knee, ankle, Babinski's reflex
10. fundoscopy.

Investigations

ESR to exclude temporal arteritis.

Treatment

Patients suspected of having acute severe pathology should be admitted to hospital as a matter of urgency. If the patient is suspected of having organic disease, such as severe vascular disease, tumour or arteritis, it is essential to refer urgently to a neurology clinic. All patients with recent onset headache should be reviewed to check that symptoms have settled and that no new signs have appeared.

Chronic headache sufferers may find it useful to keep a diary of occurrence to try to establish patterns or triggers. Encourage avoidance of known triggers. Relaxation techniques are a useful complement to drug therapy.

Choice of treatment depends on the diagnosis of the type of headache.
- Acute – analgesic therapy, depending on the degree of severity.
- Migraine – start treatment after an accurate diagnosis has been made and in agreement with the GP. Each practice has their own formulary for drug therapies. Acute migraine therapy includes analgesics, non-steroidal anti-inflammatory drugs (NSAIDs), antiemetics, anxiolytics, ergotamines, tranquillisers, narcotics and selective serotonin reuptake inhibitors (SSRIs) (Dowson 1997).

Prophylactic drugs are useful to consider for patients experiencing two or more attacks per month, and for those with less frequent but severe or prolonged attacks. Prophylactic treatment may reduce severity and frequency of episodes, but will not eliminate them; therefore the patient will continue to need acute treatment (Dowson 1997, DTB 1998). Preventative therapy includes beta-blockers, calcium channel blockers, antidepressants, serotonin antagonists and anticonvulsants.

Tension headaches. Treat with analgesics. Encourage stress relief by relaxation or exercise. Encourage the patient to have an eye test.

Cluster headaches. Systemic corticosteroids, lithium, ergotamine and calcium channel blockers can be used to relieve attacks of cluster headaches and to shorten cluster attack periods. Surgical excision of the trigeminal ganglion has proved effective in individuals for whom conventional medicine has been unsuccessful (Khunti 1997).

Temporal arteritis

Temporal arteritis should be regarded as a medical emergency. The disease was first recognised by Jonathan Hutchinson in 1890, who described the loss of pulsation in painful, swollen temporal arteries (Bannister 1992). This disorder occurs only in the middle aged and elderly, is more common in women, may affect intra- or extracranial cerebral vessels, and is sometimes referred to as cranial arteritis. The disease may be part of a more generalised arteritis and, as yet, the cause is unknown.

Affected vessel biopsies will indicate changes of granulomatous arteritis. As the disease progresses, this leads to gradual arterial occlusion which affects the temporal, occipital or facial branches of the external carotid artery, and particularly the ophthalmic branch of the internal ophthalmic artery. Apart from headache, therefore, sudden blindness can be a presenting symptom or a result of untreated arteritis due to the involvement of the ciliary arteries supplying the optic nerve and retina.

Subjective assessment

A comprehensive history is essential to elicit symptoms, their duration and frequency and associated symptoms, and to rule out differential diagnoses. The patient may complain of:
- a boring type headache or pain in the scalp, face, teeth, jaws and eyes
- claudication pain on chewing
- vague symptoms of aches in the joints and limbs
- weakness
- weight loss
- night sweats
- arthralgia
- photophobia
- diplopia
- mental confusion
- hemiparesis.

Objective assessment

1. Vital signs
2. On palpation of the face the examiner may note a thickened, tender temporal artery with painful nodular swelling and redness of overlying skin
3. There may be diminished pulsation in the thickened artery
4. Eye examination may show oculomotor paresis, ptosis and/or papilloedema.

Investigations

Diagnosis can be established by:
- checking the ESR, which will be greatly raised in temporal arteritis
- biopsy of affected extracranial artery, which will show changes of granulomatous arteritis.

Treatment

❶ As temporal arteritis is a medical emergency, treatment should be initiated as soon as the diagnosis is made. Steroid therapy, 60 mg of enteric-coated prednisolone daily, should be started and continued for up to 1 year or more, with a gradual reduction in dosage after 1 month according to symptoms and ESR. If vision is already impaired, steroid therapy may not prevent the loss of sight, but may prevent involvement of the other eye. Monthly ESR checks are necessary to monitor the disease and tailor treatment dosage.

Seizure disorders

Epilepsy is defined as 'recurrent (two or more) epileptic seizures unprovoked by any immediate cause' (Prevett & Duncan, 1998, p. 178) (Box 11.2).

Seizures starting in a localised area of the brain are known as partial seizures. They are termed 'simple' if there is no association with impairment of conscious level, e.g. jerking of a limb, and 'complex' if there is loss of awareness. When spread of seizure activity occurs, a generalised seizure may follow.

The generalised tonic clonic seizures (previously 'grand mal') are characterised by a tonic phase with stiffening of limbs and body, after which rhythmic jerking of the limbs occurs, followed by confusion and headache.

The absence seizure (previously 'petit mal'), usually starts in childhood, characterised by the child staring blankly for a few seconds; this is sometimes accompanied by fluttering of the eyelids or swallowing, and myoclonic jerks, which are brief, jerky, muscular movements.

Subjective assessment

The diagnosis of epilepsy is clinical and depends on an accurate history from an eyewitness and from the patient. Differential diagnoses include syncope, non-epileptic attack disorder (pseudoseizures), hyperventilation, panic attack, hypoglycaemia and parasomnias.

The history should include:

1. Note from whom history is taken.
2. Date of seizure, if new onset.
3. Frequency of seizures, if more than one episode.
4. The time of day and circumstances under which the seizure occurred.
5. If seizure occurred while asleep or awake.
6. Whether the patient can pinpoint any possible precipitatory factors: emotion, stress, pregnancy, menstruation, alcohol/drugs, television, fatigue.
7. If the patient experienced an aura.
8. An accurate description of the tonic and clonic phases of the seizure by an eyewitness, noting any associated symptoms such as a change in breathing pattern; change of colour, head turning; automatisms; tongue biting; incontinence; and, if jerking occurred, whether it was bilateral or unilateral.
9. Length of attack.
10. Information regarding the postictal phase – for example: confusion; headache; fatigue; sleepiness; if unconscious, how long until consciousness was regained and length of time until full recovery.
11. Past history: specifically enquire about birth injury, head injury, febrile convulsions, encephalitis, meningitis, alcoholism or psychiatric illness. Ask about the usual conditions: coronary heart disease, stroke, diabetes, malignancy.
12. Family history of seizure, diabetes, malignancy.
13. Note allergies and current medication.

Box 11.2	*Types of seizure disorder*
Partial seizures:	Simple partial seizures
	Complex partial seizures
	Secondarily generalised seizures
Generalised seizures:	Generalized tonic clonic seizures
	Absence seizures
	Myoclonic seizures
	Clonic seizures
	Tonic seizures
	Atonic seizures
Unclassified epileptic seizures:	Due to inadequate or incomplete information (Hart 1996)

Objective assessment

- Vital signs
- Full neurological assessment, including reflexes
- Eyes: fundi, extraocular movements, visual fields
- Blood tests, including blood sugar, full blood picture and ESR, liver function tests, urea and electrolytes, calcium levels and thyroid function.

Investigations carried out by the neurological specialist include an electroencephalogram (EEG), computed tomography (CT) or magnetic resonance imaging (MRI). Additional tests such as 24-h Holter monitoring to exclude other causes of loss of consciousness may be used. After all these investigations, it may not be possible to make a firm diagnosis; note that a normal EEG does not exclude a diagnosis of epilepsy.

Treatment

The patient will be encouraged to keep a seizure diary in an attempt to establish a pattern and identify triggers. The following issues must be discussed with the patient:

- driving (banned) and inform DVLA
- free prescriptions
- females require contraception and preconception counselling
- referral to specialist.

Note hazards such as bathing and swimming (which must be supervised; work-related hazards should be avoided (such as working with dangerous machinery). It is evident, therefore, that a diagnosis of epilepsy can have profound results on the life of the individual.

Diagnosis should be certain before treatment is commenced. If there is a high risk of seizure recurrence, it is appropriate to recommend an antiepileptic drug (AED) after a single seizure: however, in other patients it may be appropriate to defer treatment until after two or more seizures (Prevett & Duncan 1998, Smithson 1999). The most common treatments used for epilepsy are carbamazepine (Tegretol), sodium valproate (Epilim), phenytoin (Epanutin) and lamotrigine (Lamictal). A study comparing carbamazepine and lamotrigine showed them to have similar efficacy against newly diagnosed partial seizures, and lamotrigine was found to be better tolerated. Lamotrigine, therefore, can be considered for first-line management, but it is more expensive than carbamazepine and sodium valproate, and it is not yet known whether it is more or less teratogenic.

There is a choice of AED for different seizure types (Prevett & Duncan 1998), as set out in Table 11.1
- Prolonged loss of consciousness following a seizure – consider hospital admission.

Multiple sclerosis

Multiple sclerosis is an inflammatory disease of the central nervous system, characterised by episodes of neurological dysfunction that evolve over days and resolve over weeks, the cause being unknown. It usually presents between the ages of 20 and 50 years, with females affected by the disease more frequently than men. The pathological process results in demyelination and, at times, irreversible degeneration of axons. The spinal cord, optic nerves, brainstem and cerebral hemispheres are all involved in time.

Subjective assessment

Multiple sclerosis is often difficult to diagnose, as the symptoms are those which could apply to many other disorders. The symptoms may initially be mild to moderate, and may not be brought to the GP's attention until the second attack occurs (Kidd 1999).

The history taker must enquire about:
1. fatigue
2. numbness/tingling – usually part of a limb or one side of the face or both lower limbs
3. double vision
4. dizziness
5. eye pain – optic neuritis is a presenting complaint in 25% of cases
6. incoordination
7. weakness – usually a limb, in particular a lower limb with dragging of the foot
8. precipitancy of micturation and bowel movements
9. erectile dysfunction
10. insidious and slowly progressive weakness of one or both lower limbs
11. family history of neurological disease
12. previous episodes.

Involvement of the spinal cord, resulting in neurological symptoms, occurs in 60% of presenting cases.

Objective assessment

Objective assessment will include a full neurological motor and sensory examination and an ophthalmological assessment. When the onset is acute or subacute, the initial symptoms tend to diminish over a period of weeks or months, and either disappear completely or leave some residual disability. The findings on examination, therefore, will vary greatly, depending on the mode of onset and the stage of the disease at which the patient is examined (Bannister 1992, DeGowin 1994).

In the early stages, the diagnosis may well depend on the history, supported by slight abnormal physical signs such as:
- pallor of the temporal half of one or more optic discs
- slight sustained nystagmus on lateral fixation to one or both sides
- slight intention tremor in one or both upper limbs
- diminished or reduced abdominal reflexes
- exaggeration of the tendon reflexes
- unilateral or bilateral extensor plantar response.

Table 11.1 *AED for different seizure types (Prevett & Duncan 1998)*

Type	First–line treatment	Second–line treatment
Partial seizures:		
■ simple, partial or secondarily generalised	Carbamazepine	Acetazolamide
	Valproate	Clobazam
		Lamotrigine
		Phenobarbitone
		Phenytoin
		Topiramate
		Vigabatrin
Generalised seizures:		
■ tonic–clonic or clonic	Valproate	Acetazolamide
	Carbamazepine	Clobazam
		Lamotrigine
		Phenobarbitone
		Phenytoin
■ absence	Ethosuximide	Clobazam
	Valproate	Clonazepam
		Lamotrigine
■ myoclonic	Valproate	Clonazepam

During early remission, abnormal physical signs may be slight or absent. As the disease advances, the cumulative effect of multiple lesions results in permanent effects on the nervous system, and this is also the result with an insidious, progressive type onset of the disease.

In the insidiously progressive onset disease, the abnormal physical signs are usually spinal, such as

- spastic paraplegia
- sensory loss over lower limbs and trunk
- impaired postural sense and/or impaired vibration sense
- ataxic gait.

In the advanced case of multiple sclerosis, the following symptoms may be present:

- pallor of both optic discs, nystagmus and incoordination of lateral eye movements
- staccato speech and slurring of individual syllables
- weakness and ataxia in upper limbs
- severe spasticity, leading to painful extensor or flexor spasms
- paraplegia
- cutaneous sensory loss and/or deep sensory loss in upper and lower limbs
- incontinence of faeces and urine
- either euphoria, depression and irritability or cognitive dysfunction
- seizures occur in 3% of patients
- trigeminal neuralgia is rare, but may occur bilaterally.

Because of the nature of the symptoms that can arise from multiple sclerosis, investigations may be performed to either rule out other causes or to make a firm diagnosis. Lumbar puncture (some abnormality is found in around 80% of cases, but serial lumbar punctures are neither practical nor acceptable in multiple sclerosis), CT scan or MRI scan tests may be performed.

Treatment

There is no specific treatment: however, there are several unproven but possibly helpful treatments and therapies that may be employed, such as steroids, immunosuppressant drugs, vitamin B_{12}, avoidance of animal fat and addition of polyunsaturated fatty acids (linoleic acid), elimination of gluten from the diet, spinal cord stimulation by electrodes planted in the epidural space and hyperbaric oxygen. The patient should receive counselling and education regarding the disease.

- ❶ Numbness in both legs accompanied by back pain and saddle anaesthesia suggests cauda equina; admit to hospital as a neurological emergency.

Parkinson's disease

Parkinson's disease is named after James Parkinson, who first described paralysis agitans in 1817. It is a disturbance of motor function characterised chiefly by slowing and enfeeblement of emotional and voluntary movements, muscular rigidity and tremor (Bannister 1992). The condition is complicated and unpredictable, and affects about 100 000 people in the United Kingdom, with a slight male predominance. The disease is primarily associated with old age, with the mean age of onset at 65 years; however, one in 50 patients is diagnosed before the age of 40 (Bunce 1998, Clarke 1999).

Subjective assessment

Parkinson's disease is a progressive, neurological disorder, the exact cause of which is unknown. It results from a shortage of the chemical messenger dopamine, which together with acetylcholine, works in the basal ganglia of the brain to coordinate movement and to control muscle tone (Derbyshire & Marsden 1999). Even the experts in neurology find that differentiating Parkinson's disease from other neurodegenerative conditions can be extremely difficult. Presenting symptoms may vary considerably, and the practitioner must enquire about:

- tremor – not always present, but often seen in the hands at rest
- bradykinesia – slowness of action, difficulty in initiating movement
- rigidity – muscle stiffness in limbs results in the body being held in a fixed position
- fatigue
- dysphagia
- difficulty with balance, speech and writing.

The practitioner must note the following to help rule out other causes:

- history of cerebral trauma (boxing, stroke)
- drug-induced (phenothiazines)
- exposure to neurotoxins (MPTP, CO, Mn, Cu)
- symmetrical symptoms
- associated ophthalmoplegia, pyramidal or cerebellar symptoms
- associated autonomic dysfunction
- rapid disease progression.

Because of the difficulty in making an accurate diagnosis, all suspected cases of Parkinson's disease should be referred to the neurologist or geriatrician with a special interest in movement disorders for expert opinion.

Objective assessment

A full motor and sensory neurological examination, along with ophthalmological assessment is required. Observe for the following:

1. Facies, for unnatural immobility, slowness of movement in mastication, deglutition and articulation.
2. Speech may be slurred and monotonous.
3. Eyes, for staring appearance, tremor of eyelids on closure.
4. Attitude or stance – trunk moderately flexed, limbs moderately flexed and adducted, wrist usually slightly extended, fingers flexed at metacarpophalangeal joint, and extended or only slightly flexed at interphalangeal joints and adducted, thumb

adducted and extended at metacarpo and interphalangeal joints.

5. Tremor at rest (may not be present), usually begins in one upper limb and later involves the lower limb, same side; the other side may be affected in the same order, as the disease progresses.

6. Disorder of movement – voluntary movement may display impairment of power and will be slowly performed, handwriting deteriorates and tends to become smaller.

7. Muscular rigidity – in early stages may be limited to one upper limb and only just detectable on passive movement; often more evident on passive flexion and extension of the wrist and pronation and supination of the forearm. In advanced cases it is generalised and severe.

8. Gait – in early stages lack of swing of one arm on walking may be the only noticeable symptom; when parkinsonism is bilateral, gait is slow and shuffling, with small steps.

9. Reflexes – parkinsonism in itself does not affect pupillary reflexes, but if it is secondary to encephalitis there is impairment, especially reaction on accommodation. The tendon reflexes are not directly affected but may be difficult to elicit and reduced in amplitude, due to rigidity. The plantar reflexes are flexor unless an independent lesion involves the corticospinal tracts.

10. Sensory loss does not occur in Parkinson's disease, but in the later stages pain in the limbs and spine, restlessness, flushing, sweating, excessive oiliness of facial skin, and excessive salivation may occur in encephalitic parkinsonism. This is also the cause of 'oculogyric crises', now rarely seen, which consists of spasmodic deviation of the eyes, usually upwards, and occurs paroxysmally lasting for minutes or hours.

Treatment

The majority of patients with a new diagnosis of Parkinson's disease are concerned about the possibility of more sinister causes, and the embarrassment their symptoms create. Patients should, of course, be counselled and educated regarding the disease. The patient who has received an accurate diagnosis and prognosis, and who has had time to come to terms with the tremor, can usually manage without treatment for several years. However, treatment should be started when there is evidence of functional disability; such decisions should be taken along with the patient, the carer and the physician. In recent years, the number of new drugs for the treatment of Parkinson's disease has increased. Levodopa is the most potent and effective drug for treating Parkinson's disease: however, it contributes to the long-term complications of treatment, such as end of dose deterioration and dyskinesias. This has led to a policy of delaying treatment with levodopa for as long as possible by using less effective drugs such as selegiline,

anticholinergics or amantidine and there is now a move towards the use of the more effective dopamine agonists.

Catechol-O-methyltransferase (COMT) inhibitor prevents breakdown of levodopa, so increasing bioavailability of the drug, giving more stable blood plasma levels. This allows the reduction in the overall amount of levodopa by around 20%, and should be administered with every dose of levodopa.

Selegiline is a monoamine oxidase type B inhibitor. Since publication of the UK Parkinson's Disease Research Group study, which showed significant increase in mortality after 6 years of treatment with selegiline, prescription rates have fallen by 50%.

Amantadine, originally developed as an antiviral agent, was found to be an effective antiparkinsonian drug. Its efficacy is poor in comparison with levodopa, and tolerance develops with long-term treatment, so it is rarely used in early disease; however, it may be used in later disease as an antidyskinesic agent.

Anticholinergics such as benzhexol and orphenadrine have a useful effect on tremor. The side effects of confusion and hallucinations in the elderly have been known for many years, but more recent work indicated a high risk of cognitive impairment, especially in younger patients. Consequently, anticholinergics are used much less frequently in early disease.

Dopamine agonists, of which there are quite a few, are receiving more interest since the move away from early treatment with levodopa. Bromocriptine was initially used as an adjunct therapy in later disease. It is not as effective as levodopa and has its own significant side effects, but in monotherapy results in fewer long-term complications. Ropinirole is used in the young fit patient with significant functional disability and is licensed in the UK for adjunct and monotherapy use. Whichever dopamine agonist is used as monotherapy, eventually the patient will require levodopa.

Apomorphine is a potent D1 and D2 agonist, which is given by intermittent injections through a penject system or by continuous subcutaneous infusion. Initially it was used to help 'smooth out' motor fluctuations that were resistant to other oral treatments: however, alternate applications are being investigated in the area of use as monotherapy when other medication cannot be tolerated.

There is also a renewed interest in surgical approaches to the condition. Options are pallidotomy, thalamotomy, deep brain stimulation and fetal cell implantation.

Transient ischaemic attack

A transient ischaemic attack (TIA), is a brief episode of focal neurological dysfunction usually lasting minutes, followed by full recovery, but with a tendency to recur. By definition, if it lasts more than 24 hours, or is followed by signs of residual damage, then a completed stroke has occurred. The importance of a TIA is that it is an indicator of the risk of stroke occurring. Approximately one-third of patients with TIAs develop a stroke over the subsequent 4 years, with the incidence greatest in the month after the first TIA (Fowler & May 1985, Bannister 1992).

TIAs can arise from:

- Fibrin platelet emboli, often originating from atheromatous damage in extracranial arteries; in 30% the source is the heart (mural infarcts or valve disease)
- A drop in cerebral perfusion associated with changes in heart rate or rhythm, or a very high or low blood pressure.

Subjective assessment

Symptoms and signs associated with TIA are variable depending on the site affected and whether neurological signs are absent between attacks. TIAs can be precipitated by severe anaemia, polycythaemia and hypoglycaemia, or provoked on a mechanical basis by head turning where atheromatous vertebral arteries are compromised in their passage through the cervical vertebrae. It is therefore imperative that an accurate history be elicited.

TIAs are classified in two categories, and the following symptoms should be considered in the history:

Carotid artery TIA

- Contralateral weakness, clumsiness or numbness of the hand, hand and face or entire half of the body
- Dysarthria
- Aphasia
- Transient loss of vision in one eye (amaurosis fugax).

Vertebrobasilar TIA

- Binocular visual disturbance or loss
- Vertigo
- Dysarthria
- Ataxia
- Unilateral or bilateral weakness or numbness
- Drop attacks (sudden loss of postural tone, collapse without loss of consciousness)
- Diplopia, syncope, transient confusion or paraparesis are uncommon symptoms.

Ask the patient about possible signs of – or familial tendency for – anaemia, diabetes and cardiovascular disease. Ask about lifestyle: smoking, diet, etc.

Objective assessment

The correct diagnosis of TIA is important because it is an indication of impending serious cerebral artery thrombosis. A full motor and sensory neurological examination, along with a full cardiovascular assessment, blood pressure check and auscultation of carotid arteries for bruits, is required.

The differential diagnosis of TIA includes convulsions, syncope, migraine, focal cerebral masses, such as subdural haematoma, cardiac diseases and labyrinthine disorders.

Investigations

- Bloods tests: full blood count, PCV, ESR, lipid profile, blood sugar and VDRL or equivalent test for syphilis
- Urine: test for sugar and protein
- ECG
- X-ray: chest and skull
- Arteriography: to evaluate cerebral arteries for possible surgical correction or medical treatment.

Treatment

Management of TIA will depend on the cause. Hypertension must be controlled slowly, especially in the elderly patient. Smokers are encouraged to stop, and those with hyperlipidaemia will receive dietary or drug intervention as appropriate.

Surgery. Carotid artery TIAs may arise from a local atheromatous lesion near the origin of the internal carotid artery. Surgical obliteration may prevent further TIAs and strokes; however, of patients treated successfully by surgery, a proportion die from myocardial infarcts, confirming they have widespread arterial disease.

Anticoagulants. Their use is debatable: they have been shown as beneficial in the first 6–12 months, but with prolonged use the risk of bleeding is greater than the risk of stroke. Patients with a definite source of emboli should be treated with anticoagulants, and will require blood tests to monitor control.

Antiplatelet drugs. Aspirin appears to reduce the risk of stroke and is well tolerated.

Stroke

A completed stroke implies that an infarct has occurred, and that the symptoms have persisted for more than 24 hours. The symptoms of a cerebral infarct develop most commonly over 1–2 hours; some may develop over a few days and it is not uncommon for them to occur during sleep. Stroke, which is the third most common cause of death in the world, is the most common cause of acquired disability and affects 2.4 per 1000 people in the UK each year (Fraser 1999). Stroke in young adults is uncommon, but around 4% of all strokes occur under the age of 40 years. Causes which should be specifically considered in this age group include neck trauma, causing carotid dissection; alcohol intoxication; infarction associated with migraine; post-herpes zoster infarction; and cardiac causes, such as mitral valve prolapse, atrial fibrillation or atrial myxoma.

Subjective assessment

Symptoms may increase in severity for 24–48 hours after onset. Neurological symptoms present will depend on the area of brain involved, but as the middle cerebral artery is commonly involved in the process, a hemiplegia is the commonest presentation. Hemiplegia affects the face and limbs on the side opposite the lesion. Frequently, consciousness is preserved or there is merely some confusion; however, profound loss of consciousness can occur and is indicative of either a large area of infarction or involvement of the brainstem. The diagnosis of cerebrovascular disease depends largely on clinical history and presenting symptomatology. It is important to differentiate between a completed stroke, a stroke in evolution, a TIA, a brain haemorrhage and other related disorders such as migraines, tumours and epilepsy.

The history may need to be obtained from a witness or carer, due to the patient suffering symptoms such as confusion, loss of consciousness, aphasia or dysphasia. The practitioner should elicit and note the following:

- if onset was sudden or gradual
- epileptic fit – may occur at onset or during extension of stroke
- level of consciousness, confusion, memory loss
- aphasia, dysphasia
- dysphagia
- pain or paraesthesiae (sensation of hot water running over face) on trigeminal area of affected side
- facial or limb paralysis
- hemianopia
- incontinence
- previous episode of stroke or TIA, history of cardiac disease or diabetes
- medication
- lifestyle contributory factors – smoking, alcohol, diet, exercise.

Objective assessment

A full neurological and cardiac assessment, checking carotid and cranial arteries for bruits, will be required. Note area and degree of weakness or paraesthesiae. Check Kernig's sign: With the patient supine, flex the hip and knee each to approximately 90°. With the hip immobile, attempt to extend the knee. In meningeal irritation, this attempt is resisted and causes pain in the hamstring muscles.

Check the eyes for nystagmus, scotoma (visual field defects) and transitory amblyopia (dimness of vision) and papilloedema.

Table 11.2 will aid in analysis of signs and symptoms and findings.

Investigation

CT scan, MRI scan and EEG are assessment tools that may be employed to rule out differential diagnoses. Blood tests include full blood count, ESR, blood sugar, lipid profile and thyroid function test.

Treatment

Treatment depends on the precipitating cause, the extent of the affected tissue and clinical symptomatology.

Neurosurgery may be carried out, for example, in order to rapidly re-establish blood flow through a blocked carotid.

Vasodilatory drugs have been used, but have not been associated with improved prognosis.

Table 11.2 *Analysis of signs and symptoms and findings (Reproduced with permission from Vardaxis 1995, p. 495.)*

Condition/ features	Intracerebral haemorrhage	Subarachnoid haemorrhage	Vascular anomolies	Thrombotic stoke	Embolic stoke
Clinical setting	Hypertension, heart disease	Trauma, hypertension	Young person, no hypertension	Prodromal TIA, atherosclerosis infarct	Atherosclerosis, myocardial
Onset	Usually during, activity	Sudden severe headache	Previous history, sudden headache	Gradual onset and progression	Sudden onset of symptoms
Symptoms	Headache if conscious, hemiplegia	Transient disturbance of consciousness	Paraesthesiae, eye pain, scotoma, focal epilepsy	Consciousness maintained, hemiplegia	Consciousness maintained, hemiplegia
Signs	Epileptic fit, papilloedema	Kernig's sign	Cranial bruits	Atherosclerosis related	Atherosclerosis related
Progression	Coma, death is the most usual outcome	Preretinal haemorrhage, aphasia, hemiparesis	Retinal angiomata, preretinal haemorrhage	Paralysis, dysphasia, coma, death or gradual improvement	Paralysis, dysphasia, coma, occasionally improvement apparent
CSF	Often bloodstained	Often bloodstained	Often bloodstained	Clear	Clear
Prognosis/ survival	> 30 days 20%	> 30 days 35%	> 30 days 35%	> 30 days 65%	> 30 days 70%

Corticosteroids in high dose have been tried in acute stroke patients. Their use reduces early death rate from severe strokes; however, there is no evidence of benefit in the long term.

Anticoagulants are not used in completed strokes, but if cerebral haemorrhage is ruled out they may be used in a stroke in evolution.

- ❶ An eyewitness account that the patient looked as if he was dead on collapse, with facial flushing on recovery, is indicative of Stokes–Adams attacks which may be fatal; early diagnosis is important.

Trigeminal neuralgia

Trigeminal neuralgia or 'tic douloureux' is characterised by attacks of severe pain, usually localised in the area of the maxillary and mandibular divisions of the trigeminal nerve. Episodes may last for weeks or months, followed by long asymptomatic periods, but it is always recurrent. Later there are no remissions. It is more common in the elderly and in females, the cause being largely unknown. In younger patients trigeminal neuralgia may be a symptom of underlying pathology such as multiple sclerosis, cerebellopontine angle tumour or basilar aneurysm. In such cases there may be sensory loss and other symptoms of cranial nerve or cerebellar involvement (Fowler & May 1985, Bannister 1992).

Subjective assessment

The features of trigeminal neuralgia are classical. The practitioner should note:

- Pain – paroxysmal, usually severe, described as agonising, shooting or stabbing, brief attacks lasting for a few seconds to half a minute. Note distribution of pain in relation to trigeminal nerve.
- Triggers – touch, movement, washing, shaving, talking, nose blowing, eating or temperature.
- Facial spasm – hence the name 'tic douloureux'.
- Eyes – may be closed, excessive lacrimation.
- Facial flushing.
- Frequency of attacks – may occur many times in one day.
- Previous episodes.

Objective assessment

The diagnosis of trigeminal neuralgia is largely derived from the history. A neurological assessment should be performed to rule out differential diagnoses such as a local neoplasm. The initial stages of herpes zoster may suggest trigeminal neuralgia; however, the distinction can be made when herpetic vesicles appear on the skin or mucosa. In the case of trigeminal neuralgia there are no sensory or motor changes. The practitioner can assess which branch of the nerve is involved:

- the ophthalmic branch is rarely affected
- the second or maxillary division – most commonly involved, pain is in the maxilla, upper teeth and lip and the lower eyelid

- the third or mandibular division – pain is in the lower teeth and lip, the oral portion of the tongue and the external auditory meatus.

Treatment

Analgesic and anticonvulsant drugs used in the past have been replaced by carbamazepine. This drug was developed because of its anticonvulsant properties, but is very effective in controlling the pain of trigeminal neuralgia. Side effects of carbamazepine include nausea, dizziness and drowsiness, particularly if the dosage is increased too rapidly. The initial dose is 100 mg three times daily, gradually increased over 2–3 weeks until control is achieved. During remission the dose can be reduced or stopped. If skin rash occurs the treatment should be stopped (Bannister 1992).

Surgical procedures, such as blocking of the pain fibres of the nerve, can be achieved by alcohol injection of the trigeminal ganglion, or by surgical division of the sensory root. The alcohol injection gives relief for 18–24 months, but will need repeating, whereas, surgical intervention will give permanent relief. The patient must be made aware of adverse effects such as numbness of the face after surgical section and paraesthesiae after injection. Analgesia of the cornea may lead to neuropathic keratitis; therefore, the eye needs protection by suitable goggles after the nerve interruption.

- ❶ Trigeminal neuralgia is commonly idiopathic; however, it may have a serious underlying cause if associated with motor disturbance or other neurological symptoms
- ❶ If no obvious cause is found for persistent facial pain, refer to exclude more sinister pathology.

Bell's palsy

Bell's palsy is a lower motor neurone, usually unilateral facial paralysis of acute onset. It may occur at any age, but is more common in young adults, particularly males. It is usually attributed to a nonsuppurative inflammation of the facial nerve, causing local demyelination with a conduction block. If demyelination has occurred, recovery usually follows; and if there is evidence of this 3 weeks after onset, it is likely to be a good recovery. In approximately 15% of patients the damage is more severe and axonal degeneration of the nerve may follow. If this has occurred, repair will be by regeneration, which is slow, often incomplete and may lead to deviant reinnervation with jaw winking (mouth movement causes eye closure) (Fowler & May 1985).

Subjective assessment

The diagnosis of Bell's palsy is generally made from the classical history:

1. onset – acute (often during sleep), or developing over 24–48 hours
2. paralysis – partial or complete

3. Generally painless – there may be pain in the ear, the mastoid region or in the angle of the jaw at onset; and if the cause is an ear infection or herpes zoster, there may be pain in or behind the ear
4. eyebrow – drooped, and wrinkles of brow smoothed out
5. eyes – loss or paucity of blinking, tear spill over the lower eyelid; and in complete paralysis the eye cannot be closed, so there is danger of corneal exposure damage
6. mouth – crooked, drawn to one side
7. nasolabial furrow is smoothed out
8. cheek – flaccid, food may accumulate between the teeth and cheek; cheek puffs out in respiration
9. hyperacusis.

Objective assessment

There is an increased incidence of Bell's palsy with hypertension, diabetes and multiple sclerosis. Rarely is the palsy bilateral, but this may occur in sarcoidosis, acute polyneuritis or neoplastic infiltration. Examination of the patient will include ENT assessment, neurological assessment and blood pressure check.

- Suppurative otitis can be ruled out by examining the ears; check ear and nasopharynx for vesicles to rule out herpes zoster.
- Tongue – check taste sensation, as there is loss of taste in the anterior two-thirds of the tongue if part of the facial nerve distal to the chorda tympani is involved. Tongue may deviate to the sound side when protruded and may cause paralysis of the tongue to be suspected in error.
- Frowning and raising eyebrows is impossible.

Treatment

Analgesics may be necessary during the early stage if the ear is painful.

The role of steroids is controversial as their true value has never been established. It has been suggested that their use early in the disease may reduce swelling of the facial nerve and so prevent axonal degeneration.

Passive movement of the face by massage is encouraged, while regeneration is occurring, and active exercises started as soon as voluntary power returns. Protective eyedrops should be used if the paralysis prevents blinking. As a temporary measure with a complete facial paralysis, botulinum toxin can be injected locally to create a complete ptosis for 2–3 months, giving the eye protection.

Surgical decompression of the facial nerve in the canal and early operation is difficult to justify when most of the cases submitted to operation would recover spontaneously. When severe paralysis persists for longer than 6 months, plastic surgery may be considered as an option to improve facial appearance (Bannister 1992).

- ❶ The diagnosis of Bell's palsy is usually made from the classical history; however, check the ears for sup-

purative otitis and the ear and nasopharynx for vesicles to rule out herpes zoster.

Alzheimer's disease

Alzheimer's disease is the most common cause of dementia in the elderly. It is defined as an insidious illness, characterised by a progressive decline in global cognition function and impairment of activities of daily living (Harvey 1998). In the early stages of Alzheimer's disease, it can be difficult to differentiate its symptoms from those of normal ageing. The emergence of symptomatic treatments, together with greater accessibility of behavioural therapy and care-giver support programmes, has highlighted the need for accurate, early diagnosis. Primary care practitioners play an important role in diagnosis, management and organisation of specialist support.

Subjective assessment

Early problems in older people are usually ascribed to the effects of ageing: the patient is not usually brought for assessment by a carer until difficulties become more obvious.

In the early stages some people have insight in that they realise that their memory is failing and may consult the practitioner, fearing a more sinister cause. The history may need to be taken from both the patient and the carer, and calls for considerable sensitivity, as symptoms are extremely distressing for the patient and worrying for the carer:

- onset – insidious
- cognition – deterioration in memory, language skills, writing, reading, praxis (practical application of learning) and reasoning
- functional ability – deterioration in basic activities of daily life, dressing, bathing, elimination, walking and eating, and deterioration of complex activities of daily life, cooking, shopping, finances
- behaviour – aggression, mood swings, emotional lability, wandering, insomnia, depression and, in those patients with insight, anxiety
- medication.

In addition to taking a history regarding the patient, the practitioner must enquire about quality of life of both patient and carer, and assess the burden on the carer with a view to specialised support.

Objective assessment

Objective assessment should include blood pressure, neurological and cardiac examination to rule out other causes. The practitioner must observe and interview the patient to assess thought processes, general coherence, interaction, mood, emotional responses and behaviour. The types of dementia are now considered.

Alzheimer's disease

- Initially, orientation and memory loss, particularly memory for events

- Executive dysfunction, dysphasia and dyspraxia as disease progresses
- Insidious onset
- Progressive decline.

Vascular dementia

- Focal cognitive impairments such as expressive dysphasia
- Sudden deterioration and fluctuating course.

Dementia with Lewy bodies

- Prominent attentional deficits
- Relative preservation of episodic memory in early stages
- Executive dysfunction and visuospatial impairments, many disproportionately severe
- Fluctuating cognitive impairment
- Hallucinations and delusions are common.

Fronto-temporal dementia

- Early and severe impairment of language and semantic memory (memory of meaning and knowledge about words, objects and concepts)
- Poor performance on tests requiring mental effort.

The assessment of Alzheimer's disease in primary care is limited to 'Mini Mental State Examination', 'Alzheimer's Disease Assessment Scale', or 'Abbreviated Mental Test Schedule' (Hodkinson 1972, Folstein et al 1975, Rosen et al 1994).

Mini Mental State Examination

- Rapid and simple to use mental status examination
- Domains include orientation, memory, attention, recall and language
- 10–15 min to complete
- Scores range from 0 (lowest) to 30. Scores of 27–30 are considered normal.

Assessments look at aspects of function, reasoning, orientation, memory, arithmetic and judgement. Although these techniques are reliable, it may be necessary to refer to a specialist for more comprehensive neuropsychological testing or brain neuroimaging.

Investigation

❶ Exclude treatable causes such as vitamin B_{12} deficiency, hypothyroidism, normal pressure hydrocephalus, tumour, depression and iatrogenic. Check the following blood tests: full blood picture, ESR, thyroid function, liver function, urea and electrolytes, vitamin B_{12} and folate, calcium, MSU and blood sugar.

Treatment

Anticholinesterase drugs. The anti-dementia drugs product licences are for the treatment of mild to moderate Alzheimer's disease, which correlates to a score of 10–26 on the Mini Mental State Examination. These are new drugs, and at present we cannot predict who will

Top Tips	

1 Proficient interviewing techniques are a prerequisite to obtaining a thorough history from a client. It is important not only to employ competent interpersonal communication skills such as listening, silence and empathy but also to be aware of one's body language, position and eye contact

2 When listening to the client describe symptoms, train yourself not to jump to diagnostic conclusions, rather to gather broad information and eliminate differential diagnoses by logical reasoning, physical examination and diagnostic tests

3 Always elicit the client's own beliefs regarding his illness. This allows an opportunity to air fears and for the NP to rationally discuss issues that arise

4 Safe practice is of paramount importance. An NP does not possess all the skills of a doctor; however, she holds valuable advanced nursing skills and experience, which when married with clinical expertise, should be used as a complementary adjunct to the medical role. If in doubt – refer

5 Record accurately all consultations, including history, physical examination, clinical findings and investigations. Remember to ask your patient to return if the condition does not improve

6 Students often experience difficulty in carrying out physical assessment skills simply because they are using equipment and tools incorrectly. Know your examination instruments

benefit from treatment. Some patients will not respond; others will show no change (in Alzheimer's disease this should be considered a positive response); and, in a proportion, memory and function will improve, or there will be less aggression and agitation. Side effects include nausea, diarrhoea, agitation and restlessness.

Neuroleptic drugs. Neuroleptic drugs were traditionally the main treatment for behavioural and psychological symptoms; however, the Chief Medical Officer has recommended cautious use of these drugs in patients with dementia, as side effects include parkinsonism, tardive kinesias, drowsiness, falls and accelerated cognitive decline.

SSRIs. Around 20–40% of patients suffering from Alzheimer's disease have symptoms of depression. The diagnosis is often difficult, and many practitioners consider a therapeutic trial where there is uncertainty using SSRIs, which are among the safer antidepressants for older patients.

Glossary

AC	Air conduction
AED	Antiepileptic drug
BC	Bone conduction
CN	Cranial nerve
CO	Carbon monoxide (compound)
CT	Computed tomography

Cu   Copper
DIP   Distal interphalangeal
DVLA   Driver and vehicle licensing authority
ECG   Electrocardiograph
EEG   Electroencephalogram
ENT   Ear, nose and throat
ESR   Erythrocyte sedimentation rate
GP   General practitioner
IP   Interphalangeal
JPS   Joint position sense
Mn   Manganese
MRI   Magnetic resonance imaging
MS   Multiple sclerosis
MSU   Midstream specimen of urine
MPTP   1-Methyl-phenyl-2-,3,6-tetrahydropyridine (synthetic heroin/cocaine)
NP   Nurse practitioner
OTC   Over the counter
PCV   Packed cell volume
SSRI   Selective serotonin reuptake inhibitor
TIA   Transient ischaemic attack
UK   United Kingdom
VDRL   Venereal Disease Research Laboratory Test
WV   Whispered voice

References

Bannister R 1992 Brain and Bannister's clinical neurology, 7th edn. Oxford University Press, Oxford.

Bates B 1995 A guide to physical examination and history taking, 6th edn. J B Lippincott, Philadelphia.

Bunce C 1998 Managing care of patients with Parkinson's disease. Community Nurse November: 37–38.

Clarke C E 1999 Managing early Parkinson's disease. The Practitioner 243:39–47.

DeGowin R L 1994 DeGowin and DeGowin's diagnostic examination, 6th edn. McGraw-Hill, New York.

Derbyshire M, Marsden V 1999 Parkinson's disease. Primary Health Care 9(2):16–21.

Dowson A 1997 Migraine management: the modern approach. Doctor/Practice Nurse Supplement, April.

DTB 1998 Managing migraine. Drug and Therapeutics Bulletin 36(6). Which?, London.

Epstein O, Perkin D G, de Bono D P, Cookson J 1997 Clinical examination, 2nd edn. Mosby, London.

Folstein M F, Folstein S E, McHugh P R 1975 Mini-mental state: a practical method of grading the cognitive scale of patients for the clinician. Journal of Psychiatric Research 12:189–198.

Fowler T J, May R W 1985 Neurology: management of common diseases in family practice. MTP Press, Lancaster.

Fraser H 1999 Preventing secondary stroke: identifying the risk factors. Community Nurse February: 17–18.

Gambril E C 1994 Chronic and recurrent headache. Update, September: 317–319.

Hart Y 1996 Epilepsy: clinical management. Practice Nursing 7(19):19–22.

Harvey R 1998 Assessment in Alzheimer's disease. Geriatric Medicine Clinical Bulletin 28(11): November: 1–4.

Hodkinson H M 1972 Evaluation of a mental score for assessment of mental impairment in the elderly. Age and Ageing 1:233–238.

Khunti K 1997 Management of headache. Update April: 557–559.

Kidd D 1999 Presentations of multiple sclerosis. The Practitioner 243:24–30.

Marieb E N 1995 Human anatomy and physiology, 3rd edn. Benjamin/Cummings Publishing, Redwood City, CA.

Prevett M C, Duncan J S 1998 Epilepsy. Update February: 178–188.

Rosen W G, Mohs R C, Davis K 1994 A new rating for Alzheimer's disease. American Journal of Psychiatry 141(11):1356–1364.

Smithson H 1999 Epilepsy. Doctor May: 88–90.

Vardaxis N J 1995 Pathology for the health sciences, 2nd edn. Churchill Livingstone, London.

12

MUSCULOSKELETAL DISORDERS

Nicola Nurse and Myfanny Rimmer

Key Issues

- Rheumatic diseases place a great social and economic burden on patients, families and society at large. They account for 18.7% of all consultations in general practice

- Rheumatic disease can affect any age group; however, the greatest incidence in the UK is in females over the age of 65

- The management of chronic rheumatic disease is multidisciplinary across both secondary and primary care. Shared care protocols and a whole system approach are essential for comprehensive patient care

- Chronic conditions have a global impact on an individual's life, affecting not only physical function but also her self-esteem, role, relationships, control perspectives and level of mood

- Minor injuries can be devastating in the short term for function and daily living; incorrect management in the first instance can result in delay in healing and even permanent reduction in mobility

Introduction

Patients with musculoskeletal system problems present to the health care setting in a wide and varied way, ranging from injury to chronic illness. This in itself presents unique challenges to the nurse practitioner (NP). Knowledge of the anatomy, like any system, is important, but probably more so when trying to understand the mechanisms of trauma and, thus, the patterns of injury. A comprehensive history is vital and will often give you the diagnosis before examination confirms this.

It is vital to remember that pain presenting in joints can be referred from another joint and indeed from other systems. Injury to the hip often presents as knee pain and pain in the medial thigh and hip and knee joints can be caused by gynaecological pathology involving the pathway of the obturator nerve. In addition, systemic disease can present as isolated joint pain. Thus, patients who present with no history of trauma must have possible sources of referred pain considered. If trauma has occurred, regardless of how minor, a system of examining the joint above and the joint below the injury minimises the risk of missing something.

Making the diagnosis is a matter of taking everything – the history, the examination and the patient as a whole – into consideration. In some cases, the difference between one diagnosis and another is difficult, e.g. gout and septic arthritis, and in the initial stages only your knowledge of the patient and small factors in the history will allow this differentiation.

On top of this, the use of secondary investigation is not as high as other systems, so you must rely on your communication and examination skills. The exception to this would be NPs working in health care settings with radiology facilities; in this case, the investigation you are most likely to need in addition to your skills is taking X-rays.

Finally, remember that multidisciplinary collaboration in the management of these patients can often make a huge impact on their ability to function with chronic disease or to recover fully from injury – physiotherapists, in particular, are vital.

Assessment

Subjective assessment

An accurate history is vital. Many clues in the history, the mechanism of injury or the symptoms will give you the diagnosis, which is then confirmed on examination. The trauma involved can be so minor that the patient may not even know it has occurred and can be put down to general wear and tear. Important specific pieces of information to find out are

1. Has there been an injury? Try to obtain an accurate picture of the mechanism involved.
2. Find out how the problem has affected day-to-day activities and, indeed, the functioning of the joint or limb.
3. Is there swelling, and if so, how quickly did it occur? Bleeding into joints from trauma happens really quickly and the swelling is obvious within about 20 min; this is a good indication of significant trauma, fracture or joint injury. Swelling that happens more slowly, i.e. over night, is more likely to be less serious.

4. Has the patient injured this limb/joint in the past? After previous trauma it is sometimes difficult to ascertain what can be attributed to the injury and what is new. The patient is your best source of information.

5. Ask specifically about any recent breaks to the skin, splinters or puncture wounds, especially if there is an infection query.

6. Ask about the patient's activities, work and leisure and any recent changes.

7. Ask about the patient's occupation and dominant hand.

8. The patient's general health and past medical history is important; systemic disease can first present with musculoskeletal symptoms.

9. Is there a history of skin disease? Psoriasis can affect synovial linings of the joint. It is worth excluding this in a patient who has a swollen painful joint with a history of minimal or no trauma.

10. Specific questions about the knee include asking the patient about any clicking, locking or giving way. These are all signs of damage to the meniscus (degenerative or from trauma); there may be little else to find and you have to rely on the history.

Objective assessment

When examining the musculoskeletal system, developing a systematic approach is invaluable. In general inspect, palpate and then move. Both the passive and active range of movement should be assessed within the limits of the patient's pain.

It is good advice to exclude involvement of the joint above and the joint below any injury in your examination, as injuries often occur in patterns and pain can be referred.

Inspect

1. Swelling
What is the distribution, is it isolated or diffuse? Is it confined to the joint or extending beyond the joint margins? Swelling confined to the joint (effusion) suggests
   - build-up of synovial fluid from trauma or an inflammatory response
   - bleeding into the joint (haemarthrosis) from trauma or clotting disorder
   - pus in the joint (pyarthrosis), as in septic arthritis.
If the swelling extends beyond the joint margins, consider
   - venous or lymph drainage insufficiency
   - infection, including cellulitis.

2. Deformity
Compare with the opposite limb; look at the patient's posture, any abnormality; consider
   - fracture
   - dislocation
   - previous injury
   - congenital deformity

   - degenerative joint disease.

3. The skin
Is it intact? A small, old, puncture wound may be the portal of infection in an infected joint. If not, consider
   - compound fracture or dislocation
   - penetration of a joint capsule.

4. Muscle wasting
Muscle quickly wastes if unused. Consider causes for disuse:
   - injury causing pain
   - associated nerve injury or disorder
   - congenital disability.

5. Bruising is usually indicative of trauma. If extensive, and disproportionate to the amount of trauma, consider other causes.

6. Scars. The significance of scars usually comes up in the history; however, if not, they can trigger further questioning.

Palpate

1. Temperature of the skin. If cold compared with the opposite side, consider
   - arterial insufficiency/blood supply
   - compartment syndrome (accompanied by extreme pain).
If warm or hot compared with the opposite side, consider
   - infection
   - inflammation
   - gout
   - septic arthritis/osteomyelitis.

2. Assess neurovascular function distal to the injury, palpate pulses and check sensation and reflexes if relevant.

3. Is the tenderness diffuse around the soft tissue or localised? Is it confined to the joint or bone involved? If diffuse, consider
   - inflammation
   - soft tissue strain.
If confined to the bone or joint, then consider
   - fracture
   - infection
   - rheumatological disease.

4. Feel for crepitus. Is this associated with movement? Obviously do not try to reproduce this. If the cause is a fracture, it will cause the patient a great deal of pain. However, you should be aware of it in examination. Consider
   - fracture
   - tendonitis/tenosynovitis.

Move

1. Encourage the patient to move the joint within the limits of her pain. Assess the range of movement possible actively. A completely fixed joint can be caused by
   - dislocation
   - intra-articular fracture or foreign body

- surgical arthrodesis
- pathological arthrodesis (infection in the joint can fuse the articular surfaces).

2. Check passive and active ranges of movement. Bony injury is usually painful and restricts movement, regardless of whether this movement is passive or active. Compare with the opposite limb. If movement is greater in the affected limb, consider
   - joint instability
   - ligament rupture
   - fracture
   - previous injury.

   If passive movement is less painful and/or there is a greater range than active movement, consider
   - soft tissue injury is more likely
   - neuromuscular cause.

3. Within the limits of the patient's pain, carefully stress the limb by gentle bending or longitudinal compression. If this increases pain, consider
   - fracture
   - stress fracture
   - other causes of bony pain.

Additional examination manoeuvres for specific joints

The knee

The knee comprises three joints, the tibiofemoral (Fig. 12.1), the patellofemoral (Fig. 12.2) and the tibiofibular joints (see Fig. 12.1), and a complex combination of ligament and muscular structures that have a large contribution to the stability. These allow the knee to flex and extend with some degree of rotation in flexion only. It is when it is in flexion that the knee is most vulnerable to injury. The knee joint is stabilised by ligaments, both internal and external to the capsule (see Fig. 12.1). The cruciate ligaments stabilise the tibia from an anterior posterior perspective, and the collateral ligaments stabilise valgus and varus movements. Menisci, semi-lunar cartilage structures, act as shock absorbers within the joint. All these structures are subject to stresses and strains, bearing weights of up to $3.5 \times$ body weight when going up stairs, and are vulnerable to wear and tear.

1. Patients with knee complaints should always be examined lying down.
2. Expose both knees and the lower legs.
3. As well as palpating the knee when it is straight, it is important that you palpate the knee in the bent position to isolate tenderness over the joint line. This could indicate involvement of the meniscus or the tibial plateau and is a good indicator for X-ray.
4. Palpate for an effusion by milking down the thigh, to empty the suprapatellar pouch into the joint and then cross-fluctuate from the side of the knee. If there is an effusion, you will see fluid bulging through to the other side of the joint.

5. Examine the straight leg raise in all patients with an injured knee; they should be able to lift the leg straight up off the bed, even if it only a small distance. If you fail to do this, a rupture of the extensor mechanism, either quadriceps tendon or patellar ligament, will eventually be missed; it is easily done.

6. Check the stability of the collateral ligaments with the knee slightly flexed at about 15 degrees. Stabilise the femur with one hand and then stress the lower leg laterally to test the medial collateral and medially for the lateral collateral. You will get a better idea of any laxity if you encourage the patient to relax the quadriceps muscles while you do this. Compare knees: Is there greater movement in the injured knee?

7. Check the cruciate ligaments. There are several ways of doing this. The anterior and posterior draw tests are the easiest. With the knee bent as near 90 degrees, stabilise the foot (I usually sit on it). Then pull the tibia forward (tests the anterior cruciate, see Fig. 12.3) and back (tests the posterior cruciate) on the femur. Check for laxity, and reproduction of pain. Compare with the opposite knee.

8. Checking for meniscal damage in an acutely injured knee is difficult and often inaccurate. However, the principles are to compress the meniscus in the joint between the femur and the tibia. This involves internal and external rotation of the flexed knee, while holding the lower limb and compressing it into the joint.

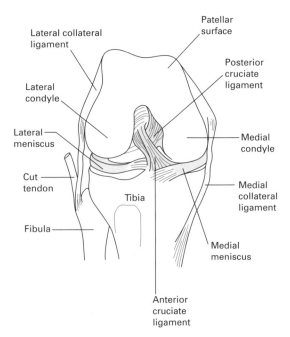

Figure 12.1 *Anterior, flexed. (Reproduced with permission from Martini 1998.)*

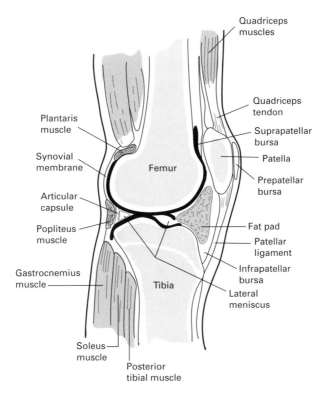

Figure 12.2 *Lateral view of parasagittal section through the right knee. (Reproduced with permission from Martini 1998.)*

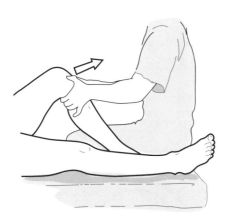

Figure 12.3 *Testing the cruciate ligament. (Reproduced with permission from Wardrope & English 1998.)*

Remember it is very difficult to make an accurate diagnosis on a painful, acutely injured knee. Many orthopaedic surgeons will review a patient after elevation, rest and ice – providing the knee is stable, the patient can straight leg raise, the knee is not locked (a block to full extension) and there is not a gross haemarthrosis. ❶ Patients who do not fit into these categories need referral.

The ankle

Essentially a hinged joint, the talus is central and surrounded by a circle of ligament complexes and bones. The distal tibial articular surface, the maleoli and the lateral and medial ligament complexes combine to lock the talus in a mortice. The lateral ligaments are longer and allow more movement in inversion and thus are more commonly injured. Medial ligaments are short and strong; injury to them usually suggests more significant trauma. The stability of the ankle depends on the integrity of all the above structures.

The tibia bears most of the weight. Dorsiflexion and plantar flexion occur at the ankle, i.e. tibiotalar joint, whereas inversion and eversion occur at the subtalar joint.

- Assess the stability of the ankle using the anterior drawer test. Place the patient's heel in one hand and *gently* pull the foot forward while stabilising the lower leg with your other hand. Pain and laxity are signs of ligament damage.
- Further ankle examination is found under the section for specific disorders.

The shoulder

The humerus is stabilised and pulled into the glenoid by a group of strong muscles (supraspinatus, infraspinatus, teres minor and subscapularis) and their associated

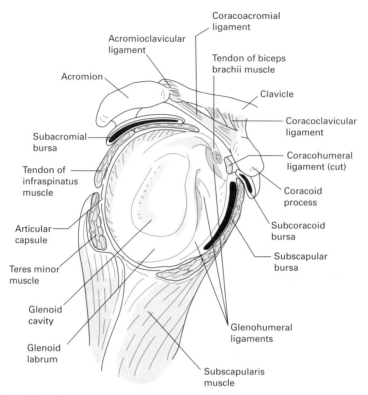

Figure 12.4 *Lateral view of the shoulder joint – humerus removed. (Reproduced with permission from Martini 1998.)*

tendons called the rotator cuff (Fig. 12.4); these facilitate the movement of what is the most mobile joint in the body. However, movement of the shoulder joint (glenohumeral joint) often involves the whole of the shoulder girdle, in other words, the acromioclavicular (A/C), sternoclavicular, scapularthoracic and subacromial joints, as well as the true shoulder joint. This concept is important as injury could involve one or a combination of these structures; however, pain in the A/C and the sternoclavicular joints tends to be localised. You must always be aware of referred pain; true shoulder pain rarely extends below the elbow, but pain can be referred from the cervical spine, elbow, lungs, heart, diaphragm, gall bladder and spleen.

Included in your examination should be

- Check for initiation of abduction to rule out complete rupture of the rotator cuff.
- Check for a painful arc (abduction from 60–100 degrees approximately). A sign of supraspinatus tendonitis and impingement syndrome.
- Check for integrity of the axillary nerve, which supplies sensation to the deltoid muscle. Injuries to this nerve, as well as to the radial, median and ulna nerves, are uncommon and involve reasonable trauma, a fracture or dislocation; however it is important not to miss them, especially when the patient will be distracted and in a lot of pain.

- Specific palpation of supraspinatus (Fig. 12.5) is only possible with the arm held in extension.

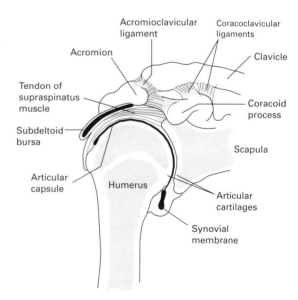

Figure 12.5 *Posterior view, right shoulder joint.*
(Reproduced with permission from Martini 1998.)

SPECIFIC DISORDERS

Septic arthritis

Although septic arthritis is an uncommon condition, it is an important diagnosis that should not be missed. If septic arthritis is not treated swiftly the joint very quickly degenerates, there is arthrodesis and, if not already, the patient becomes systemically septic.

Subjective findings

1. There is usually no history of trauma.
2. Careful questioning is vital to ascertain any penetrating injury regardless of how minor it may seem. Remember in the knee, the suprapatellar bursa extends up the thigh to end proximal and inferior to the distal end of the quadriceps. Penetration (e.g. kneeling onto a needle) into this bursa gives infection direct access to the joint.
3. The patient may complain of being systemically unwell before the pain in the joint started.
4. Ask about possible exposure to gonorrhoea.
5. Patients report pain moving the joint and an inability to bear weight.
   ❶ Beware diabetics: any hot swollen joint in a diabetic is septic unless proven otherwise by culture, even if the patient is well (Dandy & Edwards 1998).

Objective findings

- It is likely that the patient will be pyrexial and generally unwell
- The patient will have diffuse hot swelling over the whole joint and an effusion
- Check for lymphadenopathy
- Any movement of the joint is exquisitely painful and the patient will actively guard the region
- It is unlikely that the patient will be able to weight bear.

Investigations

Any further investigations can be done in secondary care.

Plan

- Offer analgesia/antipyretic
- Explain likely admission to patient.

Referral

All patients with suspected septic arthritis must be referred as soon as possible. The joint can deteriorate in 48 hours (Carr & Harnden 1999), so speed is important. They will need intravenous antibiotics and irrigation of the joint. Secondary division of the adhesions in the joint is sometimes necessary through arthroscopy (Dandy & Edwards 1998).

Bursitis

Bursa are sited over moving tissue to allow friction-free movement; so, by definition, they occur around joints. Inflammation in the bursa is usually caused by the irritation of repetitive compression or friction, e.g. frequent kneeling. This causes fluid to collect in the bursa (Cailliet 1992). There is usually no infective component; however, this must be ruled out.

It is suggested (Stell & Grandsen 1998) that patients with an infection in the bursa usually present earlier and have more severe symptoms (pain, mild fever, erythema); however, it is difficult to be 100% sure of no infective component purely on the clinical presentation (Stell & Grandsen 1998).

Subjective assessment

1. Usually the patient will have an occupation involving repeated activity, or give a history of a recent increase in the same activity. The bursa involved will depend on the type of activity: e.g. in the knee, kneeling in a clergymen (infrapatella bursa, see Fig. 12.2) and scrubbing the floors over a weekend (prepatellar bursa see Fig. 12.2); or leaning on the elbow (olecrenon bursa) all night in a bar; and in the shoulder (subacromial bursa, see Fig. 12.4), cleaning windows.
2. The patient will complain of pain and swelling over the affected area.
3. Function is not usually affected until on movement the bursa is compressed.
4. The patient reports no systemic symptoms.

Objective findings

- There will be swelling and heat, which unlike septic arthritis will be localised to the affected bursa.
- Tenderness will be localised and there should be no bony pain.
- The patient will be apyrexial.
- There will be no effusion in the joint.
- Both passive and active movements should be similar.
- In the knee, there should be full extension but flexion will get more painful past 60 degrees as the bursa is compressed (Wardrope & English 1998).
- The picture with olecrenon bursitis is similar; the patient should be able to fully extend the elbow, but pain will increase on extremes of flexion.
- Subacromial bursitis in the shoulder produces a picture of pain. It is worse on abduction, increasing in severity at approximately 60–110 degrees when the bursa is compressed between the acromion and the greater tuberosity of the humerus as the latter moves up and under the former and compresses the bursa.

Plan

- Elevation of affected limb
- Advice: avoid the precipitating factor, rest

- ❗ Patient should return if they develop any signs of infection, reduction in mobility, or if symptoms are not resolving in 7 days.

Therapeutic interventions

- In most cases symptoms settle with rest and avoidance of the causative activity. Nonsteroidal anti-inflammatory drugs (NSAIDs), usually ibuprofen 400 mg three times a day, will help, but review if not settling after 7 days.
- The bursa can be aspirated (Stell & Gransden 1998) but reoccurrence is high (Carr & Harnden 1999), and this increases the risk of introducing infection and hence a septic joint.
- Stell & Gransden (1998), in a small study, isolated *Staphylococcus aureus* as the infective component in the majority of infective bursitis, so if infection is suspected a course of appropriate antibiotics is advised.

Referral

- If there are any signs that the joint is involved, referral is indicated (see Septic arthritis)
- Occasionally, in cases that do not respond, the bursa has to be surgically removed.

Patient education

- Joints that are kept immobile get stiff very quickly; it is important to maintain mobility by gentle exercise.
- The likely cause should be discussed with the patient to avoid re-occurrence.

Tenosynovitis/Tendonitis

Tenosynovitis is inflammation and swelling of the synovium of a specific tendon sheath, most commonly the wrist and thumb extensors; it is often caused by repetitive use (Concannon 1999), but it can be triggered by minor trauma. De Quervain's tenosynovitis is thickening of the tendon sheath, which runs into the hand on the radial side of the wrist, specific to abductor pollicis longus (abducts the thumb) and extensor pollicis brevis (extends the thumb at the metacarpophalangeal (MCP) joint).

Tendonitis is similar but affects the tendon specifically; it commonly affects the shoulder. It is less commonly seen elsewhere, e.g. the Achilles tendon. In the shoulder, tendonitis most commonly affects the supraspinatus tendon (see Fig. 12.5) of the rotator cuff. This is usually secondary to microscopic tears, which heal and over time may calcify. Acute tendonitis in the shoulder tends to affect younger people, < 40 years old. Healing is quick and vigorous, and thus the pain is severe. Chronic tendonitis tends to affect older people, 40–50 years old, and there is more wear than tear and repair is slower but less painful.

Subjective findings

1. Take an occupational and social history.
2. Typically, a story of recent increased, and repetitive use and often an increase in a specific movement, e.g. carrying heavy shopping or using a hammer or a screwdriver.
3. There is usually no history of trauma; however, there may have been a very minor blow several days previously, with symptoms starting 1 or 2 days later.
4. Ask about other joint symptoms, as this can be the first presentation of rheumatoid arthritis.
5. The patient may complain of an initial pain that started as a dull ache, which has got steadily worse. The pain is worse at night.
6. The patient may report functional weakness and pain. In the wrist, gripping or lifting will be painful and there may be radiation of pain up the forearm.
7. If the wrist is affected, ask about signs of median nerve compression. There should not be any sensory signs, but the swelling of tenosynovitis can cause pressure on the median nerve (see carpal tunnel syndrome).
8. Rule out risk of tendon sheath infection. Ask about breaks to the skin.
9. Check for previous episodes.

Objective findings

- There may be subtle swelling over the area.
- There is specific tenderness, which increases on resisted movement.
- Classically, crepitus can be felt over the area as it is moved (e.g. dorsum of the wrist for the extensors) and the tendon passes through the affected sheath, but this is not always present.
- In de Quervain's tenosynovitis, resisted abduction and extension of the thumb is very painful. There will be mild swelling localised to the area with no increase in temperature. Finkelstein's test will be positive. (Ask the patient to flex the thumb into the palm and clasp it in the fingers. You then ulna deviate the wrist – in a positive test this should reproduce the pain.)
- Tinel's and Phalen's test should be negative (see carpal tunnel syndrome) (Wardrope & English 1998).
- In the shoulder supraspinatus tendonitis, tenderness on palpation will be localised to the tendon, inferior and anterior to the acromial tip over the humeral head. It may be easier to localise if the arm is extended. Typically, the patient will have pain on abduction, and particularly between 60 and 100 degrees with increased pain on resisted movements. ❗ The patient should be able to initiate abduction; if not, suspect complete rupture of the tendon and refer.
- ❗ Tendon sheath infections are rare but serious. Infection quickly spreads down the sheath and the tendon rapidly disintegrates. The flexor tendons in the fingers and hand are most vulnerable. Patients

present with rapid onset of pain, heat, swelling and reduced movement. The affected finger will be held in flexion and will be tender along the tendon sheath, with extension increasing the pain. This warrants immediate referral.

Therapeutic interventions

- The best initial treatment is to rest the affected tendon/sheath for at least 2 weeks, to interrupt the vicious circle of inflammation and swelling. For the wrist, use a Futuro splint or similar. Then review.
- NSAIDs, unless contraindicated.
- In de Quervain's tenosynovitis this involves immobilisation of the thumb and wrist: usually a splint to include the thumb (Carr & Harnden 1999, Concannon 1999) will be sufficient, but in severe or prolonged cases plaster is indicated.
- Supraspinatus tendonitis is very painful and debilitating and patients benefit from steroid injections as first-line management.

Patient education

- Rest and review of precipitating activity.

Gout and pseudogout

Gout and pseudogout are crystal-induced arthropathies, and are caused by crystal formation and deposits in the joint space: gout by uric acid and pseudogout by calcium pyrophosphate. Gout is more frequently seen, with patients falling into those who overproduce and those who undersecrete urate (Sturrock 2000), with the latter being much more common.

Traditional opinion of the typical presentation is a middle-aged, obese overindulgent man. Gout does affect more men, with a ratio of nine men to every woman (Kaplan 1999); other precipitating factors include thiazide diuretics (Snaith 1995) – however, it is suggested that loop diuretics are equally potent (Carr & Harnden 1999) – high dietary purines and other causes of hyperuricaemia.

Pseudogout often presents in patients with underlying osteoarthritis, and both conditions are more common in the elderly (Carr & Harnden 1999).

The most common presentation of gout is in the big toe at the joint of the first metatarsal and the proximal phalanx (MTP); however, there is a significant number of patients, Snaith (1995) suggests 30%, who have a first presentation elsewhere. Usually the attack is confined to one joint and is self-limiting. Pseudogout, however, most commonly presents in the knee, wrist or shoulder (Snaith 1995, Carr & Harnden 1999, Kaplan 1999). The clinical picture is similar in both conditions, regardless of the joint affected, as is the acute phase treatment; however, the differentiation between septic arthritis and gout is difficult and important.

Subjective findings

1. There will be an acute onset of a very hot painful joint. With gout this can be over matter of hours and often overnight; pseudogout tends to be less acute and less severe.
2. Exclude risk factors for septic arthritis (systemic illness preceding local symptoms, exposure to gonorrhoea or puncture wound to the skin).
3. Take a recent lifestyle and diet history. There may be evidence of a recent increase in purine-rich food (liver, kidney, red meat, pulses, beer, lager, port and some wine) intake.
4. Drug history for diuretics.
5. Previous similar episode.
6. Family history.
7. There may be a history of mild fever and malaise.

Objective findings

- The joint will be hot, swollen and acutely tender to touch – so much so that the patient may not be able to tolerate footwear.
- The skin will be red and may peel (Gibson 1986, Snaith 1995).
- Movement in the joint will be extremely painful, both actively and passively.
- In more chronic cases there can be deposits of urate crystals subcutaneously. Tophi, which are pale creamy deposits, form, commonly on the pinna, olecranon bursa and along the Achilles tendon (Gibson 1986). These lesions can ulcerate, which then predisposes infection.
- Generally, the patient is systemically well, but mild pyrexia is not uncommon.

Investigations

- Blood urate levels are not always raised in an acute attack, so this is not reliable diagnostically in the acute phase; however, they will provide information to assess risk for further attacks and can be taken at follow-up.
- Urea and electrolytes, to exclude a renal cause of hyperuricaemia.
- Inflammatory indicators (raised ESR, leucocytosis) will be abnormal, depending on the severity of the attack

Plan

Making the diagnosis can be helped by criteria suggested over 30 years ago (Bennet & Wood 1968), which are still applicable today (Sturrock 2000). These include two episodes of painful hot joint swelling which resolve within 2 weeks, the presence of tophus and resolution of symptoms within 48 hours of starting colchicine: saying that, there will be many patients with first attacks who do not fit all the criteria, so

- treat the acute phase

- assess, adapt contributory factors (drugs, diet, renal function, weight)
- establish risk of reoccurrence to consider long-term prophylaxis
- patient advice
- arrange follow-up.

Therapeutic intervention

1. It is generally accepted that in the acute attack the treatment of choice for both gout and pseudogout is large doses of NSAIDs (Gibson 1986, Snaith 1995, Sturrock 2000). Snaith (1995) recommends initial doses of naproxen (1.5 g) or indometacin (150 mg), with subsequent reduction over the next 12 hours.
2. Patients who have contraindications to NSAIDs can be treated with colchicine (0.5 mg every 3 hours for 12 hours) in acute attacks (Snaith 1995, BNF 2000). It can be used for patients on anticoagulants. The elderly do not tolerate the drug well (Sturrock 2000), and can have problems with diarrhoea.
3. For gout, prophylactic allopurinol can be prescribed, usually after the patient has had two episodes and only after at least 1 month after the acute phase is over. This drug can precipitate an acute episode during the first few months of treatment and so should be given in conjunction with NSAIDs (not aspirin) or colchicine.
4. Although allopurinol is not indicated for treatment in an acute attack – indeed it can prolong and increase the severity in the first instance – patients who are on long-term prophylactic allopurinol therapy should continue the drug through subsequent acute phases.
5. There is no prophylaxis for pseudogout.

Referral

- If there are any signs of an infective component and that the joint is involved (see Septic arthritis section)

Patient education

- If risk factors are identified within the patient's diet, small changes can prevent long-term allopurinol therapy. Patients will often prefer to make these changes.
- Initial management of gout with NSAIDs is much more effective if started early in the attack. So advice regarding self-management, before medical opinion, will reduce the severity and duration of attacks.

Collateral ligament sprains of the knee joint

Collateral ligament sprains are a common injury in the sports person, particularly in rugby and football players. The medial collateral ligament is the most commonly injured, as the player's leg goes out for a tackle and takes a blow from the lateral side.

Subjective findings

- A typical history is the knee taking a blow when in a bent position and at its most vulnerable
- The patient will present usually the next day and complain of swelling, pain on the medial aspect of the joint and difficulty walking
- In simple collateral sprains there should be no clicking or locking.

Objective findings

- There may be swelling.
- There should be no obvious new deformity.
- Bruising may be present on either the lateral side, where the blow was taken, or medially, but often this takes a day or two to appear.
- There will be tenderness along the collateral ligament, in particular at its insertion into the femoral condyle.
- There should be no bony tenderness along the joint line.
- There is usually no effusion.
- The patient should be able to bear some weight. They may be walking with a straight leg and be nervous of bending the knee.

❶ A large effusion will suggest involvement of other structures internal to the joint capsule. *Note*: if there is complete rupture of the medial collateral ligament, there will be a rupture of the joint capsule and thus no effusion (Wardrope & English 1998). This will be coupled with gross laxity of the joint on examination, and the patient will be unlikely to be able to walk. In this case referral is indicated.

- Actively, the patient should be able to fully extend the knee, give or take 5 degrees. It is unlikely that they will be able to flex past 90 degrees with a slight improvement on passive movements.
- There will be pain, pain and laxity, or gross laxity when stressing the collateral ligament depending on the degree of injury.

Therapeutic intervention

Collateral ligament injuries are graded and treated according to the degree of laxity.

- *No laxity, but pain on stressing.* Generally these heal well, with analgesia, early mobilisation and quadriceps exercises to prevent wasting of the muscle.
- *Slight laxity and pain on stressing.* These patients really benefit from active physiotherapy and follow-up. They may need crutches, support on the knee and regular analgesia. They are often referred for an X-ray initially as it is difficult to rule out bony tenderness.
- *Gross laxity.* ❶ These patients have an unstable knee. It is possible that they will have also injured the anterior cruciate ligament and the medial meniscus. They will not be walking and it is likely that they will present in the first instance to Accident and Emergency. They need X-ray and specialist referral.

Patient education

- Quadriceps exercises are vital for all knee injuries. The muscle quickly wastes with reduced use and this contributes further to instability.

Advise the patient to do each exercise 10 times at least daily. Sit on the floor or a firm surface:

1. Press the back of the knee onto the floor and dorsiflex the foot; hold for 10 seconds and relax.
2. With the leg held straight, lift the foot 12-inches off the floor; move the leg up and down 10 times.
3. Sit on the side of the bed, with the knee bent; now straighten the leg and hold for 10-seconds.

Referral

- Any gross laxity of the collateral ligaments or instability of the joint should be referred to an orthopaedic surgeon.
- Any bony tenderness should be referred for an X-ray.

Ankle sprains

Ankle sprains are common; in particular, injury to the lateral ligaments caused by twisting and, in particular, inversion. The most common lateral ligament to be injured is the anterior talofibular, which runs between the lateral maleolus and the talus. Despite their frequency of occurrence, these injuries are relatively difficult to assess and the decision whether to X-ray is not easy. However, there is useful research to facilitate the decision process (Stiell et al 1992).

Subjective findings

- The patient gives a history of going over on the ankle (usually inversion).
- Cracks or other noises heard at the time are not that helpful diagnostically, as they do not necessarily indicate bony injury.
- More important, inability to weight bear both immediately and at the time of examination are more reliable signs of significant injury.
- If the injury is a few days' old the patient may complain of pain radiating up the leg. This is often due to walking awkwardly; however, rule out bony tenderness of the proximal fibula (see Objective findings).
- Other important factors in the history are speed of swelling and previous injury, both of which increase the possibility of a more serious injury.

Objective findings

1. Patients presenting within a few hours of injury will have a very distinctive large egg-like swelling over the anterolateral aspect of the ankle. This quickly diffuses, so often overnight it becomes less defined.
2. There is commonly bruising, which becomes dependent, i.e. around the heel, if presentation is late.
3. There may be bony tenderness. Check particularly the inferior tips and posterior margins of the maleoli.
4. Palpate the base of the fifth metatarsal to rule out an associated fracture.
5. A fracture of the proximal fibula should be ruled out by palpating for pain in this area, particularly if the patient has pain on the medial side of his ankle.
6. The patient should be able to bear some weight with difficulty and pain, depending on the severity of the sprain.
7. There may be some reduction in movement, again depending on severity.
8. Sprains are graded according to severity:
   - Grade 1 – minor. There are microscopic tears of the ligament but there is no laxity or instability.
   - Grade 2 – moderate. There is disruption of the ligament with some laxity on anterior drawer test but the ankle is functionally stable.
   - Grade 3 – severe. Complete disruption of the ligament, and the ankle is unstable.
9. ❶ Gross laxity on the ankle anterior drawer test indicates ligament rupture and an unstable ankle.

Plan

- Advise patient of the rational for X-ray or not as the case may be.
- Advise of expected healing times – all but the most minor ankle sprains can take 4–6 weeks to settle.

Investigations

Plan to refer for X-ray if (adapted from Stiell et al 1992)

- there is bony tenderness on the inferior tip or posterior margin of either maleoli
- there is bony tenderness on the base of the fifth metatarsal or the proximal fibula
- the patient cannot walk (four steps) both immediately after the injury and when you see them
- the patient is over 55 years old.

Therapeutic intervention

Common practice continues to be rest, ice compression and elevation (RICE). The compression has traditionally been the application of an elasticised cylindrical bandage. However, there is significant evidence (Cooper et al 1997) from as far back as 1981 (Brooks et al) and discussion (Kennet 1996, Wilson & Cooke 1998) to suggest that this is not the most beneficial management option. However, patients have come to expect and sometimes demand this bandaging. Usually, investing time to explain that exercises, early mobilisation, ice and elevation have been shown to have better effects will result in a happy patient.

Referral

- Refer bony tenderness for X-ray
- Gross instability (grade 3) needs stabilisation and orthopaedic follow-up
- All grade 2 and the more serious grade 1 sprains all benefit from early physiotherapy assessment and management.

Patient education

1. Along with the appropriate use of ice and elevation, exercise plays a large part in rehabilitation after a sprain. It keeps the joint mobile to prevent stiffness and muscle wasting and will speed up recovery.
2. Exercises are best done little and often and preferably after the application of ice.
3. Advise the patient:
   - to move the foot up and down at the ankle
   - to move the foot slowly round in a circle one way then another
   - to try to walk normally, putting the heel down first and walking through the foot.
4. It is important to give the patient realistic expectations regarding recovery: symptoms should start to improve over 7–10 days but there may be intermittent swelling and discomfort even 4 weeks later, particularly at the end of a day on his feet.

Carpal tunnel syndrome

Carpal tunnel syndrome is a median nerve compression neuropathy. It is caused by pressure on the median nerve as it passes through the carpal tunnel. This tunnel is bordered dorsally by the carpal bones and on the palmar aspect by the transverse ligament; small changes in the available space can mean that pressure is applied to the nerve. This increase in pressure can be due to a number of causes – essentially anything that decreases the space in the carpal tunnel:

- direct pressure – mass, e.g. flexor tenosynovitis, tuberculosis, rheumatoid arthritis, bone or connective tissue tumour
- indirect pressure – swelling, e.g. pregnancy, obesity, diabetes, oral contraceptive pill, hypothyroidism.

Subjective findings

1. Take a careful health history to exclude signs and symptoms of any systemic condition.
2. Exclude pregnancy.
3. In the initial stages of the condition, patients give a history of intermittently being woken at night with burning pain and tingling in the thumb, index, middle and ring fingers – the little finger is not affected (sensory distribution of the median nerve). They then have to shake the hand and the symptoms settle. This is caused by flexion at the wrist at night, which narrows the tunnel even further.
4. As the condition progresses, there is involvement of the motor function of the nerve. Patients will complain of clumsiness, reduced dexterity and grip strength as well as increased pain when using the hand all the time.
5. At the chronic stage, there is muscle wasting and gross functional impairment due to axonal death.
6. Ask about previous wrist fractures: carpal tunnel syndrome is relatively common after a Colles' fracture.

7. Take a careful social and occupational history. Repetitive and continuous hand movements can cause an inflammatory swelling, e.g. cashiers, computer operators, assembly line workers and jackhammer operators are at risk.

Objective findings

Inspection

- There will be little to see, except in chronic cases where there will be some wasting of the thenar muscles.

Palpation

- Test sensation and two-point discrimination to median nerve distribution
- Tinel's test is positive if tapping on the volar part of the wrist over the transverse ligament and the median nerve reproduces the paraesthesia
- Phalen's test is positive if pain and paraesthesia are produced by holding the wrist in flexion while the forearms are held vertically for 1 min (Belamonte 1996).

Move

- Test function of the thenar muscles.

Investigations

Depending on history, any that are needed to exclude systemic cause. These may include

- investigations to rule out systemic conditions and pregnancy
- thyroid function tests
- blood sugar
- urinalysis.

Therapeutic intervention

To some extent this does depend on the cause, which should be treated if known. In the first instance, when symptoms are mild and intermittent, non-invasive methods are best. This is particularly the case when the cause can be addressed, or is relatively short lived (e.g. pregnancy).

These interventions include

- Modification of activity if related (see advice).
- Wearing splints at night. Use a Futuro or similar splint.
- NSAIDs.
- Monitoring the patient closely, with review after approximately 2 weeks
- Diuretics.

If symptoms are less than mild, including frequent pain and weakness or they are not responding to first-line management, then consider

- Steroid injections. These have an 80% response rate, but 80% of patients have a relapse within 2 years (Carr & Harnden 1997). This may involve referral to the GP or specialist clinic.

Patient education

1. Self-help is vital.
2. If this injury is work related, advise patients to contact their Occupational Health Department.
3. For computer workers, advise keeping the wrist at neutral (Belamonte 1996) when working on a keyboard. This will involve
   - Positioning of the keyboard away from the desk edge, so the forearm rests on the work surface. This minimises further pressure on the carpal tunnel, as the wrist presses on the desk edge.
   - Minimal slant on the keyboard, which will reduce hyperextension of the wrist.
   - Trimming long fingernails.
4. General advice should include
   - frequent rests
   - diversification of tasks, so that repetitive movements are kept to a minimum.

Referral

Some patients will need to have surgical division of the transverse ligament. Refer all cases of
- persistent symptoms after 3 months of non-invasive management
- constant sensory impairment
- thenar wasting
- Dandy and Edwards (1998) suggest referral if symptoms persist after three steroid injections.

RHEUMATIC DISEASE

Introduction

This section of the chapter will focus on the conditions of the musculoskeletal system prevalent in primary care whereby diagnosis, management and support provide the main context and focus of care.

The term 'rheumatic disease' is used to describe many conditions that affect the musculoskeletal system. These conditions can affect bones, joints, soft tissue and muscles, and range from the milder soft tissue rheumatism, such as tennis elbow, to inflammation of joint linings and destruction of joints, as in rheumatoid arthritis (RA).

Osteoarthritis

Osteoarthritis (OA) is the commonest condition to affect synovial joints. Characterized by local cartilage loss and accompanying reparative bone response, OA is the single most important cause of locomotor disability. It can be a painful disabling condition, occurring infrequently in those under 45 or of black or Asian ethnic origin. Prevalence of OA increases up to age 65 when at least half of the people have radiographic evidence of OA in at least one joint (Jones & Doherty 1995).

There are no interventions known to prevent disease progression. Individual treatment programmes are aimed at relief of pain and to maximise and/or improve function. The aetiology of OA may be related to a genetic factor, trauma or a previous joint disease.

Subjective findings

- Pain assessment.
- Explore the history of the pain: Is it related to movement? Is it present at rest?
- Assess the pain severity: it may be severe and unremitting, especially if the hip is affected.
- What are the aggravating and relieving factors?
- Timing – is the pain unremitting or intermittent?
- Stiffness of joints. Is it relieved by movement?
- Are any joints swollen and inflamed?
- Assess the patient's ability to perform acts of daily living.
- Ask about the patient's sleeping pattern and assess any factors associated with sleep disturbance.

Psychological aspects of chronic disease may well be an aspect of presenting problems:
- ask about the patient's level of mood
- establish how this person may feel about himself
- enquire whether the condition had any impact on relationships
- assess change in coping mechanisms
- have major changes in lifestyle had to be made
- if so, assess impact on dynamics of home life, employment, etc.
- establish the use of medication, including over-the-counter (OTC) preparations
- enquire about any non-medical interventions the patient has tried, and if these were helpful.

Objective findings

Before starting any articular assessment, the nurse must give a full explanation of the procedure and work in full cooperation with the patient in control. Many movements may be painful and the patient must feel confident to direct the process.
- Observe the hands (Fig. 12.6). Heberden's nodes are a common manifestation of OA. These are enlarged, initially painful nodes on the distal interphalangeal joints (DIP), and can result in painless stiffening with occasional instability. Less common are bony swelling of the proximal interphalangeal joints (PIP), known as Bouchard's nodes. OA frequently causes pain at the base of the thumb in the first carpometacarpal joint, resulting in squaring of this joint.
- Assess grip strength – this can be done with a hand-size sphygmomanometer cuff, recording in millimetres of mercury (mmHg). The range of readings can be from 30 to 300 mmHg.
- Examine any affected joints for their range of movement. Observe any swelling, crepitus, bony enlargement, deformity, instability and presence of any

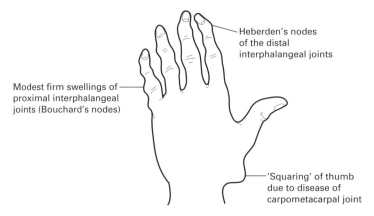

Figure 12.6 *The hand in generalized osteoarthritis.*

effusion. Joints enlarged due to bony deformity do not count as swollen joints.
- Assess the level of pain based on information in the history.
- Type of severity and the nature of the pain can be assessed with the help of a visual analogue scale (Fig. 12.7).
- Assess any evidence of joint locking.
- Any sudden deterioration, consider sepsis.
- Assess level of mobility and disability. Observe for any muscle wasting.

- Observe for generalised pain and sleep disturbance – consider fibromyalgia or depression.
- Check weight/body mass index (BMI). Discuss diet and alcohol consumption – predisposing factors of gout?
- Assess for signs of depression. The Hospital Anxiety and Depression (HAD) scale can be very useful (Le Gallez 1998).

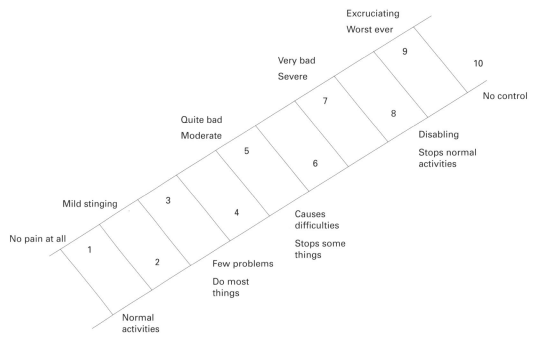

Figure 12.7 *Visual analogue scale.*

Plan

Management of OA must be focused upon the relief of pain, interventions to maximise mobility and to make necessary appropriate referrals.

Investigations

The focus for investigation is targeted locally to the affected area. This is not a systemic disease.

- An X-ray will define the cartilage loss by observing the joint space narrowing. Bone involvement is determined by the presence of osteophytes and sclerosis. This will define the main criteria for diagnosis; however, it will not determine early minimal change and, thus, early disease.
- Full blood count (FBC) – NSAIDs can cause peptic ulceration – may show a fall of haemoglobin levels. This form of anaemia is not associated with disease activity and would indicate the need for further investigation.

Therapeutic intervention

- Pain relief
- Nonpharmacological
- Hot and cold packs – reduces inflammation
- Rest – counselling about the importance of rest, addressing any emotions of guilt that might be associated here
- Relaxation
- Joint protection
- Balneotherapy – hydrotherapy or spa therapy.

Pharmacological

NSAIDs have been widely used as treatment for patients with OA; however, these agents are associated with significant toxicity, particularly in the elderly population. Also of concern are the possible adverse effects of NSAIDs on the metabolism of articular cartilage (Townheed et al 1997). Therefore, a step approach with OA is taken:

1. Paracetamol – very effective in mild to moderate OA.
2. Compound analgesics – combinations of aspirin/paracetamol with opioid agent, usually codeine phosphate.
3. NSAIDs – side-effect profile needs careful monitoring, e.g. epigastric pain, indigestion or nausea. Patients must be informed to stop the drug and consult if symptoms occur.
4. COX-2 (cyclo-oxygenase 2) inhibitors (rofecoxib) could eliminate the risk of gastrointestinal bleed and, if they fulfil the expectations, could revolutionise the use of NSAIDs in rheumatic disease.
5. Referral for intra-articular steroid injections is helpful in reducing inflammatory exacerbations.
6. In major disease, with severe joint destruction, joint replacements are undertaken surgically, especially the hip and knee.
7. Maintaining maximum mobility.

8. Address weight if appropriate. Weight-bearing joints that are already inflamed or damaged by disease will be further stressed by carrying excess weight.

Any psychological/social manifestations of the implications of chronic disease need to be addressed:

- the treatment of any depression
- financial implications – benefits may have to be assessed
- the impact of social isolation.

Linking seamless referrals to all services of the professions allied to medicine (PAMs) at the appropriate time requires a systemic approach to monitoring patients with rheumatic disease.

General practice needs to ensure systems are in place, for example

- disease registers
- systematic recall
- skilled and knowledgeable practitioners
- shared care protocols.

The organizational structures of primary care groups (PCGs) and primary care trusts (PCTs) are working towards a comprehensive whole systems approach to the management of complex pathology with multifaceted needs. This could ensure smooth appropriate and cost-effective pathways within the system.

Patient education

To give patients knowledge and understanding of their disease and treatment is to empower them to participate in their care. This would encompass:

- disease process – aetiology, symptoms and any investigations
- drug therapy – effects, side effects and usage
- exercise – effects, how and when to do, ways of assessing effect
- joint protection – what it is, use of splints, lifestyle alterations
- fatigue – causes and energy conservation
- dietary effects on health
- information on complementary therapies – many practices now have access to acupuncture, contacts with hydrotherapy activities, etc.

Referral

This must be fluid, flexible and seamless across the system, linking with a regular assessment and monitoring programme across secondary and primary care. Key players are consultant rheumatologist, specialist rheumatology nurse, GP, nurse practitioner, practice nurse, district nurse, physiotherapist, occupational therapist, podiatrist/chiropodist, dietician, social worker and voluntary organisations

Complications

- Gastrointestinal bleed from toxicity of NSAIDs
- Deformity of joints
- Immobility.

Rheumatoid arthritis

Introduction

Rheumatoid arthritis (RA) is a systemic chronic inflammatory disease affecting the musculoskeletal and many other systems of the body. Inflammation of the synovium, joints and tendons results in pain, swelling and restricted movement and eventually leads to radiological changes and deformity. RA patients show a reduction in joint flexibility, muscle strength and aerobic capacity compared with healthy persons. Furthermore, many patients experience restricted performance of daily tasks. The focus of management is to slow progression of the disease by early diagnosis and suppression of the inflammatory process before structural irreversible damage occurs. RA occurs worldwide with variable incidence and severity. It affects 1–3% of the population, with an overall 3:1 female preponderance in the younger age group, equalling out in the elderly population.

The aetiology of RA is unclear, but there is evidence of a genetic predisposition to the disease. The presence of the human leucocyte antigen HLA-DR4 is significantly commoner amongst suffers of RA who are of white ethnic origin (Akil & Amos 1995).

It is anticipated that the reader will read this section in association with the section on Osteoarthritis, as much of the content applies to both of these chronic rheumatoid conditions.

Subjective findings

- Insidous onset
- Vague history of pain, swelling and stiffness, gradually getting worse
- Bilateral findings
- Usually starts in small joints of hands (proximal interphalangeal (PIP) or MCP joints) or metatarsal/phalangeal joints of the feet
- Tiredness
- Lethargy
- Stiffness
- Loss of strength in grip
- Difficulty in walking
- Pain
- Ask about what aggravates or relieves the pain
- Establish level of pain
- Sites and radiation of any pain
- Persistency of pain
- Timing of pain – worse at night or day? With activity or rest?
- Check for any difficulties in sleeping
- Enquire about any difficulties performing the acts of daily living.

Psychological factors are very relevant in an holistic assessment of chronic disease. Explore feelings of

- low mood
- loss of self-esteem

- increased anxiety levels
- depression
- fear of loss of control and destiny.

The presentation of the patient with RA could be anywhere along a continuum from symptoms leading to diagnosis to coping with complications and severe disability. Chronic illness has been defined as an altered state of health that will not be cured by a single surgical procedure or a short course of medical therapy (Miller 1992 as quoted in Hill 1998).

Objective findings

The purpose of the objective assessment is to confirm and to measure quantitatively the severity and extent of the patient-centred problem. It must be linked with the subjective findings and history.

Observe

- General demeanour, facial expression, tone of voice, etc.
- For any deformities
- Posture
- Gait
- Any functional difficulties.

Palpation

Palpation of joints and surrounding tissue:

- confirms abnormality
- ensures normality
- helps to localise and to differentiate the exact structure or site of the lesion
- observe presence of warmth and tenderness – indicator in active pathology
- differentiate joint swelling, e.g. joint effusion mobile and soft to palpate whereas synovial hypertrophy has a 'boggy' feel to it
- observe for any muscle wasting around inflamed joints.

Assessment of pain

Read in conjunction with the Osteoarthritis section.

1. Assess the level of pain, based on subjective history. Type, severity and nature of pain can be assessed with the aid of a visual analogue chart (see Fig. 12.7).
2. Pain due to nerve involvement can be due to peripheral nerve entrapment, as in carpal tunnel syndrome, or to spinal nerve compression due to atlanto-axial subluxation or vertebral subluxation causing compression of spinal nerves and thus pain along the dermatome. See Chapter 11, p. 174 for examination skills of the nervous system.
3. Examination of movements. See p. 201–204 for examination techniques of the musculoskeletal system.
4. This procedure must be performed with the full cooperation and support of the patient. Patients know best how to hold their limbs, the pressure to apply and the tolerable range of movement. Constant communication is essential.

5. By passively gliding and sliding or compressing the joint surfaces in different directions, it is possible to determine whether the movement is normal, excessive or restricted and whether this contributes to the patient's symptoms.
6. By recording degrees of flexion, extension, adduction, abduction, rotation, pronation and supination in the affected joint/limbs, any deterioration or progress can be monitored and assessed.
7. Examination of the hands – In RA, the PIP and MCP joints are predominantly affected: rarely, the distal interphalangeal (DIP) joint, as in OA.
8. Observe for rheumatic nodules on the elbows, scapula, Achilles tendon and sometimes the sacral area. These can also form internally in the lungs and myocardium with serious consequences.
9. Where psychological problems have been identified in the subjective history, assessment of anxiety, mood, depression and coping mechanisms need to be addressed. The HAD, scale is a quick, effective useful tool (Le Gallez 1998).

Extra-articular features presenting RA:
1. Sjögrens syndrome – presents with dry gritty eyes and dry mouth.
2. Pericarditis, pericardial effusions and amyloidosis.
3. Hepatomegaly – caused by amyloid deposits.
4. Vasculitis – causing nail fold infarcts and leg ulcers. These are serious implications.
5. Osteoporosis – causing fractures of the vertebra, neck of femur and wrist. Be alerted if taking oral steroids past or present.
6. Fibrosing alveolitis and pleural effusions.
7. Felty's syndrome – serious presentation. Splenomegaly associated with vasculitis, anaemia, thrombocytopenia and lymphadenopathy.

Plan

Except in the mildest cases, one specialist in isolation from others cannot manage RA. It is very much a team approach, with the patient participating fully in his or her own health care and management plan.
■ Determine any investigations required
■ Plan liaison with other professionals
■ Ensure systems are in place to monitor and manage therapy.

Investigations

The X-ray shows swelling of soft tissue, loss of joint space or periarticular osteoporosis. Erosions typical of RA develop within 3 years of the start of the disease in 90% of patients (Akil & Amos 1995).

The magnetic resonance imaging (MRI) may hold the key to identify early disease process. Polysynovitis is the predominant clinical feature of early disease; it is not detectable on X-ray. Identification with MRI could identify early disease and influence management decisions. Access to MRI scanning is predominantly via secondary

care consultants; therefore, early diagnosis and referral is essential.

Laboratory findings in RA can include
■ anaemia – normochromic, hypochromic or normocytic (if microcytic consider iron deficiency)
■ raised ESR
■ raised C reactive protein concentration
■ raised ferritin concentration or acute phase protein
■ thrombocytosis
■ low serum iron concentration
■ low toxic iron-binding capacity
■ raised serum globulin concentration
■ raised serum alkaline phosphase activity
■ presence of rheumatoid factor in 80% of patients; 20% remains zero – negative.

Therapeutic intervention

The aims of treatment in RA are
■ relief of symptoms
■ preservation of function
■ prevention of structural damage and deformity
■ maintenance of patient's normal lifestyle.

The general practitioner and nurse practitioner in primary health care have a key role in the early recognition of disease symptoms; however, once established disease is diagnosed shared care protocols are the key feature of monitoring and management with seamless referrals between appropriate professionals as symptoms occur. The secondary care rheumatology consultant is the professional who initiates drug therapy aimed at modifying the course of the disease. Monitoring and management being key features with seamless referrals between appropriate professionals as symptoms occur. The secondary care rheumatologist initiates drug therapy aimed at modifying the course of the disease.

Disease modifying antirheumatic drugs (DMARDS)

DMARDS have potentially dangerous side effects that require safe and effective monitoring; however, they are both powerful and effective treatments. The commonly used drugs in this group are azathioprine, methotrexate, sulfasalazine and sodium aurothiomalate (Myocrisin).

Methotrexate. Regular monitoring of blood includes FBC, urea and electrolytes (U&Es) and liver function tests (LFTs). Adverse reactions of thrombocytopenia, neutrapenia, agranulocytosis and fatal marrow suppression have been reported. Methotrexate can also cause abnormal liver function and hepatic fibrosis. The liver enzyme aspartate transaminase (AST), when persistently elevated, is the best guide to toxicity. Methotrexate is given orally as a weekly dose.

Azathioprine. Regular monitoring of blood includes FBC weekly for the first 8 weeks, then monthly once stable. LFTs are carried out monthly throughout course of treatment. U/Es are checked to monitor kidney function to prevent drug accumulation. Adverse reactions include bone marrow suppression, hepatic dysfunction and renal insufficiency. Azathiaprine is given orally, daily.

Sulfasalazine. Regular monitoring of blood includes FBC 2 weekly and LFTs 4 weekly for the first 12 weeks; thereafter 3 monthly. Adverse effects include potentially fatal leucopenia, aplastic anaemia and thrombocytopenia, renal heamaturia, proteinurea and nephrotic syndrome and hepatic injury. Sulfasalazine is given orally as a daily dose.

Sodium aurothiomalate (Myocrisin). Regular monitoring FBC and urinalysis at time of each injection. Adverse reactions include skin reactions, renal disease and blood dyscrasia. Myocrisin is given intramuscularly into the gluteal muscle.

General guidelines for monitoring
- Inspect skin for rashes – enquire about pruritus.
- Assess for mouth ulcers, sore throat and loss of taste.
- Inspect skin for bruising.
- Assess for any undue bleeding, e.g. epistaxis and bleeding gums.
- Any flu-like symptoms?
- Any breathlessness or persistent cough?
- Perform urinalysis if on Myocrisin. Proceed if free of protein.
- Blood taken for relevant investigations.
- General assessment – see Objective findings, p. 214.
  - Address the management of pain – see Osteoarthritis section p. 213.
  - Psychological support – see Osteoarthritis section p. 213.
  - Team support – see Osteoarthritis section p. 213.

Surgical intervention

Orthopaedic surgery plays a major role in minimising deformity and maintaining independence and mobility

Patient education

The focus here with RA patients must be on empowerment. Most patients cope better if they understand their condition and have realistic expectations of the benefits and disadvantages of treatment. See Osteoarthritis section.

Referral

- Must be seamless across disciplines as problems arise.
- Early diagnosis and referral from PHC – improved prognosis.
- During regular monitoring any aspects of drug toxicity requires referral
- Any acute exacerbations.

Complications

See Box 12.1.

Box 12.1	*Complications of rheumatoid arthritis*
■ Cardiac	Pericarditis
■ Mitral valve disease	Conduction defects
■ Pulmonary	Pleural effusion
	Fibrosing alveolitis
	Rheumatic nodules
■ Skin	Vasculitis
	Palmar erythema
■ Deformity	
■ Eye	Sjögrens syndrome
	Scleritis
	Episcleritis
■ Neurological	Entrapment of peripheral nerves
	Nerve root compression of spinal cord
■ Amyloidosis	A complication of RA, whereby waxy starch-like glycoprotein (amyloid) accumulates in tissues and organs
■ Complications of medical and surgical treatment	

Osteoporosis

Osteoporosis is recognised by the World Health Organization (WHO) as a major worldwide health problem. An imbalance between bone resorption (removal) and bone formation (replacement) eventually results in osteoporosis. Osteoporosis is characterised by low bone mass and a micro-architectural deterioration of bone tissue, leading to an enhanced bone fragility and consequent increase in risk of fracture (WHO 1994; definition).

In the UK there are 200 000 fractures each year linked with osteoporosis. Fractures of the spine and wrist cause much morbidity; however, most serious consequences arise in patients with hip fracture, which is associated with a significant increase in mortality. It is these three sites of fracture that are affected by osteoporosis. There are two types of bone: cortical and trabecular. Trabecular is the filigree-like structure inside many bones. It looks like a honeycomb and is more porous and found mostly in the vertebrae, pelvis and at the end of long bones. Trabecular bone is lost rapidly during the female menopause, while both men and women lose cortical bone slowly after mid-life.

Osteoporosis is characterised by micro-architectural deterioration of bone tissue and low bone mass, resulting in increased bone fragility and silent insidious disease that does not cause symptoms until a fracture occurs. The condition occurs predominantly in females; however, men can also be affected. Bone mass density (BMD) can be measured and bone is considered to be osteoporotic when the BMD is 2.5 standard deviations or more below the young adult mean value.

Secondary causes of osteoporosis can be linked to endocrine disorders, e.g. hypothyroidism or hypogonadism in males. It can be drug-related, as in prolonged use of corticosteroids, anticonvulsants, thyroxine and alcohol. Immobilisation, malignancy and gastric surgery can also be predisposing factors.

Subjective findings

1. Acute presentation with wrist fracture (Colles' fracture) and hip fracture (head of femur).
2. Sudden severe back pain radiating around the thorax and abdomen.
3. Chronic back and neck pain – crush fractures of vertebrae can cause prolapsed intervertebral disc (PID) with nerve root compression.
4. It is important to assess patients presenting in primary health care for risk factors of osteoporosis; this can be done systematically in organised prevention clinics or opportunistically in routine consultation contacts with patients.
5. Family history – first-degree relative – mother, brother or sister.
6. Alcohol excess – over 14 units for women, over 21 units for men – carries a risk.
7. Hyperthyroidism and hyperparathyroidism. Thyroid hormones are involved in bone reabsorption and remodelling.
8. Anorexia.
9. Amenorrhoea for more than 6 months can result in a reduction in oestrogen levels. A predisposing factor in osteoporosis.
10. Malabsorption.
11. Smoking – smokers can experience an earlier menopause and tend to have lower BMI.
12. Establish a comprehensive drug history – a prolonged course (greater than 3 months) of corticosteroids can cause osteoporosis.
13. Immunosuppressant drugs. Many transplant patients are on lifelong treatment.
14. Anticonvulsant drugs – affect metabolism and absorption of oestrogen.
    Establish a past history of disease:
- chronic inflammatory bowel disease
- kidney disease
- chronic liver failure
- myeloma
- hypothyroidism
- Cushing's syndrome.
All carry risk of osteoporosis.

Objective findings

Osteoporotic bones are not tender and feel normal until a fracture occurs. Assess for

- loss of height
- observe for signs of vertebral kyphosis (dowager's hump)
- observe any difficulty in raising head and maintaining eye contact
- assess pain – often experienced when standing and resting; following acute episode of vertebrae fracture; may be acute, becoming chronic after 6–8 weeks.

Plan

- Refer if evidence of any Colles' fracture or fracture of the femur
- Discuss necessary therapeutic intervention
- Arrange any investigations
- In preventative circumstances, implement appropriate nonpharmacological or pharmacological interventions and health promotion advice.

Investigations

1. Spontaneous fracture can also be significant of other underlying pathology. May be necessary to check.
2. Alkaline phosphatase to exclude myeloma and metastases.
3. Calcium (corrected) plus alkaline phosphatase to exclude osteomalacia or primary hyperparathyroidism.
4. Thyroid and LFTs for underlying dysfunction.
5. Plasma biochemical profile to exclude metastases.
6. Serum testosterone in men, which may identify undetected hypogonadism.
7. Immunoelectrophoresis of serum and urine to exclude myeloma.
8. ESR or plasma viscosity to exclude multiple myeloma or skeletal metastases.
9. X-ray will identify evidence of post or present fracture.
10. Bone densometry can be measured with a DEXA scan. This is not available as a screening tool under the NHS. However, guidelines and indications for DEXA scan under the NHS have been drawn up locally in many areas. They include:
    - Clinical osteoporosis
      low trauma fracture
      osteopenia noted on X-ray
      loss of height
      kyphosis (after radiographic confirmation of vertebral deformities)
    - Oestrogen deficiency
      menopause before 45 years (patients not taking hormone replacement therapy (HRT))
      prolonged secondary amenorrhoea (greater than 1 year)
      primary hypogonadism
    - Prolonged corticosteroid therapy
    - Chronic disorders associated with osteoporosis, as defined earlier
    - BMI less than 19.

Therapeutic intervention

1. Treat pain according to severity:
   - paracetamol is effective, with few side effects
   - paracetamol and codeine
   - NSAIDs are sometimes prescribed
   - opiates may be necessary if pain due to fracture is severe
   - fentanyl patches can be effective
   - local nerve blocks may also help to control pain.
2. HRT, if taken at the menopause (natural or surgical), is the most effective therapy against osteoporosis. (See also Chapter 14, p. 261)
3. In established osteoporosis the bisphosphonates are powerful antiresorptive agents. They inhibit osteoclasts by coating the bone surfaces, but allow osteoblasts to continue to form new bone. These drugs may increase bone density by about 5% over 4 years. This form of treatment can be used for osteoporosis in men and women.
4. Calcium supplements have been shown to slow bone loss in postmenopausal women; however, there is little convincing evidence that it reduces fractures. Calcium combined with vitamin D significantly reduces fractures in elderly patients (National Prescribing Centre 1999).
5. Patients on corticosteroids and other at-risk groups consider bone sparing therapy, HRT or bisphosphonates.
6. Rehabilitation programmes in severe cases, particularly the elderly, help to maintain independence and support community care.

Patient education

- Promote weight-bearing exercise. It has a positive effect on several risk factors for osteoporosis, including femoral neck, lumber spine, muscle strength and balance (Heininen et al 1996).
- Encourage smoking cessation. Earlier menopause and lower BMI in smokers.
- Accident prevention – hip protectors.
- Support multidisciplinary approach – family planning, health visiting, district nursing, GP, practice nursing, NP, and areas within secondary care, particularly Accident & Emergency Department.

Referral

- Acute fractures
- Established disease with complications
- Other members of community team, e.g. physiotherapist, occupational therapist and chiropodist.

Complications

- Disability and deformity
- Morbidity – pain and immobility
- Loss of independence.

Polymyalgia rheumatica/giant cell arteritis

In recent years giant cell arteritis and polymyalgia rheumatica have increasingly been considered as closely related conditions. The two syndromes form a spectrum of disease and affect the same types of patient. They may occur independently or may occur in the same patient, either together or separated in time.

Both are diseases of the elderly and are rarely diagnosed in persons younger than 50 years of age. They are almost always confined to white people, with the incidence higher in northern Europe than in Mediterranean peoples.

Giant cell arteritis presents in many different forms, affecting any of the arteries within the body. The temporal artery is frequently affected. The arteries become inflamed, enlarged and nodular with ensuing narrowing of the lumen.

Subjective findings

The onset is usually acute. Because of the diverse nature of presentation, a classification of symptoms has been devised (Swannell 1997).

Systemic

1. Explore symptoms of malaise, anorexia, fever, night sweats, weight loss and depression.
2. Observe for myalgic pain in neck, shoulders and pelvic girdle that is aggravated by movement and often worse at night.
3. Observe any involvement of arteries. This may produce pain, swelling, erythema and tenderness over the affected artery. Partial occlusion can present as 'claudication-like' symptoms, whereas total occlusion presents as ischaemia and necrosis of structures supplied by the affected vessel.
4. Define any presence of headache, particularly those described as feeling outside the head.
5. Take a history of visual disturbances and be alerted for any painless loss of vision.
6. Explore any pain in the mouth and throat when chewing, tingling of the tongue and loss of taste.
7. Assess any sleep disturbance.
8. Check history for any scalp tenderness around temporal and occipital arteries.
9. Enquire about any recent history of illness. There is often a distinct prodromal event resembling influenza; viral studies are negative.

Objective findings

- Vital signs – the temperature may be raised.
- Predominant feature is stiffness.
- Affected structures feel tender.
- Shoulder movement may be restricted if diagnosis is delayed.

- Muscular pain is often diffuse and accentuated by movement.
- Muscle strength is unimpaired; however, pain makes interpretation of muscle testing difficult.
- Transient synovitis may occur; however, persistent synovitis is uncommon. Suggests a differential diagnosis, of perhaps rheumatoid arthritis.
- Temporal artery swollen and visible in giant cell arteritis. May have reduced or absent pulsation.
- Headache, jaw pain, (exacerbated by chewing), vertigo, deafness and facial pain may all be symptoms associated with partial occlusion of relevant arteries.
- Fundal examination may show optic disc oedema with retinal haemorrhages (see p. 68 for examination technique).

Differential diagnosis of polymyalgia rheumatica

- Myeloma
- Neoplastic disease
- Joint disease
- Osteoarthritis, particularly of cervical spine
- Rheumatoid arthritis
- Connective tissue disease
- Muscle disease
- Polymyositis
- Myopathy
- Infections
- Dental conditions
- Trigeminal neuralgia
- Sinus disease
- Otological conditions
- Retinal vascular accident.

Plan

Diagnosis is often made as a process of elimination:
- consider differential diagnosis
- order laboratory investigations
- discuss therapeutic interventions.

Investigations

Polymyalgia rheumatica

- ESR is usually significantly raised but not always
- Acute phase proteins are usually raised
- FBC
- Biochemical profile – alkaline phosphate is often raised in polymyalgia rheumatica.
- Bence Jones proteins are raised in myeloma.
- Thyroid function – to exclude hypothyroidism
- Chest X-ray – to exclude tuberculosis
- Rheumatoid factor.

Giant cell arteritis

1. ESR is raised.
2. C reactive protein is raised.
3. FBC – patients may have normocytic anaemia.
4. LFTs – alkaline phosphatase is often raised.

5. Referral for this condition is frequently sought and a temporal artery biopsy is sometimes considered. This is
   - most useful within 24 hours of starting treatment
   - a negative result does not exclude giant cell arteritis
   - a positive result helps to prevent later doubts about diagnosis, particularly if treatment causes complications.

Therapeutic intervention

Treatment with corticosteroids is mandatory for polymyalgia rheumatica and giant cell arteritis to prevent vascular complications, particularly blindness, as well as for rapidly relieving symptoms – improvement noted within 72 hours.

Polymyalgia rheumatica

Initial dose 15–20 mg prednisolone daily. Based upon ESR monitoring levels, a maintenance dose of about 10 mg daily is achieved by 6 months and 5–7.5 mg daily at 1 year. Most patients require treatment for 3–4 years but withdrawal after 2 years is worth attempting. This will depend on the clinical picture.

Giant cell arteritis

Initial dose 20–40 mg daily for 8 weeks. Patients with ocular symptoms may need up to 80 mg daily. Reduce dose by 5 mg every 3–4 weeks until dose is 10 mg daily, then as for polymyalgia rheumatica. A maintenance dose of 3 mg daily may be required. Reoccurrence of symptoms requires an increase in prednisolone dose.

Long-term steroid therapy is a risk factor for osteoporosis. A bone-sparing drug should be prescribed alongside steroid therapy, i.e. HRT for women, bisphosphonates for men.

Patient education

It is important that the patient understands
- the aetiology of the disease, the prognosis and the importance of regular medication
- symptoms associated with the disease and when to consult for follow-up, i.e. any visual disturbance or painless loss of sight
- the importance of review
- the side effects and adverse effects of steroids; also, the importance of not suddenly stopping the drug
- the risk of osteoporosis and the protective and preventative element of treatment – a bone mass density scan (DEXA) may be indicated.

Referral

- Any sudden painless deterioration of vision
- Changes in visual acuity
- Any changes on fundal examination
- Any signs of claudication or ischaemic changes
- No response to treatment.

Complications

- Severe infections and fractures – steroid therapy side effects
- Blindness
- Ischaemia.

Top Tips ✓

1 A good history of the mechanism of injury is invaluable in an injured joint. It will virtually give you the diagnosis provided you have a good understanding of the underlying anatomy. Trauma, no matter how minor, often precedes musculoskeletal problems, so be specific in your history taking; it may have occurred some time ago

2 Ask yourself, is the amount of pain appropriate? If the answer is no, then ask yourself, what am I missing. Beware of referred pain

3 Examining limbs gives you the advantage of having a control (except in exceptional circumstances); it is always helpful to compare the injured with the uninjured. Develop a system of examination: this will help to reduce omissions

4 Giving patients an estimated time for recovery and advice as where to go if things do not settle is a good way of picking up occult problems, reducing anxiety and preventing unnecessary returns

5 Physiotherapists are an extremely valuable resource: don't underuse them

6 Be very sure what you are doing when treating hand injuries. Hands are the means by which we communicate, nourish ourselves, earn a living, etc.; a minor injury not treated correctly can have devastating results

7 For patients with chronic rheumatoid conditions, give due consideration to patients' views of individual symptoms. They have often lived with their illness for a long time and their 'felt' and 'expressed' needs often present a differing scenario to that of the medical profession

8 While the best available clinical evidence from research can inform a diagnosis, the individual's professional experience, conscientiousness and use of such evidence can also exert influence. Not all diagnostic criteria produce a diagnosis, even for rheumatologists

9 Do not focus on one symptom. Asking the right leading questions can reveal underlying behavioural and psychological influences, e.g. poor sleep pattern, learned helplessness

10 Pre-empt prevention strategies that may alleviate a deteriorating condition, e.g. the patient on long-term steroid therapy which may warrant a bone-sparing pharmacological intervention, HRT or a calcium supplement to prevent further osteoporosis.

Glossary

Abduction Used to describe movement of joints, commonly the hip and shoulder, away from the midline sideways (opposite of adduction)

Adduction Used to describe movement of joints, commonly the hip and shoulder, towards the midline sideways (opposite of abduction)

Amenorrhea The absence of menstruation

Anorexia Lack or loss of appetite resulting in the inability to eat

Arthrodesis Fusion of a joint either surgically or by adhesions

Arthropathy Disease or condition affecting the joint

Arthroscopy Examination of the interior of the joint, commonly the knee, using an endoscope. Used for diagnostic reasons, e.g. meniscal damage, or for treatment, e.g. the removal of loose bodies

Compartment syndrome Arterial and nerve compression caused by increasing pressure, often bleeding, in a confined space, e.g. the compartments of the lower leg

Dorsiflexion Movement of the foot up towards the anterior tibia (opposite of plantar flexion)

Effusion Extra fluid in the joint capsule

Eversion Opposite of inversion. A movement at the subtalar joint in the foot. The plantar surface of the foot twists to face more laterally

Extension Straightening of the joint. In the shoulder and hip, extension is moving the limb backwards (opposite of flexion)

Flexion Bending the joint, or decreasing the angle between articulating bones. In the shoulder and hip, flexion is moving the limb upwards and anteriorly (opposite of extension)

Haemarthrosis Blood in a joint

Hyperparathyroidism An abnormal endocrine condition characterised by hyperactivity of any of the four parathyroid glands with an excessive secretion of parathyroid hormone, increased resorption of calcium from the skeletal system and increased absorption of calcium by the kidneys and gastrointestinal system

Hypochromic A red blood cell with less than normal colour. It characterises anaemias associated with decreased synthesis of haemoglobin

Hypogonadism A deficiency in secretory activity of the ovary or testes.

Hypothyroidism A condition characterised by decreased activity of the thyroid gland

Inversion Opposite of eversion. A movement at the subtalar joint in the foot. The plantar surface of the foot twists to face more medially

Lateral A descriptive term to place an aspect of the body which is furthermost away from midline in the saggital plane (see also medial)

Lymphadenopathy Enlarged palpable lymph node

Medial A descriptive term to place an aspect of the body nearest to the midline in the saggital plane. The wrist and forearm are usually described as having radial and ulna borders rather than lateral and medial to avoid confusion caused by pronation and supination

Menopause Strictly the cessation of menses but commonly used to refer to the period of the female climacteric

Metacarpophalangeal joint In the hand, the joints between the metacarpals and the phalanges, i.e. the knuckles

Metastases The process by which malignant tumour cells spread to distant parts of the body

Microcytic Pertaining to abnormally small erythrocytes often occurring in iron-deficiency anaemias

Normochromic Pertaining to a blood cell having a normal colour caused by the presence of an adequate amount of haemoglobin

Normocytic Pertaining to an ordinary, normal, adult red blood cell

Neuropathy Degeneration or inflammation of peripheral nerves

Osteomalacia An abnormal condition of the lamellar bone. It is characterised by a loss of calcification of the matrix, resulting in softening of the bone, accompanied by weakness, fracture, pain, anorexia and weight loss. The condition is a result of an inadequate amount of phosphorus and calcium available in the blood for mineralisation of the bones

Plantar flexion Movement of the foot down towards the ground (opposite of dorsiflexion)

Pronation The rotation of the forearm so that the hand faces downward and backward and the lowering of the medial edge of the foot by turning it outward and through abduction movements in the tarsal and metatarsal joints

Pyarthrosis Pus in a joint

Rheumatic nodule Aggregations of fibroblasts and lymphoid cells that may accumulate in soft tissues and over bony prominences of patients afflicted with rheumatoid arthritis and rheumatic fever

Rotation The rotation of a bone around its axis, i.e. the central axis around which the atlas turns, or the movement of the radius on the ulna during pronation and supination of the hand

Supination Rotation of joints, such as the elbow and wrist, which allows the palm of the hand to turn up

Synovium The inner layer of an articular capsule surrounding a freely moveable joint

Two-point discrimination A test to establish integrity of a sensory nerve, it is described as the smallest distance between two points where the patient can discriminate between being touched by one point or two. An open paperclip is often used. The distance between the ends is measured and then with eyes closed the patient is asked to tell if they are being touched by one end of the clip, or by both. If they are unable to make the discrimination, the distance between the points is widened until the patient is accurate. Comparison with the unaffected limb is important to establish the norm: normal two-point discrimination for the finger tip is 0.5–0.6 cm

References

Akil M, Amos R S 1995 ABC of rheumatology: rheumatic arthritis – 1. Clinical fracture and diagnosis. British Medical Journal 310:587–590.

Belamonte K 1996 Carpal tunnel syndrome. Journal of the American Academy of Nurse Practitioners 8(11):511–517.

Bennet P, Wood P 1968 Population studies of rheumatic diseases. Excerpta Medica 457–458.

BNF 2000 British National Formulary. British Medical Association and Royal Pharmaceutical Society of Great Britain, London.

Brooks S, Potter B, Rainey J 1981 Treatment for partial tears of the lateral ligament of the ankle: prospective trial. British Medical Journal 282:606–607.

Cailliet R 1992 Knee pain and disability, 3rd edn. Davis, Philadelphia.

Carr A, Harnden A 1999 Orthopaedics in primary care. Butterworth-Heinemann, Oxford.

Concannon M 1999 Common hand problems in primary care. Hanley & Belfus, Philadelphia.

Cooper D, Moran C, Everett M, Longstaff P, Riddle W, Hulbert D 1997 Treatment methods for lateral grade 1 ankle injuries. Emergency Nurse 5(4):21–23.

Dandy D, Edwards D 1998 Essential orthopaedics and trauma, 3rd edn. Churchill Livingstone, New York.

Gibson T 1986 Rheumatic diseases: an introduction for medical students. Butterworth, Norwich.

Heininen A, Kannus P, Stevanem H et al 1996 Randomised controlled trial of high impact exercise on selected risk factors for osteoporotic fractures. Lancet 348:1343–1346.

Hill J 1998 Rheumatology nursing: a creative approach. Churchill Livingstone, Hong Kong.

Jones S A, Doherty M 1995 ABC of rheumatology: osteoarthritis. British Medical Journal 310:457–460.

Kaplan J 1999 www.emedicine.com\EMERG\topic\zzl.htm.s\1\01.18.02.

Kennet J 1996 Tubigrip, ibuprofen and home? The nurse's role in the care of patients with ankle sprains in the Accident and Emergency Department. Accident and Emergency Nursing 4(3):121–124.

Le Gallez P 1998 Rheumatology for nurses: patient care. Whurr, London.

Martini F 1998 Fundamentals of anatomy and physiology, 4th edn. Prentice Hall, New Jersey.

Miller J F 1992 Coping with chronic illness overcoming powerlessness, 2nd edn. F A Davies, London.

National Prescribing Centre 1999 Prevention and treatment of osteoporosis. MEREC Bulletin 10(7).

Snaith M 1995 ABC of rheumatology: gout, hyperuricaemia, and crystal arthritis. British Medical Journal 310:521–524.

Stell I, Gransden R 1998 Simple tests for septic bursitis: a comparative study. British Medical Journal 316:1877–1880.

Stiell I, Greenburg G, McKnight R, Nair R, McDowell I, Worthington J 1992 A study to develop clinical decision rules for the use of radiography in acute ankle injuries. Annals of Emergency Medicine 21(4):55–61.

Sturrock R 2000 Gout: Easy to misdiagnose. British Medical Journal 320:132–133.

Swannell A J 1997 Fortnightly review: polymyalgic rheumatica and temporal arteritis diagnosis and management. British Medical Journal 314:1329.

Townheed T, Shea B, Wells G, Hochberg M 1997 Analgesic and non aspirin non steroidal anti-inflammatory drugs for osteoarthritis of the hip. The Cochrane Library Review – 2000, Issue 2.

Wardrope J, English B 1998 Musculo-skeletal problems in emergency medicine. Oxford University Press, Oxford.

Wilson S, Cooke M 1998 Sacred cows to the abattoir. Double bandaging of sprained ankles. British Medical Journal 317:1722–1723.

World Health Organization 1994 Technical Report and Series 843. WHO, Geneva.

Further reading

American Society for Surgery of the Hand 1990a The hand: examination and diagnosis 3rd edn. Churchill Livingstone, New York.

American Society for Surgery of the Hand 1990b The hand: primary care of common problems, 2nd edn. Churchill Livingstone, New York.

13

GENITO URINARY CONDITIONS

Claire Pratt

Key Issues

- Working in primary care provides many opportunities for staff to identify patients of all ages suffering with genito urinary (GU) conditions, as well as those at particular risk of catching a sexually transmitted infection (STI)

- GU conditions are not limited to age, gender or ethnic background, neither is sexual activity

- Patients of all ages can be affected by abnormalities, disease, infection or abuse

- Always remember that GU conditions are not always related to sexual activity

- Good history taking is the key to achieving an accurate diagnosis

- When exploring areas of sexual history, sensitivity and skilled communication are essential (see Chapter 14)

- Older people may be reluctant to discuss sexual issues

Introduction

GU conditions involve the male and female reproductive organs as well as the urinary system. Symptoms can be acute or chronic, with or without recurrences, and vary depending on the causative organism and sight of infection.

This chapter consists of three sections: sexually transmitted infections, urinary problems and male health issues.

Working in primary care provides opportunities for opportunistic screening, health education and assessment for GU conditions. However, many patients, particularly the elderly (Grigg 2000), find questions about their genitalia and sex life embarrassing. It is therefore suggested that when taking a history, the sexual history should not be left until last, as the patient may feel that the professional is embarrassed to discuss such issues. A general health assessment should be undertaken, fol-

lowed by more specific questions assessing for GU problems (see Chapter 14).

❶ Never assume a teenager is too young to have sex. Never assume an elderly person is too old for a sexual relationship and consider signs and symptoms as being related to a sexually transmitted infection. Questions to include can vary: however, they need to be flexible and worded appropriately, taking into account the age and understanding of the patient, with the aim being to help focus the assessment and aid diagnosis. Focused questions can be open or closed and may include the following:

- How is your health?
- Do you have any problems with passing urine?
- Do you ever experience any 'leaking' of your urine?
- Is there anything you would like to discuss concerning sexual issues?
- Are you currently sexually active?
- How has your health/medication affected your sex life?
- Can you tell me about the kind of protection you and your partner use?
- Do you use a condom some of the time, all of the time, or not at all?
- How many partners have been casual relationships?
- Are you currently having sex with more than one partner?
- How many partners have been male. How many have been female?
- Have you ever had a sexually transmitted infection, or been sexually involved with someone with an STI?
- Tell me about the problems you are getting with your libido
- Do you have any concerns about erections, ejaculation, penetration or orgasm?
- Have you ever had, or do you have, a discharge, rash or sores in the genital area? (Letvak & Schoder 1996, Munro & Edwards 1995)
- Could you describe the symptoms you are getting for me?
- Female patients (see Chapter 15) also need to be asked questions about their menstrual cycle, pregnancies, contraception, smoking and previous cervical treatment (Steadman 1998).

The physical examination of women must include the external genitalia, vulva, pubic hair, surrounding skin and perianal area. Internal examination of the vagina includes using a speculum to visualise the cervix, the posterior and anterior fornix and the vaginal walls (see Chapter 15).

The physical examination in men includes an examination of the penis, scrotum, pubic hair, surrounding skin and perianal area (see Male Health Issues section, pp 237–240). Be wary of examination findings that do not support the history and consider abuse: for example, a child with a bruised perineum, or slits around the anus in a child who has supposedly fallen.

SEXUALLY TRANSMITTED INFECTIONS

Acquired immune deficiency syndrome (AIDS)

AIDS and HIV are distinct from each other. AIDS is an illness characterised by a series of severe and potentially fatal opportunistic infections (indicator diseases). It is the end stage of a disease process, beginning with primary human immunodeficiency virus (HIV). HIV is a unique virus, using the CD4 cell surface receptor on the T lymphocytes (helper cells) for attachment, and then infection of cells. This leads to a depletion of T lymphocytes, resulting in increasing immunosuppression. Once depleted, T lymphocytes are inefficient, as specific antibodies are not produced. Both the function and the activities of cytotoxic CD8+ T lymphocytes (killer cells) are impaired. This process can lead to an absolute reduction of helper (T4) cells, which is the most devastating immunological defect for those with AIDS (Pratt 1995).

By December 2000, new guidelines will be requiring all antenatal patients to be routinely offered screening for HIV and hepatitis B (NHSE 1999) with a minimum uptake of 50% achieved.

HIV is transmitted:

- by blood, saliva, cerebrospinal fluid, tears
- sexually by unprotected penetrative anal or vaginal sex
- iatrogenic transmission (Pratt 1995, Steadman 1998).

Amongst children, the most common cause of transmission worldwide is vertical transmission, either in utero or by breast feeding. Homosexual men are the largest infected group and within the group of heterosexual men and women the incidence is rising (Csonka 1990).

Subjective findings

HIV

Signs and symptoms of non-specific illnesses include malaise, fever, headache, visual disturbance, joint pain, skin lesions, night sweats, abdominal pain, diarrhoea, weight loss, cough, chest discomfort and/or shortness of breath.

AIDS

A compromised immune system enables opportunistic infections to become established. Signs and symptoms may include

- memory loss, apathy, impaired concentration
- diarrhoea
- skin lesions
- shortness of breath
- common presentations in children include failure to thrive.

Objective findings

HIV

- Minor opportunitistic infections can include oral candidiasis, oral hairy leucoplakia, herpes zoster, recurrent oral or anogenital herpes simplex, tinea, impetigo and malnutrition (Alder 1998, Steadman 1998)
- In chronic HIV, one-third of patients experience persistent generalised lymphadenopathy, especially in the cervical and axillary nodes and more widespread skin lesions or tumours, e.g. lymphoma or Kaposi's sarcoma (Alder 1998).

AIDS

There are three main organ systems affected by AIDS. These are the respiratory, the gastrointestinal and the central nervous system.

The respiratory system

1. Pneumonia caused by, e.g. *Pneumocystis carinii* or *Aspergillus*. *P. carinii* is one of the commonest life-threatening opportunistic infections in patients with AIDS (Alder 1998).
2. Tuberculosis caused by, e.g. *Mycobacterium tuberculosis*. *M. tuberculosis* infection constitutes a diagnosis. Objective findings include
   - increased respiration rate
   - cough with sputum
   - pyrexia and tachycardia.

The gastrointestinal system

1. oesphagitis caused by, e.g. *Candida albicans*. Oral and oesophageal candidiasis is the commonest cause of dysphagia or retrosternal chest pain. Herpes simplex may cause ulceration of the gut from mouth to anus
2. diarrhoea caused by, e.g. *Giardia lamblia*, *Salmonella*, *Shigella flexneri* or *Cryptosporidium*. Objective findings may therefore include:
3. dehydration due to diarrhoea and malabsorption.

The central nervous system.
Chronic HIV is associated with several syndromes affecting the nervous system. AIDS-related dementia, now referred to as HIV-associated motor cognitive complex, occurs in 10–40% of patients with symptomatic disease (Alder 1998).

Other objective findings include

- skin conditions caused by, e.g. herpes simplex, herpes zoster

- malignancies, e.g. Kaposi's sarcoma, invasive cervical cancer
- lymphadenopathy caused by, e.g. Epstein–Barr virus
- meningitis and encephalitis
- in children findings include failure to thrive, progressive neurological disease, delayed development, secondary bacterial infection (meningitis or pneumonia), lymphoid interstitial pneumonitis and chronic diarrhoea (Csonka 1990).

Assessment

Assessment needs to be divided into HIV screening and diagnosis of the condition.

In the UK it is generally recognised that individuals requesting or being recommended HIV/AIDS testing should be counselled about the implications, and advantages and disadvantages to consenting to a test. If this is undertaken in general practice all information must be recorded in the patient's notes. Insurance companies may request information from such records at a later date. If the counselling is undertaken in a Genital Urinary Medicine (GUM) clinic the information remains confidential to that clinic and insurance companies do not have access to these records. These two options have obvious implications for the patient. Patients therefore need to be advised about the choices available to them. Pre-test counselling includes

- a sexual history
- risk factors are established and discussed
- implications for life insurance and mortgages
- coping strategies are explored
- support networks are discussed
- meanings and implications of negative, equivocal and positive results
- the advantages and disadvantages of testing
- confidentiality is assured (Steadman 1998).

If a patient presents with symptoms suggestive of HIV a full medical and sexual history is needed. Physical examination, including vital signs (temperature, pulse, respiration, blood pressure), an assessment of the respiratory and abdominal system, and neurological assessment for hyperflexia, hypotonia, and frontal release sign is required.

- Consider sputum and stool for culture.
- Serology tests, due to malnutrition and multiorgan involvement, include tests for CD4 viral load, HIV and hepatitis B and C antibodies, full blood count (FBC), liver function tests (LFT), and urea and electrolytes (U&Es).

Plan

Therapeutic intervention

There is no cure for HIV or AIDS at present. Antiviral drugs can help control replication of the virus itself, with most patients being managed on an outpatient basis through the GUM clinics.

Antiretroviral therapy, using a combination of three or four drugs, is important in the prevention of opportunistic infections and other conditions associated with HIV, but they are not without their side effects.

Monitoring was, until recently, performed by counting the CD4 lymphocyte level. More recently, the HIV viral load test has been hailed as a more successful marker (Steadman 1998). Both tests can be undertaken in primary or secondary health care arenas.

Patient education

Psychological support is a vital part of management, often involving a multi-agency approach for the patient, their partners, families and carers.

Indications for referral

Pre-test counselling can be undertaken by GUM clinics if the nurse is not trained and experienced in HIV/AIDS counselling.

Immediate referral to other health care professionals is required if the diagnostic tests confirm HIV, e.g. to secondary care either as an inpatient or to the GUM clinic. Additional investigations may include X-ray and endoscopy. Follow-up: It is essential that a multiagency approach is developed, with networking between such groups as primary and secondary care, GUM clinics, community nurses, social workers, schools, dietetics, physiotherapists and complimentary therapists (Hale & Sutton 1997).

Complications

Complications include multiorgan involvement, pregnancy and allergy to drug regimens (Alder 1998).

Atrophic vaginitis (AV)

This GU condition is due to falling oestrogen levels, causing the vaginal mucosa atrophy. This leads to a decrease in the glycogen available for bacterial metabolism. As a result, lactic acid levels decline, the vaginal pH rises, increasing the woman's susceptibility to infection, and AV can occur (Rutishauser 1994).

With decreasing oestrogen levels, atrophic changes also occur in the lower urinary tract. Women may therefore present with vaginal and/or urinary problems.

Subjective findings

Vaginal

- discomfort
- itching
- dryness
- dyspareunia.

Urinary

- urgency
- frequency
- incontinence (Boulton 1995).

Objective findings

Most commonly, postmenopausal women are affected, but pre- and perimenopausal women may also be symptomatic.

Assessment

A full medical and sexual history is required, including psychological and sociological factors, on how relationships, lifestyle and clothing choice have been adapted. A relaxed atmosphere is essential, as often older women find it difficult to discuss their sexuality and related physical symptoms. Physical examination of the external and internal genitalia using a warm, lubricated speculum, to identify any abnormality, i.e. prolapses, vaginal infection, incontinence is carried out (see Chapter 15).

High vaginal swabs are required if an infection is suspected, plus a urine sample for sugar, microscopy and culture.

Plan

Therapeutic intervention

The sooner that treatment for AV is commenced, the better; this can include
- appropriate systemic or topical hormone replacement therapy (HRT)
- additional infections should be treated, i.e. urinary tract infection
- adequate support and counselling is needed, as treatment often takes many months.

Patient education

This should include advice on
- lubricants to aid intercourse
- avoidance of vaginal deodorants
- pelvic floor muscle exercises may also be appropriate
- psychological support.

Indications for referral

Incontinence and vaginal prolapses require referral to the physiotherapist, continence advisor or gynaecologist.

Complications:

Other related conditions, as discussed above.

Bartholinitis

Bartholinitis or Bartholin's abscess is an infection in the glands of Bartholin and can be a complication of gonorrhoea and *Chlamydia trachomatis* (Csonka 1990).

Subjective findings
- Labia pain
- Labia swelling
- Difficulty in walking.

Objective findings

Physical examination of genitalia shows a tender, roughly spherical, inflammatory mass in the lower third of the labia (Csonka 1990).

Assessment

A full medical and sexual history, including vital signs (temperature, pulse, respirations, and blood pressure). An abscess may form, causing swelling of the vulva area and associated pain (Oates & Csonka 1990). Pressure on the Bartholin's duct may result in pus being expelled.

Plan

Therapeutic intervention

Swabs are required from the duct (if draining), cervix and urethra for microscopy and culture to isolate gonococcus and *Chlamydia trachomatis*.

If caught early, antibiotics, e.g. penicillin, can be successful. Analgesics are often required for pain relief (Oates & Csonka 1990).

Patient education
- Psychological support and explanation of treatment options are required
- Lifestyle and sexual health education.

Indications for referral
- If an abscess has formed, urgent surgical referral for drainage and marsupialisation of the gland is required (Oates & Csonka 1990).
- For diagnosis of coinfections and contact tracing of sexual partners, refer to the GUM clinic.

Complications

(None found in the literature.)

Candidiasis

Genital candidiasis (see Plates 26 and 27) is caused by one of several fungi, the most common being *C. albicans*. This common condition is better known as thrush, and historically as *Monilia* (Steadman 1998).

Subjective findings

In women

Common symptoms in women are
- vulva and vaginal itching, soreness and irritation
- sometimes perianal itch
- thick, whitish, curdy vaginal discharge, with little or no odour
- dysuria and sometimes dyspareunia.

In men

Symptoms are less common, but can include

- itchiness and erythema of glans and subpreputial area of penis
- in circumcised men, red scaly patches on the glans.

Objective findings

Women

- Inflammation of the vulva area, sometimes leading to swollen labia
- Redness and swelling of the vagina, together with white adherent plagues
- Vaginal discharge can be thick and profuse, watery or even absent.

Assessment

❶ A full medical and sexual history, including a physical examination of external and internal sex organs, is required. If a woman has genital warts, always check her cervical smear history. Consider predisposing factors, i.e. antibiotic therapy, pregnancy, diabetes, anaemia, steroid drugs and thyroid disease.

Take high vaginal and vulval swabs in women, and urethral swabs in men for microscopy and culture. If a recurrent problem, consider serology for FBC, ferritin levels for anaemia and urinalysis to exclude diabetes, plus the need to screen partner.

Plan

Therapeutic intervention·

Antifungal treatments (either local or oral) are available over the counter (OTC) or on prescription. Awareness of local sensitivities to drugs is essential and can be obtained from the local public health department.

Alternative therapies

Live natural yoghurt in the vagina helps to restore the lactobacilli levels (Steadman 1998).

Patient education

To help prevent further infections, education can include advice on avoiding
- vaginal deodorants
- bubble baths
- tights and synthetic underwear
- tight trousers or jeans
- general sexual health issues
- consider treating male partner
- reassure patients this is not a true STI and that it does not ascend into the uterus and pelvis causing pelvic inflammatory disease, infertility or blocked tubes.

Indications for referral

If the diagnosis is in doubt, or other STIs are suspected, refer to the GUM clinic.

Complications

(None found in the literature.)

Chlamydia trachomatis and pelvic inflammatory disease (PID)

Chlamydia trachomatis is one of the most prevalent, treatable STIs in the United Kingdom (Boag & Kelly 1998), affecting both genders and all ages. The socio-demographic factor most strongly associated with *Chlamydia* infection is young age, with prevalence being at its highest amongst sexually active adolescent girls. It causes a wide range of diseases. In particular, *Chlamydia* is a major cause of PID in women. PID is a syndrome resulting from the spread of ascending micro organisms to the endrometrium and fallopian tubes (CDCP 1997).

However, symptomatic *Chlamydia* infection in males and females is the exception rather than the rule, thus raising questions for the need for a national screening service. *Chlamydia* is neither a true bacteria nor a true virus but appears to show characteristics of both and appears to infect only ciliated, columnar or cuboidal epithelium; hence its preference for the
- conjunctiva
- endocervix
- urethra
- rectum
- endometrium
- fallopian tubes (Steadman 1998).

Subjective findings

In women

- Often asymptomatic
- Vaginal discharge (green/yellow)
- Dysuria and frequency
- Intermenstrual bleeding, with oral contraceptive pill
- Painful, swollen labia with abscess
- Low abdominal pain, malaise, dyspareunia, vaginal discharge
- Infertility.

In men

- Asymptomatic
- Discharge from urethra
- Dysuria
- Unilateral scrotal pain, swelling and tenderness
- Fever
- Infertility.

In neonate

- Unilateral or bilateral discharging, red, sore eye
- Chest infection at 1–3 months of age.

Objective findings

In women

- Hypertrophic ectopine cervix (ectopy oedematous, congested and bleeds on contact)
- Bartholinitis
- Fever, abdominal tenderness, cervical motion tenderness, mucopurulent discharge.

In men

- Nongonococcal urethritis typically 1–3 weeks after exposure
- Unilateral epididymitis.

In neonate

- Conjunctivitis between first and third week following delivery
- Pneumonia at 1–3 months of age
- Less commonly, otitis media, bronchiolitis and gastroenteritis (Ferreira 1997).

In child

- Sexual abuse needs to be considered when a child presents with this organism as no other mode of transport is understood.

Assessment

1. PV exam, including the Valsalva's manoeuvre, to assess cervical tenderness, vaginal bleeding, friable os (see Chapter 15)
2. Endocervical swabs for gonorrhoea into standard transport medium for culture, followed by endocervical swab for *Chlamydia*
3. Urethral swab taken 4 hours after voiding, passing swab 2–4 cm into the urethra to obtain an adequate sample
4. Urine: always suspect *Chlamydia* in women if sterile pyuria reported on a midstream specimen of urine (MSU) (Hay 1998)
5. Abdominal examination, if symptoms of low abdominal pain (see Chapter 15)
6. Samples for microscopy include urethral, urine, endocervical and eye, depending on symptoms.

Plan

Therapeutic intervention

Antibiotics for *Chlamydia* infections include broad-spectrum antibacterial drugs, depending on local patterns of sensitivity. If PID or gonorrhoea are diagnosed in addition to *Chlamydia*, treatment regimes require additional antibiotics (Hay 1998). Specific detail can be obtained from the local public health department.

Patient education

- Explanation of disease and treatment
- Importance of contacting partners
- Refrain from intercourse during antimicrobial therapy
- How to lessen reinfection rate, including health education on condom use
- Advise bed rest if acute PID
- Education to pregnant mums as regards *Chlamydia* infections in babies' eyes and need for follow-up at 3 months

Indications for referral

- Differential diagnosis of PID is ectopic pregnancy or appendicitis
- Pregnancy (urine sample should be obtained to exclude pregnancy)
- If acute abdominal pain, refer to GP or district general hospital as an emergency
- If *Chlamydia* positive, refer to GUM clinic for further screening and contact tracing
- Suspected child abuse requires immediate referral to a paediatrician or to social services.

Complications (see Plate 28)

Complications of *Chlamydia* are
- one of the major causes of PID, chronic pain, female infertility, ectopic pregnancy, spontaneous abortion, and stillbirth, postpartum endometriosis (Ferreira 1997)
- responsible for a high proportion of non-specific urethritis and
- unexplained male infertility (Greendale et al 1993)
- epididymitis, orchitis and prostatitis (Hay 1998)
- neonatal pneumonia can lead to chronic lung disease (Ferreira 1997)
- rarely, Reiter's syndrome of sexually acquired reactive arthritis (Hay 1998).

Folliculitis

Folliculitis is infection of the hair follicles, on or near the genitals.

Subjective findings

- Multiple painful lesions are found on the genitals (Alder 1998).

Objective findings

- White papules on the genitals, which may burst, leaving a small ulcer
- Enlarged inguinal lymph nodes.

Assessment

A full medical and sexual history is required to exclude other causes of ulceration. Diagnosis will depend on the clinical appearance. For female genital examination, see Chapter 15; for male genital examination, see p. 237.

Plan

Therapeutic intervention

If papules become infected, antibiotics are required and may include a combination of sulphonamides and trimethoprim. However, regard for your local policy on drug sensitivity is essential. Details can be obtained from your local Public Health Office.

Patient education

- Saline baths may relieve symptoms.

Indications for referral

Refer to the GUM clinic if other causes of ulceration are suspected, i.e. herpes simplex.

Complications

(None found in the literature.)

Genital warts (condylomata acuminata)

Genital warts (GWs) are caused by the human papillomaviruses (HPV), of which there are 70 types (Clarke 1998). ❶ If a man has genital warts, consider female partner as regards cervical smear screening. The wart virus flourishes in warm moist conditions, particularly if a discharge or other infection is present (Alder 1998). HPV type 1, 2, 3 and 4 are particularly associated with skin warts in adults (Clarke 1998), where as 90% of GWs are caused by HPV types 6 and 11. HPV types 6, 11, 16, 18, 31, 33 and 35 are linked with intraepithelial cervical neoplasia and cervical cancer (Alder 1998). Up to 70% of mild abnormalities caused by these types return to normal, with many patients suffering numerous ongoing recurrences (Husband 1997). The disease can progress to severe abnormalities or neoplastic change after 1–4 years (Steadman 1998).

Subjective findings

Women (see Plate 29)

- Painless warts occurring at fourchette, labia minora, clitoris, labia majora, perianal area, vagina, cervix, urethra (and, uncommonly, in the mouth)
- Itching as wart develops
- Bleeding after intercourse.

Men (see Plate 30)

- Often symptomless warts, occurring on the coronal sulcus, frenum, prepuce, shaft of penis, scrotum, anal and perianal areas, urethra, mouth
- Dysuria
- Urethral discharge
- Urethral bleeding.

Children

- Vulva and perianal warts are more common than penile warts.
- Controversy surrounds the relative risk of transmission by a variety of means in children, including autoinoculation, heteroinoculation, vertical transmission, fomite spread from underwear infected by an adult or sexual transmission (Clarke 1998).
- Sexual abuse must be considered, especially if anogenital warts (AGW) are present; however, their presence is not proof of abuse (Oriel 1988).
- Screening for other STIs may be required.

- HPV 1, 2, 3 and 4 are associated with skin warts in adults. In children they are associated with skin and AGW and could, therefore, be transmitted by a variety of routes (Clarke 1998).

Objective findings

- Warts around the genital area
- Urethral discharge
- Vaginal discharge.

Assessment

A full medical and sexual history is required, including a cervical smear history for female patients; genital examination includes speculum examination in women. The consultation must be adapted according to whether a child or adult is being examined. Differential diagnosis includes condylomata latum, molluscum contagiosum, sebaceous cyst or tumours (Alder 1998).

Plan

Therapeutic intervention

Refer adults to the GUM clinic where diagnosis is made by painting 3–5% acetic acid onto the warts. Female patients should always be asked about the possibility of pregnancy before any treatment is commenced, and advised not to become pregnant while undergoing treatment. Prescription only medication, podophyllin paint or podophyllotoxin (both contraindicated in pregnancy) is applied by specialist nurses. Other treatments include chemotherapy, electrocautery, 5-fluorouracil, laser or surgical excision.

Response to treatment is affected by:

- the number and size of warts
- the site and length of time present and
- hormonal factors (i.e. pregnancy).

Patient education

Psychological support is important, as
- patients often show high levels of anxiety about their condition
- treatment takes many weeks requiring patients to take time off work
- anxiety can be reduced by GPs and nurses giving accurate information about the disease and by the local GUM clinic (Chandler 1996).
  Advice is needed on
- encourage smoking/passive smoking cessation to reduce risk of cervical neoplasm
- annual cervical smear to monitor for the presence of neoplastic changes
- safe sex: male condoms do not provide complete protection against genital warts
- teach regular vulva self-examination (see Chapter 15).

Indications for referral

- Presence of GWs or diagnosis of wart virus on cervical screening is an indication for referral to the GUM clinic; for screening of other STI, contact tracing and treatments.

■ Children must be referred to GP.

Complications

HIV and other immunodeficiency conditions, including pregnancy, lessen the individual's ability to control the virus. During pregnancy, GWs should be closely monitored as they can grow rapidly and become macerated with the development of secondary infection; they should be treated accordingly.

Laryngeal papillomatosis can occur in late infancy and is a significant condition as it may lead to malignancy.

A rare complication of AGW, causing extensive tissue damage, is a tumour called giant condylomata (Oriel & Walker 1990).

Gonorrhoea

Gonorrhoea is a highly infectious venereal disease that affects the lower genital tract in both sexes (Oates & Csonka 1990). There is a statutory requirement to report the infection to the Centre for Disease Surveillance and Control. The specific aetiological agent of gonorrhoea is *Neisseria gonorrhoeae*. The bacteria attacks mucous membrane, has a predilection for columnar epithelium, causing inflammation, and commonly affects the urethra, cervix, rectum and oropharynx; rarely, it affects the blood, skin, joints and conjunctiva.

Transmission occurs by sexual intercourse or close physical contact, and less commonly by autoinoculation or heteroinoculation from genital to eye, or by vertical transmission (Handy 1997).

Subjective findings

Women

Up to 40% may be asymptomatic; others may report
■ vaginal discharge, soreness and or itching
■ dysuria and frequency
■ urethral discharge
■ abdominal pain and backache
■ swollen painful labia due to bartholinitis
■ intermenstrual bleeding
■ locally painful and discharging eye, often unilateral.

Men

A small proportion of men with gonorrhoea are asymptomatic. Others may complain of various symptoms, depending on the site of infection:
■ urethral discharge, often profuse, purulent and yellow/green
■ dysuria, often described as 'like trying to pass broken glass'
■ perianal itch, soreness and discharge
■ sore throat
■ locally painful and discharging eye, often unilateral.

Infants and children

■ Sticky eyes at birth or within 21 days of birth
■ Stained underwear due to discharge
■ Penile discharge
■ Local soreness, itching and dysuria.

Objective findings

Women

■ Normal cervix or cervicitis may be noted
■ Vaginal discharge (yellow/green)
■ Urethral discharge
■ Bartholinits.

Men

■ Urethral discharge, often profuse, purulent and yellow/green
■ Swollen meatus
■ Inflamed inguinal lymph nodes
■ Proctoscopy often shows a reddened appearance of the mucous membrane
■ Throat examination may show no abnormality, mild tonsillitis or pharyngitis
■ Oedematous eyelid, intensely inflamed reddened conjunctiva, yellow purulent discharge.

Children

■ Reddened vulva with purulent discharge.

Assessment

Careful sexual history taking should include sensitive questioning to determine whether there are any oral or anal symptoms. It is important to note the incubation period is 3–7 days after exposure to infection, but symptoms may present 1–14 days after exposure. Gonorrhoea strains originating in Africa, Southeast Asia and the Caribbean may be resistant to penicillin; therefore, the sexual history should include a history of any recent foreign travel.

Rapid and accurate diagnosis is of great importance, as gonorrhoea is highly infectious. Correct specimen collection and transportation to the laboratory is essential.

Female

1. The combination of urethritis and cervicitis is suggestive of gonorrhoea.
2. Cervical and urethral swab are required (Handy 1997). Reported figures for detecting gonorrhoea from the cervix vary from 50 to 65% (Oates & Csonka 1990) to 66.7% (Edwards & Dockerty 1993).
3. Speculum, warmed with warm water only, should be used, as exploration creams have been shown to kill gonococci (Mardh & Danielsson 1990).
4. The urethra may need milking by placing one finger in the vagina and stroking the urethra upwards and outwards to encourage the expulsion of exudate (Handy 1997).

Male

1. Urethral swab is sent for microscopy. Figures for detecting gonococci range from 91.7% to 98% of infections.
2. The patient should not have passed urine for 2 hours before the examination (Steadman 1998)
3. Rectal, throat and urethra swabs are required from homosexual men (Handy 1997).

Children

1. Girls are more frequently affected than boys
2. Transmission of vulvovaginal infection can be from nonsexual contact with parents, from shared flannels and towels (Oates & Csonka 1990)
3. Sexual abuse must be considered in prepubertal children (Gutman & Wilfert 1990)
4. Urethral gonococcal infection in boys is indicative of sexual activity (Steadman 1998).

Plan

Therapeutic intervention

The drug of choice, usually consisting of the broad-spectrum antibiotics, will depend on a number of factors, i.e. presence of coinfections, pregnancy, age, site of infection, drug resistance, drug allergy, cost and ease of administration (Oates & Csonka 1990) plus a recent history of foreign travel.

Patient education

- Health education and safer sex advice is essential to prevent reinfection.
- Social and cultural factors are important considerations for health advisers and need to be taken into account when health education is being discussed.
- Follow-up appointments for repeat swabs are essential to prevent further spread or reinfection of gonorrhoea.

Indications for referral

- For accurate specimen collection, diagnosis of coinfections and contact tracing, refer to the GUM clinic.

Complications

In women

- PID, peritonitis, endometriosis, bartholinitis or perihepatitis (Fitz-Hugh–Curtis syndrome) (Steadman 1998).

In pregnant women

- Premature birth or low birth weight babies.

In men

- Epididymitis, cowperitis and tysonitis, prostatitis, urethral stricture and periurethral abscess.

In children

- Corneal ulceration and blindness.

Herpes genitalis

Genital herpes (GH) is caused by herpes simplex virus 1 and herpes simplex virus 2. Until recently it was believed that genital herpes was usually caused by HSV 2 and herpes on the mouth was caused by HSV 1. More recently, it has been demonstrated that genital herpes can be caused by HSV 1 and HSV 2 (Steadman 1998). GH is transmitted

- sexually
- by vertical transmission
- by autoinfection
- with asymptomatic viral shedding being the most frequent mode of transmission between sexual partners (Chard 1998).

Subjective findings

Findings differ for primary and recurrent attacks.

Primary attack

Symptoms of infection with HSV 2 are milder if the individual has a history of HSV 1 infection. Lesions begin with small vesicles, which can join to form large ulcerative legions after about 5 days. The lesions crust over and eventually resolve within 2–4 weeks. They can be extremely painful.

Primary infection may present as a severe illness (Chard 1998) and be accompanied in women by

- symptomatic or asymptomatic genital blisters
- itching
- vaginal discharge
- pain
- dysuria
- oedema.

In both sexes, a primary infection may be accompanied by flu-like symptoms (fever, malaise, myalgia), backache, dysuria, impotence, sacral anaesthesia, urinary retention, constipation, and swollen lymph glands (Steadman 1998).

Gay men who practice anal intercourse may complain of rectal pain.

Recurrent attacks

Recurrent attacks are

- less painful
- with vesicles appearing in only one area at a time.

Factors that appear to trigger outbreaks include stress, fatigue, sunlight, sexual intercourse, menstruation and conditions that compromise the immune system. Patients often experience prodromal symptoms. Around 50% of individuals never experience a recurrence (Chard 1998).

Objective findings

Vesicles, ulcers or crusty lesions are noticed in men and women.

Women

- Vulva

- Vagina
- Cervix
- Perianal area
- Inner thighs.

Men (see Plate 31)

- Lesions on shaft of penis
- Lesions on glans
- Urethra, causing dysuria
- Anal and perianal areas
- Non-specific urethritis.

Assessment

- A full medical and sexual history, including a detailed history to determine the frequency and severity of the attacks, plus a physical examination (see Chapter 15, and male genital examination p. 237).
- Clinical diagnosis must be confirmed by viral culture of swabs from the blisters
- Goggles should be worn when incising blisters (Chard 1998)
- Referral to the GUM clinic for sampling and investigation of coinfections
- Speculum examination (if not too painful) is required for HSV culture.

Plan

Therapeutic intervention

It is important to commence treatment promptly, especially with a primary attack. Oral antiviral agents are the drugs of choice for both primary and recurrent attacks. The specific regime will depend on local policy. Analgesia may also be needed to alleviate painful symptoms.

Patient education

GH is an infection often associated with stigma and embarrassment. Psychosocial, psychosexual and psychological disturbances associated with frequent outbreaks of herpes may occur (Chard 1998). Its chronic unpredictable nature may have a profound psychological effect on some individuals (Davkvist & Wahlin 1995), which can be made worse by the fact that there is no cure for the infection.

To achieve maximum physical and psychological health gains, care needs to include

- psychological care
- accurate information (verbal, written and telephone help lines)
- advice on relieving symptoms, including dysuria, i.e. bathing three or four times a day
- partners should be encouraged to attend for screening
- homeopathic remedies may relieve symptoms in recurrent attacks (Chard 1998)
- counselling as regards future sexual relationships

- psycho-educational interventions on sexual health risk in young adults (see Chapter 14) have been shown to improve knowledge and the use of condoms and spermacides (Swanson et al 1999).

Indications for referral

- Acute retention of urine due to sacral nerve involvement requires hospital admission
- Primary attack at the time of delivery requires Caesarean section to be considered.

Complications

GH can cause proctititis, herpetic pharyngitis, meningitis, herpes encephalitis and eczema herpeticum.

In immunocompromised individuals, anogenital herpes can cause viraemia.

In pregnancy, transmission of the virus, during the passage through the birth canal, can be life threatening; hence, the need for Caesarean section. Risk of preterm delivery is increased if the first episode of GH is acquired in pregnancy (Chard 1998). It was thought that HSV 2 and cervical cancer were linked; thus, women were recommended to have regular smears (Steadman 1998), but the HPV (not HSV) virus is now thought to be responsible (Posner 1998). Therefore, women are no longer referred for more regular smear tests.

Nongonococcal urethritis (NGU)

NGU, a condition resulting in inflammation of the male urethra has many causative agents, not all of which are sexually transmitted. NGU, which is one of the commonest STIs in men in the UK, is also known as non-specific urethritis and occurs more commonly in heterosexual than in homosexual men. Peak incidence is in the 20–24 age group; men are more often Caucasian, married and of a higher socioeconomic group.

Causes include *Chlamydia trachomatis, Ureaplasma urealyticum, Trichomonas vaginalis, Mycoplasma genitalium*, herpes simplex, urinary tract infections, allergies, warts and trauma (Handy 1997).

Subjective findings

- Often asymptomatic
- Urethral discharge, sometimes only first thing in the morning
- Dysuria, sometimes only first thing in the morning
- Mild penile irritation or discomfort.

Objective findings

- May be recurrent
- Oedematous end of penis
- Variable degrees of pyuria
- Often suspected on clinical grounds and confirmed by microscopy (Csonka 1990).

Assessment

A physical examination (see Chapter 15, and male genital examination p. 237), and a detailed history of events prior to the infection, aids diagnosis. Various factors may be relevant:

- previous history of NGU
- new partner or resumed intercourse with untreated partner
- recent alcoholic or sexual excess
- chronic prostatitis.

NGU is difficult to diagnose because of its multifaceted nature. Diagnosis is by urine and urethral samples for microscopy, at least 2 hours after voiding. If symptoms only occur early in the morning, swabs will need to be done early in the day, prior to voiding. Investigations should include sampling for *Chlamydia* and *Neisseria gonorrhoea*.

Plan

Therapeutic intervention

Treatment will depend on the bacterial cause of NGU, with reference to local policy on drug sensitivity.

Patient education

- If untreated, symptoms usually resolve within weeks, but reoccur later
- Pharmacological management is only moderately effective
- Drug management will depend on the causative agent
- Compliance of treatment is important
- Follow-up appointment 1 week after commencing treatment (Csonka 1990).
  Advice should also include issues on:
- basic hygiene
- avoidance of lotions which may irritate
- the use of condoms.

Indications for referral

Recent work has shown that many men with NGU self-treat with their own and other's medication before attending GUM clinics (Carlyon & Barton 1995), which makes accurate diagnosis, treatment and contact tracing difficult. Female partners should be contacted and screened for *Chlamydia* and treated simultaneously.

Complications

Complications are rare, but include

- periurethral abscess, tysonitis and abscess formation of the Cowper's gland
- acute epididymitis, prostatitis and urethral stricture may result
- Reiter's disease is a systemic complication
- persistence and reoccurrence may be part of its natural history, as NGU is not always curable (Handy 1997).

Trichomonas vaginalis (TV)

This is the most common nonviral sexually transmitted infection (Petrin et al 1998) and is often described as a concurrent STI, being diagnosed in association with other infections, i.e. *Chlamydia, Candida* or gonorrhoea. Therefore the incubation period is difficult to gauge, but generally occurs between 3 and 21 days (Csonka 1990). Women are more commonly affected than men, as the male carriage of TV may be transient (Csonka 1990). There appears to be no evidence of sexual transmission between homosexual men or women.

TV is a motile protozoan. Recent research by Cohen et al (1997) shows that TV infections may assist the transmission of HIV 1.

Subjective findings

Women (see Plate 32)

- Asymptomatic
- Vaginal discharge
- Vulvovaginal soreness and itching
- Cystitis-like symptoms
- Worsening of symptoms during and after menstruation.

  Less commonly, offensive vaginal discharge, dyspareunia, dysuria, and low abdominal discomfort are symptoms (Davis 1998).

Men

- Asymptomatic
- Discharge from penis
- Dysuria or frequency
- Testicular pain or tenderness
- Low abdominal pain.

Objective findings

In women

- Excessive vaginal discharge
- Frothy green/yellow vaginal discharge
- Inflamed vaginal walls
- Strawberry appearance of cervix and vaginal walls
- Excoriation of surrounding skin (Csonka 1990).

In men

- Nongonococcal urethritis.

Assessment

A careful medical and sexual history should be taken plus a genital examination (see Chapter 15; for male genital examination, p. 237). A high-risk profile for TV would be similar to other STIs, including

1. a recent change in sexual partner
2. multiple sexual partners
3. recurrent symptoms
4. symptoms in partner
5. general symptoms, i.e. dysuria, dyspareunia, abdominal pain, menstrual problems (Davis 1998).

6. speculum examination to obtain vaginal, cervix and posterior fornix swabs for microscopy and culture
7. urethral swabs in women and men (however, urethral or urinary samples in men are often inconclusive)
8. TV may be diagnosed in men through other STIs, i.e. nongonococcal urethritis (Phillips et al 1988).

Plan

Therapeutic intervention

The prescribing of antibacterial drugs needs to follow local policy on drug sensitivity. Information can be obtained on local patterns from public health departments. Follow-up testing at 7 and 30 days to test for efficacy of treatment is necessary (Csonka 1990).

Patient education

Advice should include the following:
- avoidance of intercourse until the infection has been treated successfully
- contact tracing and screening for other STIs is important, with male partners of infected women being treated to reduce the risk of reinfection and the spread of infection (Csonka 1990)
- education on safer sex and condom use.

Indication for referral

- Contact tracing and investigation of coinfections requires referral to the GUM clinic.

Complications

- Chronic untreated TV may lead to cervical malignancy (however, TV and cervical cancer have not been controlled for the presence of the human wart virus, which could be a more likely cause of cervical cancer (Csonka 1990)).

URINARY CONDITIONS

Enuresis

Enuresis is nocturnal urinary incontinence, or bedwetting, without organic disease, after the age when bladder control is usually attained. Doley (1977) defined enuresis as 'persistent wetting occurring during sleep in the absence of neurological or urological pathology'. It occurs most often in children, but may continue into adulthood (White 1997). It is important to make the distinction between day and night-time incontinence, as the latter is not normally associated with urinary dysfunction. Wetting may also occur during the day when the person is asleep.

For children to attain continence they need to have attained the appropriate level of physiological maturity, communication skills, mobility and social skills (Lukeman 1997). Most children become dry between 18 and 36 months old, with night-time dryness occurring later.

Subjective findings

1. Primary nocturnal enuresis:
   - child has never been dry.
2. Secondary nocturnal enuresis:
   - loss of control after a significant period of being dry, i.e. 12 months or more, beyond the age of 3 years
   - nocturnal enuresis in adolescence and adulthood.
3. Diurnal enuresis (day wetting):
   - giggling/sneezing incontinence
   - urinary tract infection.

Objective findings

- Family tensions, leading to behavioural changes
- Gender: twice as many boys as girls over 5 years are enuretic
- An equal number of boys and girls are enuretic between the ages of 13 and 15 years.

Assessment

A thorough assessment is required to understand the factors contributing to enuresis. History taking can be considered under four headings: physical factors, child factors, family factors and the history of the problem (Lukeman 1997).

Physical factors

1. Genetic factors might include a family history of bedwetting, possibly as a result of attitudes and interactions within the family.
2. Bladder capacity and function: a small bladder capacity along with a delay in development of speech and language may slow down the process of bladder control in some children (Shaffer 1994).
3. Urinary tract abnormalities: referral for a medical opinion is necessary, to exclude rare conditions, if diurnal enuresis occurs with or without nocturnal enuresis.
4. Urinary tract infection and diabetes needs to be considered, particularly when there is an onset of secondary enuresis.
5. Sleep patterns: enuretic and nonenuretic children do not have differing sleep patterns. Wetting seems to occur approximately 4 hours after onset of sleep or a previous wetting incident.

Child factors

1. Chronological age of the child must be assessed in relation to parental/carer expectations. This is more relevant to younger children.
2. Physical development: disability in the young, or a history of disability in the older child that has led to a dysfunctional learned pattern can cause enuresis.
3. Cognitive development: developmental delay affecting learning can slow down the process of learned continence.
4. Emotional/social factors: assessment needs to include whether emotional factors are causing the

wetting or is the wetting causing emotional factors? This may be particularly important in secondary enuresis.

5. Behavioural: this includes observing the child's self-esteem, his parents/carers, and the school for indications of behavioural problems causing enuresis.
6. The child's understanding of the problem. Lukeman (1997) believes this is very important in the treatment of children who have resisted any form of intervention. Butler et al (1990) found that when children understand the psychological outcomes of their enuresis they are more likely to be treated successfully.

Family factors

1. Family history (see above).
2. Environmental factors: poor housing conditions and fear of the dark may be obstacles to children reaching the toilet.
3. Stressful life events: Jarvelin et al (1990) found separation and divorce increased the risk of nocturnal enuresis in children. This may be due to a change or deterioration in housing conditions or to the psychological effect.
4. Family attitudes and expectations: if maternal tolerance was high to the problem of enuresis, then there is little motivation to seek treatment (Morgan & Young 1975). A mother who has low tolerance to the problem often seeks help sooner, but her anger can lead to a withdrawal from treatment. In both situations, children may feel unsupported.
5. Parent/child relationship: child abuse needs to be considered. Although enuresis alone is not necessarily an indication of child abuse, children are at increased risk of abuse when there are negative attitudes towards them (Brown et al 1988). Parents may also not seek treatment if they have a need or unwillingness to see their child as an independent individual.

History of the problem

Questions that need to be asked include:
- When has the situation been at its best or worst?
- Is it worse with particular situations/events/days of the week?
- What methods of treatment or management have been tried already?
- What methods have worked or not worked?
- How does the situation compare with 6 or 12 months ago?
- MSU for microscopy and culture, and glucose.

Plan

Therapeutic intervention

Drugs can be used when nonpharmacological methods have been unsuccessful. The two main types of medication available are (Smith 1997) antidiuretic hormones and tricyclic antidepressants.

Antidiuretic hormones. However, note that
- the relapse rate on withdrawal is high
- the patient must be monitored for fluid overload
- the drug should be withdrawn for 1 week every 3 months to assess the situation (BNF 1998).

Tricyclic antidepressants (from 7 years of age). These drugs inhibit micturitions; however, note that
- the relapse rate on withdrawal of the drug is also high
- they are useful for short periods of management, i.e. holidays (BNF 1998).

Patient education

- Houts et al (1994) reviewed the literature on the treatment of children with enuresis and found that psychological support was often more effective than pharmacological management, especially if the follow-up care was on a regular basis and was on a longer basis
- Involvement of the whole family/carer on general issues, including practical measures to minimise distress within the family, i.e. using mattress covers, laundry facilities, personal hygiene, adequate night-time lighting
- Parents and children are asked to record baseline measurements of wet and dry nights or days for 2 weeks to obtain an accurate picture and to monitor progress once treatment starts
- Fluid intake should not be reduced to avoid wetting
- Other nonpharmacological management may depend on the age of the child and can include psychological support, i.e. star charts and reward systems, and enuresis alarms
- Support groups can be helpful, e.g. Enuresis Resource and Information Centre (ERIC).

Indication for referral

- Day wetting is frequent
- Nonpharmacological management has proved unsuccessful or
- If sexual abuse is a concern, medical referral is indicated
- Department of Social Services may help with the cost of equipment.
  Multiprofessional involvement may include:
- health visitor, school nurse, continence advisor, social worker, psychologist
- more difficult cases are referred to paediatricians, child psychiatrists or psychotherapists.

Complications

The majority of children who are enuretic do not suffer from emotional or behavioural problems. However, normal socialisation is often affected (e.g. children and adolescents do not sleep away from home with friends or relatives), thus affecting the quality of life of the patient, their families and friends.

Incontinence of urine

Continence of urine is the ability to store urine in the bladder and to excrete voluntarily where and when it is socially appropriate. Incontinence is seen as a deviation from this (White 1997). It affects people of all ages (see Chapter 18), from all social and cultural backgrounds. Over the last decade national incontinence days, public advertising of incontinence products and a greater political awareness have all contributed to incontinence becoming less of a taboo subject. A small study found that GPs find it a difficult problem to treat and often avoid dealing with the problem of incontinence in women (Grealish & O'Dowd 1998). Embarrassment, shame, anger, guilt and frustration are emotions often felt by those affected. Lifestyles can be profoundly affected and individuals are often reluctant to admit there is a problem.

Subjective findings

Individuals or their carers/partners may complain of a variety of symptoms, including
- urinary leakage on exercise
- 'toilet seeking' when in town
- long distance journeys being broken by frequent toilet stops
- sore, chapped skin due to urine leakage
- offensive odour.

Objective findings

Causes of incontinence are varied and can include physical or mental disability, trauma, chronic disease, neurological dysfunction, obesity, childbirth or be as a result of hormone depletion postmenopausal.

Assessment

Time and privacy are needed, as often it is the first time the individual has admitted to the problem. The use of language is particularly important in assessing incontinence, as some people will deny being 'incontinent' but will admit to 'leaking' or 'being caught short'.

Careful questioning is needed to determine which of the six categories of incontinence the symptoms fall within:
- genuine stress incontinence
- urge incontinence
- overflow incontinence
- reflex incontinence
- continuous incontinence and
- functional incontinence (Grimshaw 1998).
  Useful questions (Getliffe & Dolman 1997) include
- When did the problem begin and how has it changed over time?
- How much urine is lost and how often?
- What events precipitate the loss? i.e. exercise, coughing, getting up from a chair?
- Are there any urinary symptoms, e.g. frequency, sensation of not emptying bladder, nocturia, difficulty in initiating flow, pain on micturition, postmicturition dribbling?
- What is the usual pattern of voiding, including day and night frequency?
- Are there any current coping strategies, e.g. use of pads, not going out?

In addition,
- a urine sample should be obtained for glucose, microscopy and culture
- abdominal examination may reveal a distended bladder
- a rectal examination may be required to assess for constipation or faecal impaction
- women should undergo an internal physical examination to assess for prolapses and pelvic floor muscle tone (see Chapter 15)
- history taking should include any surgery to the prostate and examination of the prostate gland (see male genital examination p. 237).

Assessment should include a visual observation of movement of the vaginal introitus during pelvic floor movement. A subjective assessment of pelvic floor movement can be made by placing a gloved and lubricated index and middle finger into the patient's vagina and asking them to demonstrate pelvic floor contraction (Rigby 1999). The Oxford scale of muscle strength (Barger & Woolner 1995), an identified graded system, an integral part of this assessment, is used by experienced clinicians; the scale is 0= nil, 1= flicker, 2=weak, 3= moderate, 4= good and 5= strong muscle movement.

Plan

Therapeutic intervention

Treatment will depend on the findings of the assessment. Nonpharmacological interventions including patient education, referral to continence advisors may be commenced as a first-line approach (see below and also Chapter 18).

Patient education

1. A multidisciplinary team approach is often required (see referral list below).
2. Health education on diet to reduce obesity and constipation.
3. Women may need advice and education on pelvic floor muscle exercises.
4. For women with a prolapse, education on lifting may be helpful.
5. A number of new devices are available through the continence specialist nurses, e.g. weighted vaginal cones to encourage pelvic floor exercises, stimulation techniques to stimulate muscle fibres, or 'Femassist', a device sits by suction over the urethra, and can be worn by women who experience stress incontinence during exercise.
6. Support groups can be beneficial by providing psychological support.

Medication

- Antimuscarinic drugs are used to treat urinary frequency. They help to increase the bladder capacity by diminishing the detrusor contractions. Side effects include dry mouth, blurred vision and the drugs may precipitate glaucoma. Care should be taken in the elderly.
- Tricyclic antidepressants are sometimes effective because of their antimuscarinic properties
- Antibiotics are indicated if urinary frequency or incontinence is due to a urinary tract infection (see below)
- Hormone replacement therapy (HRT) can be considered for menopausal and postmenopausal women.

Indication for referral

Referral to the continence advisor, district nurse, physiotherapist, GP or urologist may be required (Getliffe & Dolman 1997) if

- specialist advice and support is needed
- the assessment is inconclusive
- a complex problem is indicated
- potential risks to health, e.g. haematuria, is highlighted
- further investigations, i.e. cystoscopy, ultrasound scan, urodynamic assessment, prostate biopsy are required
- referral to gynaecologist for, i.e. repair of vaginal prolapse.

Complications

Complications can include biological, psychological and social factors.

Urinary tract infections (UTI), cystitis, pyelonephritis

A UTI is an infection of the upper renal tract (kidneys) or the bladder and is usually caused by Gram-negative bacteria. Women are more often affected than men. Cystitis is not the same as a UTI, but it is often the term used by women to describe their symptoms. Cystitis can have noninfective causes, i.e. atrophic urethritis due to oestrogen deficiency. Only half of all patients suffering from cystitis have a positive MSU (Mead 1998).

Subjective findings

- Dysuria
- Frequency
- Urgency
- Loin pain (pyelonephritis).

Objective findings

- Urine positive to nitrates and leucocytes strongly suggests an infection
- Haematuria
- Vaginal discharge.

Assessment

There is a double peak in the prevalence of UTI in women (Cardozo et al 1993):

- 30–40 age group: predisposed by intercourse
- 55–65 age group: related to oestrogen status.

History taking should include details on contraceptive choice, as ill-fitting contraceptive diaphragms, spermicidal gels or condoms may also cause UTIs.

A sexual history, including questions about recent change in sexual partners or sexual practices, should also be established (Getliffe & Dolman 1997).

An abdominal examination is required to diagnose loin tenderness (pyelonephritis).

An MSU should be collected from all men, children, pregnant women and those with suspected pyelonephritis.

Plan

Therapeutic intervention

1. Home treatment for mild UTI:
   - sodium bicarbonate – Dose: 1 teaspoon into a tumbler of water, three times in 1 hour
   - potassium citrate – dose: 3 g in water three times a day
   - cranberry juice (research continues to investigate the benefits and contraindications of this historical remedy) – dose: At least three glasses during an acute phase or a glass daily for prophylactics (Getliffe 1996).
2. OTC products, including Cymalon, Cystoleve and Cystopurin help by alkalising the urine.
3. Prescription only medication
   Uncomplicated UTIs in adult, nonpregnant women include 3-day courses of antibacterials. Resistance to amoxicillin is widespread, so should not be used routinely.
4. Special cases: men, children, pregnant women, immunosuppressed or patients with impaired renal function require a 7-day course of antibiotics.
5. HRT should be considered for menopausal, postmenopausal, noninfective symptoms caused by atropic vaginitis (Mead 1998).

Patient education

Patients need to feel comfortable in the consultation to enable them to discuss recent sexual intercourse and their choice of contraception (especially diaphragm use), which might be the cause of the UTI.

Historically, this should consider

- the female anatomy
- personal hygiene (i.e. wiping 'front to back')
- tight clothing
- bath additives and deodorants which have been voiced as risk factors for UTIs; but such statements are often not evidence-based, and have been found to be insulting to women (Rink 1998).

Reattendance figures for cystitis can be reduced by using patient leaflets (Banks & Howie 1998), which include advice on increasing fluid intake and voiding frequently.

Indication for referral

- Men and children with UTIs
- Pyelonephritis (pain in the loin is often accompanied by dysuria and sometimes rigors (Munro & Edwards 1995)
- Patients with gross haematuria should be referred for further investigation.

Complications

In men

- Kidney disease, bladder disease and prostatic disease.

In children

- Enuresis needs to be investigated.

MALE HEALTH ISSUES

Introduction

Men are more vulnerable to serious illness than women (Bradford 1995), but women visit their GPs three times more often than men, either for themselves or with other family members.

The 1992 MORI (Market and Opinion Research Institute) poll found men had more knowledge about the function of the ovaries than the prostate gland (Bower 1993) and the 1994 MORI found that about half of all men won't visit the GP unless their female partners make them (Bradford 1995).

In today's environment of separation and divorce, health care professionals need to increase their awareness of and promote male health issues in a way that appeals to men.

Epididymitis

Acute or chronic inflammation of the epididymis is caused by a bacterial infection either as a result of sexually transmitted infections (i.e. *Chlamydia trachomatis*, nonspecific urethritis or *Neisseria gonorrhoeae*) or by nonsexual infections following, e.g. a UTI or prostatitis (Oates 1990).

Epididymitis can occur at all ages after puberty, with the infection reaching the epididymis by the bloodstream, via the lymphatics or from the prostatic urethra and seminal vesicles (Laker 1994).

Subjective findings

- One-sided pain and swelling of the scrotal sac
- Urethral discharge
- Dysuria.

Objective findings

- Tender swelling of the epididymis (see below).

Assessment

A full medical and sexual history is required (see Chapter 14).

A physical examination of the male genitals is required to assess for prostatic disease. Examination of the male genitalia includes:

- Examine the penis and scrotum.
- Carefully palpate both the testes the epididymis and vasa deferentia (the left testis usually lies lower than the right).
- Assess for any scrotal swelling, paying particular attention to the position of any abnormality in relation to the testes. Note size, shape, tenderness, movement, consistency, texture, margin and any associated swellings.
- Confirm that any swelling originates in the scrotum and is not an inguinal hernia (Munro & Edwards 1995).

A rectal examination to assess for prostatic disease is carried out. Digital rectal examination of the prostate gland is performed to ascertain the size, shape and feel of the gland. The normal prostate is smooth and firm, with lateral lobes and a central groove (Munro & Edwards 1995). An enlarged prostate gland that is smooth, and slightly elastic and possibly no central groove suggests benign prostatic hyperplasia. A hard irregular gland, sometimes without a medial groove, suggests prostatic carcinoma. Tenderness accompanied by a change in consistency of the gland may be due to prostatitis or an abscess.

Urethral swabs (including *Chlamydia*) and MSU should be sent for microscopy and culture.

Plan

Therapeutic intervention

- Analgesics
- Antibiotics if a causative organism is identified.

Patient education

This includes advice on

- bed rest
- good scrotal support
- psychological support.

Indication for referral

- To exclude differential diagnosis of torsion of the testicle or malignant neoplasm, refer to GP
- If STI is suspected, refer to the GUM clinic.

Complications

- Infertility can occur in bilateral disease
- Acute epididymitis may be caused by pulmonary tuberculosis
- Chronic or recurrent epididymitis (Oates 1990).

Erectile dysfunction

Normal erectile function requires coordination of vascular, cavernosa and psychological factors. Erectile dysfunction is an inability to achieve or maintain an erection sufficient to complete sexual intercourse or another sexual activity, as a result of insufficiency in anyone of these areas (Christopher 1998). It is estimated that 10% of the male population suffer from impotence.

Subjective findings

- Generalised anxiety about health
- Tiredness, stress, depression
- Poor libido
- Overt or covert complaints of impotence.

Objective findings

- Depend on cause (see below).

Assessment

A full medical and sexual history is required, including physiological, psychological and social factors.
  Physiological contributing factors include
- vascular disease, i.e. diabetes, hypertension, hyperlipidaemia, heavy smoking
- neurological problems, i.e. spinal cord injury, multiple sclerosis
- peripheral neuropathy due to diabetes or alcoholism
- endocrinology, i.e. hyperprolactinaemia
- drug-induced impotence, i.e. antihypertensives, antidepressants.
  Psychological factors may include
- infertility investigations
- fears and misguided beliefs postvasectomy
- female partner suffering from ill health, i.e. breast cancer, cervical abnormalities
- infidelity
- dyspareunia, e.g. postmenopausal partner
- men are often embarrassed to discuss their feelings and personal problems; therefore, attention must be paid to the atmosphere surrounding the consultation.
  Social factors may include
- anxiety at work or home
- recent significant life event, e.g. bereavement.
  Questions are required to determine whether the erectile dysfunction is organic or psychological in origin and should include
1. Is the onset gradual (organic) or rapid (psychological)?
2. Is there a consistent lack of erection (organic)?
3. Have the nocturnal or early morning erections stopped (organic)?
4. Is there an underlying disease or medication contributing to the symptoms?
5. Has the patient or partner had a recent major life event? (Christopher 1998).

A physical examination may include pulses, reflexes, testing for gynaecomastia, penile or testicular abnormalities and prostate examination.

Investigations should include blood pressure, urinalysis, blood tests for testosterone, prolactin, thyroid function and prostate-specific antigen (Hurn 1998). An organic cause should be eliminated in patients over 55 years of age.

Plan

Therapeutic intervention

- Penile injections, e.g. Caverject or Viridal
- MUSE (urethral pellet containing alprostadil)
- Sildenafil (Viagra) taken orally before sexual activity (BNF 1998).

Patient education

- Psychological support is an important part of care.
- Inclusion of the partner can be beneficial to some couples.
- Nondrug treatments can include sex therapy, vacuum pumps and penile implants (Scott 1998).

Indication for referral

- If the problem is organic, referral to the GP is required
- Psychosexual factors may need to be referred to an appropriate counsellor.

Complications

Psychological well-being can be affected.

Benign prostatic hyperplasia (BPH)

From the age of 45 years the number of cells in the prostate gland often increase and the gland enlarges, causing BPH. The exact cause of this increase in cells is unknown but is thought to be linked with the conversion of testosterone to a more powerful androgen – dihydrotestosterone. Incidence increases with age as follows:

- 14% of 40 year olds
- 40% of 70 year olds
- 80% of 80 year olds (Brewer 1998).

Subjective findings

- Straining or difficulty when starting to urinate
- Weak urine stream, which may stop and start
- Nocturia
- Dysuria, urgency, and/or frequency
- Dribbling urinary incontinence
- Feeling of not having emptied the bladder
- Erectile dysfunction (Brewer 1998).

Objective findings

With further questioning it might become apparent that the patient's lifestyle has been affected, e.g. avoidance of social occasions, restriction of fluid intake, poor self-esteem.

Assessment

A physical examination of the male genitalia and rectal examination is required (see p. 237). Other investigations should include:

- urinalysis – test for glucose and blood and send for microscopy and culture
- blood for urea, electrolytes and creatinine
- bloods for prostate-specific antigen.

A medical history should be followed by a physical and digital rectal examination of the prostate gland.

Plan

Therapeutic intervention

A variety of prescription-only medication drugs are available including

Alpha-blockers. Treatment should be continuous, as the prostate gland will enlarge again if medication is stopped. However, they are not without their side effects, including sedation, hypotension and impotence (BNF 1998). If patients are to use hormonal drugs, condoms should be advised to protect their partners.

Patient education

Watching and waiting may be all that is required following the initial diagnosis. Advice on self-help measures can include:

- avoiding constipation
- an adequate fluid intake
- a high protein diet, rich in complex carbohydrates (Bradford 1995).

Natural plants

Alternative therapies for mild-to-moderate symptoms have been shown to improve symptoms of BPH without the side effects of low sex drive or impotence (Brewer 1998). In addition, extract of rye has undergone clinically controlled trials and has been approved for medical use in many countries (Bradford 1995).

Surgical treatments

Transurethral resection of the prostate (TURP), or surgical options to shrink the prostate with heat, freezing it or by using laser or ultrasound energy, are also an option (Brewer 1998).

Indication for referral

- If prostate disease is suspected, refer to GP for physical examination
- If symptoms become progressively worse, referral to urologist for further investigations is recommended.

Complication

Cancer of the prostate.

Testicular cancer

Testicular cancer is the commonest cancer in men aged between 15 and 35 years (Laker 1994). The cause is unknown, but the incidence is highest in professional and nonmanual workers. Survival rates are high if the cancer is detected early.

There are four types of testicular malignancy:

1. teratoma, which is prevalent in young children and infants
2. seminoma, which is the commonest tumour and carries the best prognosis
3. embryonal cancer, which is characterised by rapid growth and spread
4. choriocarcinoma, which carries a poor prognosis (Laker 1994).

Testicular self-examination (TSE) is an important technique that can detect testicular abnormalities early and should be discussed with men. Tugwell (1996) found that 83% of men would perform TSE if taught how.

Subjective findings

- Dull ache in the lower abdomen or groin
- A feeling of heaviness in the scrotum
- Pain in the testicle
- Swelling or lump in the testicle
- Very occasionally breast swelling (Bradford 1995).

Objective finding

Swelling or lump in the testicle.

Assessment

A history of undescended testicles increases the risk of testicular cancer, but only 10% of patients will have a history of this (Mead 1992). There is no evidence to suggest that vasectomy leads to an increased risk of testicular cancer (Stanford 1987).

Prompt diagnosis is important. If teratoma is suspected, blood samples are collected for alpha-fetoprotein (AFP) and human chorionic gonadotrophin (HCG) levels. Either or both will be raised. Liver function tests (LFTs) and bone marrow function tests are performed to detect for metastasis (Tugwell 1996).

Plan

Therapeutic intervention

Treatment depends on the stage and type of cancer, and includes chemotherapy and radiotherapy.

Patient education

Psychological support is important, as the affects of testicular cancer can be paralleled to a women following a mastectomy.

- feelings of fear and embarrassment are often experienced
- relationship problems, lethargy, reduced libido, feelings of being inadequate or incomplete may follow diagnosis and treatment (Tugwell 1996)

- family members may also need support
- men are advised not to father children while recovering from chemotherapy or for 2 years after radiotherapy
- sperm banking can be offered prior to surgery.

Indication for referral

- Differential diagnosis is epididymoorchitis; however, an incorrect diagnosis will delay referral to a urologist
- Urgent referral to urologist for surgery and radiotherapy or chemotherapy.

Complication

Infertility can occur as a result of surgery or treatment.

Glossary

Coinfection   Infection caused by more than one bacteria or virus

Contact tracing   Identifying and treating recent partners who have been in contact with an STI

Fomite spread   Route of transmission of infection from an object to a person

Indicator disease   A series of potentially fatal opportunistic infections associated with AIDS

Prodromal   The time between the first symptoms of an infectious disease and the development of a rash or fever

Vertical transmission   Route of transmission of infection from mother to child

Viral load   New marker for monitoring the disease process in HIV and AIDS.

References

Alder M W 1998 ABC of sexually transmitted diseases, 4th edn. British Medical Journal Books, London.

Banks J C, Howie J G R 1998 Reducing consultations for symptoms of cystitis using a health education leaflet. British Journal of General Practice 48:1595–1596.

Barger M, Woolner B 1995 In: Rigby D 1999 Assessment and management of genitourinary tract disorders. The Journals of Nursing and Midwifery. March–April 40(2):231–245.

Boag F, Kelly F 1998 Screening for *Chlamydia trachomatis*. The case for screening is made, but much detail needs to be worked out. British Medical Journal 316(7143):1474.

British National Formulary (BNF) 1998 No. 36. British Medical Association and Royal Pharmaceutical Society of Great Britain.

Boulton A 1995 Hidden signs of ageing. Practice Nurse 19 May:427–430.

Bower H 1993 Is machismo a barrier to health. Practice Nurse 15–31 March:823–824.

Bradford N 1995 Men's health matters. The complete A–Z of male health. Vermillion, London.

Brewer S 1998 Symptoms of prostate disease. Practice Nurse 15:333–336.

Brown K, Davies C, Stratton P (eds) 1988 Early presentation and prediction of child abuse. John Wiley, Chichester.

Bulter R J, Redfen E J, Forsythe W I 1990 The child's construing of nocturnal enuresis: a method of inquiry and prediction of outcome. Journal of Child Psychology and Psychiatry 31:447–454, cited.

Cardozo L, Cutner A, Wise B 1993 Basic urogynaecology. Oxford Medical Press, Oxford.

Carlyon E M, Barton S E 1995 How common is self treatment in non gonnococcal urethritis? Genitourinary Medicine 71(6):400–401.

CDCP (Centre for Disease Control and Prevention) 1997 Case definitions for infectious conditions under Public Health Surveillance. MMWR 46(10):1–55.

Chandler M 1996 Genital warts: a study of patient anxiety and information needs. British Journal of Nursing 5(3):174–197.

Chard S 1998 Diagnosing and treating genital herpes. Nursing Times 94(46):58–62.

Christopher E 1998 Understanding erectile dysfunction. Practice Nurse 16:622–626.

Clarke J 1998 How did she get these warts? Anogenital warts and sexual abuse. Child Abuse Review 7:206–211.

Cohen M S et al 1997 Reduction of concentration of HIV-1 in semen after treatment of urethritis: implications for prevention of sexual transmission of HIV-1. Lancet 349:(9096): 1868–1873.

Csonka G W 1990 Non gonococcal urethritis and post gonococcal urethritis. In: Csonka G W, Oates J K (eds) 1990 Sexually transmitted diseases: a textbook of genitourinary medicine. Baillière Tindall, London.

Davkvist J, Wahlin T B 1995 Herpes simplex and mood: a prospective study. Psychosocial Medicine 57(2):127–135, cited.

Davis A 1998 Trichomonas vaginosis: signs, tests and treatment. Nursing Times 25(94):58–59.

1 Genito urinary health covers a wide range of personal as well as social issues

2 Genito urinary health care involves a multiprofessional, multiagency approach

3 It is important to put all patients at ease and to be nonjudgemental

3 It is vital to discuss safer sex issues with all patients, including the elderly

4 Referral to the GUM clinic for diagnosis of coinfection and contact tracing of partners

5 Patients wishing to be screened for HIV should be refered to the GUM clinic

6 Incontinence does not have to be part of longevity

7 Sexual abuse should be considered in children presenting with STIs, repeated UTIs and enuresis

8 Male health issues need to be promoted in a way that appeals to men

9 Testicular self-examination can reduce the mortality of testicular cancer

10 Men may approach the subject of erectile dysfunction overtly or covertly

Doley D M 1977 Behaviour treatments for nocturnal enuresis in children; a review of recent literature. Psychol Bulletin 84:30–54, cited.

Edwards S, Dockerty G 1993 Diagnosis of gonorrhoea by microscopy. Genitourinary Medicine 71(3):98–101, cited.

Ferreira N 1997 Sexually transmitted *Chlamydia trachomatis*. Nurse Practitioner Forum 8(2):70–76.

Getliffe K 1996 Urinary incontinence; assessing the problem. Primary Health Care 6(8):31–38.

Getliffe K, Dolman M (eds.) 1997 Promoting continence: a clinical research resource. Baillière Tindall and Royal College of Nursing, London.

Grealish M, O'Dowd T 1998 General practitioners and women with urinary incontinence. British Journal of General Practice 48:975–978.

Greendale G A, Haas S T, Holbrook K et al 1993 The relationship of *Chlamydia trachomatis* infection and male infertility. American Journal of Public Health 83(7):996–1001, cited.

Grigg E 2000 Sexually transmitted infections and older people. Nursing Standard 14(39):48–53.

Grimshaw R 1998 Incontinence treatment using physiotherapy. Practice Nurse 15:203–206.

Gutman L T, Wilfert C N 1990 Gonorrhoea disease in infants and children. Cited in Sutton A, Payne S (eds) 1997 Genito urinary medicine for nurses. Whurr, London.

Hale J, Sutton A 1997 HIV and AIDS. In: Sutton A, Payne S (eds) Genito urinary medicine for nurses. Whurr, London.

Handy P 1997 Gonhorrhoea and non specific urethritis. In: Sutton A, Payne S (eds) Genito urinary medicine for nurses. Whurr, London.

Hay P 1998 *Chlamydia* infections: who is at risk? The Practitioner 242:704–710.

Houts A C, Berman J S, Abramson H 1994 Effectiveness of psychological and pharmacological treatments for nocturnal enuresis. Journal Consult Clin Psych 62:737–745.

Hurn W 1998 Erectile dysfunction: causes and treatment options. Community Nurse Sept:33–35.

Husband P 1997 Genital warts. In: Sutton A, Payne S (eds) Genito urinary medicine for nurses. Whurr, London.

Jarvelin M R, Moilanen I, Vitevainen-Tervonen L, Huttunen N P 1990 Life changes and protective capacities in enuretic and non enuretic children. Journal of Child Psychology and Psychiatry 31:763–774.

Laker C 1994 Urological nursing. Scutari Press, London.

Letvak S, Schoder D 1996 Sexually transmitted disease in the elderly: what you need to know. Geriatric Nursing July–Aug:156–160.

Lukeman D 1997 Mainly children. Childhood enuresis and encopresin. In: Getliffe K, Dolman M (eds) Promoting continence. A clinical and research resource. Baillière Tindall and Royal College of Nursing, London.

Mardh P A, Danielsson D 1990 *Neisseria gonorrhoeae*. Cited in Sutton A, Payne S 1997 Genito urinary medicine for nurses. Whurr, London.

Mead M 1992 Testicular cancer and related neoplasms. British Medical Journal 304:1327–1429.

Mead M 1998 Drugs for urinary tract infection. Practice Nurse 16:39–40.

Morgan R T T, Young G C 1975 Parental attitudes and the conditioning treatment of childhood enuresis. Behav Res Ther 13:197–199, cited.

Munro J, Edwards C (eds) 1995 Macleod's clinical examination, 9th edn. Churchill Livingstone, Edinburgh.

NHSE 1999 Reducing mother to baby transmission of HIV (HSE 1999–183). Department of Health, London.

Oates J K 1990 In: Csonka G W, Oates J K (eds) Sexually transmitted diseases: a textbook of genitourinary medicine. Baillière Tindall, London.

Oates J K, Csonka G W 1990 Gonorrhoea and syphilis. In Csonka G W, Oates J K (eds) Sexually transmitted diseases: a textbook of genitourinary medicine. Baillière Tindall, London.

Oriel 1998 Anogenital papillomavirus infection in children. British Medical Journal 296:1484–1485, cited.

Oriel J D, Walker P G 1990 In: Csonka G W, Oates J K (eds) Sexually transmitted diseases: a textbook of genitourinary medicine. Baillière Tindall, London.

Petrin D, Delgaty K, Bhatt R, Garber G 1998 Clinical and microbiological aspects of *Trichomonas vaginalis*. Clinical Microbiology Review 11(2):300–317, cited.

Phillips M, McGlynn C, Fagan B 1988 Bacterial vaginosis, candidiasis and trichomoniasis cited in Sutton A, Payne S 1997 Genito urinary medicine for Nurses. Whurr, London.

Posner N 1998 Herpes simplex. The Experience of Illness Series. Routledge, London.

Pratt R 1995 HIV and AIDS. A strategy for nursing care, 4th edn. Edward Arnold, London.

Rigby D 1999 Urinary incontinence. Primary Health Care Feb, 9(1):17–21.

Rink E 1998 Risk factors for urinary tract symptoms in women: beliefs among general practitioners and women and the effect on patient management. The British Journal of General Practitioner 48:1155–1158.

Rutishauser S 1994 Physiology and anatomy. A basis for nursing and health care. Churchill Livingstone, Edinburgh.

Scott L 1998 A miracle drug? Practice Nurse 16:267–269.

Shaffer 1994 Enuresis. In: Rutler M, Taylor E, Hersor L (eds) Child and adolescent psychiatry; modern approaches. Blackwell, Oxford, cited.

Smith M 1997 Drugs for incontinence. In: Getliffe K, Dolman M (eds) Promoting continence. Baillière Tindall and Royal College of Nursing, London.

Stanford J 1987 Testicular self examination, teaching, learning and practice by nurses. Journal of Advanced Nursing 12:13–19.

Steadman T 1998 Sexually transmitted infections. Nursing care and management. Stanley Thornes, Cheltenham.

Swanson J, Dibble S, Chapman L 1999 Effects of psychoeducational interventions on sexual health risks and psychosocial adaptation in young adults with genital herpes. Journal of Advanced Nursing 29(4):840–851.

Tugwell M 1996 Testicular self examination. Primary Health Care 6(5):18–21.

White H 1997 Incontinence in perspective. In: Getliffe K, Dolman M (eds) Promoting continence. Baillière Tindall and Royal College of Nursing, London.

Further reading

Love S.T.I.NGS 1999 A beginners guide to sexually transmitted infection. Family Planning Association, UK.
This new publication, aimed at teenagers and young adults, provides information in a humorous and colourful cartoon booklet. The use of colour, language and terminology is excellent.

Munro J, Edwards C (eds) 1995 Macleod's clinical examination, 9th edn. Churchill Livingstone, London.

This book is aimed at medical clinicians to complement medical and surgical textbooks. It is particularly relevant to nurse practitioners in that it brings together the skills of good history taking and physical examination. Normal findings and abnormal signs are discussed. Investigations, key points, and illustrative case studies run throughout the chapters.

Sutton A, Payne S 1997 Genito urinary medicine for nurses. Whurr, London.

I was recommended this book as a key reference for this chapter by my local GUM clinic health advisor. It is well written and has proved to be a useful resource, suitable for nurse practitioners in primary health care as well as for specialist nurses working in GUM clinics.

14

CONTRACEPTION, SEXUALITY AND THE MENOPAUSE

Sue Reed and Myfanwy Rimmer

Part 1: Contraception and Sexuality

Sue Reed

Key Issues

- Giving contraceptive advice provides an opportune time for health promotion concerning sexual health, cervical screening, fertility awareness and preconceptual care

- Nurse practitioners in primary care are ideally placed when seeing young people as a matter of routine, to check out contraceptive awareness and discuss risk factors associated with unprotected sexual intercourse

- Awareness of the range of contraceptive choices and possible side effects can aid patient compliance

- The choice of a suitable method of contraception may change at different stages of the life span, as personal circumstances change

- Although hormonal methods of contraception may be more reliable, barrier methods will also maintain sexual health

- This chapter represents an overview of contraceptive options and is not intended as a substitute for the training and knowledge base of an experienced family planning trained nurse.

Introduction: sexual history

Free family planning services have only been widely available in general practice since 1975. Even though community clinics provide an excellent service, many women, and men, may prefer the anonymity, accessibility and convenience of their doctor's surgery. Therefore,

it seems like a good idea for the nurse practitioner in primary care, who is not family planning trained, to have knowledge of contraception and sexual health in general. Explaining different methods to patients can help them to make informed choices about their reproductive health. Evidence has shown that when it is easier to access services that provide a range of contraceptive choices, there is an improvement in contraceptive compliance (Belfield 1999).

Nurse practitioners are also in an ideal position to work with the adolescent age group, who are often at risk of pregnancy and may need nonjudgemental support and guidance from a health professional to maintain sexual health and well-being.

❶ Be alert for child protection issues.

Recent guidelines allow young people under the age of 16 to be prescribed contraception and to be given confidential advice: if it is judged to be in their best interests as they intend to pursue sexual activity, if they show sufficient maturity and understanding and if they have considered informing their parents (Department of Health 1990).

To avoid embarrassment with such a sensitive subject as sexual health, it is often more comfortable for the patient to provide the relevant information through answering open questions such as: 'What kind of contraception have you been using?' and 'How do you feel about using condoms?'.

The contraceptive history is particularly important in any consultation involving contraception. This will provide a lot of information about which methods are acceptable, previous contraceptive problems, and should promote the opportunity for encouraging safer sex. Young people often welcome the opportunity to talk about concerns with their sexuality, relationships, contraceptive choices, parental attitudes and any health problems. Discussion about the risks of smoking, the importance of a healthy diet and regular exercise can also be stressed at this time. ❶ Be alert for hidden agendas when taking contraceptive history.

For all methods of contraception, a gynaecological history should be taken, which encompasses:

- Age of menarche. How old were you when your periods started?
- Frequency, regularity and duration of the cycle.
- Amenorrhoea. Have you missed any periods recently?
- Premenstrual problems. Do you get bloated, irritable or have sore breasts before your periods start?
- Dysmenorrhoea. Do you get backache or stomach ache before or during your periods?
- Any abnormal discharge, tenderness or lesion in or around the pubic area?
- Previous history of pelvic inflammatory disease (PID).
- Dyspareunia. Do you experience pain with intercourse?
- Cervical smear status (if appropriate).

When working with young people, it is also important to use sensitivity in determining how long they have been sexually active, and whether they have had many sexual partners. There is evidence that early age of sexual intercourse, particularly if this leads to a number of different sexual partners, can be a risk factor for future cervical cancer (Singer & Szarewski 1988, Guillebaud 1997). Whereas a positive correlation has also been found between smoking and cervical cancer (Barton et al 1988), women need to be aware that it can still occur without a history of these risk factors. ❶ Being aware of risk factors for sexually transmitted diseases and cervical cancer.

Knowledge of the patient's medical history, with particular reference to cardiovascular risk, is mandatory for hormonal contraception, and useful for other methods. It should include:

- headaches, especially migraineous attacks, and whether or not focal symptoms are present
- varicose veins and any circulatory problems, especially previous thromboembolism or phlebitis
- allergic skin disorders and known allergic reactions to copper, rubber, latex, or to spermicide containing nonoxinol '9'
- epilepsy
- depression that has needed treatment
- current medication
- past history of serious illnesses (e.g. hepatitis)
- any previous abdominal or gynaecological operations
- personal or family history of diabetes
- family history of circulatory problems or heart disease
- personal or family history of cancer
- smoking habits
- basic observations – blood pressure (BP), weight, height, body mass index (BMI).

The efficacy of contraceptive methods is given in Box 14.1.

Hormonal methods of contraception

The combined oral contraceptive pill

'The Pill' was introduced in the early 1960s as a combination of ethinyloestradiol (oestrogen) and a progestogen. It prevents pregnancy by inhibiting ovulation, causing the endometrium to be unfavourable for implantation and making the cervical mucus impenetrable to sperm. 'The Pill' revolutionised women's lifestyles by enabling them to control their fertility in a convenient way, with the additional benefit of relieving any dysmenorrhoea, menorrhagia or premenstrual symptoms.

The combined oral contraceptive (COC) pill now contains much less oestrogen than when it was initially introduced in the early 1960s, with the result that many side effects have been significantly reduced. The Family Planning Association and The Faculty of Family Planning and Reproductive Health Care advise that to minimise any long-term adverse effects, 'the pill of

Box 14.1	*Efficacy of contraceptive methods* *(Reproduced with kind permission from FPA Contraceptive Handbook, T Belfield (1999) Family Planning Association.)* *% of women per year*

Methods that have no 'user' failure	
Injectable contraception	over 99% effective
Implants	over 99% effective in first year (over 98% per year over 5 years)
Intrauterine system (IUS)	over 99% effective
Intrauterine device (IUD)	98–over 99% effective (depending on IUD type)
Female sterilisation	over 99% effective 1 in 200 lifetime failure rate
Male sterilisation (vasectomy)	over 99% effective 1 in 2000 lifetime failure rate

Methods that have 'user' failure	
Combined oral contraceptive	over 99% effective
Progestogen-only oral contraceptive	up to 99% effective
Male condom	up to 98% effective
Female condom	up to 95% effective
Diaphragm or cap + spermicide	up to 96% effective
Natural family planning: ■ combining two or more fertility indicators	up to 98% effective
■ new technologies (Persona)	up to 94% effective

Note Efficacy rates of methods with 'user' failure reflect use when used absolutely correctly and consistently. Where methods are used less well, lower efficacy will be seen.

choice should be the one containing the lowest suitable dose of oestrogen and progestogen which:

- provides effective contraception
- produces acceptable cycle control
- is associated with the fewest side-effects
- has the least-known effect on carbohydrate and lipid metabolism and homeostatic parameters' (NAFPD 1984).

Combined oral contraceptive pills may be monophasic, biphasic or triphasic. Monophasic pills include Brevinor, Cilest, Eugynon 30, Femodene, Loestrin 20, Loestrin 30, Marvelon, Mercilon, Microgynon 30, Minulet, Ovranette and Ovysmen. These pills are the most commonly used and consist of a single strength of the hormones oestrogen and progestogen, whereas with biphasic pills, such as BiNovum, half the pills contain one strength of the two hormones, and half another strength. These are now rarely prescribed since the introduction of triphasic pills (Logynon, Synphase, Trinordiol, TriNovum and Tri-Minulet), which produce better cycle control with lower doses of hormones given in three different strengths during the cycle (Guillebaud 1998).

All contraceptive pills contain one of the following progestogens: levonorgestrel, norethisterone, norgestimate, gestodene or desogestrel. Of these, the last two were the subject of the 1995 'pill scare', in which it was claimed that pills containing gestodene or desogestrel increased the risk of venous thromboembolism (CSM 1995). Subsequent research has suggested that they can reduce the risk of arterial disease through their beneficial effects on lipid metabolism (Lewis et al 1997).

However, more recent research has found no difference in cardiovascular outcomes when any combined oral contraceptive is used, unless its use is also associated with additional risk factors such as smoking, hyperlipidaemia, diabetes, obesity, hypertension or a family history of myocardial infarction (Dunn et al 1999).

On the other hand, gestodene and desogestrel are less androgenic than levonorgestrel or norethisterone, so tend to be more suitable for women who experience problems with acne, hirsutism and weight gain (Guillebaud 1998). Alternatively, Dianette, which is an anti-androgen/oestrogen pill, can be used if either acne or hirsutism is a problem, as it also has contraceptive benefits. However, as Dianette is not licensed for contraceptive use, the manufacturers recommend that it be discontinued once the skin condition has completely cleared (Schering Data Sheet 1999), after which a regular hormonal contraceptive pill could be introduced.

Most combined pills consist of a 21-day regime with a 7-day break before the next packet is started. It should be stressed during the initial consultation that the pill-free interval is only safe if all the pills in the last packet are taken and the new packet is started exactly on time. Some pills are taken every day (e.g. Femodene ED, Logynon ED, Microgynon ED, TriNovum ED) for 28 days, with the last seven pills being inactive, for those who have trouble remembering to take their next pack on time.

With consistent use, the pill is over 99% effective (Guillebaud 1999) when pills are taken correctly on time, every day, in the right sequence (Fig. 14.1),

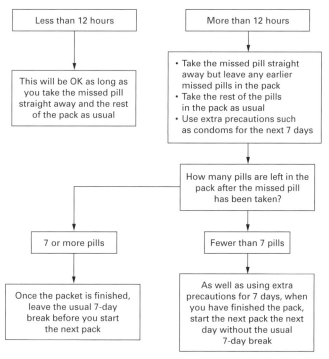

Figure 14.1 *Missed pill guidelines. What to do if you forget a pill.*

without concurrent antibiotic medication and no history of severe diarrhoea or vomiting (see disadvantages).

Instructions on pill taking need to be clear, user-friendly and supported by appropriate literature to avoid increasing the failure rate. As the pill does not protect against sexually transmitted diseases, concurrent use of condoms should be encouraged, which has the added benefit of enhancing contraceptive efficacy.

Advantages (Belfield 1999, Everett 1997, 1998)

- Reliable, convenient and easily reversible
- Relieves dysmenorrhoea and menorrhagia
- Reduces premenstrual symptoms – monophasic pills are more likely to be beneficial than triphasic pills (Guillebaud 1999)
- Reduces risk of iron-deficiency anaemia due to lighter periods
- Reduces risk of benign breast disease
- Reduces pain from endometriosis
- Fewer ectopic pregnancies, as the COC prevents ovulation from occurring
- Reduction of ovarian cysts and fibroids
- Less PID
- Protects against endometrial and ovarian cancer
- Protects against osteoporosis
- Protection from the more severe forms of rheumatoid arthritis
- Improvements in skin and hair – an oestrogen-dominant COC is often prescribed as a treatment for acne
- In suitable women with no contraindications, a low-dose COC may continue to be used up to the menopause, with the advantage of offering protection against osteoporosis during this time (Guillebaud 1997).

Disadvantages (Everett 1998, Belfield 1999)

- It needs to be taken carefully, consistently and regularly. Extra precautions may be necessary for missed pills or any taken more than 12 hours late for the next 7 days.
- Severe diarrhoea and/or persistent vomiting may preclude absorption of the pill, so extra precautions will be necessary for the duration, as well as for the following 7 days.
- Some drug interactions may reduce efficacy – extra precautions need to be taken if antibiotics are required, for the whole course of treatment + another 7 days. ❶ Be aware of drug interactions with combined pills.
- Does not protect against sexually transmitted diseases (STDs) and HIV.
- Increased risk of circulatory problems, including migraines, hypertension, arterial disease, venous thrombosis and pulmonary embolism.
- Increased risk of liver disorders, such as cholestatic jaundice, gallstones and liver adenoma.
- May affect the incidence of breast cancer.
- Unsuitable for smokers over the age of 35.

Before the pill can be prescribed, a comprehensive medical history should be taken (see above) to exclude possible contraindications.

Absolute contraindications (Everett 1997, 1998, Belfield 1999)

1. ❶ Suspected or confirmed pregnancy.
2. ❶ Breast feeding, as the COC will inhibit milk production.
3. ❶ Undiagnosed vaginal or uterine bleeding.
4. ❶ Increased risk of blood clotting disorders:
   - past history of venous or arterial thrombosis
   - hereditary thrombophilia (e.g. factor V Leiden)
   - cardiovascular or ischaemic heart disease
   - history of cerebral haemorrhage or transient ischaemic attacks
   - 2–4 weeks before major or leg surgery.
5. ❶ Disorders of lipid metabolism.
6. ❶ Focal or crescendo migraine, or migraine requiring ergotamine treatment.
7. ❶ Active liver disease, e.g. malignancy, history of cholestatic jaundice, gall bladder disease, unexplained jaundice or impaired liver function tests (LFTs), although the combined pill may be given 3 months after LFTs have returned to normal (Guillebaud 1999).
8. ❶ Oestrogen-dependent tumours, e.g. breast cancer.
9. ❶ Serious medical conditions which are either related to previous use of COC or affected by sex steroids, e.g. porphyrias, hypertension, pemphigoid gestationis, otosclerotic deafness, systemic lupus erythematosus, Stevens–Johnson syndrome, trophoblastic disease, acute pancreatitis, chorea.
10. ❶ Obesity (BMI > 35) can lead to an increased risk of all side effects.
11. ❶ Severe diabetes mellitus with complications.
12. ❶ Acute episodes of ulcerative colitis or Crohn's disease.
13. ❶ Smokers over 35 years of age.

The combined pill should be given with caution, under specialist advice, to women who have a family history of a first-degree relative with arterial or venous disease below the age of 45 years.

Relative contraindications (Everett 1997, 1998)

- Sickle cell disease.
- Severe depression or psychosis.
- Inflammatory bowel disease (e.g. Crohn's disease, ulcerative colitis) in remission.
- Splenectomy.
- Diseases where high-density lipoprotein (HDL) is reduced, e.g. diabetes, hypertension.
- ❶ Diseases whose drug treatment affects the efficacy of the combined pill, e.g. epilepsy, tuberculosis. Be aware of drug interactions with combined pills.

- Diabetes mellitus, although healthy, young, non-smoking diabetics without complications may be given a low-dose combined pill.
- Long-term immobilisation.
- Obesity with BMI 30–35.

Side effects (Everett 1997)

1. Nausea can occur in the first few cycles of starting the pill. It usually settles after three packets of pills and can be avoided by taking the pills with or after food. Should it occur in an established pill user, pregnancy will need to be excluded.
2. Breast tenderness or bloatedness will usually disappear after three pill packets have been taken, but if it persists the pill may need to be changed to a lower-dose oestrogen or different progestogen.
3. Break-through bleeding may occur in the first few months but does not interfere with efficacy. It is important to check that the pills are being taken correctly, and that none have been missed, that there has not been any diarrhoea or vomiting, or that any drugs, which may interfere with the pill, have been taken. If the bleeding persists, a vaginal examination and swabs should be taken to exclude infection and disease. Bleeding can then be controlled with a higher-dose pill, a different progestogen or a triphasic pill.
4. Depression and loss of libido are progestrogenic side effects that can be overcome by changing to a pill with a higher dose of oestrogen.
5. Weight gain may occur initially, but if it continues despite a healthy diet and regular exercise, a different pill can be considered.
6. Contact lenses may become uncomfortable, but this is usually only a problem associated with hard lenses and high-dose pills.

The progestogen–only pill

The progestogen-only pill or POP has also been commonly known as the 'mini pill'. However this misnomer should not reflect its efficacy, as if taken correctly and consistently, and preferably a few hours before intercourse, prevention of pregnancy can be as high as 99%. The POP is a microdose of one of the progestogens, levonorgestrel or norethisterone, which is taken at the same time each day, or within 3 hours, without the usual break from pill taking. As the POP mainly prevents pregnancy by thickening the cervical mucus so that it is impenetrable to sperm, its effectiveness is greatest a few hours after ingestion, and lowest when the new pill is due to be taken (Everett 1997). It also renders the endometrium less favourable for implantation, reduces fallopian tube function and, in some women, it will also suppress ovulation.

It is a useful alternative for women who wish to use oral contraception but are unable to tolerate oestrogen, or where oestrogen is contraindicated, as in breast-feeding

mothers. It is also suitable for women over 35 years who smoke, those with cardiovascular risk factors or where there is a history of thrombophilia. For a full range of contraindications to COC, see the previous section.

Efficacy will be affected by severe diarrhoea, or if vomiting occurs within 3 hours of ingestion and a replacement pill is not taken. In this case, and if a pill is taken late or completely forgotten, extra precautions will be needed for the duration of the diarrhoea and vomiting as well as for the next 7 days.

Advantages (Everett 1998)

- Suitable for breast-feeding mothers, as it does not inhibit lactation
- Suitable for women for whom oestrogen is contraindicated
- Suitable for women with diabetes or focal migraines
- No evidence of increased risk of hypertension
- Does not need to be stopped prior to surgery
- Reduction in dysmenorrhoea
- May relieve premenstrual symptoms
- The thickening of the cervical mucus may protect against salpingitis and PID
- Is not affected by antibiotics unless the antibiotic is an enzyme-inducer (e.g. rifampicin, griseofulvin – see relative contraindications) (Guillebaud 1999).

Disadvantages (Everett 1998)

- Must be taken at a regular time, or within 3 hours of it, to achieve optimum effectiveness.
- May cause irregular bleeding pattern, with increased spotting, breakthrough bleeding or amenorrhoea.
- A small number of women may develop spontaneously reversible functional ovarian cysts.
- There may be a slight increase in risk of ectopic pregnancy if the pill fails.
- There may be an association between weight over 70 kg and increased failure rate (Vessey et al 1990). Two POP pills taken together will provide better efficacy (Guillebaud 1999), but this treatment is not licensed. ❶ Be aware of excess weight with POP users.

Absolute contraindications (Everett 1997, 1998; Belfield 1999)

- Suspected or confirmed pregnancy
- Previous ectopic pregnancy
- Any abnormal vaginal or uterine bleeding
- Past or present severe arterial disease
- Severe lipid abnormalities
- Recent trophoblastic disease until elevated human chorionic gonadotrophin (hCG) levels have returned to normal
- Current liver disease, cholestatic jaundice, liver adenoma or cancer
- Serious side effects with the combined pill not linked to oestrogen.

Relative contraindications (Everett 1997, 1998; Belfield 1999)

The POP may be given to women with relative contraindications but they will need careful monitoring:

- Concurrent medication with liver enzyme-inducing drugs, such as rifampicin, carbamazepine or phenobarbitone, as these drugs will reduce the effectiveness of the POP. ❶ Be aware of drug interactions.
- History of jaundice in pregnancy.
- Functional ovarian cysts which have required hospitalisation.
- Any history of breast malignancy or other sex steroid cancers.
- Risk factors for arterial disease, such as lipid abnormalities, may be exacerbated by the POP.

Side effects (Everett 1998)

- Menstrual irregularity
- Breast tenderness
- Bloatedness
- Fluctuations in weight
- Depression
- Nausea
- Amenorrhoea
- Functional ovarian cysts.

Injectable contraception

There are two injectable contraceptives licensed in the UK: Depo-Provera (depo medroxyprogesterone acetate or DMPA) and Noristerat (norethisterone enanthate). Since 1995, Depo-Provera has been licensed as a first-choice method of contraception. It is more widely used than Noristerat, which is licensed for short-term use only when two consecutive injections may be given 8 weeks apart if a highly effective method is required for a short period of time, such as following a partner's vasectomy or after rubella immunisation (Belfield 1999).

Similarly to the POP, injectables prevent pregnancy by thickening the cervical mucus, causing the endometrium to be unreceptive to implantation, and reducing fallopian tube function. However, their primary objective is to suppress ovulation. With an efficacy of 99–100%, they are a highly efficient form of contraception, with reduced failure rates since women do not need to remember to take a pill, and its efficacy is not affected by diarrhoea and vomiting. For immediate contraceptive protection, DMPA should be administered within the first 5 days of a menstrual period. On the other hand, Noristerat needs to be given on the first day of a period, otherwise extra protection will be needed for 7 days.

Advantages (Everett 1997, 1998)

- Highly effective with low user failure rate since women do not need to remember to take a daily pill
- Lasts 8–12 weeks

- Ideal method for adolescents as it is discrete
- Less premenstrual symptoms in some women
- Reduced dysmenorrhoea and menorrhagia, so less anaemia
- Suitable for breast-feeding women
- Less PID
- Possible reduction in endometriosis due to thickened cervical mucus
- DMPA is method of choice in sickle cell disease and may reduce crises (Khoiny 1996)
- Efficacy not reduced by diarrhoea, vomiting or broad-spectrum antibiotics.

Disadvantages (Everett 1998)

- Irregular bleeding, spotting or amenorrhoea – 60% of women have amenorrhoea at the end of the first year
- Delayed return of fertility for up to 1 year
- Some users experience weight gain of up to 2 kg
- Depression and loss of libido occurs in some women
- Galactorrhoea may occur
- Possible increased risk of osteoporosis with long-term use, although recent research suggests that there are no significant adverse effects on bone density (Gbolade et al 1998)
- Once given it cannot be reversed, so its effects last 2–3 months
- Does not offer protection against HIV infection.

DMPA will need to be given at 10-week intervals instead of the usual 12 weeks when there is concurrent administration of enzyme-inducing drugs. Enzyme inducers include anticonvulsants (phenytoin, primidone, carbamazepine, topiramate), antitubercule (rifampicin), antifungal (griseofulvin), diuretic (spironolactone), hypnotic (dichloralphenazone) and tranquilliser (meprobamate). ❶ Be aware of drug interactions.

Absolute contraindications (Everett 1998, Belfield 1999)

- Suspected or confirmed pregnancy
- Undiagnosed vaginal or uterine bleeding
- Cancer of the breast or undiagnosed breast lump
- Present or past severe arterial disease, or severe lipid abnormalities
- Recent trophoblastic disease until elevated hCG levels have returned to normal
- Active liver disease, liver adenoma or cancer
- Serious side effects on COC that are not due to the oestrogen.

Relative contraindications (Everett 1998, Belfield 1999)

- Chronic systemic disease
- Risk factors for arterial disease, as lipid abnormalities may be adversely affected by the POP
- Progestogen-sensitive migraine
- Severe depression

- Obesity
- Those who cannot accept menstrual irregularity
- Any woman wishing to conceive immediately after using an injectable method.

Side effects (Everett 1998)

- Irregular bleeding
- Amenorrhoea
- Headaches
- Bloatedness
- Depression
- Weight gain
- Mood swings.

Implants

These are inserted subdermally to release a set amount of a progestogen over a predetermined period of time. Norplant was the first contraceptive implant that became available in the UK in 1993. Although it is a safe and effective form of contraception, Norplant has now been withdrawn from the market for commercial reasons. Any woman who still has the Norplant in place can be reassured that it can remain until it is due for removal within 5 years of insertion.

Whereas Norplant consists of six thin flexible rods each containing levonorgestrel, the new implant, Implanon is a single non-biodegradable rod containing the progestogen etonogestrel. Similarly to Norplant, it is inserted on the inner aspect of the upper arm by a trained professional. It is designed to provide contraceptive protection for up to 3 years by suppressing ovulation and increasing the viscosity of the cervical mucus, thus preventing sperm penetration. Implants can be inserted within the first 5 days of the start of menstruation without additional contraceptive methods being necessary.

Advantages (Everett 1997, Belfield 1999)

- Highly effective
- Long lasting
- Reduces menstrual bleeding in 80% of women
- Easily reversed with no effect on future fertility
- Requires little medical attention other than at insertion and removal.

Disadvantages (Everett 1998, Belfield 1999)

- Insertion requires a minor operative procedure
- Irregular menstrual bleeding may occur in 10–20% of women
- Amenorrhoea
- Slightly increased risk of ectopic pregnancy
- Slightly increased risk of asymptomatic functional ovarian cysts
- Following removal of Implanon, there may be a delay in return of normal periods for up to 3 months.

Contraindications

These are similar to other progestogen-only methods.

Side effects (Everett 1998)

- Acne, although in some cases acne has improved
- Breast pain
- Headache
- Weight gain.

Barrier methods of contraception

Male condom

Apparently, the name of the condom originated from the Earl of Condom, who was personal physician to King Charles II, and fashioned a device to protect the king from syphilis in the 17th century (Everett 1997). In the 18th century, Casanova called his condoms 'English Riding Coats', and used them not only to prevent infection, but also to avoid impregnating his many women friends (Durex 1993). It is therefore not only one of the oldest methods of family planning, and the only reliable one under the control of the male, apart from male sterilisation (vasectomy), but if used correctly and consistently it is still an effective contraceptive method and a means of providing safer sex.

On its own, the condom can provide up to 97% protection against pregnancy. However, ideally it should be used in addition to another effective method of contraception, which is known as 'double Dutch', or the 'belt and braces approach'.

Method of use

- The expiry date on the packet should always be checked, and the packet opened carefully to avoid damaging the condom.
- Male condoms prevent pregnancy by providing a physical barrier so that sperm are not released into the vagina, thereby ensuring that fertilisation does not take place.
- The condom should be rolled on to an erect penis before genital contact is made. Many males do not realise that pre-ejaculate can contain sufficient sperm to initiate a pregnancy.
- The closed or teat end of the condom is squeezed to expel any air, which leaves about 1 cm to collect ejaculated semen.
- After ejaculation, the condom should be held in place at the rim, and the penis is withdrawn gently to prevent spillage of semen.
- Modern male condoms should only be used once, unlike in previous times where they were washed and reused (Durex 1993).

Advantages

1. If used consistently there is up to 50% less risk of sexually transmitted infections and PID
2. They may protect against cervical neoplasia
3. They can be useful for men with premature ejaculation

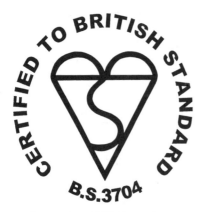

Figure 14.2 *Illustration of BSI kitemark.*

4. There is a wide range of latex condoms to suit most requirements:
   - extra strong
   - sensitive
   - teated vs. non-teated
   - flavoured, scented, ribbed and coloured
   - lubricated with spermicide (nonoxinol '9') or sensitol for those allergic to spermicide.
5. They should conform to the British Standards Institution specification (BSI) and bear the kitemark (Fig. 14.2), which signifies reliable quality products
6. They are readily available from chemists, supermarkets, barbers and vending machines.

Disadvantages (Everett 1998, Belfield 1999)

- Use requires forward planning and may interrupt sexual spontaneity, although this can be overcome by incorporating it into foreplay.
- They need to be used carefully as breakage can occur as a result of trapped air, careless opening of packet, snagging with fingernails or poor lubrication.
- Slippage and leakage are also common problems if the male does not withdraw as soon as he has lost his erection. ❶ All condom users should be aware of emergency contraception.
- Should not be used with oil-based lubricants (e.g. baby oil, Vaseline, massage oil, ice cream, butter, etc.) as they can cause deterioration of the condom. Useful lubricants are spermicidal cream/jelly or a water-soluble lubricant (e.g. KY jelly), which can increase sensitivity if inserted into the teat of the condom.
- Certain vaginal and rectal medications (e.g. Ortho Dienoestrol, Gyno-Daktarin, Nystan cream, Cyclogest and similar preparations) should not be used concurrently as they may damage the latex.
- There is usually only one size available, which may cause tightness in some men. However, there is now a larger polyurethane condom (Avanti), which is less

likely to be affected by oil-based lubricants, is stronger, more durable and has less of an odour.
- There may be loss of sensitivity during intercourse.
- Condoms should be disposed of carefully and not flushed down the toilet.

Contraindications (Everett 1998, Belfield 1999)

- An allergic reaction, irritation or sensitivity to latex or spermicide
- Failure to obtain an erection during intercourse.

Female barrier methods

Whereas the male condom can be used as a suitable ongoing method of contraception, it can also provide maximum protection for both sexual health and pregnancy when combined with another method of contraception.

On the other hand, apart from the female condom (Femidom), female barrier methods are not as effective at providing protection from sexually transmitted infections; nor are they recognised as a suitable method of reducing HIV infection. However, by creating a barrier across the cervix, they prevent sperm from entering the upper genital tract, thereby offering some protection against cervical cancer, some STDs and PID.

The main female barrier method that has been available for most of the 20th century is the diaphragm. This is a round device, consisting of a soft latex rubber dome, reinforced by a flexible circular coiled or flat spring. It is usually known as 'the cap', which may be confusing as cervical caps, vault caps and vimules are also available, although not as widely used, due to difficulties with fitting and being easily dislodged.

Until hormonal methods of contraception and the intrauterine device (IUD) were introduced, the diaphragm was the most popular form of female contraception. Diaphragms come in a range of different sizes and should only be fitted by an appropriately trained nurse or doctor. When properly in place, the diaphragm covers the cervix, and is held in place by the vaginal muscles and the tension of the sprung rim.

However, the reliability of this method is entirely user-dependent. It can be from 92–96% effective when used carefully with a spermicide.

Advantages (Everett 1998, Belfield 1999)

- It can be put in at any convenient time before intercourse, so does not interfere with spontaneity
- There are no health risks or systemic side effects
- It may give some protection to the cervix against cervical cancer and STDs
- It is under the woman's control
- It does not interfere with lactation
- Spermicide provides extra vaginal lubrication
- It can be used during menstruation
- The Femidom is lubricated with a non-spermicidal lubricant, so a spermicide may be added.

Disadvantages (Belfield 1999)

- Women need to be fitted and taught how to use and care for it
- It should be checked for deterioration and replaced regularly
- It requires forethought to avoid inhibiting spontaneity with intercourse
- It may cause vaginal irritation and can increase the incidence of urinary tract infections
- It must be used with spermicides which may appear 'messy'
- It should not be used with vaginal medications or oil-based lubricants, e.g. Vaseline, bath oil, massage oil, cold cream or salad dressing
- Size can vary with weight loss or gain of 3 kg or more
- Ideally, it should not be used until 6 weeks postnatally to allow muscle tone to return.

Contraindications (Everett 1998, Belfield 1999)

1. Poor vaginal muscle tone or prolapse
2. Congenital abnormalities, e.g. vaginal septal wall defect
3. Irritation, sensitivity or allergy to rubber, latex or spermicide
4. Infection within the vaginal or pelvic area, or recurrent urinary tract infections
5. Undiagnosed genital tract bleeding
6. Past history of toxic shock syndrome, which is more common in women who have left the cap in situ for longer than 30 hours
7. Lack of hygiene or privacy for insertion and removal
8. Aversion to touching genital area
9. It should not be used if there is a strong suspicion of pregnancy.

Emergency contraception

Failure of barrier methods may precipitate a need for emergency contraception, also known as postcoital contraception. It is a safe and highly effective method of preventing an accidental pregnancy in the following circumstances:

- after unprotected sexual intercourse (UPSI) or coitus interruptus (withdrawal)
- failure of a barrier method due to a broken or slipped condom
- a poorly fitted or dislodged diaphragm
- complete or partial expulsion of an IUD mid-cycle
- if two or more COC pills have been missed at the beginning or end of a packet, or there is concurrent medication with antibiotics, or severe diarrhoea and vomiting when supplementary precautions fail or are neglected
- if any POPs are completely missed or taken more than 3 hours later than the usual time, since ovulation is not inhibited by the POP in many women.

There are two types of emergency contraception: hormonal methods or the insertion of an IUD. Until very recently the Yuzpe method, marketed as Schering PC4, was the most widely used form of hormonal emergency contraception. However there is now a progestogen-only formulation known as Levonelle-2 that appears to have greater efficacy and fewer side effects (WHO Task Force 1998).

Hormonal methods of emergency contraception

- The Yuzpe method comprises four tablets, two to be taken within 72 hours of a single act of unprotected intercourse, followed by a further two tablets taken 12 hours later.
- Levonelle-2 follows the same guidelines, except that there are only two tablets of 750 μg of the progestogen levonorgestrel, each of which is taken 12 hours apart.
- In cases of multiple exposure, it needs to be started within 72 hours of the first episode of unprotected intercourse.
- It is important to take the first dose at a time that would enable the second dose to be taken at a convenient time during normal waking hours, as some women have been known to sleep through an alarm despite good intentions.
- The WHO research found that hormonal emergency treatment appeared to be more effective the earlier it was given (WHO Task Force 1998). Therefore, the public's insistence on naming the method 'the morning after pill' may not be far short off the mark after all!
- Levonelle-2 has all the advantages of Schering PC4 with few of the disadvantages. It is better tolerated, as there is less nausea or vomiting than with Schering PC4, and no known side effects, apart from porphyria or an allergy to the product (J Guillebaud, personal communication, 2000).

Advantages

1. There are no limits to the number of times a woman can use emergency contraception, but any woman who uses it as an ongoing method runs a higher risk of pregnancy than she would have if an established regular contraceptive method failed (Kubba & Wilkinson 1998).
2. A request for emergency contraception gives an opportunity to discuss future contraceptive requirements.
3. There are no upper or lower age limits for any of the methods.
4. In the 1998 WHO trial, the progestogen-only emergency contraceptive regimen prevented 86% of expected pregnancies when treatment was initiated within 72 hours of unprotected intercourse, whereas the combined oestrogen–progestogen regimen prevented 57% of expected pregnancies. However, if treatment was initiated within 24 hours of

unprotected intercourse, the efficacy rose to 95% and 77%, respectively (WHO Task Force 1998).

5. Depending at which point in the menstrual cycle it is given, it can prevent or delay ovulation, prevent fertilisation or implantation of an egg.

Disadvantages (Everett 1997)

1. It does not provide future contraception, so there is no contraceptive cover from it for the rest of the cycle.
2. Nausea can occur in up to 50% of women using Schering PC4 (Kubba & Wilkinson 1998), but only 23% using Levonelle-2 experienced nausea (WHO Task Force 1998). If nausea is found to be a problem, an antiemetic such as domperidone 10 mg may be prescribed at the same time or just before each dose. Nausea and vomiting are believed to be less troublesome if the method is taken with or after food.
3. Vomiting may occur in up to 20% of those using the Yuzpe method, but only 5.6% of women using Levonelle-2 reported vomiting (WHO Task Force 1998). If the patient vomits within 2 hours of taking the pills, she should return to the surgery and either take further pills with an antiemetic or consider having an IUD inserted.
4. The next menstrual period may be early or delayed. If a woman is more than 7 days late with her period, she should return for a pregnancy test.
5. Some women experience headaches, dizziness or breast tenderness.

Absolute contraindications for Schering PC4 (Everett 1997, 1998)

- Pregnancy
- Migraine at presentation in a woman with a history of focal migraine
- Past history of thromboembolism
- Pre-existing hepatocellular jaundice (Guillebaud 1997)
- Sickle cell crisis (Guillebaud 1997)
- Pre-existing active arterial disease (Guillebaud 1997)
- Active porphyria (Guillebaud 1997)

Absolute contraindications for Levonelle-2 (Schering Data Sheet 1999)

- Pregnancy
- Unexplained vaginal bleeding
- Active breast cancer
- Hypersensitivity to any ingredients in the product.

Relative contraindications for Schering PC4 (Everett 1998)

- History of arterial disease (Guillebaud 1997)
- Family history of venous thrombosis
- Previous ectopic pregnancy
- Breast-feeding if not well-established
- Unprotected sexual intercourse that has occurred more than 72 hours previously.

Relative contraindications for Levonelle-2 (Schering Data Sheet 1999)

- Severe hypertension
- Diabetes mellitus associated with vascular disease, nephropathy, retinopathy or neuropathy
- Ischaemic heart disease or stroke
- Past history of breast cancer.

Figure 14.3 illustrates the management of patients requesting emergency contraception.

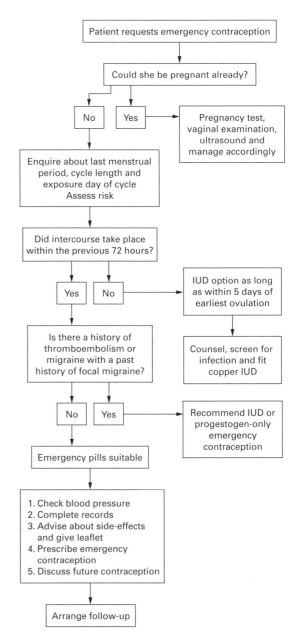

Figure 14.3 *Management of patients requesting emergency contraception.*

The emergency IUD

The insertion of a copper IUD is a viable alternative to hormonal postcoital treatment. The IUD can be fitted up to 5 days after unprotected intercourse. According to recent guidelines (Kubba & Wilkinson 1998), it can also be inserted up to 5 days after the earliest calculated ovulation day in the cycle. However, the use of the levonorgestrel-releasing intrauterine system (IUS) is not recommended for this purpose.

As it is the most effective of any of the emergency contraceptive methods, insertion of an IUD should be the preferred choice when efficacy is a priority. It also protects against pregnancy for the rest of the cycle, and can remain in situ providing ongoing contraception, assuming there are no contraindications to its long-term use.

The IUD works almost instantaneously due to the interceptive anti-implantation effect of the copper ions on the endometrium. Thus, it can be said that it does not act as an abortifacient, since neither implantation nor subsequent pregnancy can occur until at least 5–7 days following fertilisation (Kubba & Wilkinson 1998).

Absolute contraindications (Everett 1998)

- Suspected pregnancy.
- Untreated vaginal, cervical or pelvic infection unless screening is given for sexually transmitted infections and full antibiotic cover is provided. These precautions should also be taken if an IUD is inserted following sexual assault.
- Undiagnosed bleeding of genital tract.

Relative contraindications (Everett 1998)

- Past history of ectopic pregnancy, although the IUD should be removed at the next menstrual period
- Past history of pelvic infection
- Heart valve replacement or previous history of bacterial endocarditis, unless the IUD is inserted with antibiotic cover.

Side effects

These are similar to those pertaining to the IUD in general (see below). However, any side effect would be limited to that cycle as there is an option of removing the IUD once menstruation has commenced.

Intrauterine contraception

This includes the copper bearing IUD, the intrauterine contraceptive implant marketed as GyneFix and the evonorgestrel intrauterine system (IUS), or Mirena.

The IUD

The IUD is a small, flexible polyethylene and copper device containing monofilament threads for removal, and to allow women to check regularly that it is still in position. It comes in various shapes and sizes; the newer devices contain barium sulphate in the polyethylene, which means their position can be located by X-ray or ultrasound.

The IUD is inserted into the uterus through the cervical canal, usually at the end of a menstrual period when the cervix is marginally more dilated, although it can be inserted any time up to 5 days after the earliest calculated ovulation day in the cycle (or day 19 in a 28-day cycle). Ideally, screening for *Chlamydia* and other STDs should be done pre-insertion.

Mode of action

The IUD causes a foreign body reaction in the endometrium, with subsequent increased numbers of leucocytes and phagocytes. This reaction is enhanced by the copper, which may also inhibit sperm transport. The viability of the sperm and ovum are impaired through alteration of the uterine and fallopian tube fluids. These endometrial changes thus interfere with implantation at an early stage.

Advantages (Everett 1998, Belfield 1999)

1. Failure rate can be as low as or less than 1% with the newest IUDs containing a high copper content. Other copper devices have a failure rate of 1–2%.
2. It provides long-term, highly effective, rapidly reversible contraception.
3. Contraception takes effect immediately after fitting.
4. Efficacy is not related to sexual intercourse.
5. There are no drug interactions.

Disadvantages (Everett 1998, Belfield 1999)

1. There is an increased risk of pelvic infection within the first few weeks after insertion. Young, nulliparous women, those with a previous history of PID and those with multiple partners have a greater than average risk of infection.
2. Menstrual irregularities of menorrhagia, intermenstrual bleeding, vaginal discharge or lower abdominal pain may occur.
3. There is a slightly increased risk of ectopic pregnancy in the event of IUD failure, but it appears that this risk is less than in women not using any or minimal contraception (Guillebaud 1999).
4. It may be expelled spontaneously, become displaced or perforate the uterus, bowel or bladder in very rare instances.

Absolute contraindications (Everett 1997, 1998, Belfield 1999)

- Known or suspected pregnancy
- Previous ectopic pregnancy in a nulliparous woman
- Recent PID
- Any untreated pelvic or vaginal infection
- Undiagnosed abnormal bleeding from the genital tract

- Distortion of the uterine cavity due to congenital abnormalities (e.g. bicornate uterus), or large fibroids
- Allergy to copper and Wilson's disease
- Heart valve replacement or previous history of bacterial endocarditis, because of an increased risk of infection
- HIV and AIDS due to reduced immune function and increased risk of infection.

Relative contraindications (Everett 1998)

- Previous ectopic pregnancy
- History of pelvic infection
- Fibroids and endometriosis
- Dysmenorrhoea and menorrhagia
- Penicillamine treatment for Wilson's disease or rheumatoid arthritis may reduce the contraceptive effect of copper (Guillebaud 1999).

GyneFix

This is a frameless intrauterine device consisting of six copper beads threaded on to a length of non-biodegradable suture thread. The device is inserted by implanting the knot at the upper end of the thread into the fundal myometrium, where it acts as an anchor to keep the system in place. It works in the same way as all IUDs by preventing fertilisation, and should be effective for 5 years. However, it can only be fitted by a medical professional with specialist training.

The IUS

This relatively new intrauterine device was introduced from Finland in 1995. It consists of a T-shaped frame containing the progestogen, levonorgestrel, in a hormone reservoir around the stem. It is inserted and removed in the same way as the IUD, and marketed under the name of Mirena.

The IUS prevents pregnancy by much the same mechanism as the IUD, but it has the added benefit of the levonorgestrel, which is released slowly and helps to make the cervical mucus impenetrable to sperm. The endometrium becomes less favourable for implantation, and fallopian tube function decreases. In some women, it may also prevent ovulation. With most of the benefits of hormonal and uterine methods of contraception and few disadvantages, it is becoming an increasingly popular method.

Advantages

1. It has a high safety rate of 99.5% effectiveness against pregnancy. It should be fitted within the first 7 days of the start of a period and is effective immediately. If fitted after this time, additional precautions need to be used for 7 days.
2. There is reduced risk of infection, which may be due to the effect of the progestogen on the cervical mucus, menstrual loss or cervical thickness.

3. There is reduced dysmenorrhoea and less menstrual blood loss, so it can be an effective treatment for menorrhagia.
4. It is easily reversible with immediate return to fertility.

Disadvantages (Everett 1998, Belfield 1999)

1. Intermenstrual bleeding, particularly within the first 3 months
2. Amenorrhoea, which can be of concern to some women
3. Some women develop progestogenic symptoms of breast tenderness, bloating, irritability or acne in the early months of use
4. The body of the IUS is wider than the other IUDs, so the cervix may need dilatation for insertion
5. ❶ Pregnancy caused by expulsion, perforation or malposition, with a slightly increased risk of such a pregnancy being ectopic
6. It is not suitable for postcoital use
7. It is considerably more expensive than other intrauterine devices.

Absolute contraindications

These are similar to those relating to the IUD, but also include:

- sensitivity to levonorgestrel
- liver disease
- recent trophoblastic disease with elevated levels of hCG (Belfield 1999).

Relative contraindications (Everett 1998)

- Chronic systemic disease
- Past or present severe arterial disease or risk factors
- Severe lipid abnormalities
- Recurrent cholestatic jaundice
- Sex-steroid dependent cancer, e.g. breast cancer
- Functional ovarian cysts which need hospitalisation
- Past history of ectopic pregnancy.

Side effects (Everett 1998)

- Some women may develop functional ovarian cysts
- Breast tenderness
- Acne
- Headaches
- Fluid retention
- Mood changes
- Nausea.

Natural methods of contraception

After weighing up all the ifs and buts, advantages, disadvantages and contraindications of the different methods, some women opt for using natural methods of contraception. Natural methods have also been known as periodic abstinence, the safe period and the rhythm method, based on when ovulation was thought to occur.

They do not include coitus interruptus or withdrawal, which although natural, has little contraceptive benefit as sperm can escape at any time from an erect penis before ejaculation. However, even though this is the oldest method of contraception known, and is also the least satisfying for both partners, it is thought to be used by about 4% of the sexually active population in Britain. As an 'emergency' method, withdrawal is better than no method, and can be made safer by also using a simple contraceptive pessary (Guillebaud 1997).

There are four main methods of natural family planning (Everett 1997, 1998):
1. The calendar method
2. The temperature method
3. The cervical mucus or Billings method
4. The sympto-thermal method.

The calendar method

For natural family planning to be most effective, women need to have an acute awareness of their own fertility. This involves an understanding of the menstrual cycle and identifying when ovulation takes place. As most menstrual cycles are completed on average every 28 days, with a normal range of 21–35 days, ovulation will usually occur about 14 days before the onset of the next period.

At ovulation, an ovum is released into the uterine cavity and is then capable of being fertilised for up to 24 hours. However, as sperm can live within the female body for 3–5 days and have been known to survive for up to 7 days, estimation of the fertile time is based on sperm survival and deducing when ovulation will occur. This deduction can be made by looking retrospectively over the woman's menstrual cycles for a period of at least 6 months.

As stress and illness can contribute to cycle irregularities, this method is no longer recognised as being reliable on its own, but it is useful to teach women how to calculate their time of maximum fertility if they are trying to become pregnant.

The temperature method

Using a special ovulation thermometer, a woman's basal body temperature is recorded every day for a minimum of 3 min on waking. Following ovulation, the temperature will drop slightly, and then, due to the release of the hormone progesterone by the corpus luteum, it will rise by 0.2–0.4°C until the onset of the next period. After 3 days of a raised temperature, intercourse should be able to take place safely until the start of the next period.

The basal body temperature will be affected by infection, illness, disturbed sleep or any alteration to the normal time of waking. Late nights, particularly if alcohol is consumed, stress, drugs or medication such as aspirin will also interfere with normal body temperature.

The cervical mucus method

The cervical mucus varies throughout the cycle. Following menstruation, oestrogen levels are low, which causes the mucus to be scanty and dry, and known as infertile mucus. Before ovulation, increasing amounts of mucus are produced and it becomes clear and stretchy with a consistency similar to raw egg white. This is the fertile mucus. After the ovum has been released, the level of oestrogen drops, and under the influence of progesterone, the mucus becomes thick, sticky and opaque, with a sensation of dryness.

This method may be affected by vaginal infections, and some medications (e.g. for the common cold) may inhibit cervical mucus production. The increase in vaginal mucus produced by sexual arousal can also appear similar to ovulatory mucus. It is also unsuitable for perimenopausal women, whose fluctuating hormonal changes will affect the consistency of the mucus.

The sympto–thermal method

This is a combination of the calendar, temperature and cervical mucus methods. It is considered the safest of the natural methods, as it also combines an awareness of body changes such as breast tenderness, mid-cycle ovulatory pain (mittelschmerz) and the change in position and consistency of the cervix.

At ovulation, the cervix rises high in the vagina, becoming softer and the cervical os opens slightly. Locating the position of the cervix, and assessing the softness and opening of the cervical os as a daily routine requires commitment, motivation and specialist teaching. However, the combination of these methods does give good contraceptive efficacy, which can be used in reverse to aid conception.

The personal contraceptive system (Persona)

This small hand-held electronic monitor can be bought over the counter. It identifies a woman's fertile status by analysing a sample of her early morning urine. With careful and consistent use, it has been found to be between 93 and 97% effective in preventing pregnancy (Everett 1998).

However, Persona is not suitable for women with menstrual irregularities, or those with polycystic ovary syndrome. Women who have recently given birth, those who are breast-feeding, women with menopausal symptoms or women using any form of hormonal treatment cannot use this system. Neither should it be used by women with kidney or liver disease (Everett 1998).

Advantages (Everett 1998)
- No systemic effects
- Under the control of the woman
- Can be used to plan pregnancy.

Disadvantages
- Expensive

- Can only be used by women whose menstrual cycles range from 23 to 35 days and who have no hormonal irregularities.

Sterilisation

Female sterilisation

As this is the only permanent method of female contraception, with an efficacy of 99.4–99.8% (Everett 1998), it should also be considered irreversible. It is a surgical procedure that involves either excision and tubal ligation, sealing the fallopian tubes by cauterisation and diathermy, or blocking the tubes with clips or rings. The ovum is therefore prevented from travelling from the ovary to the uterus, or being fertilised by sperm on the way, even though ovulation and menstruation will continue as before. Contraception should continue to be used up until the first period following the sterilisation procedure (Belfield 1999).

Procedure

- Local or general anaesthetic
- Usually involves day-care surgery
- Abdominally by laparoscopic sterilisation or mini laparotomy
- Vaginally by culdoscopy, although this is rarely used in the UK (Belfield 1999).

Advantages

1. High efficacy
2. Immediately effective
3. Permanent method
4. Fear of unplanned pregnancy is removed.

Disadvantages

1. Involves an anaesthetic and surgical procedure
2. Is not easily reversed.

Contraindications (Everett 1998)

- Marital or relationship problems
- Uncertainty about the operation by either partner
- Ill health or physical disability, which may increase risk of operation
- Psychiatric illness.

Side effects

❶ Very rarely sterilisation may fail, depending on which procedure is used. Should this occur, there is a higher risk of an ectopic pregnancy.

Otherwise, side effects are rare, although occasionally a woman may regret her decision and experience feelings of grief and loss. This can be reduced with careful counselling before the operation takes place. It has been found that regret is more prevalent if the decision for sterilisation is made during times of crisis or stress, and should be avoided after termination of pregnancy, miscarriage or immediately following childbirth

(Guillebaud 1997). As there is increased vascularity of the tissues after a pregnancy, sterilisation is also unwise at this time due to a higher risk of failure (Everett 1998).

Male sterilisation (vasectomy)

As it is a less-invasive procedure than female sterilisation, vasectomy is becoming a more popular choice of permanent contraception for many couples. Contemplation of the procedure should always involve counselling, preferably with both partners. Men need to consider whether they would want more children should their partner die or the marriage break down.

Vasectomy is usually performed under local anaesthetic, and involves the excision or removal of part of the vas deferens, which transports sperm from the testes to the penis. It takes about 3 months for the vas deferens to be cleared of sperm, after which time the method is 99.9% effective in preventing pregnancy.

Advantages

1. Permanent method
2. Highly effective
3. Safe and simple procedure.

Disadvantages (Everett 1998)

1. Not immediately effective – contraception is still required until two consecutive clear sperm counts have been produced
2. Not easily reversed
3. Minor surgical procedure with local or general anaesthetic
4. Side effects are generally minor but may involve infection, haematoma or sperm granuloma.

Contraindications (Belfield 1999)

- Urological problems
- Any marital or relationship problems
- Indecision about sterilisation by either partner
- Psychiatric illness.

Preconceptual care

A nurse practitioner who has been involved in giving women contraceptive advice, or perhaps performing a pregnancy test on a new patient is in a very good position to provide preconceptual care. She can also give advice about the timing of intercourse to coincide with the most fertile phase of the menstrual cycle for those who are planning a pregnancy (see Natural Methods of Contraception section).

The concern of how to minimise risks to a developing baby may be the trigger needed to help some women develop healthier lifestyle choices. For many women general advice about diet, exercise, relaxation, smoking and alcohol intake may be all that is needed, although whether there are any potential inherited medical conditions will also need to be discussed.

Diet

A healthy diet is important for all women, but women planning to become pregnant should be encouraged to eat a diet which is low in fat with increased amounts of vegetables, fruit, carbohydrates and wholegrain products. Overweight women should plan to lose weight at least 3 months before conceiving so that their metabolism has a chance to stabilise before dealing with the strain of pregnancy. Those who are underweight may have difficulty falling pregnant, and are at risk of having a low birthweight baby. These babies have a higher incidence of perinatal mortality and morbidity, as well as further health problems in later life (Everett 1997, 1998).

Foods to avoid in pregnancy include undercooked meat, cooked chilled chicken and foods made with uncooked eggs (e.g. mayonnaise) because of the risk of salmonella. Pâté, cheeses made with unpasteurised milk and blue-veined cheeses should also be avoided as they may contain high levels of listeria bacteria which can result in miscarriage, stillbirth, brain damage or severe illness in a newborn baby (Everett 1997, 1998). Birth defects can also occur when there is a high intake of vitamin A, so pregnant women should avoid dietary supplements containing vitamin A and foods high in this vitamin (e.g. liver).

Folic acid

It is recommended by the Department of Health that all women planning a pregnancy should take 400 µg of folic acid daily prior to conceiving and until 12 weeks' gestation, to prevent neural tube defects (Department of Health 1992).

Smoking and alcohol

Smoking should be avoided in pregnancy, as it is associated with an increased risk of miscarriage, prematurity and intrauterine growth retardation. Smoking can also reduce fertility in both men and women. Although it is probably safest to stop drinking alcohol altogether when pregnant, it is not contraindicated in small amounts of 1–2 units once or twice a week. Heavy drinking in pregnancy can result in fetal abnormalities and low birthweight babies.

Drugs and medications

Women taking illegal drugs are often not going to admit that they have a problem. Should a woman be planning a pregnancy she needs to be advised that illegal drugs can harm the developing baby and referred for the appropriate support before conception. Some regular medications may also be contraindicated in pregnancy and need to be discussed with the doctor, dentist or pharmacist.

Rubella status

All women planning a pregnancy should be routinely screened for rubella immunity before conception, as exposure can cause fetal abnormalities. Since, currently, most females of child-bearing age have been immunised at school in Britain, those at risk are women who were educated outside Britain, and nulliparous women in their late thirties whose schooling took place before the immunisation programme began (Louden et al 1995). However, a previous history of rubella infection or vaccination does not confer automatic immunity. Any woman who is found to be susceptible to rubella needs to avoid pregnancy for at least 1 month following immunisation (Everett 1998).

Toxoplasmosis

This parasitic infection is contracted through raw meat, cat faeces, sheep and goats' milk. It causes a flu-like illness that can lead to brain damage and blindness in the fetus (Everett 1998).

Medical history

Before becoming pregnant a woman should have had a recent cervical smear and be clear of any STDs. She will need to be made aware of the importance of regular dental checkups before, during and after her pregnancy.

A family history should be taken from both partners and screening offered for any potential inherited disorders such as sickle cell disease, thalassaemia and Tay–Sachs disease (Everett 1997). Couples with a personal or family history of these conditions and other genetic disorders, such as cystic fibrosis, muscular dystrophy or Down's syndrome, may benefit from genetic counselling.

Part 2: Menopause

Myfanwy Rimmer

Introduction

The menopause is defined as the inevitable and irreversible decline in ovarian hormones that culminates in the cessation of menstruation, and thus represents a marker in the transition from a reproductive state to a non-reproductive state. Choi (1995) expands on this to include the climacteric, which refers to the transitional years surrounding the menopause during which an array of biological, psychological and social changes are taking place.

Women living in the United Kingdom (UK) can reasonably expect to have one-third of their lives postmenopausally, with the average life of a female now predicted into the eighth decade (Coney 1995). This statistic has implications for health care. The long-term effects of oestrogen deficiency have become apparent as women live longer. Prevalence and risk of coronary heart disease (CHD), cerebrovascular disease (CVD)

and osteoporosis increases with each year after the menopause.

The menopause is classified into three states:
- A premenopausal state, where periods are still fairly regular but where there maybe associated menopausal symptoms.
- A perimenopausal state, where there is decreasing frequency of periods, 3–11 months of amenorrhea, often with associated menopausal symptoms. This typically occurs in the 47–53-year-old age group.
- A postmenopausal state, where there has been a period of 12 consecutive months of amenorrhea, or where the woman is aged 54 or over.

These classifications reflect the natural physiological process. During the fertile years the waxing and waning of the anterior pituitary and ovarian hormones are regulated by a negative feedback interaction. Follicle-stimulating hormone (FSH) and luteinising hormone (LH) from the anterior pituitary stimulate ovarian follicle growth and oestrogen secretion begins. As oestrogen levels rise, a negative feedback on the anterior pituitary causes FSH and LH levels to fall (a switch effect). Once oestrogen reaches a critical concentration, it exerts a negative feedback on the anterior pituitary and FSH again begins to rise, switching oestrogen off. In this way a regular menstrual cycle is controlled (Fig. 14.4).

As menopausal oestrogen levels fall, fluctuations in cyclic activity occur. Imbalances in oestrogen and progesterone and increase in FSH levels as negative feedback is reduced all have influences on menopausal, particularly vasomotor, symptoms (Marieb 1989).

Consulting with menopausal problems can be difficult for patients. Perceived as a non-medical problem, legitimization of claiming a general practitioner's (GP's) time can hold ambiguities. The nurse practitioner (NP) may be seen as the appropriate person to consult, with her nursing role, skill of assessment and ability to diagnose and manage primary care presentations. The NP offering, discussing and advocating menopausal management is able to explore enhancing lifestyles, health behaviours and holistic counselling. In our culture there is a 'taboo' or 'cloak of secrecy' surrounding many menopausal myths. Women need time to talk, time to explore fears and expectations and time to ask questions and gain knowledge, enabling them to make decisions based on sound knowledge and not ignorance.

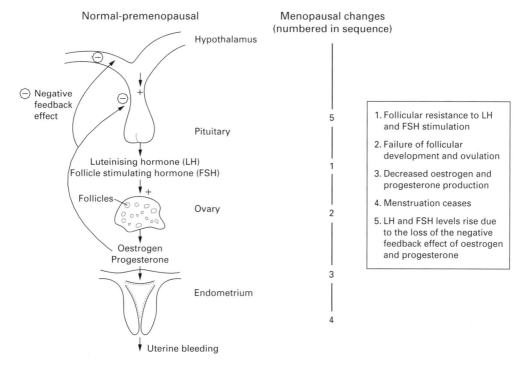

Figure 14.4 *Normal (premenopausal) and menopausal changes.*

Assessment

Subjective assessment

Presentations of menopausal problems can be classified into the following categories:
- physiological
- psychological
- social/cultural.

Taking a complete and accurate history is essential to enable patients to identify hidden agendas, explore values and beliefs and to ensure correct diagnosis and management outcomes. Many symptoms associated with the menopause present as 'by the way' or 'while I'm here nurse' situations, and in many instances prove to be the primary reason for the consultation.

Subjective findings

Vague symptoms
- Patient complains of being tired all the time
- Patient reports loss of libido.

Physical symptoms
- Irregular periods
- No periods
- Heavy periods
- Frequent periods
- Hot flushes and night sweats
- Sleep disturbance
- Headaches
- Dry vagina
- Pain on intercourse
- Urgency and frequency of micturition
- Changes in skin, hair and nails
- Joint and muscle pains
- Palpitations
- Constipation
- Bloating.

Psychological symptoms
- Low mood
- Loss of confidence and self-esteem
- Irritability
- Poor concentration
- Poor memory
- Depression.

Depression and despair have been identified as a symptom of the menopause and evidence from research studies is conflicting. Kaufert (1994), concluding from her research on samples drawn from the general population, repeatedly supports the null hypothesis that 'women may be both depressed and menopausal, but there is no significant relationship between being depressed and menopausal'.

Social and cultural

- Changes in relationships and roles: children leaving home can precipitate feelings of loss, which often presents subjectively as a hidden agenda.
- Separation and divorce.
- Fears and myths may be handed down through generations. Frequently, verbalisations of a fear of loss of mental stability are presented: 'nurse I thought I was going mad'.
- Bereavement.
- Loss of parents.
- Change of role.

Women's roles have traditionally been linked to their biological function: their gender identity has been linked to their reproductive capacity and their value judged by their youth and beauty (Choi 1995). In the light of this, the menopause in Western culture is often viewed negatively. It is this negative stereotyping and lack of status (ageism) that can precipitate a consultation, although it is not often verbalized in this way. The history taken must be approached with sensitivity, exploring these diverse perspectives.

History

Clinical history should include:

1. Discussion of presenting symptoms.
2. Past history of any serious disease: this information could influence management, e.g. past history of breast cancer or a clotting disorder help determine treatment
3. Past history of any surgical procedures: a hysterectomy, with or without conservation of the ovaries would be vital information in treatment and management.
4. Past history of episodes of depression or mental illness: a very important element of a differential diagnosis relating to psychological related presenting symptoms.
5. Date of last cervical smear: if screening has lapsed, a menopausal consultation is an ideal opportunity to explore the reasons why.
6. Date of last menstrual period (LMP): very useful in determining stage of menopause and helps identify cases of early or late menopausal status.
7. Contraceptive history: to assess any risk of pregnancy or the need to continue contraceptive protection. Assess any problems related to previous contraceptive methods, i.e. weight gain or increase in blood pressure with oral contraceptive pill. This information could influence management and follow-up.
8. ❶ A menstrual and bleeding history: symptoms of intermenstrual bleeding (IMB), bleeding after sexual intercourse (SI) or menorrhagia will need further investigation and referral.
9. Pain: any pelvic pain, dyspareunia or dysmenorrhoea needs further investigation.
10. Presence of any discharge: it is important to establish if any pathology is involved. Symptoms of itching, profuse discharge or odour need further investigation.
11. Drug history: determine any prescribed medication being taken. Calcium antagonists can cause flushing, and withdrawal from benzodiazepines may be influential in disturbed sleep patterns. Interaction with other medications can occur. Explore over-the-counter (OTC) medications and include vitamins and supplements. Explore any self-help remedies for presenting symptoms.
12. Social history: employment status. Any redundancy or unemployment could be important in establishing levels of self-esteem or financial problems. It could be important in determining any frustrations that may be linked to unfulfilled career or personal ambitions.
13. Marital status: explore, if appropriate, any feelings around relationships that may important in menopausal assessment. These may be clinical in problems such as loss of libido, or may be emotional issues such as infidelity or divorce. New relationships may have implications for sexual health education. ❶ Do not forget to explore sexual health issues when indicated with the mature adult.
14. Family:
    - Have children recently left home?
    - Does partner work late hours?
    - Is loneliness a factor?
    - Do the demands of family overwhelm and exclude self?
    - Are there elderly dependent relatives?
    - Family history – are parents alive and well? If not, what was the cause of their death? Is there any family history of heart disease, diabetes, breast cancer, fractures or osteoporosis in a first-degree relative?
15. Lifestyle history:
    - Explore dietary eating pattern. Dietary implications in CVD and breast cancer (HEA 1996, HEA 1999).
    - Smoking: as an influence on CVD, cervical cancer and osteoporosis (Law & Hackshaw 1997).
    - Alcohol: influencing factor in breast cancer (Smith-Warner et al 1998). It can cause flushing or sleep problems. Abuse is linked with liver disease. This factor could be relevant when planning management.
    - Exercise: pattern and frequency are important in assessing osteoporosis risk and prevention. Exercise enhances well-being.
    - Breast self-examination: establish pattern of practice, any recent mammograms and the patient's attitude to breast cancer.

Objective assessment

This will be directed very much from the findings of the history:

- Blood pressure. If raised greater than 140/82 mmHg, a risk factor for CVD (Hansson et al 1998).
- Weight/height. A BMI greater than 30 is a risk factor for CVD.
- Breast examination. Involve the patient and teach self-examination skills. Observe attitude. Some ladies are very reluctant to self-examine. See pages 263–264 for breast examination technique.
- Pelvic examination. This may be required if pain, discharge or abnormal bleeding has been determined from the history. See page 263 for examination technique.
- Investigations. Most likely none. In a younger person less than 45 years old, FSH levels could confirm an early menopause; however, results can be unreliable. Normal levels can be present with a menopausal state. If a differential diagnosis is suspected, thyroid function tests may be indicated, to exclude hyper- or hypothyroidism.

Management

Hormone replacement therapy (HRT)

- Any decision to start therapy must be made with the patient
- All questions or barriers to treatment should be explored
- Compliance will be poor if uncertainties or lack of support exist.

Benefits of HRT

- Improvement of menstrual symptoms
- Reduced incidents of heart attacks (Stampfer & Colditz 1991)
- Reduced incidents of strokes (Finucane et al 1993)
- Decrease in osteoporotic fractures (Breslau 1994)
- May reduce incidence of Alzheimer's disease (Tang et al 1996)
- Improved prognosis in many cancers, particularly colorectal (Grodstein et al 1998)
- Less depression (Studd & Smith, 1994)
- Improved sexuality and libido (Burger et al 1987)
- Improved quality and length of life.

Disadvantages of HRT

Side effects of oestrogen
- Feeling of bloatedness
- Breast tenderness
- Nausea
- Vomiting.

Side effects of progesterones
- Breast discomfort
- Depression
- Nausea
- Irritability
- Fluid retention
- Headaches
- Weight gain
- Sometimes irregular bleeding, particularly in the perimenopausal lady.

Absolute contraindications to HRT

- Previous history of breast cancer or endometrial cancer
- Severe liver disease
- Pregnancy
- Undiagnosed abnormal vaginal bleeding.

Special precautions to HRT

- Patients with diagnosed otosclerosis: the fear is this could be exacerbated
- Active endometriosis: oestrogen stimulates endometriosis
- Gallstones may be aggravated
- Benign breast disease: there is a slightly increased risk of developing breast cancer.

Types of HRT

1. Oral:
   - Unopposed oestrogen. Conjugated oestrogens, oestrodiol valerate and oestrodiol. For hysterectomised ladies only.
   - Sequential – 28 days continuous oestrogen plus progesterone 12–14 days per cycle. Withdrawal bleed.
   - Continuous combined therapy – oestrogen and progesterone taken daily. No withdrawal bleed.
   - Quarterly HRT – continuous daily oestrogen with progestogen for 14 days every 3 months. Four withdrawal bleeds per year.
2. Transdermal patches: oestrogen only. Combined sequential–continuous oestradiol with transdermal progestogen added for 14 days per cycle. Withdrawal bleed.
3. Subcutaneous implants.
4. Skin gels – measured amount applied daily. Oestrodiol and oestradiol hemihydrate.
5. Vaginal creams – oestrogen only.
6. Vaginal pessaries – oestrogen only.
   Recommended minimum doses for bone conservation:
   - oral conjugated oestrogens: 0.625 mg daily
   - oral oestradiol: 2 mg daily
   - in combined continuous therapy: 1 mg daily
   - piperazine oestrone sulphate: 1.5 mg daily
   - transdermal oestradiol: 50 µg patch
   - subcutaneous oestradiol: 50 mg implant every 6 months
   - tibolone: 2.5 mg daily.
   Minimum doses of progestogen necessary for endometrial protection

1. Synthetic C_{19} group – structurally related to testosterone:
   - norethisterone: 1 mg daily
   - levonorgestrel: 150 µg daily
   - norgestrel: 150 µg daily.
2. Synthetic C_{21} group – structurally related to progesterone
   - medroxyprogesterone acetate: 10 mgs daily
   - dydrogesterone: 10–20 mg daily.
3. Natural progesterone
   - progesterone: Crinone 4% vaginal gel alternate days.

The choice of HRT preparations is growing all the time. *MIMS* (*Monthly Index of Medical Specialities*) contains a table that is updated monthly identifying all current medications and classification of oestrogen and progestogen components.

Factors that influence choice:
1. Hysterectomy: patients do not need progestogen challenge.
2. Oestrogen history: past history of oestrogen side effects on oral contraceptive pill, e.g. weight gain.
3. Progesterone history: past history of contraception, e.g. many years of norethisterone without problems would influence choice. With a loss of libido C_{19} progestogen could help. Premenstrual tension problems could be improved with a C_{21} progestogen.
4. Patient preference: conjugated oestrogens are unacceptable to some patients due to the equine connection.
5. Menopausal state: Pre- and perimenopausal ladies with an intact uterus must have a withdrawal bleed to prevent endometrial hyperplasia and thus eliminate any risk of endometrial carcinoma. Ladies aged 53 or over with 12 months amenorrhoea may have combined continuous therapy. Age is no barrier. To minimize oestrogen side effects it may be necessary to start with a lower dose of oestrogen and titrate up.
6. Compliance: implants may overcome this problem; however, ladies with an intact uterus must have a progestogen challenge.
7. Skin problems: allergy to patches may be a problem with conditions such as eczema.

Patient education

- Explain HRT regime being started
- Explain expected bleeding pattern
- Explain when withdrawal bleed should occur
- Explain possible problems in early months, i.e. tender breasts and heavy withdrawal bleeds
- Provide diary card to record menstrual pattern
- Explore unreal expectations
- Advise on side effects
- Support with literature
- Organise 3-month prescription
- Arrange 3-month follow-up appointment
- Specify support mechanism for contact if problems occur.

Guidelines for follow-up:
- Check symptom control
- Check bleeding pattern
- Explore any side effects
- Check blood pressure
- Check weight
- Breast examination
- If appropriate discuss duration of treatment.

Troubleshooting

1. Bleeding early. Check compliance: Could be due to inadequate progestogen; consider increasing dose of duration. ❶ If it continues after two cycles, suspect pathology, investigate and possibly refer.
2. Heavy bleeding. Could be too much oestrogen or insufficient progestogen. Dose adjustment may be indicated. ❶ If it continues, suspect pathology and refer.
3. Spotting during cycle. Check compliance: it could be insufficient oestrogen. ❶ If it continues, suspect pathology and refer.
4. No withdrawal bleed. Check compliance with progesterone. If compliance is good, this is not uncommon in postmenopausal women: no need to investigate. It could mean too low an oestrogen dose (in younger women one would expect the majority to bleed).

Alternative therapies

While there are few women who cannot take HRT in some form, there are many women who decide not to take it. For whatever reason a women opts not to take HRT, the range of options should be explored and she should be supported in her decision.

Dietary influences

Calcium. There is a growing body of evidence that a calcium supplement of 1000–1500 mg per day will have some preventive benefit against osteoporosis (Breslau 1994).

Vitamin D. Vitamin D is essential for calcium absorption; however, people eating a Western diet probably ingest sufficient (Andrews 1997, p. 344). People at risk may be those with limited solar exposure.

Vitamin E. There is evidence to support a significant reduction in CVD in postmenopausal women taking vitamin E supplements. This is thought to be linked with antioxidant properties (Pahor & Applegate 1997). A UK daily requirement for vitamin E has not been established; however, European union (EU) labelling RDA for vitamin E is 10 mg per day. Dowden (1999) debates any efficacy at this level and reports that up to 800 mg per day as an upper safe level. This level is supported by the Council for Responsible Nutrition.

Phyto-oestrogens. These are nonsteroidal substances, found in plants, with oestrogenic activity. They are mainly present in soya bean, red clover and are a major source of isoflavonoids. The molecule is similar in structure to female oestrogen; however, it is less potent. Phyto-oestrogens have an affinity for oestrogen receptors (Stewart 1998, p. 18). Aldercreutz & Mazur (1997) in his review of the literature supports the view that they probably have some effect in limiting hot flushes and vaginal dryness and to some degree inhibit osteoporosis, However, dietary intake may be insufficient to give complete protection. No definite recommendations can be made as to the dietary amounts needed for the prevention of disease.

Breast examination

Introduction

A large body of evidence now exists supporting the benefits of HRT. As discussed earlier, HRT not only relieves climacteric symptoms but has long-term benefits in preventing bone loss, reducing the risk of cardiovascular disease, offering protection from colorectal cancer and possibly preventing the development of Alzheimer's disease. (Hart 1997) The importance of these benefits on mortality and morbidity have the potential to be quite dramatic; however, HRT remains relatively underused. It is the fear that HRT may increase the risk of developing breast cancer or stimulate the recurrence in breast cancer survivors that has led to many women refusing therapy. Bergkvist (1997) debates the epidemiological evidence and concludes that overall HRT can be considered safe with respect to breast cancer, with the exception that there is a moderate increase of risk after long-term use – defined as 10–15 years.

Achuthan et al (1997), in a reanalysis of data from 51 epidemiological studies of women taking HRT, states that, for women aged 50 not using HRT, 45 in every 1000 will have breast cancer diagnosed over the next 20 years. For women in the same age group taking HRT:

5 years of use: an extra 2 cases per 1000
10 years of use: an extra 6 cases per 1000
15 years of use: an extra 12 cases per 1000.

Many of the extra cancers will be in situ as opposed to invasive lesions, and thus will have a better long-term prognosis.

RCN (1997) guidelines for practice on breast palpation and breast awareness highlight that there is no evidence that palpation alone is effective in reducing mortality from breast cancer. The guidelines state that the nurse's role is to educate and facilitate within this area of health care and to provide information and support for women: it is not to provide a diagnosis or to imply that the nurse can in any way define whether a woman may or may not have breast cancer. It is recommended that nurses promote 'breast awareness', encouraging women to get to know their own breasts and become familiar with what is normal for them, thus enabling them to detect the abnormal. In the context of becoming familiar with her breasts, a woman may seek the help of a nurse to demonstrate how this may be achieved – including verbal and written information supporting this care.

Within the philosophy and role definition of the nurse practitioner, patients may consult with undiagnosed undifferentiated problems. Many patients choose to consult the NP as their primary contact for HRT and, sometimes, associated breast anxieties. It is within this context, and within the framework of the RCN philosophy and guidelines, that in completing a comprehensive assessment of a presenting problem, a breast examination is an essential element of management and treatment. HRT consultations are such an example.

The breasts and axillae

The female breast lies between the second and sixth ribs, between the sternal edge and midaxillary line. About two-thirds of the breast is superficial to the pectoralis major, about one-third to the serratus anterior. The nipple and areola that surrounds it are somewhat lateral to the midline of the breast (Bates 1991).

For the purpose of description, the breast may be divided into four quadrants by vertical and horizontal lines crossing at the nipple. In addition, a tail of breast tissue frequently extends towards or into the axillae. An alternative method of localising findings visualises the breast as the face of a clock. A lesion may be located and recorded by the 'time' (e.g. 4 o'clock) and by the distance in centimetres from the nipple.

The lymphatics of much of the breast drain toward the axillae. These form three main groups.
1. The pectoral (or anterior) group of nodes are located along the lower border of pectoralis major inside the anterior axillary fold.
2. The subscapular (or posterior) group is located along the lateral border of the scapula and is felt deep in the posterior axillary fold.
3. The lateral group is felt along the upper humerus.
   Lymph also drains from the central axillary nodes to the infraclavicular and supraclavicular nodes.

Techniques of examination

General approach
- Sensitivity to patient needs and feelings
- Awareness of fear, shyness and cultural issues
- Provide a safe, private and warm environment
- Ensure a screened examination couch
- Cover to avoid unnecessary exposure
- Be sure that the setting ensures confidentiality.

Inspection

Ask the patient to sit on the edge of the examination couch with her legs dangling over the edge. Inspection has four parts:
- look

- lift
- stretch
- press.

Look. Note size and symmetry. Asymmetry of size may be a normal finding. Note the contour – observe any unilateral differences, any flattening or dimpling. Note the appearance of the skin – observe differences in colour and any thickening or signs of oedema (peau d'orange).

Lift. Place hands on head – note any change in size or shape, any unilateral changes or any dimpling.

Stretch. Stretch arms above head – note any change in size or shape, any unilateral changes or dimpling.

Press. Place hands firmly on the hips and press towards them, thus contracting the pectoral muscles. Observe for puckering or dimpling on skin, especially on the underside of the breast.

Inspect the nipples. Compare their shape and size. Observe any retraction, rashes, ulcerations or discharge.

Palpation

Ask the patient to lie down. Place a small pillow under the patient's shoulder on the side you are examining and ask her to rest her arm over her head. These manoeuvres help to spread the breast tissue more evenly across the chest and make it easier to palpate any lesions. Expose the patient as little as possible: use a cover over the side not being examined.

With a relaxed flat hand, compress the tissues, gently rotating out from the nipple to the chest wall. Proceed systematically, examining the entire breast, including the periphery, tail and areola.

Note:
- consistency
- tenderness.
    Possible findings: physiological nodularity, infection or premenstrual tenderness.

Lesions. Note:
- location
- size
- shape
- consistency
- delineation
- tenderness
- mobility.
    Possible findings: cysts, fibroadenoma or cancer.
    Palpate each nipple.

Axillae. Inspect for rashes, infection and pigmentation. Palpate central axillary nodes; if suspected, palpate other axillary nodes:
- pectoral group
- lateral group
- subscapular group.

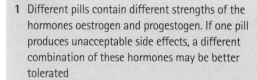

Top Tips ✓

1 Different pills contain different strengths of the hormones oestrogen and progestogen. If one pill produces unacceptable side effects, a different combination of these hormones may be better tolerated

2 Some pills may have beneficial effects on other medical conditions. For example, oestrogen-dominant COCs may reduce acne and hirsutism; combined monophasic pills can relieve the symptoms of premenstrual syndrome

3 Overweight can increase complications of contraceptive pills: a BMI > 35 is an absolute contraindication for COCs, and women who weigh more than 70 kg may find that the POP is not as efficacious

4 A thin addition of a water-soluble lubricant used inside a condom can heighten sensation

5 Hormonal emergency contraception should be taken within 72 hours, but its efficacy is enhanced the earlier it is ingested, whereas an emergency IUD can be fitted up to 5 days after the earliest calculated ovulation date in the cycle

6 Stress of any kind can trigger hormonal changes, which may make natural methods unreliable

7 Hysterectomised women may not respond to the lowest available therapeutic dose of oestrogen. Over 75% need a higher dose of hormone replacement therapy (HRT)

8 Testosterone replacement can be considered if lethargy, loss of libido and depression persist after commencement of HRT

9 Counselling, listening and support can be as therapeutic as any medical intervention for some patients

NHS Breast Screen Programme Guidelines for referral (Austoker et al 1999) define criteria for urgent referral.

Lump
- Any new discrete lump
- New lump in pre existing nodularity
- Asymmetrical nodularity that persists at review after menstruation
- Abscess
- Cyst persistently refilling or recurrent cyst.

Pain

- If associated with a lump
- Intractable pain not responding to reassurance; simple measures such as wearing a well-supporting bra and common drugs
- Unilateral persistent pain in postmenopausal women.

Nipple discharge

- Women under 50 years of age with bilateral discharge sufficient to stain clothing
- Bloodstained discharge
- Persistent single duct discharge
- All women aged 50 and over.

Glossary

Abortifacient A drug that induces abortion or miscarriage

Ageism An attitude that discriminates, separates, stigmatises, or otherwise disadvantages older adults on the basis of chronological age

Amenorrhoea The absence of menstrual periods. In primary amenorrhoea periods fail to appear at puberty, which may be due to the absence of a uterus or ovaries, a genetic disorder (e.g. Turner's syndrome) or to a hormonal imbalance. Secondary amenorrhoea occurs when normal periods cease due to disorders of the hypothalamus, deficiency in ovarian, pituitary or thyroid hormones, mental disturbance, depression, anorexia nervosa or as a result of a major change in surroundings or circumstances

Culdoscopy The direct observation of the uterus, ovaries and fallopian tubes using a tubular instrument with lenses and a light source that is passed through the wall of the vagina behind to the neck of the uterus

Diaphragm A dome-shaped rubber cap fitted inside the vagina to cover the cervix. It is a reliable form of barrier contraception when used with a chemical spermicide

Dysmenorrhoea Pain associated with menstruation. Primary dysmenorrhoea is menstrual pain that results from factors intrinsic to the uterus and the process of menstruation. Secondary dysmenorrhoea is menstrual pain that occurs secondary to specific pelvic abnormalities such as endometriosis and chronic pelvic infection

Dyspareunia An abnormal pain during sexual intercourse. It may result from abnormal conditions of genitalia, dysfunctional psychophysiological reaction to sexual union, forcible coitus, incomplete sexual arousal or hormonal changes of the menopause and lactation that result in drying of vaginal tissues. It may be associated with pelvic pathology such as endometriosis

Ectopic pregnancy The development of a fetus at a site other than the uterus. It most commonly occurs within a fallopian tube, which becomes blocked or inflamed, causing the tube to rupture and bleed.

FSH Follicle-stimulating hormone. A gonadotrophin secreted by the anterior pituitary gland, which stimulates the growth and maturation of graafian follicles in the ovary and promotes spermatogenesis in the male

Galactorrhoea Abnormal secretion of milk from the breasts, when breast-feeding is not taking place

Hysterectomy Surgical removal of the uterus

Implant A non-biodegradable rod that is inserted subcutaneously to provide the continuous administration of progestogen over a predetermined period of time

Implantation The attachment of the early embryo to the lining of the uterus. This occurs at the blastocyst stage of development, 6–8 days after ovulation

LH Luteinizing hormone. A glycoprotein hormone, produced by the anterior pituitary, that stimulates the secretion of sex hormones by the ovary and is involved in the maturation of spermatozoa and ova

Menarche The start of menstrual periods and other physical and mental changes associated with puberty

Menorrhagia Abnormally heavy or long menstrual periods

Menopause Strictly the cessation of menses, but commonly used to refer to the period of the female climacteric

Myometrium The muscular tissue of the uterus that surrounds the endometrium. It is composed of smooth muscle that undergoes small regular spontaneous contractions in response to the hormones oestrogen and progesterone, at different stages of the menstrual cycle

Oestrogen One of the group of hormonal steroid compounds that promote the development of female secondary sex characteristics. Human oestrogen is elaborated in the ovaries, adrenal cortices, testes and fetoplacental unit. During the menstrual cycle oestrogen renders the female genital tract suitable for fertilisation, implantation and nutrition of the early embryo

Osteoporosis A disorder characterised by loss of bone mass density occurring most frequently in postmenopausal women, in sedentary or immobilised individuals and in patients on long-term steroid therapy. The disorder may cause pain, pathological fractures, loss of stature and various deformities

Pectoralis major A large muscle of the upper chest wall that acts on the joint of the shoulder. Thick and fan-shaped, it arises from the clavicle, the sternum, the cartilages of the second to the sixth rib and the aponeurosis of the obliquus externus abdominis

Serratus anterior A thin muscle of the chest wall extending from the ribs under the arm to the scapula

Spermicide A cream, jelly or pessary, used in conjunction with a diaphragm or a condom, containing an agent (usually nonoxinol '9') that kills spermatozoa

References

Achuthan R, Parkin G, Horgan K 1997 Breast cancer and hormone replacement therapy: collaborative reanalyses of data from 51 epidemiological studies of 52,705 women with breast cancer and 108,411 women without breast cancer. Collaborative group on hormonal factors in breast cancer. Lancet 350(9084):1047–1059.

Aldercreutzh H, Mazur W 1997 Phyto-oestrogens and Western disease. Annals of Medicine 29(2):95–120.

Andrews G 1997 Women's sexual health. Baillière Tindall, London.

Austoker J, Mansel R, Baum M, Sainsbury R, Hobbs R 1999 Guidelines for referral of patients with breast problems. Department of Health NHS Breast Screening Programme.

Barton S E, Maddox P H, Jenkins D et al 1988 Effect of cigarette smoking on cervical epithelial immunity: a mechanism for neoplastic change? Lancet 11:652–654.

Bates B 1991 A guide to physical examination and history taking, 5th edn. Lippincott, Philadelphia.

Belfield T 1999 FPA contraceptive handbook, 3rd edn. Family Planning Association, London.

Bergkvist L 1997 Epidemiology of hormone replacement therapy and breast cancer. Gynecological Endocrinology 11(1):13–16.

Breslau N A 1994 Calcium, estrogen and progestin in the treatment of osteoporosis. Rheumatic Disease Clinics of North America 20(3):691–717.

Burger H G, Hailes J, Nelson Y 1987 Effect of combined implants of oestrodiol and testosterone in postmenopausal women. British Medical Journal 1:936–939.

Choi M W 1995 Menopause and the climacteric. Holistic Nursing Practice 9(3):53–62.

CSM 1995 Combined oral contraceptives and thromboembolism. Committee on Safety of Medicines, London.

Coney S 1995 The menopause industry. The Women's Press, London.

Department of Health 1990 Handbook of contraceptive practice. Department of Health, London.

Department of Health 1992 Folic acid and neural tube defects: guidelines on prevention. Department of Health, London

Dowden A 1999 The health matters learning file. Health Matters Supplement May:1–111.

Dunn N, Thorogood M, Faragher B et al 1999 Oral contraceptives and myocardial infarction: the results of the MICA case-control study. British Medical Journal 318:1579–1584.

Durex 1993 History of the condom. Durex Information Service, London.

Everett S 1997 Contraception. In: Andrews G (ed) Women's sexual health. Baillière Tindall, London, ch 9, p 173.

Everett S 1998 Handbook of contraception and family planning. Baillière Tindall, London.

Finucane F F, Madang J, Bush T 1993 Decreased risk of stroke amongst postmenopausal hormone users: results from a national cohort. Ann Intern Med 153:73–79.

Gbolade B, Ellis S, Murphy B 1998 Bone density in long-term users of depot medroxyprogesterone acetate. British Journal of Obstetrics and Gynaecology 105:790–794.

Grodstein F, Martinez E, Platz E A 1998 Postmenopausal hormone use and risk for colorectal cancer and adenoma. Annals of Intern Med Journal 128:705–712.

Guillebaud J 1997 Contraception. In: McPherson A, Waller D (eds) Women's health, 4th edn. Oxford University Press, Oxford, ch 6, p 128.

Guillebaud J 1998 Contraception today. A pocketbook for general practitioners, 3rd edn (revised). Martin Dunitz, London.

Guillebaud J 1999 Contraception: your questions answered, 3rd edn, Churchill Livingstone, London.

Hansson L, Zanchetti A, Carruthers S G et al 1998 Effects of intensive blood pressure lowering and low dose aspirin in patients with hypertension: principle results of the Hypertension Optimal Treatment (HOT) randomised trial. Lancet 351(9118):1755–1762.

Hart D M 1997 Current attitudes to hormone replacement therapy. Gynecological Endocrinology 11(1):9–12.

HEA 1996 Nutritional aspects of cardiovascular disease. Health Education Authority, London.

HEA 1999 Nutritional aspects of the development of cancer. Health Educational Authority. London.

Kaufert P A 1994 A health and social profile of the menopausal woman. Experimental Gerontology 29(3/4):343–350.

Khoiny F E 1996 Use of Depo-Provera in teens. Journal of Pediatric Health Care Sept/Oct:195–200.

Kubba A A, Wilkinson C 1998 Recommendations for clinical practice: emergency contraception. Faculty of Family Planning and Reproductive Health Care of the Royal College of Obstetricians and Gynaecologists, London.

Kumar V, Cotran R 1992 Basic pathology. W B Saunders, Philadelphia, p 219.

Law M R, Hackshaw A K 1997 A meta-analysis of cigarette smoking, bone mineral density and risk of hip fracture: recognition of a major effect. British Medical Journal 315:841–846.

Lewis M A, Spitzer V O, Heinemann L A J 1997 Lowered risk of dying of heart attack with 3rd-generation pill may offset risk of dying of thrombosis. British Medical Journal 515:679–680.

Loudon N, Glasier A, Gebbie A (eds) 1995 Handbook of family planning and reproductive health care, 3rd edn. Churchill Livingstone, Edinburgh.

Marieb E 1989 Human anatomy and physiology. Benjamin/Cummings, California.

National Association of Family Planning Doctors (NAFPD) 1984 Interim guidelines for doctors following the pill scare. British Journal of Family Planning 9:120–122.

Pahor M, Applegate W 1997 Recent advances in geriatric medicine. British Medical Journal 315:1071–1074.

Royal College of Nursing (RCN) 1995 Breast palpation and breast awareness: guidelines for practice. Issues in Nursing and Health 35.

Roberts J 1992 Psychosocial adjustment in postmenopausal women. The Canadian Journal of Nursing Research 24(4):29–46.

Schering Data Sheet 1999.

Singer A, Szarewski A 1988 Cervical smear test. Macdonald Optima, London.

Smith-Warner S, Spiegelman D, Yaun S et al 1998 Alcohol and breast cancer in women: a pooled analysis of cohort studies. JAMA 279(7):535–540.

Stampfer M J, Colditz G A 1991 Oestrogen replacement therapy and coronary heart disease: a quantitative assessment of the epidemiological evidence. Preventive Medicine 20:47–63.

Stewart M 1998 The phyto factor. Vermilion, London.

Studd J W W, Smith K N J 1994 Oestrogens and depression. Menopause 1:33–37.

Tang M X, Jacobs D, Stern Y et al 1996 Effect of oestrogen during menopause on risk and age at onset of Alzheimer's disease. Lancet 348:429–432.

Vessey M P, Villard-MacIntosh L, Yeates D 1990 Effectiveness of progestogen-only contraceptives. British Journal of Family Planning 10:121–126.

WHO Task Force 1998 Postovulatory methods of fertility regulation. Lancet 352:428–433.

Further reading

Clubb E, Knight J 1996 Fertility – fertility awareness and natural family planning, 3rd edn. David & Charles,

Flynn A, Brooks M 1996 The manual of natural family planning, 3rd edn. Thorsons.

Furedi A 1996 Unplanned pregnancy – your choices. Oxford University Press, Oxford.

Guillebaud J 1997 The pill, 5th edn. Oxford University Press, Oxford.

THE GYNAECOLOGICAL SYSTEM

Mary Rawlinson

Introduction

The gynaecological system presents many challenges for the nurse practitioner working in primary care. Many women are unaware, or only partly aware of the anatomy of their body and how their bodies should function through the many stages of their life. Therefore, presenting signs and symptoms, which often include the absence or increase of vaginal bleeding and pain, can be both confusing and frightening. By caring for women of all ages and ethnic backgrounds with understanding and sensitivity, the nurse practitioner will be able to achieve a rapport with her patients, which is essential when taking a detailed gynaecological history and performing a thorough examination.

The nurse practitioner needs to be able to recognise what is normal and abnormal, remembering that because of the anatomy of the female pelvis, some presenting features, which at first appear gynaecological, may be genitourinary or gastrointestinal in origin.

This chapter will undertake to explain some of the common and sometimes not so common conditions that you may be presented with in your surgery. By considering each condition subjectively and objectively through assessment, a diagnosis can be made, a plan formulated and treatment or referral carried out if necessary. However, first, it is useful to refamiliarise yourself with the anatomy of the female reproductive system. It is sometimes easier to appreciate the close relationships of the organs in the female pelvis by first looking at a diagram before considering each separate structure and its function (Figs 15.1 and 15.2).

The menstrual cycle and hormone control

From the fifth month of intrauterine life the female fetus has already begun the process of oogenesis. Through mitosis, diploid stem cells of the ovary multiply and grow rapidly and are transformed into primary oocytes. At the same time the fetus develops six to seven million follicles in each ovary (Rymer et al 1993). The oocytes begin their first meiotic division and then stop. By this process a female baby at birth already has 700 000 primary oocytes in her immature ovaries (Marieb 1995). This lifetime supply then remains in suspended animation until the wake-up call of puberty begins.

Puberty is defined as the period when secondary sexual characteristics develop and the sexual organs mature, allowing reproduction to take place (Smith 1995). Normal puberty in girls usually occurs between the ages of 10 and 15 years. Girls who start puberty before the age of 8 years, or who have not had their first period (menarche) before 17 years needs referral to a gynaecologist for investigation. However if there is no development of secondary sexual characteristics by the age of 14 years then early investigation is necessary. For a complete puberty stage guide refer to Tanner's sex maturity ratings. The most common reason, for delayed puberty although this is still a rare condition, is Turner's syndrome. Other reasons include anorexia nervosa, hyperthyroidism and Noonan's and Kallmann's syndromes (Hopcroft & Forte 1999). Before puberty, suppression of the adult female hormone cycle is achieved by small quantities of oestrogens that inhibit the release of gonadotrophin-releasing hormone (GnRH) from the hypothalamus. At puberty, as the hypothalamus becomes less sensitive to oestrogen, GnRH is pulsatingly released. GnRH then stimulates the anterior pituitary to release follicle-stimulating hormone (FSH) and luteinising hormone (LH) every 70–220 min depending on the phase within the menstrual cycle, which is itself the product of hormonal and specific organ interactions.

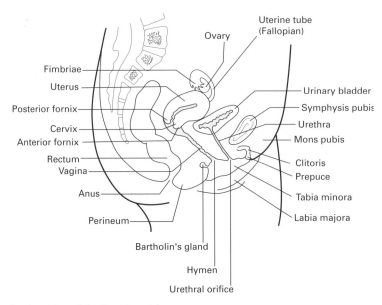

Figure 15.1 *Mid-sagittal section of the female pelvis.*

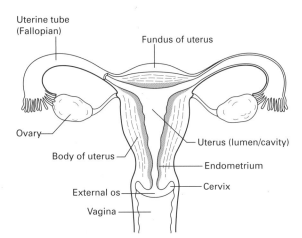

Figure 15.2 *Anterior view of the female reproductive organs.*

Normal menstruation results in interaction between the hypothalamus, pituitary, ovary and endometrium (Fig. 15.3). The cyclical production (follicular and luteal phases) of sex steroids from the corpus luteum (androgens, oestrogens and progestins) results in cyclical changes to the endometrium (proliferative and secretory phases) as it tries to achieve the monthly goal of preparing for the implantation of an embryo.

By understanding what is normal, a diagnosis is more easily achieved when the abnormal occurs. Gynaecological problems are frequently encountered by nurse practitioners in primary care, either as specific presentations by the women or as incidental findings during 'well woman' consultations; therefore, it is essential to be well prepared.

Subjective assessment

It is essential to take a thorough and accurate history from any woman presenting with a gynaecological problem, as your diagnosis will be based on 90% history and 10% examination. Always consider carefully the woman's age and could she be pregnant when taking her history, as similar signs and symptoms will lead to different differential diagnoses with these considerations.

Types of questions to ask

Initial open questions will allow the woman to describe the presenting problem. Allow her to 'tell her story': by doing so, fewer questions will be necessary and you will find the consultation easier.

- Can you tell me about the problem?
- When did it start?
- How long has it been going on?

Having learnt the general nature of the problem, go on to a more detailed history of the presenting problem:

- When was your last period? By having a date, the possibility of pregnancy or irregular bleeding can be discussed.
- Are your periods normally regular or irregular? It is important to ascertain with the woman what she understands by these terms and what her normal cycle is.
- How old were you when your periods started? This may not be relevant but is useful to remember.

Answers to the last three questions can be recorded as, for example, M.H. 12 7/30 regular, which means that menstrual history began at age 12, lasts 7 days and occurs regularly every 30 days.

- How much blood are you losing? This can be measured in number of tampons or sanitary towels used.
- Is this more or less than usual?

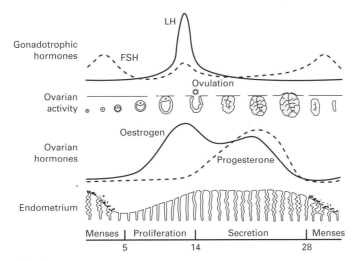

Figure 15.3 *The menstrual cycle.*

- Are you flooding and/or passing clots? Women are often very worried about passing clots and that alone can be a common presenting problem.
- Do you get pain when you have your period?
- Do you have any other pain? If so, discuss relation to periods.
- Do you have a vaginal discharge? If so, discuss colour, odour, amount and presence of blood.
- Have you had any abdominal surgery? If so, what, when and why?
- When was your last cervical smear test? This is dependent on age and may not be relevant; but, if it is, discuss the result.

If the presenting problem warrants it, a menstrual chart lasting 3 months is a very useful tool to aid diagnosis. This can highlight not only to you but also to the woman what exactly the problem is or whether the perceived problem is a normal finding.

Sexual and contraceptive history

As well as questions highlighted in Chapter 13, useful gynaecological questions are
- During intercourse do you or your partner experience any pain? If your patient has come to discuss infertility, it is important to ascertain whether intercourse is normal, the frequency and time during the menstrual cycle.
- Do you use any contraception? If so, what? Particularly, ask about the intrauterine contraceptive device (IUCD), as many are forgotten until they cause problems. This factor is important when considering, for example, ectopic pregnancy (IUCD), menstrual changes (oral contraceptive) and vaginal/vulval rash (rubber allergy from condoms).

Obstetric history

- Do you have any children? If so, what are their ages, and weights at birth?

- Were your pregnancies normal? Any antenatal, labour, delivery and postnatal problems?
- Have you had other pregnancies? Any miscarriages and/or terminations?

Taking details of past medical history, social and family history, any other current problems, plus any medication being taken, always remembering to check 'over the counter' (OTC) as well as prescription drugs, will all help to achieve a comprehensive assessment of your patient.

Objective assessment

General approach

Your objective assessment will be dependent on what you have learnt from your history taking. Many women coming to you with a gynaecological problem will be expecting to be examined, but for some, especially the younger woman experiencing her first examination or the elderly woman, it can be an acutely embarrassing and uncomfortable process (Lewis & Chamberlain 1990), as well as the fear about what the nurse or doctor will find (Bates 1995).

- Before starting your examination ask the woman to empty her bladder. Obtain a urine specimen for general analysis as it can save time later.
- While relaxing your patient and explaining the procedure to her, general observation of colour/pallor of her skin should be noted.
- Check her vital signs – temperature, pulse and blood pressure.
- If at any time you are told or you are suspicious that your patient has recently been raped then do not examine her. Once her permission has been gained, inform the doctor.
- Be prepared to examine other systems as clinically indicated. For abdominal examination refer to Chapter 9, pp 137–140.

The cervical smear test

Many women wrongly assume that the cervical smear is a diagnostic test and not a screening tool (Nottingham 1999). It is important to give your patients the information so they can make an 'informed choice' about screening, always remembering that 20% of all smear tests taken produce false negative results. This is either because of the smear reader in the hospital laboratory or the poor technique of the smear taker (Adams et al 1998). Muir Gray (1997) and Slater (1998) suggest that false negative results are an unavoidable part of any screening programme. This may be true but it never harms to audit your own smear-taking results and, if necessary, review your technique:

- Warm Cusco's speculum in tap water to body temperature. Lubricate sides if necessary but not the end of the speculum.
- Inspect the vulva (see 'Inspection of vulva, vagina and cervix' opposite).
- As the speculum is inserted, note any discomfort the woman experiences.
- Always visualise the cervix. To achieve this, if necessary, change the woman's position, or a rolled-up towel or the woman's hands under her buttocks can help.
- Before taking the smear, note the position of the squamo-columnar junction.
- Using an Ayre's spatula insert into the os and rotate twice through 360°. Ensure that the transformation zone is sampled, especially if it is away from the os.
- If the transformation zone is well into the os, as in postmenopausal women, it may be helpful to use a brush as well as a spatula.
- Once the material has been transferred evenly onto a labelled slide, flood the slide with fixative and leave for at least 5 min.
- Tell the woman how and approximately when she will receive her result. All smear takers have a legal responsibility to ensure women receive their results and it is not enough to tell them 'no news is good news' (Austoker et al 1997).
- If possible take a cervical smear test mid-cycle.
- Sexual intercourse within 48 hours of the smear being taken will increase the chances of the result being inadequate.
- Vaginal discharge/blood may make a smear test more difficult to read, leading to an inaccurate result.
- If a suspicious area is seen on the cervix, the woman should be referred regardless of the smear test result.

Pelvic examination

As with all physical examinations, a pelvic examination should only be performed if you have been instructed on the procedure and assessed as competent.

A pelvic examination should not be carried out if you suspect:

- An ectopic pregnancy with or without vaginal bleeding: refer urgently.
- Any vaginal bleeding in a pregnant woman: refer to the GP who may do a vaginal examination if suspecting a threatened miscarriage to determine if the os is open or closed. If 24 weeks or more refer urgently.

The woman can be lying in any one of several positions for the examination, but the most commonly used are

- Lateral or dorsal position – good for bimanual palpation.
- Semi-prone or Sim's position – particularly good for examining the cervix and anterior vaginal wall.
- Lithotomy position – rarely used in primary care, but is useful to discuss with women who you are referring to a Genito Urinary Medicine (GUM) clinic or will have certain procedures, e.g. colposcopy.

Inspection of vulva, vagina and cervix

1. Look for signs of vaginal discharge: if present, note colour, texture, consistency and odour.
2. Inspect labia and clitoris for signs of infection, ulceration, growths or swellings.
3. Inspect urethral orifice. Note any urethral discharge.
4. Inspect Bartholin's ducts for swelling: if present, could indicate acute or chronic infection.
5. Ask woman to cough. Note any stress incontinence.
6. Unless already undertaken during a preceding cervical smear test, a visual examination should be undertaken using a Sim's or Cusco's speculum.

Palpation of vagina and cervix

Making sure your gloved hand is well lubricated, insert right index and middle fingers into the vagina. Your other two fingers should be flexed and your thumb drawn back. If the woman has a small vaginal opening, use one finger:

1. Palpate the vaginal walls, distinguishing between normal rugae and the abnormal findings of cysts, foreign bodies, nodules and tenderness.
2. Palpate the cervix. Note its size, shape, position and regularity of contour and consistency. Note any tears, ulcers or polyps you can palpate.
3. Hold the cervix gently between your fingers, moving it from side to side. Note mobility and sensitivity of the cervical surface. It should feel smooth, mobile and non-tender when moved or touched. Cervical tenderness with adnexal tenderness is suggestive of pelvic inflammatory disease (PID).
4. Palpate the external os. This will be a round, usually small, hole in a nulliparae and a slit in a multiparae.
5. Palpate the fornices around the cervix. Note if they are bulging, which is usually caused by a swelling inside the pelvis.

Bimanual palpation of the uterus

This examination is a means of physically assessing the pelvic organs and is carried out with the hands of the examiners palpating together. Your right-hand index and middle fingers are placed into the vagina, as described in the previous section, keeping the wrist straight so that the hand and forearm are in a straight line. The left hand is placed on the abdomen between the umbilicus and the symphysis pubis. In this way the pelvic organs can be palpated between the two hands. (Fig. 15.4).

1. Reach under and behind the cervix and lift the cervix and uterus upward towards your external hand.
2. At the same time apply gentle pressure downward with your external hand. The uterus should now be felt between your hands.
3. Note its size, shape, position, mobility and its surface regularity.
4. Size is usually estimated in weeks of gestation or equivalent size in fruit. Non-pregnant = pear, 12 weeks = small orange, 16 weeks = grapefruit. If the uterus is lifting out of the pelvis, size can also be estimated by the position of the fundus on the abdomen. An enlarged uterus can suggest pregnancy, a benign or a malignant tumour.
5. Determine position by moving fingers into the anterior fornix. If the uterus can be felt when counter pressure by the left hand is on the abdomen, then the uterus is anteverted. Repeating the procedure with the internal fingers in the posterior fornix can then check this. Also remember which way the cervix was pointing when viewed. If the cervix was pointing anteriorly, then the uterus is retroverted; if pointing posteriorly, then the uterus is anteverted. Note whether the uterus is midline or deviates to the right or left of the pelvis.
6. Determine mobility by gently balloting the uterus between your internal and external fingers. Limited movement may indicate adhesions, infection or a tumour.
7. Identify any masses or tenderness of the uterus: the uterus should feel firm to touch due to its muscular composition and unless the woman is menstruating

should be non-tender. If a mass is felt, note its size, shape, consistency, mobility and whether it is attached to the uterus. If it is unattached, it probably arises from a fallopian tube, ovary or bowel (Lewis & Chamberlain 1990). A loaded colon can be confused with a pelvic mass, but if faecal will indent on pressure. Go on to do a rectal examination to confirm.

8. Lastly, examine the right and left adnexal fornices for the ovaries and fallopian tubes. Starting with the right fornix, move your internal fingers deeper inward and upward towards your external hand, which is now placed on the right lower abdominal quadrant. The ovary and any masses should now be felt between your hands. The procedure should then be repeated on the left side. Normal ovaries can be recognised as small almond-shaped smooth organs, about 4–6 cm in diameter, which are firm, smooth and sensitive to palpation. Ovaries should not be palpable in prepubertal girls or postmenopausal women: if felt, consider an ovarian cyst or tumour. Normal healthy fallopian tubes are not usually palpable, but it is sometimes possible to feel the round ligaments as cord-like structures. These can be mistaken for the fallopian tubes.

Rectovaginal examination

It is sometimes essential (but not often performed in primary care) to do a rectal examination at the same time as a vaginal examination. This is particularly important in examining behind the cervix and may detect a rectovaginal pouch tumour. A finger in the rectum can extend further into the pelvic cavity than a finger in the vagina (Lewis & Chamberlain 1990). A rectovaginal examination is performed by repeating the procedures of the bimanual examination but with the hands palpating between the rectum and the vagina.

Diagnostic tests

The diagnostic tests you carry out or order will be wholly dependent on your subjective and objective findings. It is sometimes tempting to over investigate in the hope that the diagnosis will become obvious. However the most commonly used and helpful investigations include:

- Full blood count (FBC) – will indicate anaemia and thrombocytopenia. Helpful in menorrhagia and severe systemic illness. White blood cells (WBC) are increased in pelvic inflammatory disease (PID).
- Erythrocyte sedimentation rate (ESR) – increased in PID and severe systemic illness.
- Urea and electrolytes (U&E) – if considering adrenal disorders or severe systemic illness.
- Thyroid function tests (TFTs) – if considering causes for amenorrhoea, although hypo/hyperthyroidism is not a common cause.
- Follicle-stimulating hormone (FSH), luteinising hormone (LH) and testosterone.

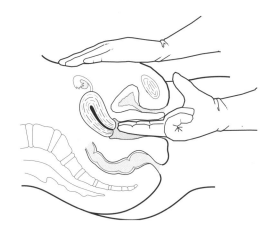

Figure 15.4 *Bimanual palpation.*

- Prolactin levels – If considering causes for amenorrhoea. Levels high in prolactinoma and with some drugs (phenothiazines).
- Liver function tests (LFTs) – check if suspicious of liver disease.
- International rate (INR) – check if there is a clinical history of other bleeding or bruising as well as vaginally.
- Urinalysis/urine culture.
- Pregnancy test – consider regardless of contraception used or if the woman has been sterilised, especially if considering ectopic pregnancy.
- Vulval/vaginal/cervical swabs.
- Endocervical swab – if considering *Chlamydia* infection.
- High vaginal swab (HVS) – sometimes useful in chronic PID if discharge is present.
- Ultrasound – to detect pregnancy, ovarian cysts, fibroids and tumours.
  If referred, diagnostic tests may also include:
- CT (computed tomography) imaging – if suspecting prolactinoma or other pituitary tumour.
- Dilatation and curettage (D&C) – not used so much now
- Endometrial sampling
- Hysteroscopy
- Colposcopy
- Laparoscopy – if suspecting PID, endometriosis, polycystic ovary syndrome (PCOS).

Differential diagnoses

The presenting features of many gynaecological conditions will lead you to consider a variety of differential diagnoses. Many of these will be gynaecological in origin, but some will lead you to also consider other systems. These may include:

1. Chronic pelvic pain – PID, endometriosis, intrauterine contraceptive device (IUCD), mittelschmerz, dysmenorrhoea, prolapse, fibroids, cysts, tumour, bowel obstruction, diverticulitis, irritable bowel syndrome (IBS), low back pain (LBP).
2. Acute pelvic pain – miscarriage, ectopic, PID, ovarian cyst, endometriosis, pelvic abscess, pelvic congestion, fibroids, cancer, IUCD, urinary tract infection (UTI), strangulated hernia, referred bowel spasm.
3. Dyspareunia – endometriosis, vulvovaginitis, PID, dryness, atrophic vaginitis, pelvic pain syndrome, fibroids, pelvic adhesions, cancer, psychogenic spasm, cystitis, congenital abnormality, unruptured hymen, anal fissure, haemorrhoids, perianal abscess.
4. Menorrhagia – dysfunctional uterine bleeding (DUB), endometriosis, puberty, perimenopause, fibroids, IUCD, PID, contraceptive pill, hormone replacement therapy (HRT), polyps, hypo/hyperthyroidism, liver disease (especially if alcohol induced), clotting disorders, cancer.
5. Irregular vaginal bleeding – DUB, breakthrough bleeding (contraceptive pill/injection, HRT), polyps,

cervical erosion, PID, atrophic vaginitis, perimenopause, cancer, bleeding in pregnancy (first trimester, miscarriage, ectopic).
6. Amenorrhoea – pregnancy, menopause, PCOS, stress (especially in younger women), anorexia nervosa, excessive exercise, drugs (phenothiazines, metoclopramide, valproate, cytotoxics), thyroid disorders, severe systemic illness, adrenal disorders.

If presented with the following you should also consider several gynaecological conditions:

7. Low back pain – PID often presents this way
8. Anorectal pain – endometriosis, ovarian cyst or tumour.

As demonstrated, many conditions have more than one presenting feature, which aids the differential diagnosis.

The following section covers some of the more common conditions, that you may be presented with in primary care.

SPECIFIC DISORDERS

Fibromyomata – more commonly called fibroids

Fibroids are the commonest tumour in women affecting 2% of females. The exceptions are Afro-Caribbean women, in which fibroids occur three times more frequently and at an earlier age (Lewis & Chamberlain 1990). Fibroids are also more common in nulliparous women or in those women who had their pregnancies many years previously.

Fibroids first present once menstruation has established but rarely give any problems before the age of 25. New fibroids do not form after the menopause. Fibroids arise from the muscular uterine wall and comprise smooth muscle and fibrous tissue. They vary in size from tiny seedlings to enormous tumours filling the entire abdomen and pelvis and can be single or multiple.

Subjective findings

- Women often present with menorrhagia, which has increased in amount and duration over a period of time. It is important to determine how long it has been going on.
- She may complain of passing clots.
- Intermenstrual bleeding is uncommon. It is important to establish whether bleeding is cyclical or acyclical.
- She may feel very tired and even short of breath if anaemia is severe.
- If the fibroid is large, the woman may notice a hard non-tender abdominal swelling.
- The woman may complain of her tummy getting bigger and clothes not fitting.
- She may describe a feeling of local discomfort and heaviness.

- The woman will not be in pain unless there is an added complication, e.g. endometriosis, PID, torsion.
- She may have frequency or difficulty in passing urine.
- She may have stress incontinence.
- Women do not complain of bowel problems, as the rectum is rarely affected by any pressure from a fibroid (Lewis & Chamberlain 1990).
- They are often older and appear to be late for the menopause: if postmenopausal bleeding, refer urgently.
- The younger woman may present after several miscarriages, as a fibroid may cause implantation difficulties (Clubb & Knight 1992).
- In the younger woman, infertility may be the initial presenting symptom.

Objective findings

1. Vital signs are normal, except in
   - red degeneration (necrobiosis), which occurs more often during pregnancy, and is also associated with sudden increase in tumour size, pain and vomiting
   - torsion – acute abdominal pain, vomiting and shock
   - infection – high fever, tenderness and foul discharge.
2. Observe the woman for signs of anaemia and, less commonly, pain.
3. Abdominal examination:
   - abdomen may look swollen
   - on auscultation, a uterine souffle (similar to pregnancy) may be heard
   - a hard, irregular, usually central, mass may be palpated
   - the abdomen is non-tender.
4. Pelvic examination:
   - cervix may be pushed down or displaced to one side
   - normal outline of the uterus may be difficult to detect.

Investigations

- FBC: anaemia is common
- U&E: if urinary output is disrupted
- Hormonal assay: some laboratories will automatically include TFT in with the usual FSH and LH
- TFT: thyroid dysfunction can sometimes cause abnormal bleeding
- Urinalysis: if urinary symptoms are present
- Ultrasound of pelvis and abdomen.

Management

Once fibroids have been positively diagnosed, treatment is very dependent on how debilitating the woman's symptoms are: if necessary, treat anaemia with iron supplements.

Referral should be made if the bleeding is unmanageable for the woman, or other more worrying signs and symptoms are present.

Polycystic ovary syndrome or Stein–Leventhal syndrome

It is estimated that out of all women with menstrual dysfunction, 50% have PCOS, and 3% of the population have the condition (Hagan & Knott 1998). This makes it one of the commonest female endocrine disorders, with several recently discovered metabolic tendencies (Hopkinson et al 1998).

The aetiology of PCOS is still in question, but it is known that if there is any imbalance of the menstrual system, then loss of ovulation can result. Then, if chronic anovulation results for any length of time, it has been suggested that PCOS can develop. Two-thirds of anovulatory women have PCOS (Hagan & Knott 1998).

However, the condition has also been recently associated with an underlying insulin resistance (Hopkinson et al 1998). Excess ovarian androgen production is stimulated by the resultant hyperinsulinaemia. These women as well as having insulin resistance also have dyslipidaemia, a predisposition to non-insulin dependent diabetes and cardiovascular disease as they get older.

At laparoscopy a polycystic ovary is enlarged and smooth (oyster ovary), with a thickened tunica albuginea and multiple cystic follicles. These vary in size but rarely exceed 0.5 cm in diameter.

Subjective findings

- A quarter of women will present with secondary amenorrhoea (Conway 1996).
- They may present with irregular periods, having previously had a normal onset of menarche, a year or two of regular periods, then irregular periods until they eventually stop.
- They may present with abnormal uterine bleeding, but particularly menorrhagia. This occurs because, as there is a failure of ovulation, when oestrogen is increased by the ovarian follicles it is unopposed by progesterone.
- Infertility may be the presenting problem.
- Fifty per cent of women with PCOS have hirsutism (Hopcroft & Forte 1999).
- Acne is also a common problem.
- Alopecia – male pattern balding.
- Reduced libido.
- Patients may present wanting to lose weight: 50% are obese and most of those have central obesity (Hopkinson et al 1998).
- Acanthosis nigricans: hyperpigmentation of vulva, axillae, neck and extensor surfaces of joints.

Objective findings

- Vital signs are normal.
- Body mass index (BMI) >30, with increased waist/hip ratio (Edwards 1999).
- Hirsutism in male distribution sites (Hopcroft & Forte 1999).

- Abdominal examination is normal.
- Pelvic examination is usually unremarkable.

Investigations

Initial investigations should be aimed at determining any disorders of the hypothalamic–pituitary–ovarian axis that would cause ovulatory disturbance, and then to confirm the diagnosis of PCOS:

1. FSH and LH – if possible, take day 2–6 of the menstrual cycle; FSH will be normal, LH will be raised.
2. Testosterone levels – to assess degree of hyperandrogaemia. In PCOS, levels rarely exceed 5 nmol/l. If greater, it needs further investigation.
3. Prolactin – 20% have high levels of prolactin. If serum prolactin >1000 mU/l plus oestrogen deficiency, patient must have an MRI (magnetic resonance imaging) scan of the pituitary fossa to exclude pituitary adenoma.
4. Sex hormone-binding globulin (s-HBG) – levels will be reduced.
5. Urinalysis/blood glucose levels.
6. Fasting lipids.
7. Transvaginal ultrasound – used to confirm diagnosis, as biochemical tests alone are unreliable diagnostically (Hagan & Knott 1998).

Management

Clinical management of women with PCOS should be concentrated on controlling the symptoms and problems specific for each individual woman. However, all symptoms are exacerbated by obesity (Conway 1996, Hopkinson et al 1998).

- A weight-reducing diet and exercise plan is the single most important therapy.
- Restoration of menstrual function – often achieved by losing weight.
- Reversal of hirsutism and acne. At present some of the contraceptive pills are useful treatment options, as they will improve several symptoms as well as acting as a contraceptive.
- For women with androgenic symptoms – Dianette (ethinyloestradiol and cyproterone) is good first-line therapy.
- For women with no androgenic symptoms but who have amenorrhoea – a cyclical progesterone can be used, using the least androgenic.
- The combined pill exacerbates insulin resistance and therefore continuation of this treatment for PCOS is in question (Hopkinson et al 1998).
- For some women a beautician's advice for excess hair removal may be appropriate.
- If needed, referral to an infertility specialist centre.
- As a last resort treatment, laser or electrocautery of the ovary is performed in some centres.
- Suggested treatment in the future may be aimed at lowering insulin resistance, with the aim of restoring menstrual function and improving lipid profile (Edwards 1999).

Complications

Women who have PCOS have got a greater risk of contracting endometrial and breast cancer because of the increased levels of oestrogen without having the opposing progesterone.

Endometrial cancer

Most endometrial cancers are adenocarcinomas. It is a disease that occurs equally through all socioeconomic groups, but a woman is more at risk if there is an excess of oestrogen (Lewis & Chamberlain 1990), e.g. late menopause, PCOS, obesity, unopposed oestrogen therapy HRT.

Subjective findings

- Predominantly the woman will be postmenopausal, with peak incidence at 50–70 years; 20% will be premenopausal.
- She will usually present with vaginal bleeding: at first slight, but it will eventually become heavy and continuous.
- If premenopausal, the woman may present with irregular intermenstrual bleeding.
- She may have a watery discharge.
- If presenting at a later stage, discharge may be offensive.
- She may be very tired, due to anaemia or severe systemic disease.
- She may be in pain: rectal as well as abdominal.

Objective findings

1. Vital signs are normal in early stages.
2. Observe for signs of anaemia and pain.
3. Abdominal examination:
   - normal in the early stages
   - later stages, tenderness and enlargement of the uterus may be present. Less likely in the older woman.
4. Pelvic examination:
   - blood may be seen in the cervical os
   - uterus may be enlarged and fixed, depending on stage of tumour.

Investigations and management

These may be carried out if at first you are considering DUB (see p. 276), but if postmenopausal refer urgently.

Cervical cancer

While it is always hoped to check cancer of the cervix in its advance by detecting it at its premalignant stage, 4000 new cases present every year in England and Wales. These are mainly attributed to women who have not participated adequately in the cervical screening programme (Austoker et al 1997).

Subjective findings

- The woman is usually premenopausal
- She will often present with intermenstrual or post-coital bleeding
- Micturition or defecation may bring on the vaginal bleeding
- She will often have bloodstained discharge, which may be foul smelling
- She may be in pain if the disease has spread or metastasised
- She may have bowel or bladder symptoms if the disease has spread.

Objective findings

- Vital sign are normal in the early stages
- Observe for signs of anaemia and pain
- Usually visible on the cervix: early stages may look like a nodule, a small ulcer or a large erosion
- When touched, the area will bleed easily and often heavily.

Investigations and management

- If you see a suspicious area do not take a smear test – refer urgently
- If a smear test has already been taken, do not wait for the result – refer urgently
- Do not assume a recent negative smear test result means there is no disease.

Ovarian cancer

Ovarian cancer accounts for 4000 women dying each year in the United Kingdom. It is now the commonest cause of death from the female genital tract (Lewis & Chamberlain 1990). Unfortunately, women often present once the disease has spread, as symptoms in the early stages are few.

Subjective findings

- Women often complain of vague gastrointestinal symptoms in the early stages.
- They may feel generally very tired and unwell.
- They may have loss of appetite.
- There may be urinary problems, either frequency or retention.
- There may be bowel problems caused by pressure from the tumour.
- The abdomen may be very distended if there is a large tumour or ascites. This is always a late, sinister sign.
- There may be pain in the later stages. Pain is not usual unless there are complications of torsion, rupture, haemorrhage or infection.

Objective findings

1. Vital signs are normal in the early stages.
2. Abdominal examination:
   - the abdomen may be grossly distended
   - be aware of any shifting dullness on percussion, caused by ascites.
3. Pelvic examination:
   - be suspicious if you can palpate the ovaries in post-menopausal women
   - on bimanual examination, non-tender cancer deposits may be felt in the rectovaginal pouch: if tender, more likely to be endometriosis.

Investigations and management

If suspicious, refer urgently.

Chronic pelvic pain

One of the commonest reasons for a woman to present at a surgery is for pelvic pain. As listed on p. 276 of this chapter, chronic pelvic pain, which to diagnose must be present for at least three cycles, can be caused by many conditions, both gynaecological and non-gynaecological in origin. A thorough history taking is again the key to a successful diagnosis.

To aid diagnosis, the pain will be more suggestive of a gynaecological problem if:

- it is cyclical
- the woman is aged 15–45 years
- there is menstrual disturbance
- the pain is at level T10 or below (below anterior superior iliac spines)
- the woman experiences dyspareunia.

Dyspareunia

Dyspareunia is defined as difficult and painful intercourse, which women will rarely seek help with unless directly asked (Sarazin & Seymour 1991). Primary dyspareunia occurs during sexual intercourse, while secondary dyspareunia occurs after initially having pain-free lovemaking.

There are many causes for dyspareunia, including PID, pelvic or abdominal surgery, adhesions, endometriosis, tumours including fibroids, IBS, UTI and ovarian cysts. However, a more common reason is positional, and suggesting a change of position to left lateral during lovemaking can help many couples. It would also be of benefit to suggest the use of lubricates (KY jelly or Senselle), or oestrogen cream if appropriate and the woman is not on HRT.

A more complicated cause, however, is vaginismus, for which referral is needed to a counsellor specialising in sexual problems. The woman as well as experiencing pain, also has a deep-seated fear of intercourse which causes an involuntary spasm of the pubococcygeal and surrounding muscles of the lower third of the vagina, making penetration impossible. This also causes difficulty in using tampons and failed gynaecological examinations, which leads to the woman feeling frustrated and humiliated.

Endometriosis

This is a condition in which ectopic endometrium is found in other areas than the lining of the uterus. Most commonly it is found on the ovaries, rectovaginal pouch/septum, uterosacral ligaments and the uterine wall. However, it is possible to have patches of endometriosis in many more obscure places.

Subjective findings

- Women usually present between the ages of 25 and 40 years.
- Most commonly, the woman presents with pain exacerbated before and during menstruation. However, endometriosis can be painless (Forbes 1998).
- The woman can present with deep dyspareunia if rectovaginal pouch/septum or uterosacral ligaments are involved.
- There may be a history of infertility.
- The woman may experience heavy and often frequent periods.

Objective findings

1. Vital signs are normal.
   How helpful a physical examination is will depend on the sites of the endometriosis.
2. Abdominal examination:
   - may reveal sites of tenderness.
3. Pelvic examination:
   - may be painful
   - may reveal a fixed cystic ovary, felt in the rectovaginal pouch
   - may be difficult to separately identify the uterus, which may be retroverted and held by adhesions.

Investigations

- FBC – raised WBC in PID and UTI
- Urinalysis/midstream specimen of urine (MSU)
- HVS for bacteria including gonococcus
- Endocervical swab for *Chlamydia* if purulent or clear discharge is present
- Ultrasound if there is a palpable mass, but otherwise unhelpful (Forbes 1998).

Management

Many women will have already tried a variety of remedies, even before presenting, and are often happier continuing along the simple non-hormonal treatments once a diagnosis by laparoscopy has been made. However,

- it is worth suggesting anti-inflammatory drugs, e.g. diclofenac
- for some women, complementary therapies can help in pain relief
- exercise and relaxation can also be beneficial.
  However, for many, referral is needed to help control the pain and other symptoms.

Dysfunctional uterine bleeding

Dysfunctional uterine bleeding (DUB) is defined as abnormal uterine bleeding when no pathological cause can be found, but there is usually a hormonal dysfunction. One in 20 women suffer from DUB and it is found more commonly in women who are within 5–10 years of their menarche or their menopause.

Subjective findings

- The woman presents with a change in her normal menstrual bleeding.
- She will usually present with menorrhagia: blood loss of 80 ml or more per period. The normal mean blood flow per period is 35 ml.
- Sometimes, the woman presents with intermenstrual bleeding and/or spotting.
- She may complain of associated dysmenorrhoea.
- She may present with tiredness due to anaemia.

Objective findings

- Vital signs are normal
- Observe the woman for signs of anaemia: menstrual blood loss of >80 ml per period will cause iron deficiency (Prentice 1999)
- Bimanual pelvic examination will be normal.

Investigations

Investigations are aimed at determining if there is an underlying cause for the abnormal uterine bleeding:
- FBC: to check for anaemia
- Clotting screen, if there is any suspicion of abnormal coagulation (Olah 1999)
- TFTs, if clinically indicated
- FSH and LH
- Cervical smear test, if indicated
- High vaginal swab (HVS), if associated with abdominal pain and vaginal discharge
- Pregnancy test, if associated with a missed/late period
- Ultrasound of pelvis and abdomen.

Management

Once it has been determined that there is no known cause for the uterine bleeding, then treatment is dependent on how problematical the bleeding is to the woman. Treatment is aimed at reducing or regulating the blood flow to an acceptable level for each woman (Tothill 1998).

Hormonal treatments

Combined oral contraceptives (COC). They are useful if contraception is needed, and also provide cyclical control.

Progestogens. Norethisterone, although a commonly prescribed drug, has been shown to be an ineffective treatment (Tothill 1998). Dydrogesterone (Duphaston) and medroxyprogesterone acetate (Provera) are sometimes helpful in treating DUB, but should not be used in ovulatory menorrhagia (Tothill 1998).

Intrauterine progestogens. Mirena (levonorgestrel-releasing intrauterine system) causes high local tissue concentrations within the endometrium, leading to atropy. This can lead to 90% reduction in menstrual flow (Prentice 1999).

Non-hormonal treatments

Antifibrinolytics, e.g. tranexamic acid (Cyclokapron). They are useful if the woman has menorrhagia with regular ovulatory cycles, especially if she is wanting to conceive or cannot tolerate hormonal treatment. They work rapidly, within 2–3 hours, need only be taken during menstruation and reduce blood flow by 45–60% (Tothill 1998).

NSAIDs (non steroidal anti-inflammatory drugs), e.g. mefenamic acid (Ponstan), ibuprofen, naproxen, diclofenac. These drugs need only be used during menstruation. They can also be used if menorrhagia is associated with IUCD, and are also helpful if there is associated dysmenorrhoea. They can reduce menstrual loss by 25–33% (Prentice 1999).

Ethamyslate (Dicynene). They are used by some doctors, but recent RCOG (Royal College of Obstetricians and Gynaecologists) guidelines suggest it is an ineffective treatment.

Danazol (Danol). High side effects of this treatment often makes it unacceptable.

Referral. If the uterine bleeding is uncontrollable, then referral may be necessary.

Gonadorelin analogues (Zoladex). Prescribed by the gynaecologist prior to surgery to thin the endometrium.

Bacterial vaginosis

Bacterial vaginosis (BV) is one of the commonest causes of vaginal discharge. In women of child-bearing age, 1 in 10 will have BV at some time.

It is not sexually transmitted, but more common in women who are having a sexual relationship. It is also more common in women who have an IUCD and those who smoke.

Bacterial vaginosis is not caused by poor hygiene but rather by an alteration of the balance of normal bacteria in the vagina, resulting in a loss of lactobacilli and an overgrowth of anaerobic bacteria and *Gardnerella* (what BV used to be called) (Cooling 2000).

Subjective findings

1. The woman usually presents with a vaginal discharge that 'smells fishy'.

2. She may report that the discharge is heavier just before or just after a menstrual period.
3. She may complain that the discharge is worse after sexual intercourse.
4. The woman may present with another problem:
   - wanting to change her contraceptive pill – it is important to establish why she wants to change, especially if there have been several requests, as she may assume wrongly that her vaginal discharge is pill-related
   - requesting a smear test before it is due – she is hoping that the nurse will notice the discharge without her having to say anything.

Objective findings

1. Vital signs are normal.
2. Vaginal/pelvic examination:
   - vulval soreness is absent
   - there is a grey-yellow, frothy, fishy discharge
   - the vaginal mucosa and cervix appear normal
   - if you suspect pelvic infection, then a bimanual examination should be performed.

Investigations

HVS for culture. Some laboratories will make a Gram-stained slide of the swab if BV is suspected, as many cases are missed by culture alone. Microscopically characteristic 'clue cells' are seen. Also, the vaginal pH is higher than usual at 4.7.

Endocervical swabs for *Chlamydia* and gonococcus. If a sexually transmitted disease (STD) is diagnosed, refer to a GUM clinic.

Management

- Fifty per cent of cases of BV are asymptomatic (Hosker 1997) and are discovered as an incidental finding. These women only need treating if they are due to have a vaginal surgical procedure, to reduce the risk of PID.
- Metronidazole (Flagyl) 400 mg twice daily for 5 days or 2 g as a single dose. Patients should be advised not to drink alcohol during the course.

Unfortunately, in approximately half of successfully treated women, BV will recur within 3 months. Simple self-help ideas can be suggested to the woman and, although they are not proven, appear to help prevent recurrences in some cases.

- Advise stopping smoking.
- Advise that excessive washing or douching may make BV worse. This is thought to be because washing will alter the vaginal acidity, possibly leading to an alteration of the vagina's normal bacteria.
- Advise not to add bubble bath, oils, etc., to bath water.

If a woman has recurrent BV, then advise that her partner is tested for nonspecific urethritis at the local GUM clinic.

Complications

- BV is a risk factor for morbidity following gynaecological surgery.
- It can be the cause of the development of PID and endometritis following a birth, an abortion/miscarriage or Caesarean section.
- There is a possible association between BV and miscarriage and premature labour.

Genitourinary prolapse

A prolapse occurs when there is weakness of, or damage to, the supporting structures of the pelvic organs, causing them to descend from their normal positions and eventually herniate through the vaginal opening (Lewis & Chamberlain 1990).

The most common cause is childbirth, especially if there is a history of large babies and/or long labours (Jackson & Smith 1997). Other causes include obesity, chronic respiratory disease, pelvic mass, poor postnatal exercise regimen, hysterectomy, intra-abdominal pressure and connective tissue disease.

Subjective findings

- The woman often presents with 'a feeling of something coming down.'
- She may feel a lump in the vagina.
- She may experience a dragging ache in the lower back, worse at the end of the day, and especially if standing a lot.
- There may be coital problems, including loss of sensation and orgasm.
- She may present with dyspareunia.
- She may experience vaginal flatus.
- The woman may have stress incontinence. Only 50% of these women have a cystocele, and therefore this finding should be considered separately (Jackson & Smith 1997).
- The woman may present with recurrent UTIs.
- She may have difficulty in or sensation of incomplete defaecation – rectocele.
- She may experience difficulty in keeping tampons in.
- She may present with bloodstained discharge if prolapse is beyond the introitus and ulceration has occurred.

Objective findings

Genitourinary prolapse is diagnosed clinically on pelvic examination:

- Prolapse can usually be seen, but it is sometimes helpful to examine the woman standing to reproduce symptoms.
- Ask the woman to cough and observe the rate of descent.
- Note any stress incontinence.
- If prolapse is present, use a Sim's speculum to examine vaginal walls, fornices and cervix.
- Perform a bimanual examination to exclude a rare pelvic mass.
- If necessary, go on to perform an abdominal examination.

Investigations

Investigations are only needed to investigate associated symptoms, e.g. recurrent UTI, pelvic mass.

Management

1. If prolapse found on routine pelvic examination with no symptoms, it needs no treatment.
2. If the woman is experiencing mild symptoms,
   - teach pelvic floor exercises
   - consider referral to a physiotherapist
   - advise losing weight, if appropriate
   - consider other symptoms, e.g. chronic cough, and treat.
3. If the woman is experiencing moderate to severe symptoms, referral for surgical opinion:
   - Some GP's will instigate the use of pessaries/rings to alleviate symptoms while waiting for an appointment or if surgery is declined.
   - If the woman is fitted with a ring, it should be changed every 6 months. The size is measured by estimating the distance from the posterior aspect of the symphysis pubis to the posterior vaginal fornix.
   - If prolapse is causing discomfort and erosion, oestrogen cream, if appropriate, can help.

Infertility

Infertility, which affects 1 in 7 couples at some point during their reproductive lives (Chambers 1999), is defined as the inability for a couple to achieve conception after 1 year of regular unprotected intercourse (Rodriguez-Armas et al 1998). This can be further subdivided into primary infertility, when pregnancy has never been achieved by either partner, and secondary infertility, when a pregnancy has been achieved in the past.

The causes of infertility are varied and involve both partners although it is still perceived to be a 'woman's problem'. However, as 22% of infertility is caused by the man and a further 21% by a combination of both partners, it is considered to be good practice to interview both partners together.

History taking of a couple failing to conceive:

- Age – in women, fertility is at its height from late teens to early 20s, then drops after age 35
- Smoking status
- Alcohol intake
- Occupation: in men fertility can be affected if working with some chemicals or heat
- Drug history – in particular, note NSAIDs, cannabis and chemotherapeutics
- Extent of any stress

- Extent of exercise – note if overstrenuous
- Systemic or debilitating illness – e.g. anorexia nervosa
- Menstrual history
- Previous abnormal smear and subsequent treatment
- Length of unprotected sexual intercourse
- Frequency of sexual intercourse
- Previous pregnancies with the same or different partners
- Previous relevant diseases, e.g. sexual, pelvic, varicocele
- Previous relevant surgery, e.g. pelvic, abdominal, urogenital

Initial investigations

- Two sperm samples, which should be sent to the same laboratory as the infertility clinic uses
- Serum progesterone in mid-luteal phase to confirm ovulation
- Rubella status of the woman
- Endocervical swab to test for *Chlamydia*
- Any tests which are necessary after history taking and examination of either partner
- It is not necessary to carry out TFTs or test for prolactin levels in the woman unless she has galactorrhoea or symptoms of thyroid disease.

Management

Initial management

1. If either partner smokes or takes recreational drugs, advise stopping.
2. Advise women to drink no more than 1–2 units of alcohol once or twice a week.
3. Advise men to drink no more than 3 units of alcohol per day.
4. If the woman's BMI>30, then advise on weight reduction.
5. If the woman is rubella seronegative then vaccination should be advised. You should also advise her not to get pregnant for 1 month after vaccination.
6. If the man has defective spermatogenesis, then advise on the wearing of loose-fitting underwear and avoid situations which might cause testicular hyperthermia.
7. Advise the couple to have regular sexual intercourse throughout the cycle.
8. Discourage the use of temperature charts and LH detection methods to time intercourse as there is no improvement of outcome (RCOG Infertility Guidelines).
9. Advise the woman to take folic acid, 0.4 mg daily, while trying to conceive and during the first 12 weeks of pregnancy. If the woman has already had a baby with a neural tube defect or she has epilepsy and she is taking medication, advise folic acid, 4 mg daily.

Further management

Recent published guidelines from the RCOG suggest that clomifene (Clomid) should not be prescribed without ultrasonic monitoring to determine dose and reduce the risk of multiple pregnancy. Therefore, referral is appropriate before any medication is given (Chambers 1999).

Referral should be to a specialist fertility centre for couples who have been trying to conceive without success for at least 18 months. Early referral should be if the woman:

- is over 35 years old and trying to conceive for 1 year
- has amenorrhoea or oligomenorrhoea
- has had previous abdominal/pelvic surgery
- has a history of PID or STD
- has had an abnormal pelvic examination
- has had abnormal results to investigations carried out
- has been *Chlamydia* positive in the past.
  Early referral should be if the man:
- has a low sperm count or quality
- has had previous or current genital pathology
- has had previous urogenital surgery
- has a history of STD
- has a significant varicocele
- has significant systemic illness.

Premenstrual syndrome

Premenstrual syndrome (PMS) is a disorder of unknown aetiology for which there are many different symptoms. It has been suggested that during their reproductive lives 50–90% of women will experience some symptoms of PMS at some stage (Clemoes 1995). Of those 3–5% will have such severe symptoms that not only are their lives affected but also those of their families as well (Clemoes 1995, Andrews 2000).

Subjective findings

Symptoms will always be cyclical, usually beginning mid-cycle and relieved when menstruation starts. Symptoms are often multiple and can be any combination of the following:

Physical symptoms

- Many women experience weight increase, bloating and oedema. Some women may gain 1 kg or more due to salt and water retention.
- The woman may also complain of breast tenderness.
- Premenstrual headache/migraine may be a presenting symptom.
- Pelvic pain/backache can also be associated with PMS.
- Dysmenorrhoea is often present along with other symptoms.
- The woman may experience hot flushes/skin rashes.
- She may complain of dizziness.
- She may be aware of appetite fluctuations and food cravings.
- She may admit to changes in libido.

Physiological symptoms

The following symptoms are usually easier to assess if you see the woman when she is feeling at her worse. It may be helpful to use some questions in your history taking which you would normally use when considering depression.

- She may have very low self-esteem
- She may feel apathetic
- She may be experiencing extreme mood swings and, even though she is aware what she is doing and how she is behaving, is unable to stop
- She may feel very irritable and tense
- She may feel she cannot cope and keeps crying
- If she has severe PMS, she may have suicidal thoughts.

Behavioural symptoms

- She may complain about loss of concentration and decreased performance
- She may have impaired judgement
- She may admit to more accidents
- She may avoid any social activities.

Investigations

- There are no accepted tests to help diagnose PMS
- Use of a menstrual chart recorded over 3 months will be an invaluable diagnostic aid.

Management

Many women will have already tried many self-help remedies when they seek help, as they usually have the more severe symptoms (Andrews 2000). It is important to establish what the woman's main symptoms are, as treatment should be directed towards relieving those symptoms.

General advice

1. For all women suffering from PMS then, understanding and reassurance to the woman that she cannot help what is happening is vital.
2. Explaining to a partner/family (if permission has been granted) can sometimes help with home situations.
3. Discuss the woman's normal diet with her:
   - Advise eating small amounts of carbohydrates (e.g. 1/2 slice of bread) every 2–3 hours. PMS symptoms tend to get worse if blood sugar levels drop.
   - Advise reduction of salt and fluids if the woman feels very bloated.
   - Advise reduction of caffeine, alcohol, dietary fat and 'fast foods'.
   - Advise reduction of tobacco.
4. Encourage relaxation and exercise, as natural endorphins will be released to help combat pain.
5. Discuss social life, work and family issues and suggest coping strategies.

Top Tips ✔
1 Vaginal bleeding with unilateral pelvic pain and late period could be an ectopic pregnancy. Admit urgently
2 Severe pelvic pain is not necessarily gynaecological in origin. Also consider other differential diagnoses, e.g. renal colic, UTI, inflamed appendix, labour
3 Postmenopausal bleeding is always abnormal and should be investigated fully
4 Do not assume that 'break through bleeding' is caused by hormonal contraception or HRT. Always investigate and refer if it continues
5 Every woman's idea of heavy bleeding is different. Ask about numbers of pads, tampons used as a guide. Also ask about clots and flooding
6 When considering amenorrhoea, consider anorexia and thyrotoxicosis
7 If there are other symptoms as well as amenorrhoea, especially early morning headache with visual disturbance, there could be possible intracranial pathology. Refer urgently
8 Remember 20% of smear tests taken can be false negatives. If in doubt, refer for colposcopy
9 Remember to test for *Chlamydia* if cervix looks inflamed and there is purulent or clear discharge is present. Also refer to local GUM clinic
10 Remember the forgotten tampon or IUCD

6. Suggest contacting local self-help groups and give telephone number/address.
7. Some women will find complementary therapies beneficial and many surgeries now have connections with different therapists. Always encourage checking that the therapist is trained in their particular skill.

Medical treatments

Pyridoxine/vitamin B6. This is the most common OTC treatment. Although there is no evidence to its efficacy, many women appear to find it helpful.

Evening primrose oil. Another common OTC treatment that is sometimes helpful for premenstrual mastalgia.

Efamast. Evening primrose oil on prescription, which is expensive and needs 8×40 mg daily to be effective.

Diuretics. These are helpful if the woman feels very uncomfortable with fluid retention.

Combined contraceptive pill. If the woman also needs a contraceptive, then it may be helpful.

Progesterone and progestogens. A common treatment in several forms, e.g. Cyclogest. However, research has shown that it is no more effective than a placebo (Andrews 2000).

Danazol. It may be useful to treat premenstrual mastalgia, but not helpful with other symptoms. It also has an androgenic side effect.

Oestrogen therapy. If given as patches or subcutaneous implants, then symptoms can be significantly improved. Doses have to be higher than in HRT, with a protective progestogen also prescribed.

Gonadotrophin–releasing hormone analogues. These are usually used to treat endometriosis. As they suppress the ovaries, they can be used short term to treat PMS. It may be necessary to give HRT as well.

Selective serotonin reuptake inhibitors (SSRIs). These are useful if the woman has underlying depression. Fluoxetine (Prozac) is the only drug licensed in the UK to treat depression associated with PMS.

Hysterectomy with bilateral salpingo-oophorectomy. For some women with very severe symptoms it may be the only solution.

Glossary

Amenorrhoea   The absence of menstruation

Cystocele   Prolapse of bladder and anterior vaginal wall

Dysmenorrhoea   Painful periods. **Primary** – painful periods after the menarche when the periods have become ovulatory. Characterised by colicky, central, lower abdominal pain radiating to the back and upper thighs. **Secondary** – due to organic disease, e.g. endometriosis, PID. Often associated with menorrhagia

Dyspareunia   Painful sexual intercourse

Menarche   Onset of menstruation

Menopause   Cessation of menstruation

Menorrhagia   Excessive blood loss during menstruation: usually 80 ml or more.

Mittelschmerz   Mid-cycle iliac fossa pain at ovulation. More common in women under 30 years

Multiparae   Many vaginal deliveries

Nulliparae   Never delivered vaginally

Oligomenorrhoea   Periods infrequent or blood loss scanty

Polymenorrhoea   When the menstrual cycle is less than 22 days

Rectocele   Prolapse of rectum and posterior vaginal wall

Rugae   Small ridges running concentrically around the vaginal wall

References

Adams M, Evans A S, Peet E 1998 Gynaecological cancers. Update March 18:510–524.

Andrews G 2000 Alleviating the misery of premenstrual syndrome. Community Nurse 5(12):23–24.

Austoker J, Davey C, Jansen C 1997 Improving the quality of the written information sent to women about cervical screening, NHSCSP, Publication No 6, Cancer Research Campaign.

Bates B 1995 A guide to physical examination and history taking, 6th edn. J B Lippincott, Philadelphia.

Chambers R 1999 Infertility. Family Medicine 3(7):16–17.

Clemoes H 1995 Premenstrual tension. Practice Nurse Nov 17:461–465.

Clubb E, Knight J 1992 Fertility: A comprehensive guide to natural family planning. David & Charles.

Conway G 1996 Treatment options in secondary amenorrhoea. Prescriber 7(23):25–29.

Cooling H 2000 Bacterial vaginosis. Update Feb 17:251–252.

Edwards M 1999 Know the symptoms and the risks of PCOS. Practice Nurse Nov 5:502–506.

Forbes P 1998 Diagnosis and treatment of chronic pelvic pain. The Practitioner 242:120–125.

Hagan P, Knott P 1998 Diagnosing and treating polycystic ovary syndrome. The Practitioner 242:98–106.

Hopcroft K, Forte V 1999 Symptom sorter. Radcliffe Medical Press, Oxford.

Hopkinson Z E C, Sattar N, Fleming R, Greer I A 1998 Polycystic ovarian syndrome: the metabolic syndrome comes to gynaecology. British Medical Journal 317(7154):329–332.

Hosker H, 1997 Vaginal discharge. Update Oct 22:521–528.

Jackson S, Smith P 1997 Diagnosing and managing genitourinary prolapse. British Medical Journal 314(7084):875.

Lewis T L T, Chamberlain G V P (eds) 1990 Gynaecology by ten teachers, 15th edn. Edward Arnold, London.

Marieb E N 1995 Human anatomy and physiology, 3rd edn. Benjamin/Cummings, California.

Muir Gray J M 1997 Evidence-based healthcare. Churchill Livingstone, Edinburgh.

Nottingham J 1999 False-negative cervical smears are 'inevitable'. GP Feb 12:17.

Olah K 1999 Menorrhagia. Family Medicine 3(10):13–15.

Prentice A 1999 Menorrhagia: a guide to rational prescribing. Prescriber 10(7):89–97.

Rodriguez-Armas O, Hedon B, Daya S 1998 Infertility and conception. Parthenon, London.

Rymer J, Davis G, Rodin A, Chapman M 1993 Preparation and revision for the DRCOG. Churchill Livingstone, London.

Sarazin S K, Seymour S F 1991 Causes and treatment options for women with dyspareunia. Nurse Practitioner 16(10):30,35–38,41.

Slater D N 1998 False-negative cervical smears: medico-legal fallacies and suggested remedies. Cytopathology 9:145–154.

Smith T (ed) 1995 The British Medical Association complete family health encyclopedia, 2nd edn. Dorling Kindersley, London.

Tothill S 1998 Diagnosis and treatment of menstrual problems. Prescriber 9(18):91–95.

16

MENTAL HEALTH AND THE NURSE PRACTITIONER IN PRIMARY HEALTH CARE

Ruth Davies and Deborah Humble

Key Issues

- The role and responsibilities of the nurse practitioner in working with people with actual/potential mental health problems

- Assessing yourself and developing relevant knowledge, skills and attitudes

- Supervision in clinical practice.

Introduction

As nurses we are all bound by the United Kingdom Central Council for Nurses, Midwives and Health Visitors' Code of Professional Conduct (UKCC 1992a). This clearly states that no action or omission should be detrimental to or harm the patient. We can also extend our practice to work within the parameters laid down by the scope of professional practice (UKCC 1992b). Given this, and the increasing demands on the primary health care team to work with people with mental health problems, the aim of this chapter is to help you refresh or enhance your understanding of people with possible mental health problems in order that your assessment and management is appropriately focused and that your practice develops and, ultimately, patient care is enhanced.

We assume that most of you are not trained mental health nurses and that most frequently following assessment you will be making decisions regarding who you can manage yourself versus the need for referral (sometimes balanced with the patient's wish not to be referred) to either a general medical practitioner or to specialist services. For this reason we will be focusing on key processes such as assessment of mental health within this chapter.

It is quite inappropriate to work beyond your expertise and to assume that you can safely and competently manage someone who may be mentally ill; hence, we will be writing about principles of practice, including the need for supervision, rather than specific mental illnesses. Some common presenting issues will be explored through case studies and we suggest further reading and resources at the end of the chapter.

Why do nurse practitioners in primary care need to know about mental health?

A key feature of nurse practitioner (NP) practice is that NPs see patients who present for a wide variety of reasons, often undifferentiated and undiagnosed. The NP should be able to take a full history, form a diagnosis (or at least a working hypothesis) and discuss and agree management and/or treatment with the patient. This may include referral to other colleagues or agencies. Dowrick (1992) suggests that 'up to 40% of patients attending their general practitioner for any reason have a probable psychiatric disorder' (Dowrick 1992: 382), whereas Armstrong (1995) working on figures from 1980, suggests that mental illness in the community appears at a rate of 250–315 per 1000; 230 per 1000 consult their GP and 101.5 per 1000 have mental illness actually detected by the GP. Only about 10% of patients, who tend to be the most ill, are referred to psychiatric outpatients.

Whatever the actual figures, it is apparent that much primary care work concerns people who may have mental health problems and, more importantly, that many such people go undiagnosed and therefore unhelped. Craig & Boardman (1997) suggest that 'about a quarter of patients with probable mental disorder in the general population will consult in any two week period' and they continue to tell us that 'poor outcome is associated with delayed or insufficient initial treatment, more severe illness, older age at onset, comorbid physical illness and continuing problems with family, marriage or employment' (Craig & Boardman 1997: 1609).

It is clear, therefore, that any history taking must consider the patient as a person within their whole environment, including domestic, occupational and leisure aspects. The NP must ensure that she is able and willing to take a holistic history and not fall into a reductionist model of care. Hannigan (1998) writes about the contribution of non-specialist nurses to mental health care and suggests that in the future practice nurses could be actively managing people with depression, phobias and obsessional disorders. It is quite likely that many of you, as NPs, are already actively involved in the management of people with depression and anxiety at the very least.

What is mental health? What is mental illness?

The word mental means pertaining to the mind. Within psychology there is great current debate regarding the mind – What is it? Where is it? Where is personality located? Is the mind a physical entity? Is there such a thing as a soul? Where is consciousness located? are some of the questions within this debate. When we speak of mental health or illness, we are referring to the state of mind of a person and this can be simply taken to include their cognitions (attention, perception, memory, thought, speech), emotions and behaviour. It may also include the soul or spirit or self of a person if this is a meaningful concept to you. What is apparent, though, is that mind is more than cognition; it includes emotion and behaviour at the very least, and a mental health assessment should, in turn, include all of those aspects.

Before trying to define mental health, it is worth considering what you mean by health generally. Is health the absence of disease or illness? Is health – ill-health a continuum or a clear step? Can you be or feel healthy when you have proven pathophysiology? Can others allow you to be or feel healthy when you have proven pathophysiology? Can you be physically healthy but mentally unhealthy? Does this mean you are not healthy? Does being mentally unwell make you mentally ill? What is perfect mental health? Many of these questions are unanswerable; they can only act as a catalyst for discussion and debate.

This leaves us as nurses in a difficult position. There are few rules for mental health – for defining and differentiating between the normal and the abnormal. The definition of abnormal is problematic; the definition of normal is even more so in relation to mental status. Atkinson et al (1987) write very clearly about this, explaining how to use a purely statistical definition of normal to define the abnormal is insufficient. They suggest that deviation from social norms, maladaptive behaviour and personal distress are included.

Imagine, then, two people who actively wish to die. One is a young man, in work and in a relationship, with a concerned and loving family, with no apparent reasons to be suicidal. He is statistically abnormal (most young men are not suicidal, although as a group they are at higher risk than the rest of the population). He is abnormal in so far as his peer group thinks and behaves; his suicidal behaviour is certainly maladaptive (has adverse effects on the individual or society) and he is deeply distressed. The other is a middle-aged man, in work, in a relationship and with a concerned and loving family, but dying a slow, sometimes physically painful and inevitable death. He too is statistically abnormal (most middle-aged men are not suicidal). He is abnormal in so far as his peer group thinks and behaves; his wish to die is certainly maladaptive and although he was deeply distressed at being told his diagnosis, he is not so now, and has apparently come to terms with both his diagnosis and his prognosis.

Are either of these men mentally ill? Would you refer either of them to psychological or psychiatric services? The likelihood is that you would refer the first man but not the second – the differences being that the second man has a reason to think and feel as he does (implying rationality) and that he may also have a group around him, or accessible to him who do think like him, i.e. there is a tentative societal norm. Furthermore, the second man is not currently distressed. However much we may disagree with a person's opinions and feelings, this alone does not make them mentally ill. Our own feelings towards these two men are also likely to influence our management of them. Craig & Boardman (1997) suggest that patient characteristics which influence the decision to refer include male sex, younger age, severe disorder and suicidal ideation or attempt. Thus, we may be more likely to refer the first patient due to his age and continue to manage the second within the primary care setting.

If it is difficult to define the abnormal; defining the normal is even more challenging. Statistically, many of us will have gone through periods where we felt anxious, depressed and overwhelmed and where our feelings, thoughts and emotions were different from our own personal norms. Were we mentally ill at that time? How did we know? Were we aware? So many people have similar periods that, although they are abnormal to us, statistically within the overall population, they are so frequent as to be normal. A parallel in physical terms might be the common cold. In a maladaptive, physiological sense, this is an abnormal event, but in a statistical sense it is so common that it might be abnormal not to have a cold one winter.

All this illustrates is that to think of mental health in terms of normality and abnormality is highly problematic; yet that is the challenge facing us. As nurses in primary care, we have to make assessments and then management decisions regarding the mental health of the patient with us. We are required to somehow identify how and when someone is mentally ill.

Atkinson et al (1987) tell us that there is general agreement among psychologists that the mentally healthy person displays particular tendencies or traits to a greater degree than the person who is mentally unwell. The first of these concerns the efficient perception of reality, where the individual is accurate and realistic both in self-perception and in other/world perception. For example, the healthy person will set himself attainable goals, being aware of what he is capable of doing. He will consider being challenged in this but expects to rise to the challenge. Someone less healthy in terms of self-perception might aim too high or too low or not at all: for example, in perceptions of what they can achieve as a working mother (a group increasingly reported as feeling they never do anything well). Most of us will be able to tell when we have misperceived something, or hold different views from others. Some people however, will hallucinate (perceive something for which there is no external stimulus) or perhaps think that the television or radio is speaking to them or about them (ideas of reference): the primary care team visited one man, who had become increasingly withdrawn, to discover that every piece of electrical equipment in his house was turned to the wall. In addition, some people may be deluded and hold an enduring belief which is fixed and false and defined as so by the person's culture. Some of the most common delusions relate to feelings of persecution, or paranoia.

The second trait is self-awareness: for example, of how we think, feel and behave. The aware person is able to reflect, to identify patterns, to have insight into their behaviour and then have choice about how to behave or intervene in a situation. The aware person will also have some sensitivity to others' feelings, thoughts and behaviours. Someone less healthy might be quite lacking self-awareness, unable to identify how or why they behave in a particular way. A patient I saw recently came in with a marked tremor, a fearful expression and in clothes which hung off him, a marked change in the man I knew. He could not, however, articulate what the problem was and having excluded any obvious physical cause for this I began to explore his wider environment. He denied any idea about what was wrong, or concerns about his impending retirement but could not talk about how he felt about retiring – 'It's just going to happen' – although I knew he loved his job and the life which went with it. One hypothesis was that his current way of coping was to unconsciously deny the anxiety his retirement could cause, but in so doing, the symptoms of anxiety were present in other ways. He had little awareness other than to know at some level that he needed help, hence the presentation.

Thirdly, the healthy individual is able to exercise voluntary control over his behaviour. This does not exclude occasional impulsive behaviour, where choice is still available to that individual. It does, however, exclude those whose behaviour is obsessive or compulsive in some way, who feel that they have no control over what they do. Such people may obsessively check

that they turned off the gas ring, compulsively wash their hands three times instead of once, or compulsively vomit after eating, or have intrusive repetitive thoughts which enter their heads. Other people may be phobic in some way, unable perhaps to leave the house, although they wish to go out. De Silva & Rachman (1998) write clearly about the relationship of obsessive–compulsive disorder to other problems, and various assessment and management strategies.

The fourth trait is that healthy people have a sense of self-worth and respect for themselves and equally for others around them. They feel accepted as part of a group and are comfortable in social situations. They do not have to agree with everyone around them or conform in order to be liked. By contrast, many people who are anxious or depressed feel worthless and dread getting things wrong, even though they may not be able to articulate what they might get wrong. They may also feel that no one wants them or that they are a burden to others who would be better off without them. In some ways, this relates to the first trait in that persistent negative, intrusive thoughts can be considered a thought disorder. Cognitive behavioural techniques are often very useful in the management of these thoughts and a referral could be worthwhile.

The healthy individual is able to form lasting affectionate and satisfying relationships, in which mutual respect and sensitivity is a feature. Part of this includes having the confidence to be yourself, to not have to act in a way to please or manipulate others, but to be able to make and refuse requests, to state opinions and to be assertive. Some people may fear intimacy and this may concern them. Others might not realise that this is a difficulty. Consider how many people present with relationship difficulties that they know are affecting or will affect their general well-being.

Finally, the mentally healthy person is able to be productive and active. This might include paid employment or voluntary activity and certainly includes the ability to use leisure time actively or creatively. The person who is tired all the time may fail to meet this criteria of mental health, and when any possible organic causes have been excluded (Gambrill & Mead 1994) we might consider exploring their psychological life in more depth.

So, can we begin to define mental health or mental illness? It would seem to become increasingly problematic, particularly when the traits identified above help us to consider our own mental health status. Just as few of us are in peak physical shape and fitness, the same may be true of mental health. Gillis (1988) suggests that, in addition to the above, mentally healthy people get satisfaction from simple everyday things, have a tolerant easy-going attitude and can laugh at themselves. This is probably a helpful idea, particularly in a social and work climate where audit, scrutiny, criticism and a focus on output feature highly and where demand exceeds supply. It is refreshing to notice (or be able to notice) the flowers on the desk at reception, to feel joy with a patient, to identify what we have enjoyed about our work each day and to laugh at ourselves. This helps us to keep a balance and a perspective on life.

Assessing mental health

If we cannot define normal and abnormal mental health, how do we go about assessing someone's mental state? We may have a picture of someone who is mentally ill in a florid way – perhaps, hallucinating and withdrawn, unable to engage in coherent conversation – but what of all those people who present in a less extreme or borderline way? What follows are some principles by which you might assess, some tools and resources which you might use and key pointers for common mental health diagnoses. What matters is that you can identify whether or not you need to refer and with what degree of urgency. The fine-tuned diagnosis is for the expert clinician to make. For example, it is important that you can identify someone who is clinically depressed and the depth of their depression, and then take appropriate action.

Some resources that you might find useful on a regular basis are the decision trees in Armstrong (1995), regarding the assessment of depression, suicide risk and antidepressant follow-up, the diagnostic and statistical manual (DSM-IV) of the American Psychiatric Association (1994), which includes criteria for all psychiatric diagnoses and therefore prompts areas of questioning to consider, and for those of you who give depot neuroleptic medication to people with severe enduring mental illness, the practice guidelines from the Royal College of Nursing (1994).

The principles of mental health assessment are no different from those of physical health assessment and indeed the two are inseparable if we work within a holistic model of health. In any history taking a structured and systematic approach is necessary in order that all possible information is gained upon which to formulate a diagnosis or working hypothesis and upon which to base the subsequent management and treatment. Various tools and models exist for assessment and management of mental disorders and at the end of the chapter is a brief list of resources which you might use in addition to those mentioned above. You should have access to these as a minimum, and be familiar with the presenting features of common mental disorders, particularly depression and anxiety.

The two most important assessment tools we have are the skills of observation and of listening, both of which can be developed so that we become more astutely observant and more acutely aware of what is being said and how. Before we begin to observe and listen, though, we must be aware of our own willingness to do so. Stuart & Sundeen (1987) suggest that nurses may well have the knowledge base and skills with which to undertake a mental health assessment but their uneasiness with mental health problems might prevent them from exploring such issues. It is quite possible that the patient is not helped at all in such situations. Armstrong (1995) makes a similar point with GPs, commenting that they know how to take a psychiatric history but avoid doing so through fear of being overwhelmed by their workload. A fear of 'opening a can of worms' is not unusual, but continued avoidance or blocking of someone's attempts to get help for mental distress may not be ethical or even adequate professional practice.

Observation and listening

A willingness and ability to relate to people in such a way that they can tell their story provides the framework for observing and listening. These two processes enable us to gather information about a person prior to forming a hypothesis about what might be happening. It is almost impossible to separate out these two skills as we listen and observe simultaneously. We observe a person from the minute we meet them. For those of you who go out to greet a patient and walk back to your room with them you can notice how they move, the speed, the ease, the gait, the posture. For those of you who call people to your room you can take note in addition of the time it takes the person to actually get to your room, the sound of the knock on the door, the apparent confidence with which they enter your room and sit down. Do they make eye contact with you? Do you make eye contact with them?

The likely course of the interview will then be for you to introduce yourself if necessary and give a broad opening in order to ascertain the reason for attending today. Then, just as in a physical consultation, you can let the patient tell the story before focusing on a line of inquiry. It is important to ascertain whether the patient has any ideas about or understanding of what is happening or why they are feeling or behaving or thinking as they are; also, what it is that has brought them specifically today. Have they had to build confidence to consult you. Have they had to wait until they could attend secretly or without children in attendance? Have symptoms suddenly got worse, for example? What are their concerns? Some people with recurrent or chronic illness may know when they are getting worse and present early enough to get help while they still have some insight. Sackett et al (1997) suggest using the framework of ideas, concerns and expectations (ICE) when history taking. A middle-aged lady with a long history of manic depression always sought help when she found herself speeding up with filing at work. This particular lady had an idea of (insight into) what was happening to her in that she was sufficiently aware of her own behaviour to notice a change; she was concerned that it did not deteriorate into a major psychotic episode (of which she had previous experience) and her expectation was that we and she could prevent this from occurring by altering her psychotropic drug dosages. One important feature of this was that we could trust each other – she knew us well enough to present early, with an idea and concern, prior to any more florid symptoms developing, and as health professionals we were willing to believe her and be guided by her own assessment of her mental state and act both quickly and appropriately to prevent a relapse.

Observation and listening are the key skills in history taking, but not all patients are able or willing to talk about what is happening. Some do not have the vocabulary; someone profoundly depressed may be almost silent; others may deny any psychological difficulties, insisting that 'if you could just give me something to sleep, I'll be all right'. Where a patient is unable, for whatever reason, to tell a story, we may need to be both more lateral thinking and more focused in our approach, and ask questions which might enable the person to say more.

A framework for history taking sometimes used in counselling and psychotherapy practice asks patients about four main areas – their occupation (paid or unpaid), their leisure time, their relationships and their spirit. The theory is that the healthy person has a balance between these four areas of their existence, and an imbalance may indicate a need for help, and the type of help which might be indicated.

For example, a young woman may be a 'frequent attender' presenting with minor physical complaints which she or the children experience. This pattern of attendance can be considered as conveying a message of sorts. What is happening that she needs frequent contact with health services? Does she need help in some way that she cannot overtly express, or of which she is not conscious? Next time she presents, you attempt to ask different questions and discover initially that she is apparently happily occupied caring for her children, her relationship with her partner is OK, she feels all right in herself (she knows she is not ill) but she gets no leisure time at all and she feels exhausted. Exploring this avenue, enables her to say that although she is generally content with her life, she used to be far more active and is now gaining weight. She misses adult company. She feels all her time is spent being a wife and mother and is too tired to want sex with her partner. Having identified this, it can be relatively straightforward to problem solve such a situation, although this might take a couple of sessions with her or even her seeing a counsellor. Her partner, meanwhile, might be feeling that his life is dominated by work – he equally has no leisure, he is not relating to his children, other than to shout at them, and he feels quite unwell. Further inquiry elicits that he feels (and is) solely responsible for the financial income of the family, that his job is insecure and that he feels under constant threat of losing his job, to the extent that he puts in extra hours to make himself indispensable. He

knows this is not how he wants to live, he sleeps poorly and is irritable, and that it is not a healthy way to live. On further questioning, it appears that he is mildly depressed, although this is not a label he has used. He is, however, not surprised when this is offered as a hypothesis, and he goes away to think about the various forms of help on offer. Again, the relationship with the nurse has been such that he has been able to tell his story and be taken seriously. Someone has listened to him, and by doing so, has helped him to listen to himself. Men will often express an increase in irritability or a change in drug or alcohol use rather than low mood, but the former may indicate depression.

A structured and systematic approach to assessing a person's mental state does not necessarily mean filling in a form or checklist. As identified above, engaging in conversation will provide much of the information you require. However, a complete mental state assessment includes the following, which are widely discussed and described in many psychiatric reference books and manuals. Kates & Craven (1998) provide the following structure and make the point that the mental state examination is only the first part of the overall assessment. It is important that you pay attention to any changes which you observe or the patient reports and your previous knowledge of the patient is important here, as is your ability not to jump to conclusions.

Kates & Craven (1998) suggest that the mental state examination includes consideration of general appearance and behaviour, particularly with reference to social norms and participation in the interview, i.e. are you able to relate, make contact with the patient? Is eye contact achievable? Does the patient appear suspicious? Be aware also that adolescents and adults may use a different language and posture, for example. Does the patient appear to be taking care of him/herself in terms of hygiene and dress? What is normal for that patient? The same applies for mood (how the patient feels) and affect (expressed emotion). Are these congruent? If someone says they're OK, do they look OK (explore what they mean by this) or do they look tired, seem angry or sad? Mental state also includes thought content and processes, by which we mean what a person is actually thinking (for example of committing suicide, that someone is poisoning them) and the processes of how they actually think – fluently and ordered, jumping around, is this under their control? A person might express ideas of reference where they relate external events (e.g. on television, radio, newspapers) directly to themselves. Any such disorder in thought content or process is worthy of further sensitive probing with referral in mind.

Speech gives clues to thought content and process, as often we speak as we think, so pay attention to the rate, volume, coherence (does what is said make sense?). For some people speech will be difficult: someone severely depressed may hardly speak at all. Enquire also into the presence of hallucinations or delusions. Sometimes these will be apparent as a patient is interrupted by an auditory or visual hallucination, or will tell you that they are being controlled by something else, or that they are really the son or daughter of someone very important and are being followed. Try to explore this without being judgemental, as sometimes the voices may be telling the patient to harm himself, or the patient may be so distressed by his symptoms that self-harm seems the only way out.

Finally, mental state examination includes cognitive functioning, i.e. memory, attention, perception, concentration, orientation, etc. You may be accustomed to assessing for orientation (date, time, place) and memory as part of over 75 health checks and you might consider how easily depression can mimic Alzheimer's disease. Accurate diagnosis is important and we recently referred a 60-year-old man for further assessment which indicated that he had an early onset dementia rather than depression.

Kates & Craven (1998) state that the above complete the mental state examination and the next important consideration concerns the severity and impact of the problem. Essentially this concerns the level of functioning and the level of distress and, in practice, this is often the most important factor in terms of management, treatment and referral. You must consider whether there is a risk of self-harm or harm to others as part of this, and consider an immediate referral if necessary. Otherwise, inquire about the impact on daily life. Is the patient continuing to work, to parent, to care for self and others and to what degree of 'normal' for them? Ask also about previous history. Have they felt like this before? What happened? Did they get worse or better? What helped (if anything)? A useful question to ask is, 'What are you like at your worst?', as this can give an indication of future risk or prognosis. Include any precipitating factors – the 'Why now' question – and anything else which might indicate vulnerability. For example, a man may become depressed when made redundant from his job, but he is additionally vulnerable if his ability to cope is influenced by his lack of social support. Equally, the presence of social support may be a resource for the patient to draw upon, and should also be included, although not depended upon in place of professional care – family and friends also have their own needs and concerns when a loved one is unwell.

Other areas to consider as part of mental health assessment will include gaining information at times from other family members and friends, or agencies, and remaining aware of any physical conditions. For example, it is easy and cost-effective to exclude some physiological problems that may have a psychological presentation. These include people who present with tiredness and lethargy (exclude anaemia and hypothyroidism) and overactivity (exclude hyperthyroidism). Consider also that a person who is confused may be either depressed or presenting with a possible early onset Alzheimer's disease or have some other physiological (sometimes toxic) reason for this presentation. Remember that medication for physical conditions may have iatrogenic effects, e.g. a beta-blocker may cause tiredness, lack of libido, which in turn effects the relationships, work, leisure and self of the person taking it. Steroid-induced psychosis is rare but does occur and some people with postnatal depression may respond to treatment with oestrogen. Too often, medical and psychiatric services fail to see the whole person, which does not serve the patient at all well.

Management and treatment decisions should always be made in conjunction with the patient. Kates & Craven (1998) recommend that you reach agreement on what the problem is and negotiate treatment plans and goals. As Sackett et al (1997) recommend: if you can remember to inquire about their expectations of you and how they think they can best be helped, you are more likely to form a successful working alliance with them. Many people presenting in primary care will manage with support from the primary care team, without referral to secondary services or counsellors. However, share your limitations and practice guidelines with the patient. The following case studies illustrate some of these points.

Case studies

We now consider the role of the NP in primary care regarding assessment and management of people with mental health problems.

As discussed earlier, it is becoming increasingly likely that people with mental health problems will be assessed and managed within the primary care setting without referral to community psychology and psychiatry. In this section we consider, through case studies, some decisions we have made where we had a choice of whether or not to refer. Part of working as an NP in primary care is that patients can choose whether they wish to see the GP or the NP, who is often more able to fit them in urgently. As such, the NP will not necessarily know the reason for presentation and has to start with an open mind.

The case studies which follow are based on a combination of real events and people. Detail has been altered at times to provide anonymity or to make clinical or teaching points.

Case study 1   Can I manage this person myself?

Jill, aged 30, presented to me one morning as an emergency patient. We had not met prior to this and as I greeted Jill in the waiting room, I noticed that she was sitting huddled up in her coat; she looked pale and unhappy. Once in my room, she kept her coat on and made minimal eye contact with me. She fiddled with a handkerchief. She told me that she felt like she had flu for the last 4 days; she had taken paracetamol and now didn't know what to do with herself, she felt so awful. At this stage I noted this comment and asked if I might examine her. She agreed and examination of her ears, nose, throat and thorax revealed nothing to suggest a different diagnosis. I told her this and she said she actually felt better than she did yesterday.

At this stage I could summarise Jill as having flu-like symptoms for 4 days, which she had treated herself, quite appropriately. Why then had she consulted today? I was mindful of her comment about feeling awful and not knowing what to do with herself, and this along with her lack of eye contact caused me to think broader. I told her that she was managing her symptoms in the way I would recommend. Then I added: 'But you seem unhappy or worried about something. Is that the flu or is there something on your mind?' Jill proceeded to tell me that she had recently frequently felt tearful and hated living by herself. She had a 9-year-old son and had separated from his father 2 years ago, at which time she had been depressed and had seen a counsellor. I asked if she had had any relationships since her separation and at this point she began to cry. I sat with her and stayed silent until she was ready to talk. She told me this was how she was a lot of the time. At this stage my hypothesis became one of possible depression and when I invited her to tell me more, it became apparent that although she was still able to go to work (as an insurance clerk) she had felt low for several weeks, and she felt that she was just existing and had nothing to look forward to. She had lost about 4 kg weight and found it difficult to get to sleep at night. Importantly, she had no suicidal thoughts or plans.

At this stage, it was clear that Jill was clinically depressed. She met the major criteria of low mood for more than 2 weeks and the secondary criteria of weight change and insomnia. I did not say this to her, preferring instead to get more history. I asked her what had prompted her visit today. She was physically improving, but she did indeed feel awful. She had been having an affair with a married colleague at work, who said he had left his wife, but only met Jill when it suited him. She did not know whether to believe him and felt increasingly low, used and frustrated by this situation, while simultaneously finding that some attention was better than no attention at all. This was complicated by hearing only a few days

earlier that her sister, to whom she was very close, was planning to emigrate.

I asked Jill what she thought about how she was feeling, and she was immediately able to say that she thought she was depressed and she felt similar to how she had a couple of years ago. She also recognised that her sadness about her sister emigrating was normal but harder to deal with because she felt depressed anyway. As part of my assessment I asked her what she had been like at her worst when she was depressed before. She said she cried continually, she could not work and she slept badly. She had not felt suicidal at all. We talked about treatment and management options. Jill did not want to take antidepressant medication, saying she hadn't needed to before and she wasn't that bad. She did not want to be referred to a counsellor but asked if she could continue to see me instead. I told her that I could offer her support but that I was not a counsellor and that if I or she felt referral should be considered in the future, we should say so. We agreed to this and met as and when she needed.

Several issues arise from this: not least that if Jill were clinically depressed, should I have referred her to a specialist? I did not, for the following reasons:

- I liked Jill and felt we had established a rapport over the course of the consultation. As part of this, we were working towards a shared management strategy, and I trusted her to come back to me. I think she also trusted me to want to help her.
- I have a personal interest in mental health and further training in counselling skills. I also have access to supervision within the work setting, from the practice counsellor, so I am well prepared for and supported in work at this level (mild depression using DSM-IV criteria).
- I had ascertained that she was not suicidal.
- She did not want to see a counsellor and I could continually assess her if I saw her.
- She was not sufficiently ill to merit referral to local psychiatric services (neither did she want this). As a non-urgent presentation, an assessment with them would take up to 8 weeks.
- Some research (Gournay & Brooking 1994, Ridsdale 1995) supports the role and input of practice nurses in terms of mental health outcomes.

Jill saw me three times after this consultation, during which I listened to how she was. She finished the affair with her colleague, grieved over her sister's departure and began to think about ways she could make her life more interesting. This included going out with her son more.

Anxiety and depression often coexist, although this was not the case with Jill. However, the same principles of assessment apply, with attention being paid to the nature, severity and frequency of symptoms, the impact of the symptoms on daily life, any identifiable precipitants or patterns, attempts at self-management and why now. There are several forms of anxiety – e.g. panic disorders, generalised or specific anxiety and phobias – and referral to psychological services

may be indicated. However, as identified earlier, it is increasingly likely that you may work with many people with anxiety under the supervision of a psychologist.

David, a 22-year-old labourer, booked a routine appointment with me. It is practice in the surgery that the receptionists ask all patients who they wish to see. David and I had not met before and when I went to call him from the waiting room, I noticed that he was of average height and weight (slightly thin, if anything) and had apparently come straight from work as his clothes were dirty and he wore heavy boots.

I invited him to sit down and tell me the reason for his visit. He spoke audibly but hesitantly, needing prompts. He said he had been experiencing a thumping chest, which his mother told him was palpitations, for the last 2 months. He was extremely concerned that there might be something wrong with his heart and his uncle had recently survived a heart attack. David also had difficulty sleeping at night and said this was when he had most palpitations, although they could occur at any time of day and seemed to do so without warning. Each episode lasted probably 2–3 min. He had no ideas what might be causing them: work and social life were fine. Life was pretty good except for this worry. At this stage, I had elicited a concern, but I did not have enough spoken material with which to hypothesise. I asked him about his previous medical history, which was uneventful, with no similar previous episodes and tonsillitis as a child. He was not taking any prescribed or over-the-counter (OTC) medication. What was apparent, though, was that he appeared agitated. As he spoke, he continually moved, tapping his fingers, fiddling with his hair, inspecting his nails, scratching his cheek, feet tapping the floor. He made eye contact inconsistently. These were clues to me to continue.

I held four hypotheses:

■ anxiety/depression
■ primary cardiac dysfunction
■ thyroid disease
■ something else.

I was not sufficiently sure about the first three, mainly because of his age and these being unlikely in a 22 year old who says life is generally good. I asked him to tell me more about himself: that work seemed OK. What did he do in the evenings and weekends? He said he went to pubs and clubs with his mates and they watched videos and hung out at each others' homes. I asked about whether alcohol and drugs featured in this

and he told me that he and his mates all used cannabis and took ecstasy, which was easily available. They had used cannabis for years, and ecstasy for the last few months. Ecstasy, methylenedioxymethamfetamine (MDMA), can lead to anxiety, depression, panic, insomnia and psychosis. At this stage I thought that ecstasy use was the likely cause of his symptoms, but I still wished to exclude any physical cause. An examination showed his cardiovascular system to be normal, and I also ordered an electrocardiogram (ECG) and blood tests for thyroid function and anaemia.

I suggested to David that ecstasy use was the most likely cause of his symptoms. He was surprised at this. He thought ecstasy was safe so long as he didn't drink alcohol at the same time. He had very limited knowledge of the effects of drugs generally and was happy to take home details of the local addiction prevention counselling service, which offers a drop-in service. He returned to me a week later for his ECG and blood results (all normal) and said he was going to see a counsellor to support him through stopping his drug use, which he anticipated being quite difficult.

Technically, I invited David to self-refer to the clinic. I did this because:

■ All people with drugs-related issues in our area are asked to self-refer or are referred to the specialist service.
■ Self-referral would indicate motivation on his part to find out about the effects of drugs and withdrawal programmes.
■ He seemed surprised by what I told him and wanted to find out more (his uncle's history may have compounded this).
■ I do not have much experience or knowledge regarding drug use.
■ I had ascertained that his drug use had occurred over several years and I did not know if he was addicted or not.
■ I would not know how to best help him, or what strategies were available should he wish to cease using drugs.
■ In this way I was working within my limitations and according to local practice. I was pleased that I had been sufficiently confident to ask about drugs and alcohol, as these can be difficult areas to broach at times.

Case study 3 — A referral

Jason came to the surgery with his mother as an emergency appointment. On appearance, he looked like a healthy 10-year-old boy. His family unit consisted of himself, his brother aged 8 and his mother aged 30. His presenting complaint was of a headache. His mother said that he had experienced several over the last 3 weeks and that this morning he had woken saying that he had another one. Her ideas about it were that she didn't think it was serious and she thought he didn't want to go to school. She was, however, concerned to get it checked out. I tried to use a PQRST framework to gather more information, but it was scant and no patterns could be identified. I suggested that Jason have his eyes checked, as his last eye check was at age 5 at school. At school Jason was doing well. He told me he was in the top groups for maths and English, he liked school and there were no problems such as bullying. His voice was quiet and flat.

I had little firm material on which to begin to hypothesise. The headaches had no apparent cause or pattern; school was fine. What else might be going on? His mother had a tendency to talk for him, but this is quite typical of most parents bringing in their children. I asked what Jason did after school and he said, `not much'. His mother told me that he was spending more time on his own at home: this had happened over the previous few months. She volunteered that she had a 6-month period of depression and, during that time, Jason had taken on a lot of the responsibility for his younger brother and also for shopping and meals. She had felt better for the last 3 months and was now back to her normal self. She was genuinely concerned for Jason but didn't know what to do. Jason could not say

how he was, but this could have been because his mother was there, he did not know me or he just did not have the words.

One tentative hypothesis was that Jason himself might be depressed. He had been responsible for the family until a few weeks ago and, thinking in symbols, the headaches might be his only way of expressing his disease. With this in mind, I tentatively suggested to Jason and his mother that they had all been through a hard few months and that it might be worth the health visitor, GP and Child and Family Service being involved. They agreed to this and ultimately attended some family therapy sessions.

I referred because:

- I was reasonably confident that Jason's headaches were not due to any underlying physiological cause.
- It was possible that he was depressed but unable to use such words.
- His headaches could be his way of asking for help.
- If the latter two were the case, then specialist professionals would be able to give an expert opinion and help him (and possibly the family unit) appropriately.
- Jason's mum agreed that she needed some help and support. In some way, this referral `felt' appropriate.

It is important to note here that had Jason been a few years older (late teens) I would have added in to my hypothesis a possible early onset psychotic episode, particularly because of the behaviour change and withdrawal over the last few months. In this case I would have referred to the Child and Adolescent Community Mental Health Team, with some degree of urgency.

Case study 4 — A crisis

Jenny and her husband Brian presented one evening for an urgent appointment. I knew Jenny slightly and was surprised to see her husband too. When I called them to my room, it was immediately apparent that Jenny was very distressed – her eyes were red, she had been holding back tears in the waiting room but sobbed as soon as my door was shut. She had a stack of tissues in her pocket. Her husband looked pale and shaken and was clearly concerned about Jenny. He had his arm round her to support her and made sure she sat down first, pulling his own chair next to hers.

In situations such as this, waiting a few seconds before launching into conversation is important. Generally people have come in because they need help of some sort and they anticipate talking, which will happen in due course. Letting someone cry until they are ready to talk is also likely to mean that the story is more coherent when it does come, but it also means

that as a nurse I have to be willing to let someone feel distressed without compulsively trying to make them feel better.

Jenny looked at me after maybe 30 seconds and I invited her to talk when she was ready. Haltingly she told me that she and her husband were having in vitro fertilisation (IVF); she has been pregnant for 3 weeks but had started bleeding yesterday and today the clinic confirmed that the baby had died. At this point she cried bitterly again and there was little I could do other than sit quietly with her and Brian. Over the next few minutes it transpired that this was their third IVF attempt and the previous two had followed the same pattern. They had come to see me this time because Jenny could not stop crying; she hurt everywhere, she wasn't eating or drinking, she felt so unhappy, such a failure; it wasn't worth living like this. Brian was close to tears as Jenny spoke and when I asked him how he was, he said his main concern was for Jenny, who was taking this so much worse than previous times. They were both concerned that Jenny might be 'cracking up' and needed some treatment, particularly as she seemed unable to stop crying.

A feature of people in crisis is that often they are experiencing a normal reaction to an event which is critical to their well-being (Stone 1993). Emotions may be very strong and seem long lasting, particularly as in this culture we tend to be encouraged not to express emotion, or certainly not for too long. Being distressed does not necessarily mean someone is mentally ill, but the extent of distress may be frightening to some people, or concerning at the very least. As identified earlier, if you can elicit what the patient's expectations of you are, you can address these, but sometimes people in crisis are, by its nature, disorientated and less able than usual to formulate questions and ideas.

I gently said to Jenny and Brian that it was clear that this was a very sad and worrying time for them both but what they, and particularly Jenny, were experiencing and feeling was quite normal at this early stage. I did not think Jenny was mentally ill or depressed and I would not at this stage recommend anything other than some time at home with supportive people around them both. This information seemed to help. Brian visibly relaxed and Jenny again made eye contact with me. I used this opportunity to mention that she had said she felt a failure, that it wasn't worth it and could she say a bit more about what she meant. She said she thought IVF wasn't worth it if it made her feel so awful and such a failure to Brian. They really wanted children. I probed a bit further and asked specifically whether feeling a failure and so awful included any thoughts of harming herself. She said no, not at all; she just felt awful. I accepted this but wanted to keep in touch with Jenny and Brian in order to monitor any possible deterioration in her mental state. I suggested that they come back to see me together or individually in a couple of days and again a few days later, and advised them that I would be available tomorrow if they needed me then.

Jenny came back 2 days later, still very sad but much calmer, and 2 weeks later Jenny and Brian returned together. They had both gone back to work but were exhausted, irritable, sad, not eating or drinking properly and not sleeping well. When I asked them how I could help, they wanted to know if this was still normal. They thought they could get through it together but wondered how long it would take. This of course, is unanswerable. They thought this was all a reaction to the loss of the baby, with which I agreed, and at this stage I told them that the likely course would be of good days and bad days, with slow improvement overall. I asked them to come back if they had any further concerns about their health and that I would phone them in a further fortnight if I did not hear from them.

Depression can be diagnosed at a minimum of 2 weeks' duration of symptoms, using DSM-IV criteria, but Jenny's and Brian's symptoms were better accounted for by bereavement, in which case a 2 month window is used as a guideline. At the end of 2 months, Jenny and Brian described themselves as more or less back to normal, still sad at times, and anticipating that the period around the due birth date might be difficult. They asked me about likely support then and I again invited them to return to me any time with a view to seeing me or for a referral to counselling if they felt that would be helpful.

In this situation, I decided not to refer Jenny and Brian to other colleagues or agencies, because, as in the first case study, I felt able to manage the situation due to my knowledge and experience and also because I could again take this to supervision. Key features too were that Jenny had support and company, they both had insight into what was happening and confidence in their own abilities to heal. They had also been through this before, although emotions this time had been more overtly expressed and perhaps more deeply and painfully felt. Occasionally you will meet people in crisis to whom nothing bad has ever happened before. They may need more structured help, more frequent contact and more information or help with problem solving in the acute phase.

The case studies above illustrate, we hope, that not only must we be aware of our own interests and abilities but also of the scope of the local services, both statutory and voluntary, with whom we might work and cross-refer. Armstrong (1995: 137) provides useful guidelines for compiling a local directory, using common problems as headings. This is well worth considering, if you have not already done so. We have also made reference to supervision, which we will discuss briefly below.

Supervision

The final issue we wish to address is that of supervision. There are a variety of models of supervision in use today, with many interpretations of the purpose of supervision and how it is practised. The UKCC (1996) in its position statement on clinical supervision for nursing and health visiting tells us that

Clinical supervision assists practitioners to develop

skills, knowledge and professional values throughout their careers. This enables them to develop a deeper understanding of what it is to be an accountable practitioner and to link this to the reality of practice more easily than has previously been possible.

They go on to state (UKCC 1996: 2):

Potential benefits are not thought to be limited to patients, clients or practitioners. A more skilled, aware and articulate profession should contribute effectively to organisational objectives.

In a different vein, Barker (1992: 6) writes:

Supervision in psychiatric nursing has two main aims: to protect people in care from nurses and to protect nurses from themselves.

He is concerned with nurses who think they know best, those who practice 'benign paternalism' and those who need help to explore how they are as a result of their work. Supervision is a planned, purposeful activity, and the supervisor has a clear responsibility to ensure that patient or client care is appropriate and of a high standard. In addition, the supervisee may need help to talk about their own distress or concern at the content or process of a consultation. Combining the ideas of UKCC and Barker, it is possible to see how supervision can have benefits for the patient and the nurse as well as for the profession as a whole.

Hawkins & Shohet (1989) describe four functions or forms of supervision: educative, supportive, managerial and consultancy. The educative function is concerned with 'developing the skills, understanding and abilities of the supervisee' through reflective process. The supportive function is concerned with exploring our own reactions to our patient's distress in order that we do not become overwhelmed by emotions. The managerial function provides 'the quality control function in work with people' (Hawkins & Shohet 1989: 42). The consultancy form of supervision occurs where the supervisor has no direct responsibility for service management or care delivery, i.e. is not related to your own work setting. This can be very useful at times when your manager or a colleague is not the best person, for whatever reasons, to provide your supervision. The consultancy supervisor will, however, still work to a code of practice and will educate, support and provide quality control as part of the process.

The decision as to who can be a supervisor is delegated by the UKCC (1996) to local policy makers. Supervisors should be skilled in supervision, and need not necessarily be nurses. Some psychiatric nurses have as their supervisors social workers or psychologists and act as supervisors themselves to these groups. The UKCC, however, make it clear that where supervision is offered by someone from a different discipline, this 'would normally be in addition to supervision from a fellow practitioner' (UKCC 1996: 4). With regard to working with people with mental health problems in primary care, it is essential that you have appropriate supervision, both for clinical

and personal support. Some of you may receive supervision from your practice counsellor or a GP with specific expertise, in addition to participating in other forms of supervision. Some of you may not have a supervisor and, if this is the case, you might wish to consider how to establish this activity.

Reflection and supervision are both structured, purposeful activities and, as stated earlier, reflection can and does usefully occur within supervision. Boud et al (1985) are clear that reflection brings together the intellect and the affect and proposes the structure of returning to the experience, attending to feelings and re-evaluating the experience. They describe the outcomes of reflection as 'a personal synthesis, integration and appropriation of new knowledge, a new affective state, or the decision to engage in some further activity' (Boud et al 1985: 21). For example, having described the slow progress of a patient who is depressed, and my own feelings that I must be either omitting something or doing something wrong, it may become apparent through discussion that I am picking up the patient's feelings, or I am somehow tied in to one of my own expectations of myself (omnipotence, benign paternalism, feeling responsible for others) or that it is early in this patient's process, or that medication may be indicated. A possible outcome is that I am reminded that people with depression may take 1–3 years to recover and that I will feel more at ease with my own interventions and the pace of the work. Sometimes supervision gives permission to try something different, to ask the unaskable questions, knowing that we are supported in this and having explored how to do this, perhaps through role play. In such a way, practice develops and both patient and nurse are supported. Supervision is not an optional extra: it is crucial to maintaining and supporting our own mental health.

Conclusion

We hope we have met some of your needs as you read this chapter and that the case studies have provided you with some insight into the processes and encounters which we meet regularly in clinical practice. We can only stress the importance of being willing to be pro-active, to ask people how they are in themselves and to listen to what is said both verbally and non-verbally. Further, do not be afraid to ask for advice from other colleagues or to consult a book or paper if you are uncertain about what to ask the patient. Use the resources you have available to you. One major principle in working with people with mental health problems is that early diagnosis is highly significant in relation to prognosis and the impact on the patient and their whole family and social system. A willingness to look at yourself and to use supervision is also important in maintaining and developing an ability to help these people. We wish you and your patients well.

References

American Psychiatric Association 1994 Diagnostic and statistical manual of mental disorders IV (DSM-IV) 4th edn. American Psychiatric Association, Washington, DC.

Armstrong E 1995 Mental health issues in primary care: a practical guide. Macmillan, Basingstoke, Hampshire.

Atkinson R L, Atkinson R C, Smith E E, Hilgard E R 1987 Introduction to psychology, 9th edn. Harcourt Brace Jovanovich, San Diego.

Barker P 1992 In: Butterworth T, Faugier J (eds) Clinical supervision and mentorship in nursing. Chapman and Hall, London.

Boud D J, Keogh R, Walker D 1985 Promoting reflection in learning: a model. In: Boud D J, Keogh R, Walker D (eds) Reflection: turning experience into learning. Kogan Page, London.

Craig T K J, Boardman A P 1997 ABC of mental health: common mental health problems in primary care. British Medical Journal 314:1609–1612.

De Silva P, Rachman S 1998 Obsessive–compulsive disorder – the facts, 2nd edn. Oxford University Press, Oxford.

Dowrick C 1992 Improving mental health through primary care. British Journal of General Practice 42:382–386.

Gambrill E C, Mead M 1994 Tired all the time. Update Sept 1:233–235.

Gillis L 1988 Human behaviour in illness, 4th edn. Faber and Faber, London.

Gournay K, Brooking J 1994 Community psychiatric nurses in primary health care. British Journal of Psychiatry 231–238.

Hannigan B 1998 Mental health: the difference non-specialist nurses can make. Community Practitioner 71(6):210–212.

Hawkins P, Shohet R 1989 Supervision in the helping professions. Open University Press, Milton Keynes.

Kates N, Craven M 1998 Managing mental health problems: a practical guide for primary care. Hogrefe and Huber, Seattle.

Ridsdale L 1995 Evidence based practice – a critical reader. W B Saunders, London.

Royal College of Nursing 1994 Guidelines for practice nurses re depot neuroleptic medication. Royal College of Nursing, London.

Sackett D, Richardson W S, Rosenberg W, Haynes R B 1997 Evidence based medicine: how to practice and teach EBM. Churchill Livingstone, London.

Stuart G, Sundeen S 1987 Principles and practice of psychiatric nursing. Mosby, St Louis.

Stone H 1993 Crisis counselling: caring for people in emotional shock. London SPCK.

United Kingdom Central Council for nurses, midwives and health visitors 1992a Code of Conduct. UKCC, London.

United Kingdom Central Council for nurses, midwives and health visitors 1992b The scope of professional practice. UKCC, London.

United Kingdom Central Council for nurses, midwives and health visitors 1996 Clinical supervision. UKCC, London.

Further reading

American Psychiatric Association 1994. 4th edn. Diagnostic and Statistical Manual of Mental Disorders, IV. American Psychiatric Association, Washington, DC.
This is worth having readily available as it contains the key symptoms and diagnostic criteria for all mental illness. A quick reference guide is available.

Armstrong E 1995 Mental health issues in primary care: a practical guide. Macmillan Basingstoke, Hampshire.
A very useful and practical book with flowcharts for questions and follow-up for people with mental health problems in primary care. Easy to read and understand.

Goldberg DP 1978 Manual of the General Health Questionnaire. NFER/Nelson, Slough.
You may already use this or a version of it in practice.

Levi MI 1998 Basic notes in psychopharmacology, 2nd edn. Berkshire Petroc Press, Newbury.
A handy guide to psychopharmacology.

McFarland G K, Wasli E, Gerety EK 1997 Nursing diagnoses and process in psychiatric mental health nursing, 3rd edn.
This comprehensive book is based on DSMIV criteria and includes likely outcomes and nursing interventions with rationale.

Martin A C, Davis L L 1989 Mental health problems in primary care: a study of nurse practitioners' practice. Nurse Practitioner 14(10):46–55.

RCGP Defeat Depression.
Your GP should have a copy of this pack which includes assessment and management tools and patient information leaflets.

Royal College of Nursing Guidelines for practice nurses on depot medication.
A useful booklet, informative and practical.

Other resources

In addition, there are many useful websites which you will find if you subject search on depression, anxiety, schizophrenia, etc.

The Royal College of Psychiatrists' own site (www.rcpsych. ac.uk) is useful, depending on what you need.

www.mental health.com is a comprehensive site which includes a rating scale.

www.mind.org.uk provides lists of publications and help sheets for the general public, all of which are highly relevant.

www.futur.com/edu-info provides an excellent source of information about schizophrenia, as does www.nsf.org.uk for the National Schizophrenia Foundation.

17

CARE OF THE CHILD

Katie Barnes and Debra Sharu

Key Issues

- *Listen* to children and their parents; you are all working together to impact the health and well-being of the child within a familial context

- A child's age and developmental level are the foundation upon which the nurse practitioner's (NP's) approach to the physical examination, normal physical exam findings and the differential diagnosis of illness is based; a solid understanding of these age and developmentally determined characteristics is imperative for the NP who is often caring for children

- Important components to be considered in the *subjective* assessment of an ill child include order of appearance and timing of associated symptomatology; history of exposures; previous interventions/treatments; and the caretaker's perception of the child's illness

- Important components to be considered in the *objective* assessment of an ill child include age-appropriate vital signs; presence or absence of fever (and degree of elevation); head to abdomen physical examination; and a careful check for skin rashes and mucous membrane lesions

- Key indicators in the evaluation and potential referral of an ill child include astute observation of child's appearance (ill or well); the child's interaction with the environment (playfulness, appetite and consolability/irritability); and the child's respiratory effort, degree of hydration and perfusion status (e.g. capillary refill)

- Premature infants and those less than 90 days are at increased risk of serious bacterial infection

- It is important to think laterally with regard to your differential list of potential diagnoses in children; the patient's age and other epidemiological features of different illnesses should be carefully considered

- Management plans for ill children should always consider the following: additional diagnostics; pharmacotherapeutics; behavioural interventions (including interventions for the child to implement); and patient education

- Adults and children respond differently to drugs and, as such, there are numerous issues to be considered with regard to medication use in children. Variable pharmacokinetics and differences in dosages, formulations and frequencies impact not only the NP's recommendation of a specific medication but also on patient adherence and education.

Introduction

Nurse practitioners (NPs) working in primary care will routinely care for paediatric patients and, as such, they must possess a working knowledge of the differences that separate the care of children from that of adults. More specifically, this includes

1. an understanding of the developmental platform upon which the history and approach to physical examination of children are built
2. an appreciation of the general anatomical and physiological differences that impact a child's ability to grow, develop and cope with illness
3. an understanding of the link between a child's age and the list of aetiologies to be considered on a differential list.

This chapter will provide a starting point for your primary care management of children and their families. However, it must be emphasised that it is not intended to be a definitive guide to the ambulatory care of children; rather, the NP is referred to the References and Further reading at the end of the chapter for information to assist in further investigation. Please note that due to the complex configurations of many families, the terms 'care' and 'parent' will be used interchangeably. The chapter comprises:

- a developmental approach to the assessment of the child within the family context
- anatomical and physiological differences intrinsic to the care of the paediatric client

- an outline of commonly occurring paediatric illnesses in relation to their typical presentations in primary care
- pharmacological considerations in the care of infants, children and adolescents.

Assessment of the child within the family context

A family's visit to the primary care provider should be a positive experience that fosters understanding and empowerment of personal health. This is especially important for the child who is formulating concepts and perceptions of the world that will potentially last a lifetime. Contact with the NP should provide children and their families with a valuable experience in which healthy life decisions can be promoted along with the development of a trusting relationship. It is therefore essential that your knowledge base incorporates a developmental approach to assessment and management of children within the family context.

The episodic visit

> *Angela has this rash on her stomach. She has had a fever and runny nose for 2 days now.*
> *Jonathan has been up all night with this cold. He has been tugging at his left ear and is extremely irritable.*

The main agenda in an episodic visit in primary health care involves a patient presenting with one or more signs and symptoms that are perceived either by the patient or the patient's caregiver as being outside of the norm. Concerns related to the implications of these symptoms are often also communicated. It is up to the practitioner to determine the depth and level of assessment needed to promote sound clinical reasoning and decision making. This should be dictated by the type of presentation, the individual child and the family.

Certain basic concepts can be applied to all paediatric patients, while others are particularly relevant to the individual's developmental status, personal situation and presentation. General points to consider in relation to history taking include the following:

1. The paediatric history (like an adult history) should be a time in which trust and a positive rapport is developed and fostered; this can then be built upon during the physical assessment.
2. The interview (with the possible exception of the adolescent) involves at least two historians, the parent and child. Good communication with both individuals is the key to a successful encounter.
3. The history is often the parent's interpretation of the patient's signs and symptoms; so if the child is old enough, ask him/her for a history as well, and consider both accounts. Remember there may be a hidden agenda, such as parental fears or guilt, in addition to a long-standing pattern of parent–child interaction that will influence what you are told.

When taking an episodic history for a paediatric complaint it is important to have an appreciation of the more general history of the child. This basic history should incorporate biographical information such as date of birth, ethnicity and primary provider. Other important points to assess include any special circumstances; past medical history (including immunisations); personal/social history and family history/dynamics; and a general review of systems to ascertain whether there is something additional that the family would like assessed.

The episodic history should explore the presenting complaint(s), including the history of the present illness, prodrome, associated symptoms and relevant characteristics such as quantity/severity, aggravating/relieving factors, location, character/quality and parent/child's perceptions of what is occurring. Situational factors such as other ill members of the family and parental coping with the illness should also be assessed. In addition, a brief discussion of the child's current status (nutrition, growth and development, elimination, sleep patterns and behaviour) may provide clues to the severity of the illness.

While a cooperative child allows for a more efficient assessment, it is important to incorporate general principles of physical examination with age-specific techniques to be used with all children. Certain basics to consider when conducting a physical examination include:

1. *organisation:* have equipment accessible and in working order; the more organised you are the easier it will be not only to examine the child but also to incorporate health education into the exam
2. *flexibility:* it is the key to your approach in the care of infants, children and adolescents
3. *safety:* it is important to remember in any paediatric exam; be careful with electrical outlets and equipment in your examination area.

Age-specific approaches to be considered when conducting a history and physical examination of a child include developmentally related information and appropriate exam techniques. These are organised around age groups typically seen in general practice.

Infants (birth–12 months)

A birth history is particularly relevant in this age group. Issues such as premature delivery, prenatal care and intrauterine exposures may offer important information, e.g. potential vulnerability to certain conditions such as respiratory ailments. The caretaker's observations regarding the infant's growth and development in addition to his/her perception of what is potentially wrong with the infant enables the provider to assess the baby within a broader context. Family coping mechanisms and social situation (e.g. both parents employed full time with other siblings at home; recent family stresses, etc.) need to be addressed in order to formulate a realistic plan of care for the infant. Activities of daily living such as whether the baby is eating well, is using a bottle or breast-feeding and/or has any food intolerances should likewise be explored.

When examining an infant it is particularly important to provide a warm, protective environment. The infant should be undressed completely, taking care with the removal of the nappy! At the same time, remember that infants do not like to be cold and feel unprotected. Generally, the younger the infant, the easier he or she is to examine. Developmental factors such as stranger and separation anxiety play an increasingly important role when assessing children from about 7 months. Stranger anxiety tends to peak at 9 months and fear of separation from the carer peaks at 15–18 months (however, there is wide variation with both of these behaviours). Respect for the parent–child attachment is therefore a key issue.

When a baby is less than 5 months old, placement on an examining table is acceptable. When the infant can sit alone (generally around 6 months of age), the sitting position should be used whenever possible, preferably on the parent's lap. If the baby needs to be on the examination table, the parent/carer should be in full view.

The rule of employing a cephalocaudal approach to physical examination does not always apply with infants and children. Take advantage of a quiet child and auscultate the heart, lungs and abdomen first if possible. Then palpate and percuss these areas, proceeding in a head-to-toe direction. Traumatic procedures should always be done last. The parent/carer should help in restraining the baby when needed, e.g. during an ear exam. Cooperation can be obtained through use of appropriate distracters, such as rattles and a soft, high-pitched voice. Above all, avoid jerky, sudden movements and be ever vigilant in maintaining a safe environment throughout your assessment.

Toddlers (12 months–2 years)

This group is the most difficult group to examine. The toddler is increasingly independent and displays characteristic negativity and egocentrism. In addition, stranger and separation anxiety continue to influence the social interactions during toddlerhood. The toddler's fear of bodily harm is also a factor to be considered. A child of this age can communicate verbally to a limited extent and by 30 months should know between six to eight body parts. It is important to assess the caretaker's reaction to these developmental issues and this should be discussed as part of the episodic history. For example, problems coping with tantrums and negativity may influence how the family is able to deal with the irritable, ill child.

Physical examination of the toddler should start with a gradual approach in the presence of the parent. As children in this age group do not like to be undressed or touched, having the parent remove the child's clothes will avoid your implication in a power struggle. Consider what the most important aspects of the physical assessment are: focus on them and perform the examination

as quickly as possible. The use of distracters such as inspection of the equipment, finger puppets and other toys are invaluable tools in getting the child's cooperation. Child appropriate stickers can be useful distracters if stuck onto a shoe or tongue blade as it gives little fingers something to focus on. Keeping the child's hands busy while you conduct your exam minimises the opportunity for the stethoscope being pulled from your ears or the otoscope being dropped. The examination should be started distally, saving ears, mouth and anything lying down or unpleasant for last. Use restraint, with the parent's assistance, only if necessary. Praise is paramount and safety still an essential consideration.

Pre-school child (3–5 years)

Generally easier to deal with than toddlers, pre-schoolers still fear bodily harm and need to feel comfortable in the clinical environment. They like to 'help' and can follow simple instructions such as undressing themselves bit by bit and identifying most body parts (including some internal ones). Verbal communication skills should be well developed, allowing the child to make a limited contribution to the history by indicating 'where it hurts' and 'what makes it better'. Cognition is characterised by egocentricity, literal interpretations and magical thinking. The use of games such as the paper doll technique (where the child's outline is traced onto the exam table paper for teaching and developing rapport) and storytelling can be very effective in eliciting cooperation. Stickers continue to be valuable with this age group as reinforcers of positive behaviour (a.k.a. 'bribes'). Brief inspection of the equipment, with demonstration and explanation, usually proves helpful, and close proximity of the parent is desirable. If the pre-schooler is cooperative, proceed in a head-to-toe direction. If cooperation is poor, proceed as with a toddler. Modesty is important at this stage of development and genitalia should be examined last. Praise and positive reinforcement throughout the encounter will help establish a good relationship between the child and the NP.

School-age child (6–11 years)

These children are usually willing participants and curious about what you may be asking or doing. Perceptions of what the problem is should be explored with both parent and child. School-aged children like to participate in care and can understand simple scientific explanations such as cause and effect. When explaining things to them, bear in mind that they are still thinking in concrete terms. Younger school-age children may still prefer the parent/carer to be in the room, while older children may prefer privacy; stickers continue to be helpful additions for early school-age children.

A head-to-toe exam sequence should now be possible. The NP needs to be mindful that modesty continues to be important; good technique includes exposing only the area that needs to be examined, in addition to requesting that these children undress themselves and keep their underwear on. Genitalia and unpleasant procedures should be saved until last.

Adolescents (12–18 years)

This is a time in which tremendous growth and change take place. The individual becomes increasingly independent and separates easily from parents. The adolescent is future-oriented and the peer group is very important. Most adolescents have a basic knowledge of anatomy and physiology and can be active and articulate participants in their care. Now is a time when the practitioner can assist the patient not only in the care of a particular problem but also in making general 'healthy lifestyles' decisions.

The option of parental presence should always be given. Remember the adolescent may be verbally and physically cooperative but not necessarily verbally open or physically comfortable. Privacy while taking a history and conducting a physical examination should be respected and will foster a more relaxed atmosphere. Physical assessment should progress in a head-to-toe direction, again leaving the examination of genitalia and unpleasant procedures until last. Findings during the exam should be explained, with reassurance given regarding normal findings, as adolescents are particularly concerned that they are developing as they should be. A summary of the developmental issues, important history and physical examination approach in the assessment of infants, children and adolescents can be found in Table 17.1.

The 'difficult paediatric patient'

There will be times when you will encounter a child who simply refuses to be examined. There may be several explanations for this behaviour, including

Table 17.1 *Important development issues, history and physical examination approaches in the assessment of infants, children and adolescents*

Age	Developmental issues	Significant components of paediatric history	Approach to physical examination
Infant	Stranger anxiety (7–9 months) Dislikes restraints	Birth history, prenatal history and activities of daily living (feeding, elimination, sleep) Parental coping, bonding and perception of infant's growth, development and health status	Can place on exam table before 4–6 months After 6 months, infant mainly examined on parent's lap Traumatic procedures last Parent involved if restraint necessary
Toddlers	Egocentric Negativity Separation anxiety (peaks at 15–18 months) Development of autonomy Language skills starting Knows several body parts	As above Issues such as tantrums, negativity and parent's response to increasing independence	Minimal physical contact (initially) Examine close by parent Use play to inspect body parts Parent to remove clothes Restrain only when necessary Traumatic procedures last *Praise*
Pre-schoolers	Follows simple instructions Likes to help Fears bodily harm	Issues such as school readiness, discipline and sibling relations discussed as appropriate	Keep parent close by Prefers sitting or standing Sequence of exam influenced by child's behaviour Request self-undressing Use appropriate play techniques Allow equipment to be inspected *Praise*
School-aged children	Industrious Self-control increases Understanding of cause and effect develops	School performance Increasing participation of child in history	Privacy Head-to-toe exam (genitalia last) Self-undressing with gown/drape Explain purpose of equipment and procedures Educate re: body care and function *Praise*
Adolescents	Increasing independence Future orientation	Privacy Option of parental presence Issues such as work, smoking, drugs and sexual activity	Undress in private Use gown/drape Explain procedures and findings Emphasise normalcy

1. prolonged separation anxiety
2. fear of medical procedures, possibly related to traumatic health care experiences in the past
3. previous physical or sexual abuse have instilled the child with a fear of being touched or examined
4. manipulative behaviour by the child.

To deal effectively with these children you must first identify the cause of their resistance. Never personalise their distress or rush the assessment no matter how tempting it may be. The child with extreme separation anxiety should have the parent close by at all times. The child with medical fears should be given appropriate reassurance by addressing their specific fear(s). The practitioner may have to defer parts of the physical examination and should make every effort to associate visiting the clinic with a pleasant experience, e.g. using stickers or flavoured tongue blades. For very fearful children, consider a 'well' visit to the clinic to play in an attempt to decrease anxiety levels.

Differentiating a sexually or physically abused child from one that is simply fearful may not always be an easy task. Discrepancies in the history and subsequent physical examination findings may assist in confirming your suspicions. Immediate reporting and careful documentation are essential to help protect these children. The NP is referred to the numerous texts/publications that address child protection issues in more depth. However, the examination techniques used with fearful children are applicable to the examination of potentially abused children. Dealing with the manipulative child can be particularly trying if he or she throws a tantrum. It is important to protect them from injury, but at the same time capitulation in response to this behaviour should be avoided and the disruptive behaviour should be ignored.

Anatomical and physiological differences in paediatrics

There are numerous differences in the anatomy and physiology of infants, children and adolescents that are developmentally determined. These differences will be discussed in relation to the age groups outlined previously.

Infants and toddlers

The period of time from birth to 1 year of age is characterised by rapid and dramatic growth. While the growth rate slows (with a corresponding decrease in caloric requirement) during the second year of life, growth parameters (height, weight and head circumference) are key indicators that the NP should be alert to. An infant/toddler that is not growing is cause for concern and will require additional investigation. In addition, an inadequate caloric intake is often associated with deficiencies of other nutrients essential for adequate growth and development. Further complicating this picture, 90% of brain growth is complete by 2 years of age, so an infant with an inadequate caloric intake (or inappropriate representation of fats, proteins and carbohydrates) is at significant risk for future developmental sequelae. Nervous system myelinisation in infancy is dependent on an adequate intake of fats. Children under age 2 require 30% more fat for neural development; reduced fat milk should not be included in the diet of children less than 2.

Regarding body proportions during infancy and toddlerhood, the head and trunk comprise a greater percentage of total body surface area (TBSA) compared with older children. This has important implications in the assessment of the infant or toddler with thermal trauma, e.g. burns. In addition, infants have a higher percentage of water in their body fluid composition and they experience slightly increased insensible losses as a function of their higher metabolic rate and greater TBSA. Infants have a poorly developed temperature control system, and anticipatory guidance regarding ambient room temperatures and amount of clothing or 'bundling' may be needed. The renal system in young infants is less efficient in waste product excretion and, thus, is less able to concentrate, dilute or acidify urine. In addition, insensible losses in both infants and toddlers are increased in the presence of fever. Collectively, these characteristics place infants and toddlers at greater risk for dehydration and fluid – electrolyte disturbances during an acute episode of vomiting and diarrhoea. It is imperative that the NP accommodates these considerations into her management of gastroenteritis.

The infant immune system undergoes numerous changes during the first year. Young infants (premature infants even more so) are less able to localise and mount an immune response and, consequently, are at greater risk of bacteraemia. However, newborns receive significant amounts of maternal immunoglobulin, (IgG) which confers immunity (until approximately 3–6 months of age) to antigens to which the mother was immune. The infant's ability to synthesise IgG increases steadily during the first 2 years of life (40% of adult level by 1 year), while significant amounts of IgM are produced after birth and adult levels are reached by 9 months of age. Production of other immunoglobins (IgA, IgD and IgE) is much more gradual, with normal levels not achieved until early childhood. Lymphoid tissue grows rapidly after birth.

Several factors predispose infants to more upper and lower respiratory system problems, which are often more acute and more severe. The trachea, bronchi and lower respiratory structures are in very close proximity and, therefore, transmission of an infectious agent is much more efficient. In addition, IgA production in the mucosal lining is not established until later childhood, thereby increasing the susceptibility of infants to lower respiratory infection. The eustachian tubes are shorter, straighter and in close communication with the middle ear; thus, ascension of pathogens from the oropharynx is enhanced. The narrower lumen of the trachea and lower respiratory structures is more readily compromised by oedema, mucus or a foreign body.

Respiratory effort in infants is largely abdominal, therefore marked supra- or substernal retractions require further investigation. Upper airway sounds are much more easily transmitted to the chest of young children and this may make the auscultation of the lung fields especially challenging for the NP. Listening with the diaphragm of the stethoscope at the nose before moving to the chest may familiarise the clinician with the sounds coming from the upper respiratory tract and thus enable a distinction between upper airway 'noise' and lower respiratory adventitious sounds.

The heart is located higher up and more horizontally in the chest cavity in infants and toddlers. This has implications for the apical impulse (AI), which in infancy is found at the fourth intercostal space (ICS) and laterally displaced from the mid-clavicular line (MCL), while in toddlers the AI is located slightly more medially (fourth intercostal space at MCL). The heart rate during infancy and toddlerhood is increased and age-appropriate vital sign norms (respiration, heart rate and blood pressure) should be used in their assessment. Distress, excitement and fever all can have dramatic effects on heart rate. Sinus arrhythmia (heart rate increasing on inspiration, decreasing on expiration) is a normal finding.

Haemopoietically, there is a shift from fetal haemoglobin to adult haemoglobin during the first months of life that may result in a physiological anaemia until erythropoiesis is better established (6–8 months). Maternal iron stores of the infant begin to wane at 5–6 months and may contribute to an anaemia of infancy if iron intake is not adequate. It is important to obtain age-appropriate normal values in the interpretation of any haematological parameters in children.

Evidence of the immature digestive processes during infancy is manifest in the appearance of stools. Many solid foods (peas, carrots, corn) are passed incompletely digested in the faeces and, as such, an excess intake of fibre-rich foods predisposes infants to loose, bulky stools. The liver is the most immature of the gastrointestinal organs during infancy. This has implications for the conjugation of bilirubin and secretion of bile in addition to impacting the other functions of the liver (gluconeogenesis, formation of plasma proteins, vitamin storage, deaminisation of amino acids and drug metabolism). Consequently, infants and toddlers need to be fed at regular and more frequent intervals. Anatomical and physiological differences among infants and toddlers are summarised in Table 17.2.

Pre-school and school-age children

The rate of physical growth slows and stabilises in the years from 3–11. Growth gains are steady and should follow the same trajectory established in infancy and toddlerhood. Physical proportions are more adult-like with the pre-school and school-age child characteristically slender, leggy, agile and posturally erect. Most bodily systems are mature and stable, with a greater capacity to handle stress and change. The gradual increases in bone and muscle growth over these years result in a doubling of strength and physical capabilities by the end of 10 years of age. However, it must be noted that despite these gains, muscles remain functionally immature compared with adolescence and are more readily damaged by muscular overuse injuries. In addition, bone mineralisation is not complete until after adolescence and children of this age group are less resistant to pressure and muscle pull; consequently, guidance regarding age-appropriate physical activity may be necessary when young footballers or cricketers present with overuse syndromes. Likewise, attention should be given to carrying heavy loads (i.e. full book bags); backpacks should have equal weight distribution, with both straps used simultaneously.

The immune system is much more competent in its ability to localise and respond to acute infection, with lymph tissue actually hypertrophied to greater than adult size (it atrophies to adult size during adolescence). The first few years of school attendance are often characterised by several acute infections; however, this is related to increased exposure to other children rather than a less than competent immune system. By the end of the school-age period children are immune to a wide variety of pathogenic microorganisms.

The heart and respiratory rates of pre-school and school-age children are decreased (compared with their earlier values), while blood pressure increases. The heart has reached its adult position by 7 years of age; thus, the AI will be found at the fifth ICS, just medial of the MCL.

Physical maturity is evidenced in the urinary and gastrointestinal systems. Bladder capacity is greatly increased and, while it varies widely among individual children, on the whole it is generally greater in girls than boys. There are typically less episodes of stomach upset compared with infancy and toddlerhood, with better maintenance of blood sugar levels and increased stomach capacity. Therefore, school-age children do not need to be fed as frequently or promptly as younger children. Caloric needs for school-age children are less than they were in earlier years and less than they will be during adolescence.

The wide variation that is possible in physical growth and development towards the end the school-age period requires mention. These differences are due to discrepancies in physical maturation that occur across genders (girls maturing earlier than boys) and within gender (early developers as opposed to 'late-bloomers'). These differences become increasingly apparent as the child approaches the latter half of the school-age period and if extreme (or unique) can contribute to significant stress for these children and their

Table 17.2 *Anatomical and physiological differences among infants and toddlers*

System	Anatomical/physiological difference
General	Rapid and dramatic growth (height, weight, head circumference) during first 12 months of life Head and trunk comprise greater proportion of TBSA Infants with greater percentage of water in body fluid composition Infants with increased metabolic rate and increased insensible losses Infants with poorly developed temperature control
Neurological	Ninety per cent of brain growth complete by 2 years of age Nervous system myelinisation dependent on adequate fat intake
Genitourinary	Young infants with less efficient waste product excretion and decreased ability to concentrate, dilute or acidify urine
Ear, nose and throat	Eustachian tubes shorter, straighter and in close proximity to middle ear Infants are obligate nose breathers
Immune	Infants < 3 months of age less able to localise and mount an immune response; at much greater risk of overwhelming bacteraemia Rapid increase in ability to synthesise IgG (achieving 40% of adult level by 12 months of age) Significant amounts of IgM produced after birth (achieving adult levels by 9 months of age) Ability to synthesise IgA, IgD and IgE much less developed Lymph system develops rapidly after birth
Pulmonary	Trachea, bronchi and lower respiratory structures in very close proximity Poor IgA production in mucosal lining; narrower lumen of trachea and lower respiratory structures allow for easier compromise by oedema, mucus or foreign body Respiratory effort in infants is largely abdominal Upper respiratory 'noise' easily transmitted to lower respiratory areas (infants < 12 weeks of age are obligate nose breathers)
Cardiovascular	Heart is higher up and more horizontal in the chest cavity Resting heart rate is markedly greater than adult norms (use age-appropriate values for all vital signs) Sinus arrhythmia is normal finding
Haemopoietic	Shift from fetal haemoglobin during first month of life Maternal iron stores waning by 5–6 months of age Obtain age-appropriate parameters to interpret laboratory values
Gastrointestinal	Immature digestive processes during first year of life affects digestion of fibre-rich foods and appearance of stools Liver still maturing during first year of life with implications for functions (gluconeogenesis, plasma protein production, vitamin storage, drug metabolism, etc.)

IG, immunoglobulin; TBSA, total body surface area.

families. Anticipatory guidance related to height and weight relationships, rapid or slow growth and development (or delay) of secondary sexual characteristics is important. In addition, physical maturity is often not well correlated to cognitive, social and emotional maturity and, although an 8-year-old child may look like a 12-year-old child (as well as the reverse), it is imperative to match behavioural expectations to the child's emotional, social and cognitive level. Anatomical and physiological characteristics of pre-school and school-age children are summarised in Table 17.3.

Adolescents

The fundamental biological changes of adolescence are collectively referred to as puberty. More specifically, they are changes in physical growth and sexual maturation that are triggered by neuroendocrine events and occur in an orderly and predictable sequence. The most striking of these changes are the increases in height, weight, body proportions and secondary sexual development that can give the adolescent a very adult-like appearance. The predictable sequence of secondary sexual development is well documented (Wong et al 1999).

The increased size and strength of the heart, increased blood volume and increased systolic blood pressure contribute to the adolescent's greater physical endurance and strength. The lungs increase in length and diameter, with resultant increases in respiratory volume, vital capacity and respiratory functional efficiency. Likewise, the other internal organs (kidneys,

Table 17.3 *Anatomical and physiological differences in pre-school and school-age children*

System	Anatomical/physiological difference
General	Rate of physical growth slows Steady growth trajectory established in infancy/toddlerhood should be maintained Physical proportions more adult-like and characteristically slender, leggy and posturally erect Most bodily systems mature with greater capacity to handle stress and change Frontal sinuses develop ≈ 7 years of age Broad variations in physical growth at end of school-age years related to disparity in the onset of puberty Physical maturity may not be well correlated to social, emotional or cognitive maturity
Genitourinary	Bladder capacity greatly increased (although wide individual variation)
Immune	Competent immune system that is able to localise and respond to acute infection Lymph tissue hypertrophied to > adult size during school-age years First years of school attendance characterised by several acute infections
Cardiovascular and pulmonary	Heart and respiratory rate decreased while blood pressure increased compared with infancy/toddlerhood norms Use age-appropriate normal values to interpret vital signs Heart reaches adult position by 7 years of age
Gastrointestinal	Typically fewer episodes of gastrointestinal upset compared with younger ages Improved maintenance of blood sugar levels Increased stomach capacity in school-aged children Caloric needs in school-age less than in earlier years and less than they will be during adolescence
Musculoskeletal (MSK)	Great gains in bone and muscle growth (strength and physical capacities have doubled by 10 years of age) Muscles remain functionally immature (until puberty); greater risk for overuse injuries Bone mineralisation incomplete (until puberty); less resistant to pressure and muscle pull

liver, stomach, etc.) increase in size and capacity, reaching a peak at about 14 years of age. There is maturation of the musculoskeletal system, haemopoietic system (with corresponding attainment of adult blood values) and an increase in the proliferation of neurological support cells and growth of the myelin sheath in the nervous system. This allows for faster neural processing, with corresponding improvements in coordination and more advanced cognitive capabilities. Lastly, there is maturation of the reproductive system, with the onset of menarche in girls (although this may occur during the school-age years) and the ability for seminal emissions in boys.

Pubertal changes and related concerns of the adolescent that may be expressed during a physical examination provide an ideal opportunity for health promotion and prevention regarding healthy lifestyles choices, sexual health, pregnancy prevention and risk-taking behaviours. While adolescents have been collectively described here, greater sophistication regarding the differences intrinsic to early, middle and late adolescence (that are beyond the scope of this chapter) would be important for the NP that works largely with this special group. Anatomical and physiological changes of adolescents are summarised in Table 17.4.

Commonly occurring paediatric illnesses

Nurse practitioners in primary care will inevitably care for children with an infectious disease. In the first 2 years of life it is estimated that children will have from two to four acute illnesses per year, although this number decreases with advancing age (McCarthy 1993). As a primary care provider, it will therefore be your responsibility to assess and manage these children. You will need to determine the diagnosis(es) and treatment plan; whether further evaluation, referral and/or follow-up is required; and whether additional diagnostics are necessary to augment your thorough history and physical examination.

The following section will outline some commonly occurring paediatric illnesses and include a discussion on recognition of the ill child. Please note, however, that in the interest of 'ambulatory probabilities' (e.g. the likelihood that you will have a child present with a specific illness) comments on vaccine-preventable diseases (with the exception of varicella) have been omitted. However, for information related to vaccine-preventable diseases, the NP is referred to the plethora of sources (medical and nursing texts, the Department of Health and the internet) that discuss these illnesses. In this

Table 17.4 *Anatomical and physiological differences in adolescence*

System	Anatomical/physiological difference
General	Rapid and dramatic period of physical growth, sexual maturation and cognitive, social and emotional development
	Growth events occur in an orderly and predictable sequence
	Increase in height, weight body proportions and secondary sexual development can give an adult-like appearance
	Caloric requirements increase in response to increased need
	Significant differences in cognitive and psychosocial development intrinsic to early, middle and late adolescence
Neurological	Proliferation of neurological support cells and growth of myelin sheath
	Faster neural processing (related to above), with corresponding improvements in coordination and more advanced cognitive capabilities
Genitourinary	Development of secondary sex characteristics (Tanner staging)
	Maturation of reproductive system manifested by the onset of menarche in females and seminal emissions in males
Cardiovascular and pulmonary	Increased size and strength of heart with corresponding increases in stoke volume and cardiac output
	Increased blood volume and blood pressure (adult norms by late adolescence)
	Lungs with increased length and diameter, with resultant increases in respiratory volume, vital capacity and respiratory functional efficiency
Haemopoietic	Adult values applicable as system is fully mature
Gastrointestinal	Increases in size and capacity, which assume adult levels around 14 years of age

chapter, content has been limited to include commonly presenting (or in the case of meningitis, significant) paediatric illnesses and encompasses important components of the subjective and objective findings, differential diagnoses and routine management.

Recognition of the ill child

A large percentage of paediatric illnesses are likely to have a viral aetiology, are easily managed and resolve completely (McCarthy 1993, Goodman & Brady 1996); fewer still are likely to be grave bacterial illness. However, irrespective of the aetiology, the information required for your assessment and management remains the same. In addition to the components of the episodic history as outlined earlier in the chapter, the NP should *always* carefully note the following as part of the assessment of an ill child:

Subjective findings

1. *Order* of appearance and *timing* of associated symptomatology
2. Presence, duration, pattern and height of any associated fever
3. History of exposure to others with similar symptoms, recent travel, contact with animals (or animal by-products), cravings/consumption of non-food items, consumption of raw milk or meats, medication history and possible drug use and/or poisoning
4. Previous treatment and/or medical intervention
5. Allergies, pre-existing conditions, congenital abnormalities or hereditary diseases

6. Caretaker's perception of illness and its aetiology and whether the complaint awakens the child from sleep.

Objective findings

1. Vital signs with careful observation of respiratory effort, presence or absence of fever and degree to which temperature is elevated.
2. Careful physical examination (head to abdomen minimum, with careful check for skin rashes and mucous membrane lesions). ❶ The younger the child the more astute your observations must be – if there is poor engagement with the environment or caretaker the child will require more intensive management.
3. *Age* (premature infants and those less than 90 days are at greater risk of serious infection related to their relatively poor immune response).
4. Astute observation of the child's interaction with the environment, e.g. degree of 'bright-eyed' interactiveness/ alertness, consolability/irritability, activity level, playfulness and appetite (if any of these indicators are very poor, especially in the absence of fever, consider seeking assistance in management). ❶ A child that appears extremely ill is ill, until proven otherwise.
5. Repeat observation of child after fever relief, as this often provides a different picture (either more or less reassuring).
6. Degree of hydration (skin turgor/recoil should be assessed on the abdomen of infants and young children) and perfusion (capillary refill time < 2 seconds). ❶ Symptoms of early dehydration

(dry mouth, lack of tears and urine) can be subtle and quickly progress to more serious illness.

Assessment

- It is vital to think laterally with regard to your differential list of diagnoses (e.g. assessment = fever, rule out pneumonia), considering the patient's age as an important springboard to potential aetiologies
- Be sure to include epidemiological features of different illnesses into your thinking (e.g. seasonality of some infections, likelihood of exposure, incubation periods, patient age, etc.).

Plan (and if appropriate, specific instructions for the child as well)

Additional diagnostics (if appropriate): This includes full blood count (FBC), cultures and erythrocyte sedimentation rate (ESR). Additional diagnostics are included in the discussion of managing sick children, because they should always be considered as part of the clinical decision-making process, and they should be used to confirm clinical suspicions or assist in the critical evaluation of a child. It is up to the individual NP to decide what is (or is not) appropriate/feasible given the clinical setting, resources, child's differential, clinical condition and (if appropriate) opinion of the collaborating physician.

Pharmacotherapeutics (if required). This consists of medication issues such as administration, refrigeration, scheduling and specific instructions regarding dosage and length of treatment.

Behavioural interventions. This comprises nutritional management, supportive care, special or adjuvant therapy.

Patient education. Aetiology of illness (if known) with infection control measures; the course the illness is 'expected' to take; what would be considered 'unexpected' (and a reason for a follow-up visit or telephone call); follow-up instructions; reassurance and praise for caretaker's management (if appropriate).

Referral. This is largely contingent on the NP's comfort level in managing the ill child and whether management of the child (or family) fall outside the NP's scope of practice. This is regardless of the aetiology of the illness and as such. ❶ Applies to all further discussion of specific illnesses in this chapter.

Fever

One of the most common paediatric complaints is that of an ill child with a fever. While the cause is often apparent, it is the child that presents with an acute onset of fever (less than 7 days' duration) and without a source for the fever (identified during your history and physical examination) that is a diagnostic and management challenge for the NP. The discussion of this type of presentation, fever without localising source (FWLS) will therefore be a focal point of the following section. In addition, because fever in older children (e.g. those > 36 months of age) is less likely to be a marker for serious bacterial infection (meningitis excluded) and as their immune system is better equipped to localise and mount a response, the discussion of fever will focus to a larger extent on the management of FWLS in younger children.

Fever, while commonly used as a diagnosis, is in fact, a non-specific symptom of an underlying process or condition that involves inflammation. It is generally defined as a core temperature (e.g. rectal) of at least 38°C. The fever is caused by various inciting agents triggering the release of cytokines that subsequently reset the thermoregulatory centre in the hypothalamus. Once reset, mechanisms such as shivering and cutaneous vasoconstriction are employed by the body to maintain a higher temperature. In addition, cytokine release triggers the body's own defence system (helper T cells) to proliferate, thereby improving the body's ability to fight infection (McCarthy 1998). In children who have both prolonged and acute fevers, the inciting agents are most often bacterial or viral pathogens. Less commonly (although often associated with prolonged fevers), the inciting agent may be pyrogens, released by malignant tumour cells, or circulating immune complexes, as found in autoimmune disease (McCarthy 1998). It should be noted that in neonates the pyrexic response is immature and resetting of the thermoregulatory centre often does not occur despite the presence of infection. The neonate may be septic and still be apyrexic or hypothermic.

While there are many causes for fever, they can be grouped into three categories differentiated by the absence or presence of a source for the fever and the length of time the fever has been present (Wilson 1995, Grover 1996).

- *Fever of short duration (< 7 days) with localising source:* a diagnosis is easily established through the clinical history and physical examination; laboratory tests are usually not indicated (e.g. otitis media or varicella).
- *Pyrexia of unknown origin (PUO):* a prolonged fever (> 7 days), where history and physical examination do not establish a source but laboratory tests might. Evaluation of these children will likely require consultation and collaboration with medical colleagues.
- *FWLS:* a fever of short duration (< 7 days), where history and physical examination fail to reveal a source but laboratory tests may establish an aetiology.

The NP's assessment of the child presenting with FWLS needs to synthesise the child's appearance, age and temperature risk, as fever can be a marker for serious bacterial infection (SBIs) or occult bacteraemia (OB). Occult bacteraemia is the presence of bacteria in the blood despite a benign clinical appearance, while diagnoses generally accepted as SBI include meningitis, bacteraemia, urinary tract infection (UTI), osteomyelitis, septic arthritis, pneumonia, bacterial gastroenteritis and serious skin or soft tissue infections.

However, most of the above infections (with the exception of early meningitis or UTI in young infants) will present with clinical findings that lead the astute clinician to identify the problem. Complicating SBI, however, is the possibility of OB, which may be present in approximately 3–5% of children less than 36 months of age who present with a temperature > 39°C and without a localising source (Grover 1996). In addition, approximately 50% of children subsequently diagnosed with OB originally presented as FWLS (Wilson 1995). Both OB and meningitis are discussed more fully in the differential diagnoses that the NP needs to consider in the management of a child with fever.

The goals of the assessment and management of FWLS are (1) to identify the patient at risk for SBI or OB and (2) to implement treatment options that diminish the risk of secondary complications (e.g. sequelae from a missed diagnosis, sepsis work-up, hospitalisation or antibiotic use). As such, it is essential for the practitioner to differentiate those paediatric patients who are seriously ill from those who are not. With regard to age and temperature risk, it is generally accepted that the higher the temperature and the younger the age, the greater the risk of bacteraemia (although for all children the higher the temperature the greater the risk of SBI). More specifically, children aged 1 month to 36 months can be classified into high and low risk for OB or SBI. Those considered to be at low risk are (Baraff et al 1993).

- non-toxic in appearance (without signs of lethargy, poor perfusion, tachypnoea, hyper/hypoventilation, or cyanosis)
- previously healthy with no history of prematurity, perinatal antimicrobial therapy, chronic illness or hospitalisation
- without a focal bacterial infection (otitis media excepted)
- living in a good social situation (telephone, responsible caretaker who is able to read a thermometer and lives within a reasonable distance from an Accident & Emergency Department)
- $5000 \times 10^9/l <$ WBC (white blood cells) $< 15\,000 \times 10^9/l$ with band forms $< 500 \times 10^9/l$
- urine sediment with < 10 WBCs/hpf (high power field) and negative for leukocyte esterase and nitrite on urine dipstick
- stool (if diarrhoea present) with < 5 WBCs/hpf.

Note that debate exists with regard to (1) the management of low-risk febrile infants 28–90 days of age and (2) the WBC cut-off and its relationship to risk assessment. While US-based recommendations utilise a total WBC count of $<15\,000 \times 10^9/l$ (Baraff et al 1993), evaluation of an Australian protocol that utilised a WBC cut-off of $<20\,000 \times 10^9/l$ resulted in less empiric antibiotic treatment (Browne et al 1996). In addition, the NP in the practice setting must be cognisant of the balance between consideration and action (with regard to diagnostics), which is dependent on a number of factors

(see discussion of additional diagnostics in Recognition of the ill child section above).

Children who are considered to be at high risk are the converse of the above criteria, with special consideration given to neonates and infants < 28 days of age (always considered high risk when FWLS). In the clinical setting, the NP's determination of high versus low risk has important clinical implications. For example, a child that is 30 months old with a temperature of 40°C, a WBC of $7000 \times 10^9/l$ and a non-toxic appearance is at low risk of OB or SBI. This is in sharp contrast to a child that is 9 months old with a temperature of 40°C, a WBC of $17\,000 \times 10^9/l$ and lethargic behaviour during your physical examination.

Subjective findings

1. History reveals typical complaints associated with fever (dry, hot skin with flushed cheeks and cool distal extremities; poor appetite and malaise). You should obtain information on the duration, height and pattern of fever.
2. The NP must ask about any additional physical symptoms and/or behaviours which may provide information regarding a potential aetiology of the fever.
3. It is important to obtain the carer's impression of the child's *current* appetite and activity level (e.g. playing and smiling) as compared with their *usual* patterns.
4. Table 17.5 outlines some important questions to include in your subjective history and includes possible aetiologies for the NP to consider; note that this is not a comprehensive guide and further reading is suggested.

Objective findings

1. Pyrexia of $\geq 38.0°C$ (rectally). Be careful to verify (if possible) the reported temperature, as mistakes can be made in reading a thermometer (or other device). Administration of antipyretics prior to your assessment may effect this finding.
2. Observation of the child's response to the environment is crucial. Signs of lethargy, irritability or change in mental status should be assessed. The NP must be familiar with what is developmentally appropriate in order to appraise the infant or child's response correctly. The sicker the child, the less responsive he or she will be.
3. Specific evidence of disease may be discovered on your careful physical examination (head to abdomen, minimum). These positive findings exempt a child from the diagnosis of FWLS. The NP is referred to more comprehensive paediatric texts (or the appropriate sections of this book) for discussion of the management of these conditions. Table 17.6, while not comprehensive, identifies common examination findings with their likely diagnoses.
4. Selected findings have developmental dimensions (e.g. meningeal signs may not be present in the child with meningitis that is less than 16 months old; shiv-

Table 17.5 *Potential aetiologies to be considered with regard to reported history (Used with permission from Wilson D 1995 Assessing and managing the febrile child.* The Nurse Practitioner *20(11):59–74,* © *Springhouse Corporation.)*

Complaint/reported history	Consider
Dysuria and frequency	UTI (in infants UTI may present as poor feeding and/or lethargy with possible history of irritability during urination)
Nausea, vomiting, diarrhoea, abdominal cramping, others may have similar symptoms	GI related, e.g. food poisoning, reaction to antibiotics (e.g. ampicillin or cephalosporins) or viral infection
Cough or respiratory difficulties	URTI, pneumonia, asthma or other lower respiratory tract involvement
Pain	May indicate a focal source of infection, such as pharyngitis or otitis
Abdominal pain, weight loss	Inflammatory bowel disease, appendicitis, acute non-specific abdominal pain and UTI
Steady loss of weight	Malignancy or coeliac disease
Pain in joints	Connective tissue disorders
Fever pattern is variable, e.g. once or twice a day	Occult abscess or juvenile rheumatoid arthritis
Other members in the family or peer group may have similar signs and symptoms	Infectious aetiology, children with a history of contact with *Haemophilus influenzae* or *Neisseria meningitidis* are at greater risk for bacteraemia
History of recent illness or surgery	Recurrence of previous infection or secondary infection. May be a complication of surgery
History of travel	Infectious causes, e.g. amoebiases
History of contact with pets	Dogs (brucellosis) or cats (cat-scratch disease)
Immunisation may have recently been administered or child may not be up to date on immunisations	Reaction to immunisations or infectious disease
History of having recently been medicated	Drug reaction or hypersensitivity
Medical history of immunological impairment	Greater risk of infection/bacteraemia

GI, gastrointestinal; URTI, upper respiratory tract infection; UTI, urinary tract infection.

ering is uncommon in young infants). It is useful to ask an older child to 'kiss' his or her knees (while lying prone on the examination table with knees flexed) as an aid to assessment of nuchal rigidity.

Assessment

1. The diagnosis of the acutely ill febrile child is dependent on the symptom history, clinical presentation and physical examination findings. The age of the child, degree of temperature elevation, general appearance and length of the febrile episode are contextual factors in the NP's assessment.
2. In pyrexic infants younger than 3 months and children 3–36 months old, most serious illnesses are caused by infectious agents.
3. Differential diagnoses are numerous for the many aetiologies of fever in children. In addition to the diagnoses outlined in Table 17.6 (and especially when considering FWLS as a diagnosis in children < 36 months of age), the following serious illnesses *must* be considered:
   - *occult bacteraemia (OB):* the presence of bacteria in the blood despite a benign clinical appearance. This in contrast to bacteraemia that is found in a

child with a toxic appearance, where the bacteria has spread to the bloodstream, reflecting the invasive nature of the illness. The possibility of OB should be considered in all young infants and children who present with FWLS. Common pathogens implicated in occult bacteraemia among young children are age-related and include (Grover 1996):
   - infants < less than 3 months: Group B streptococcus, *Escherichia coli*, *Listeria monocytogenes*, *Salmonella* spp. (1–3 months old) and *Haemophilus influenzae* type B (1–3 months old)
   - infants 3–36 months: *Streptococcus pneumoniae*, *H. influenzae* type B (note that the incidence has been significantly decreased by Hib vaccines) and *Neisseria meningitidis*
   - *Staphylococcus aureus* and Gram-negative enteric pathogens are some of the less common agents.

Children with OB may recover spontaneously with no sequelae, or localising signs of infection may develop (with a resultant deterioration of the child's condition). Peripheral sites of infection include the skin (cellulitis), lungs (pneumonia) and meninges (meningitis).

Table 17.6 *Diagnoses to be considered in the evaluation of fever* (Used with permission from Wilson D 1995 Assessing and managing the febrile child. The Nurse Practitioner 20(11):59–74, © Springhouse Corporation.)

Physical exam finding	Consider
Rash	Measles, varicella, roseola, enterovirus infection. May also be seen in malignancies and collagen vascular disease
Petechiae, purpura	Sepsis, meningitis, bacteraemia
Dull, red, bulging tympanic membranes	Otitis media
Lesions in the mouth such as Koplik spots, fissuring or crusting of the lips or strawberry tongue	Rubeola, Kawasaki disease or scarlatina
Sinus tenderness with poor transillumination of the sinuses and foul nasal discharge	Sinusitis (note that tenderness occurs in only 20% of children with sinusitis) or nasal foreign body
Throat inflammation and exudate	Streptococcal pharyngitis or Epstein–Barr virus
Adenopathy	Epstein–Barr virus (generalised lymphadenopathy), malignancy or toxoplasmosis (supraclavicular node enlargement), cat-scratch fever (pectoral node involvement) or local infection
Respiratory observations such as decreased or adventitious breath sounds, cough, increased rate and respiratory effort	Lower respiratory tract infection or pneumonia
Significant heart murmurs	Bacterial endocarditis
Abdominal tenderness and/or bloody diarrhoea	UTI (seen in about 7% of male infants less than 6 months and 8% of female infants less than 12 months presenting with FWLS), appendicitis, intussusception, bacterial gastroenteritis
Joint pain, skin or joint inflammation	Collagen inflammatory disorder, osteomyelitis, cellulitis, septic arthritis
CNS signs of nuchal rigidity (Kernig's or Brudzinski's signs), irritability or bulging fontanel	Meningitis
Ill appearance, anxious, drooling, leaning forward	Epiglottitis (this is a medical emergency, *do not* examine oropharynx)

FWLS, fever without localising source; UTI, urinary tract infection.

- *meningitis*: should be ruled out if the child shows signs of CNS involvement. It is *usually* an age-related infection, with the majority of cases occurring in patients aged between 1 month and 5 years (Feigin & Perlman 1998, Willoughby & Polack 1998). However, as there continues to be a number of school-age, adolescent and university-aged patients affected, meningitis should be included in the differential list of *all* patients presenting with fever, ill appearance and no localising source (FWLS).

Clinical findings exhibited by neonates and many infants are generally non-specific and non-localising (e.g. fever or temperature instability; poor feeding, lethargy, hypotonia, irritability). Older infants and children may have a prodromal mild illness which progresses to a high fever, vomiting, photophobia, headache (in older children), nuchal rigidity, listlessness or irritability, seizures and cranial nerve involvement. Skin eruptions may range from maculopapules to petechiae and purpura. The onset of meningitis can be rapid or may be sub-acute, preceded by several days of genitourinary symptoms or upper respiratory tract infection (URTI). Different pathogens can cause this condition and the child's prognosis usually depends on the nature of the organism. ❶ Any child suspected of having the disease should be discussed immediately with a physician and a determination made as to administration of antibiotics and referral to acute care. However, suspected cases of meningitis identified in the community setting are usually given benzylpenicillin (1200 mg intramuscularly (IM) for children > 10 years of age; 600 mg for those 1–9 years; 300 mg for < 1 year of age) prior to referral or transfer to the acute setting.

- *urinary tract infection (UTI)*: there is strong evidence that UTI should be considered in infants and young children presenting with FWLS as this group (1) is at increased risk for acute renal injury with UTI; (2) has an incidence of vesicoureteral reflux that is greater than older children; and (3) the severity of vesicoureteral reflux is greater in this population, with the most severe form of reflux almost exclusively limited to infants

(American Academy of Pediatrics 1999). However, clinical findings in young infants and children can be very non-specific. Consequently, if there is compromise with regard to the child's general appearance, level of hydration and ability to retain oral fluids, UTI should be included on a list of possible aetiologies.

While a urine culture obtained by suprapubic aspiration or bladder catheterisation remains the gold standard for diagnosis of UTI among infants and small children, a routine urinalysis (or dipstick) performed on a specimen obtained by the most convenient method possible can be valuable in selecting individuals for prompt intervention while awaiting culture results. More specifically, the components of the urinalysis that are the most useful include the leucocyte esterase test, nitrite test and microscopy (or detection of WBCs on a dipstick test). While a positive result on any of these tests alone lacks sensitivity (and specificity is likewise variable), when considered collectively (and especially if negative) the NP has important information upon which to base clinical decisions.

Plan

It is a good idea to consult with medical colleagues when presented with any child that is acutely febrile and without a localising source. This is especially relevant for inexperienced NPs or those without a significant degree of clinical confidence in managing ill children.

In cases where a focal infections is identified (e.g. otitis or pharyngitis), treatment is aetiology specific. However, it is important to keep in mind that (especially with young children or those with temperatures > 38.9°C) localised findings can coexist with more serious infections such as meningitis, OB or UTI.

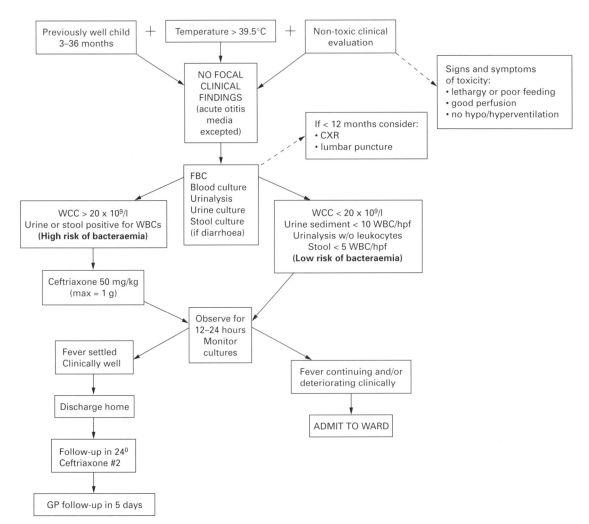

Figure 17.1 *Management of the febrile child 3–36 months; West Mead Emergency Department, Sydney, Australia. (Adapted from Browne et al 1997.)*

Further assessment and/or referral may be necessary to rule out additional problems.

A protocol for selective empiric treatment of FWLS in infants and young children (used in a university-based Accident and Emergency (A&E) Department) given in Fig. 17.1

Additional diagnostics. This is largely dependent on the clinical presentation and what type of services are available in the practice area. Many NPs will have to refer children to the Outpatient or A&E Department in order to obtain timely results if additional diagnostics are required. If the clinical appearance is worrying, an FBC provides important information. As a general guideline, among patients from 1–36 months of age (presenting with fever and no localising source) the NP should *consider* the possibility of determining the WBC count when the fever is greater than 40°C; ❶ at the very minimum this situation requires consultation with medical colleagues. Other non-specific tests of inflammation can also be considered (C-reactive protein (CRP) or ESR). Note that if the ESR and WBC counts in a pyrexic child are elevated, the risk of serious illness is twice as great as when they are within normal limits (Wilson 1995). Please note that these are not diagnostic tests, but screening values to be used to guide your clinical decision making. A urine test for protein, blood, white cells, leucocyte esterase and nitrites can usually be done in the surgery if the cause of fever is not obvious. This is particularly appropriate for girls. This should be followed up with a midstream specimen of urine (MSU) for culture if the test is positive or any urinary symptoms are reported.

Depending upon the age of the patient and the clinical presentation, additional routine cultures such as blood, throat and stool should be considered as well as the possibility of referral for lumbar puncture. If diarrhoea is present, it is sometimes possible to examine the stool for WBCs in the surgery. A positive result is one in which there are > 5 WBCs/hpf. ❶ It is likely that any child requiring more extensive diagnostics should be referred to a physician.

Pharmacotherapeutics. Treating children with acute pyrexia includes both the control of the fever and treatment of the underlying cause. Many clinicians choose not to treat fever in the otherwise normal child. Note that children with cardiac insufficiency, chronic lung disease, pulmonary insufficiency or metabolic instability may find fever stressful and therefore are prime candidates for antipyretic therapy. Antipyretics such as ibuprofen and paracetamol may be used in order to help relieve discomfort and malaise. Paracetamol is generally the drug of choice. Aspirin should *not* be used. If a focal bacterial infection is found, it should be treated with antimicrobial therapy as appropriate. As outlined previously, in the child without focal bacterial infection, the decision to empirically treat the infant or child with antibiotics is made in consultation with medical colleagues.

Behavioural interventions. Sponging/bathing with tepid water and use of light clothing will encourage heat loss and make the child feel more comfortable. Sponging can be particularly useful in children who have been overbundled, are hypersensitive to antipyretics, are dehydrated and/or have a history of febrile seizures or liver disease. However, note that sponging along with paracetamol is only slightly more effective than paracetamol used on its own and many children will find it distressing. Oral fluids and adequate nutrition should be encouraged as much as possible.

Patient education. It is important to stress to the caretaker that treating the child's fever will not change the course of the disease, and the response to antipyretic therapy is not an indicator to be considered when trying to assess the underlying cause. Care should be taught to assess the child for lack of response to antipyretics and signs of deterioration. Deterioration may happen very quickly, and it is essential for parents to be made aware of this. These signs include increasing fever, nuchal rigidity, dehydration, respiratory distress and changes in level of alertness or colour. Any deterioration requires immediate notification and possible visit to an A&E Department. Close follow-up is essential, with a return visit the following day for re-evaluation. This is particularly important for the child under 3 months of age, as the younger the child the greater the risk of SBI. Older children that are at low risk should return if their fever persists for more than 2–3 days or their condition worsens. It should be stressed, however, that most fevers will resolve without complications.

Referral. The following children presenting with an acute febrile episode should be referred:
- all toxic-appearing infants and children
- all infants under 28 days old (and likely all those < 90 days)
- all infants and children who are at high risk for OB or have a clinical appearance that is suggestive of toxicity or CNS involvement
- all children with an underlying chronic disease, such as malignancy or sickle cell anaemia
- all children whose condition deteriorates.

Varicella (chickenpox)

Varicella is a highly contagious viral disease caused by varicella-zoster virus (VZV) an antigenic strain of the herpes virus. Patients present with a pruritic, vesicular rash that appears in crops. The most commonly affected children are those between 2 and 10 years of age, but individuals of any age can contract the disease. Varicella is spread primarily by airborne respiratory secretions or contact with fluid from the vesicles. Direct contact with an individual with shingles may also cause chickenpox in a susceptible host. The incubation period ranges from 10 to 21 days (mean = 14). Patients are contagious 1–2 days before the rash appears until all the vesicles have crusted, approximately 5–7 days after the onset of the rash. Immunity from further infection is generally acquired following recovery. The virus does, however, remain latent in the nerve ganglia and re-activation by subsequent exposure can result in zoster or shingles. A vaccine is currently available.

Subjective findings

1. History of a mild prodrome consisting of malaise, headache, low-grade fever and anorexia. Adolescents may complain of a more severe prodrome, while young children will have a very mild or absent prodrome.
2. A pruritic rash which classically appears initially on the face or trunk. The rash usually spreads centripetally from the presenting lesions, potentially affecting the mucosal tissue in the mouth, oesophagus, rectum and vagina.
3. Recent exposure to chickenpox.
4. No previous knowledge of having had the disease.

Objective findings

1. Vital signs with careful observation of respiratory effort. Temperature will range from low-grade elevation to marker fever (39–40°C). For the most part, the more severe the rash, the greater the likelihood of significant elevation.
2. Physical examination reveals an exanthem occurring in stages. 'Crops' of lesions present as pink maculopapular 'spots', which progress to fluid-filled vesicles that develop a crust over 6–10 hours.
3. Possible infection of lesions may be noted.
4. Generalised lymphadenopathy may be present.
5. Heart, lungs and tympanic membranes should be normal but need to be assessed for signs and symptoms of complications such as pneumonia and/or bacterial otitis media. Likewise, lesions need to be assessed for possible bacterial suprainfection.

Assessment

- The diagnosis of varicella is a clinical decision based upon the subjective history and typical patient presentation. In many cases, the child may not need to be seen in the surgery, as the diagnosis and management may be handled by telephone (thereby reducing the risk of exposure to others).
- Differential diagnoses are dependent on your history and objective examination findings. They may include scabies, herpes simplex, folliculitis, contact dermatitis, insect bites, drug eruptions, enterovirus infections such as Coxsackie virus (no crusting on vesicles will be noted) or hand, foot and mouth disease, in addition to secondary syphilis.
- Complications of varicella, while rare, occasionally occur, and the NP must be alert to their possibility. They commonly include secondary bacterial infection of the lesions (usually caused by *Staphylococcus aureus* or Group A streptococcus) or otitis media, and

much less commonly idiopathic thrombocytopenia, CNS problems (encephalitis, seizures, Guillain–Barré syndrome) and Reye's syndrome.

Plan

Additional diagnostics. None are usually required.

Pharmacotherapeutics. Oral aciclovir can reduce the rate of acute complications if given *within 24 hours of illness*. It is not routinely recommended for healthy infants and children with uncomplicated varicella. It may be considered in healthy nonpregnant adolescents, children over 1 year of age with chronic cutaneous or pulmonary disorders or for those on short-term, intermittent or aerosolised corticosteroids; if possible, corticosteroids should be discontinued. Antihistamines such as chlorphenamine (chlorpheniramine) may be considered. Antipyretics (e.g. paracetamol) may be recommended for the symptomatic treatment of fever and discomfort. ❶ Never advise the use of aspirin. Lotions for such as calamine (needs to be kept in the refrigerator) for lesions will help to control pruritus and may be applied as required. Use of topical lotions containing steroids or antihistamines is contraindicated.

Behavioural interventions. Tepid baths with a handful of bicarbonate of soda or oatmeal may relieve itching and help prevent bacterial suprainfection. Children's nails should be cut and hands kept clean. Loosely fitted mittens padded with cotton wool may be helpful in preventing infants from further irritating lesions.

Patient education. This should incorporate teaching the child and caregiver to identify potential complications, with clear instructions regarding a return to the clinic (or telephone consultation at the minimum) if the child displays anything unexpected during the course of the illness. The child may go back to school 5–7 days after the onset of the rash once all of the lesions have crusted. Patients that have an uncomplicated disease course do not require follow-up.

Referral

High-risk children are those who are immunocompromised, pregnant adolescents, infants less than 4 weeks old and any child that develops a serious complication. Serious sequelae of varicella infection are uncommon and most children can be managed in the primary care setting.

Epstein–Barr infection
(glandular fever or infectious mononucleosis)

Glandular fever or infectious mononucleosis is an acute viral syndrome caused by the Epstein–Barr virus (EBV). It is most commonly seen in adolescents and young adults. Young children may acquire the disease (generally benign and frequently unrecognised/subclinical); mild cases are common among all age groups. Epstein–Barr infection is primarily a disease of the lymphoid tissue and peripheral blood. As such, there is enlargement of lymphoid tissue and atypical lymphocytes in peripheral blood. Almost all body organs can be involved and EBV infection is considered to be the 'great impersonator' as it can mimic so many illnesses (Goodman & Brady 1996). EBV is spread by the oropharyngeal route via saliva – hence the term 'the kissing disease'. It may also be spread via blood transfusion, but this is rare. It is thought to have an incubation period of 2–8 weeks, with a prolonged period of communicability (up to 1 year or more after the illness). The actual duration of symptomatic disease varies; however, the average uncomplicated illness lasts about 1 month.

Subjective findings

History reveals the classic EBV triad of fever, lymphadenopathy and sore throat. Patients may also have a recent history of malaise, headache, fatigue or rash. Exposure to others with EBV may be reported. Patient complaints common with EBV infection are numerous and include myalgia, arthalgia, ocular pain, photophobia, loose stool, cough and rhinitis.

Objective findings

1. Vital signs are usually within age-appropriate normal values; however, temperature is frequently elevated.
2. A thorough physical examination (including a neurological assessment) is necessary. Positive findings are numerous and potentially include:
   - *Non-specific exanthem:* can be of any form (maculopapular, urticarial, nodular, etc.), and occurs in approximately 5–15% of cases, particularly if the patient has recently been taking ampicillin or amoxicillin.
   - *Pharyngitis,* marked tonsillar enlargement, ulceration and psuedomembrane formation are common. There may be petechiae on the palate.
   - *Periorbital oedema:* common (approximately 30% of cases) and will have some swelling that may be tender.
   - *Lymphadenopathy:* palpation of the neck will reveal involvement of the anterior and posterior cervical nodes, but any lymphoid tissue can be affected. Nodes are usually firm, tender and discrete. It is important to assess for any obstruction of the upper airway by enlarged tonsils and lymphoid tissue.
   - *Splenomegaly:* occurs in approximately 50–75% of cases, although rupture is rare and this usually resolves within 1 month.
   - *Hepatomegaly:* some degree of enlargement is common and almost all patients will have abnormal liver function tests. Some patients (5–25%) may have jaundice.

Assessment

- The diagnosis of EBV infection is largely grounded in symptom history and clinical presentation. However, as clinical features are so similar to other conditions, it is likely that additional laboratory tests may be needed to be confirm your suspicions of EBV infection.
- Differential diagnoses are numerous, as EBV infection could potentially be included in almost every disease. As such, the NP would need to consider other viral syndromes, streptococcal pharyngitis, hepatitis, cytomegalovirus and toxoplasmosis.
- Complications are rare but include splenic rupture, thrombocytopenia, agranulocytosis, haemolytic anaemia, orchitis, myocarditis and chronic EBV infection. Very rarely EBV is implicated in fatal disseminated disease or B-cell lymphoma.

Plan

Additional diagnostics. The NP should consider an FBC, a monospot for the patient presenting with an acute phase illness or a Paul–Bunnell test if the patient appears to be beyond the acute stage of disease. An FBC indicating EBV infection will characteristically result in a lymphocytosis in which more than 10% of cells are atypical. The monospot and Paul–Bunell test will identify approximately 90% of cases in children over 4 years of age and adults, although patients often need to be ill for about 2 weeks for either test to be accurate. If symptoms persist after a negative result, a repeat test should be done in 7–10 days and the NP may consider the possibility of cytomegalovirus infection as the two are clinically indistinguishable. Viral culture and EBV specific core and capsule antibody testing can be done if a definitive diagnosis is required. Many patients with EBV also have streptococcal infection, and a throat swab should be considered.

Pharmacotherapeutics. This is the same as for other viral infections in that antibiotics are not required. Likewise, antiviral drugs such as aciclovir are not indicated; treatment is supportive. Over-the-counter (OTC) pain medication and salt water gargles may help sore throat discomfort. If the patient has concomitant (group A betahaemolytic streptococcus–GABHS) streptococcal pharyngitis, treatment with erythromycin or penicillin V should be considered; note that amoxicillin should be avoided.

Behavioural interventions. Increase fluids and maintain adequate food intake. Contact sports should be avoided for at least 1 month or until splenomegaly subsides. A realistic schedule of rest and play (or school work) should be planned and is dependent on the patient's condition. The patient does not need to be isolated from others but good handwashing and prevention of fomite spread is important to prevent infection of others.

Patient education. Patients and their carers should be aware that treatment is basically supportive. The importance of rest and adequate nutrition should be stressed. While complications are rare, families should be instructed to contact the surgery if children do not improve and certainly if their condition deteriorates. It is important that any patient with EBV infection should not donate blood.

Referral. Consider referral of patients with noted tonsillar enlargement and difficulty in swallowing. In addition, patients with central nervous system (CNS) complications, jaundice or any persistent symptoms of more than 2 weeks should be discussed with a physician.

Enterovirus infections

Enterovirus infections are a large group of illnesses that are caused by polioviruses, coxsackie viruses and echoviruses. They are a very common aetiological agent for a number of childhood illnesses that typically are accompanied by fever and occur during warm summer months (June–September). Enterovirus infection in children most frequently presents as (Zaoutis & Klein 1998):

1. a *non-specific febrile illness* (most common)
2. *aseptic meningitis*
3. *herpangina*
4. *hand, foot and mouth (HFM) disease*
5. *non-specific exanthems* (the enteroviral pathogens are the most common cause of viral, non-specific rashes in children).

Poliovirus, while classified as an enterovirus (and, therefore, similar in the epidemiology, pathophysiology and clinical symptomatology of enterovirus infection) is not a source of morbidity in developed countries and has been omitted from discussion.

The assessment and management of the different enterovirus infections in the following section are outlined according to the five common clinical presentations.

Humans are the only known hosts for enteroviruses and transmission primarily occurs through the fecal–oral route, although there can also be oral–oral and respiratory spread. Children less than 5 years of age are at increased risk of infection (related to their lack of prior immunity and potentially poor handwashing/infection control measures). Illness caused by enterovirus infection can range from life-threatening, with severe morbidity (rare, and usually associated with neonates or children with deficiencies of B-lymphocyte function), to mild and/or subclinical cases (approximately half of enterovirus infections are asymptomatic). Functioning humoral immunity is required for adequate response to enterovirus infection as it is thought that B lymphocytes are responsible for blocking viral entry into the CNS. There is improved immunity to reinfection after an acute episode with the same serotype, but often reinfection results in a subclinical case of the illness (Zaoutis & Klein 1998).

The incubation period for most enteroviruses ranges from 3 to 10 days. Typically, the virus begins to replicate in the lymph tissue of the upper respiratory tract and small intestine after gaining entry via oral or respiratory routes. After replication, the virus enters the bloodstream and produces a low level viraemia, which is evidenced by the onset of fever and other clinical symptoms. Further replication from secondary sites (CNS, liver, adrenal glands, skin and mucous membranes) with subsequent dissemination results in a major viraemia that offers the opportunity for increased viral seeding of the CNS (Zaoutis & Klein 1998). Coxsackie and echovirus serotypes are thought to be responsible for 80–90% of aseptic meningitis cases in which a pathogen is isolated; while non-polio enteroviruses (commonly echovirus serotype 9) are the leading cause of childhood exanthems in the summer and autumn. The fever and oral vesicles of herpangina are mainly attributable to coxsackie A virus; however, coxsackie B and echoviruses have likewise been implicated (Zaoutis & Klein 1998). Similarly, the aetiology of HFM disease is largely (but not exclusively) due to Coxsackie A16 virus.

Subjective findings

1. History reveals clinical complaints typical of viral illnesses (fever, URTI symptoms, gastrointestinal discomfort).
2. Mylagia, malaise, photophobia, headache and sore throat are commonly clustered, especially in the presentation of *non-specific febrile illness*.
3. Gastrointestinal symptoms are frequent: nausea, vomiting, abdominal pain and loose stools/diarrhoea (especially common with *non-specific febrile illness*).
4. In *non-specific febrile illness*, fever often develops in the absence of a prodrome, lasts an average of 3 days and may manifest in a biphasic pattern (fever for 1 day, then afebrile for 2–3 days, then fever for 2–4 days). It is not uncommon for the fever to last for up to 1 week.
5. With *aseptic meningitis*, the fever commonly assumes a biphasic pattern with CNS symptomatology (photophobia, nuchal rigidity and/or headache) developing with the recurrence of the fever.
6. *Herpangina* can present with fever up to 41°, especially in younger children.
7. In *HFM* disease the caretaker will describe fever, oral lesions and a 'rash' on the hands and feet (but may include arms, legs, buttocks and genitalia).
8. Presenting complaints of a *non-specific exanthem* and/or *enanthem* are commonly described with or without fever.

Objective findings

1. Ill-appearing febrile child (of any age) that will typically present in the summer or early autumn.
2. Vital signs should be within age-appropriate norms (adjusting for the slight increases in heart rate and respiration that accompany fever).
3. In *non-specific febrile illness*, physical examination findings are unremarkable (excepting fever, often 38.5–40°C) but there may be mild conjunctivitis, lymphadenitis and/or pharyngeal erythema; if an FBC is done, there is likely to be no elevated WBC count or differential shift.

4. With *aseptic meningitis*, physical examination will reveal fever (commonly in a biphasic pattern), in addition to evidence of meningeal irritation that is often seen with recurrence of the fever. In children older than 12 months, signs of CNS involvement include photophobia, nuchal rigidity, Kernig's sign (extension of knee while hips flexed elicits pain) and Brudzinski's sign (flexing chin to chest triggers resistance and pain), while among younger infants there is likely to be marked irritability rather than specific meningeal signs. Asking older children to 'kiss their knees' is an effective manoeuvre to assess meningeal irritation.

5. In *herpangina* the patient is more likely to be from 3 to 10 years old, and in addition to presenting with fever (38.5–41°C; higher temperatures more likely in younger patients); the physical examination will reveal painful punctate macules in the posterior half of the oral cavity (posterior pharynx, anterior tonsillar pillars and soft palate). The lesions (usually 2–6, although there can be up to 16) vesicate, then ulcerate, and typically are surrounded by an erythematous ring. *Lymphonodular pharyngitis* (a *herpangina* variant) presents similarly; however, the oral lesions are tiny, firm white nodules.

6. HFM *disease* more commonly affects toddlers and school-aged children. On examination they will have fever (38–39°C for 24–48 hours) and mildly painful oral lesions (vesicular with red ring progressing to ulcers). The vesicular exanthem is usually limited to the palms, soles and interdigital spaces, although it can be seen on the buttocks, proximal extremities and genitalia.

7. *Non-specific exanthems* are characteristically seen in children less than 5 years old and may be present with/without a fever and usually in combination with the physical findings associated with *aseptic meningitis* or *non-specific febrile illness*. On examination, the rash is usually pink, blanching and rubelliform (discrete maculopapular) with a distribution that starts on the head and upper trunk and spreads peripherally; less commonly, the exanthem can appear vesicular, urticarial or petechial.

Assessment

1. The diagnosis of enterovirus infection is a clinical decision based upon the symptom history, risk of exposure, seasonal presentation and physical examination findings; it is uncommon for there to be virus isolation and identification.

2. Differential diagnoses for the five most common presentations of enterovirus infection are numerous and include:
   - *Non-specific viral illness*: consider bacteraemia, septicaemia, FWLS, early appendicitis presentation, food poisoning, bacterial or parasitic gastroenteritis, toxic shock syndrome, URTI, other viral infections (respiratory syncytial virus (RSV) or gastroenteritis), UTI streptococcal pharyngitis and Lyme disease.
   - *Aseptic meningitis:* consider bacterial meningitis, tick-borne illness and arbovirus infection. The simultaneous incidence of additional enterovirus infections in the community during the warmer months (HFM disease and herpangina) may be useful to narrow the diagnosis to enterovirus infection.
   - *Herpangina*: consider herpes simplex infection (herpetic gingivostomatitis), HFM, and aphthous ulcers.
   - *HFM disease*: consider all illnesses above in addition to varicella.
   - *Non-specific exanthems:* consider roseola infantum (exanthem subitum), varicella, Lyme disease, hypersensitivity reaction, Kawasaki syndrome, erythema infectiosum (fifth disease or 'slapped cheek' disease), measles, rubella, meningococcaemia, streptococcal pharyngitis (scarlatina), tick-borne illnesses, Henoch–Schönlein purpura and Epstein–Barr viral infection (glandular fever).

Plan

Additional diagnostics. Depending on the clinical presentation, the NP may need to consider FBC, urinalysis, routine cultures (urine, blood, stool or throat), CRP or ESR, in addition to possible referral for lumbar puncture. Additional laboratory methods that can be used in diagnosis include isolation of the virus from blood, stool, posterior pharynx and CSF using cell culture; serology (paired acute and convalescent antibody titres); and PCR (polymerase chain reaction) techniques. However, with the exception of an FBC and routine cultures, these diagnostics are likely to be beyond the scope of both primary care and the NP. The child requiring these more involved investigations would likely be referred to medical colleagues. At the very minimum, consultation with your collaborating physician would be advised.

Pharmacotherapeutics. There is no effective antiviral therapy for enterovirus infections; thus, treatment is supportive and aimed at symptom relief (paracetamol or ibuprofen). Antidiarrhoeal drugs are *not* recommended for use in children.

Behavioural interventions. These comprise oral fluids, adequate nutrition, rest and light clothing to enhance heat loss. Management of nausea, vomiting, diarrhoea and abdominal pain is the same as for mild gastroenteritis (small, frequent meals of bland complex carbohydrates; osmotically balanced oral rehydration fluids; and avoidance of lactose-rich foods). Small children refusing all oral intake because of mouth ulcers may need to be especially encouraged with frozen juice or rehydration solution ice-lollies.

Patient education. Caretakers must understand that the enterovirus infection is self-limiting and care is supportive. However, especially among small children with high fevers, close follow-up contact with the family is important to be sure that a more serious diagnosis is not overlooked.

Referral. Consider referral for any child that you are uneasy about managing. In addition, the referral criteria discussed in the Fever section are applicable (e.g. children with a toxic-appearance, petechial rash, signs of meningeal irritation, febrile convulsions, prolonged high fever).

Roseola

Roseola, also known as exanthem subitum, is the most common exanthem among children less than 3 years old. It is an acute, self-limiting viral infection that predominantly affects those from 6 to 24 months (it is rare before 3 months or after 36 months), with a peak incidence in the second year of life; 80% of cases are seen before 18 months of age (Paller 1993, Goodman & Brady 1996, Boynton et al 1998).

Complications are rare, although febrile convulsions can occur and encephalitis has been reported. The causative agent is herpesvirus type 6, humans are the only known reservoir and the mode of transmission is unknown. As most 4 year olds are seropositive, it is likely that there are subclinical cases of roseola infection that do not present with the characteristic history of fever and rash. While cases of roseola occur throughout the year, they are often clustered in the spring and early summer (Goodman & Brady 1996). The incubation period is not certain, but it is likely to be between 7 and 17 days, with the period of greatest communicability probably during the febrile phase and just after the onset of the rash.

Subjective findings

1. History reveals a sudden onset of high fever (to 40.5°C) for 3–5 days, with slightly irritable behaviour possible. For the most part, however, the child does not appear extremely ill and has mild symptoms.
2. After (or just before) defervescence, a faintly pink and maculopapular (parents may describe it as 'bumpy') rash erupts. It usually starts on the nape of the neck and/or behind the earlobes and spreads mainly to the trunk (but can extend to the perineum, buttocks and thighs).
3. Often there may be concomitant URTI symptoms, complaints of 'puffy eyes' and occasionally a history of febrile convulsion.

Objective findings

1. The young child (less than 3 years of age) will appear non-toxic, engagable and only slightly cranky, despite a markedly elevated temperature ($\approx$ 40.5°C, depending on time of last antipyretic). If the rash has started, the child will likely be less playful but continues to appear *not* extremely ill looking.
2. Physical examination will commonly reveal mild oedema of the eyelids and, if the rash is present, a faintly erythematous, macular or maculopapular rubelliform exanthem with a mainly central distribution; otherwise, the examination is unremarkable.

Assessment

1. The diagnosis of roseola is a clinical decision based upon the symptom history, patient's age and typical presentation.
2. Differential diagnoses include other viral exanthems (see enterovirus infection); fever without localising signs/symptoms; UTI; bacterial sepsis; and, if a febrile convulsion has occurred or the rash is atypical, meningococcaemia.

Plan

Additional diagnostics. No specific tests are available; however, depending on the clinical presentation, an FBC may be considered. This often reveals an initial leucocytosis (first 24 hours of fever) followed by leucopenia and a relative lymphocytosis (up to 90%). In addition, a urinalysis and urine culture may be considered.

Pharmacotherapeutics. Treatment is supportive and aimed at symptom relief (paracetamol or ibuprofen).

Behavioural interventions. These comprise oral fluids, adequate nutrition, rest and light clothing to enhance heat loss. Tepid baths may be helpful as an additional strategy for the management of pyrexia.

Patient education. Carers must understand the self-limiting nature of the illness and the expected clinical course (fever for 3–5 days followed by a rash that usually disappears within 24–48 hours). In addition they will require reassurance with regard to supportive care (fluids, antipyretics and extra rest), especially as a fever to 40.5°C can be quite frightening. Follow-up instructions include the importance of telephone contact and/or a return visit for monitoring and evaluation.

Referral. See indications for fever.

Pharmacotherapeutic considerations in paediatrics

Children and adults respond to drugs differently. Issues related to the use of medications in infants and children include (1) differences in the way a drug is absorbed, metabolised, distributed and utilised by the body; (2) different presentations of adverse drug reactions and toxicity; (3) difficulties in conducting drug trials with children (with the inherent implications for an evidence-base in paediatric pharmacology); and (4) issues related to medication adherence, formulation, dosage and education with children and their families: Once again, the NP is referred to the Further reading at the end of the chapter for more information, as an exhaustive discussion of these issues is not possible. However, important considerations have been outlined.

Drug absorption

For the most part drug absorption after oral administration in children is similar to that of adults. The issues of reduced gastric acid secretion and emptying time, age and growth have little clinical significance except in the treatment of premature infants, neonates and children with gastrointestinal problems (e.g. coeliac disease or cystic fibrosis) (Rylance 1988, Walson 1997). However, the issue of drug absorption relative to meals is of considerable practical importance. With the exception of a few drugs (e.g. isoniazid and narrow-spectrum penicillins) most medications should be given with food, even if only for ease of administration and adherence. Absorption of topical medications is greater in infants (related to their thinner stratum corneum) and, to a lesser extent, in small children. In addition, both of these groups have a greater total body surface area (TBSA) to weight ratio, which has implications for the amount of drug absorbed (e.g. carefully consider use of higher-potency corticosteroids in infants with severe eczema). Lastly, plastic-coated disposable nappies can increase absorption in relation to their occlusiveness in the diaper area (Niederhausen 1997).

Drug distribution

After a drug is absorbed, its distribution is related to the body compartment size and composition, blood–brain barrier permeability and protein-binding capacity. Young children, especially infants, have a greater proportion of body water and extracellular fluid for weight and, therefore, there is an increased distribution and dilution of a drug. Since most medications used in paediatrics are water soluble, this explains the increased mg/kg dosing of many medications (as compared with adult dosages). Furthermore, in neonates the blood–brain barrier is functionally incomplete, so there may be an enhanced effect of some medications. Lastly, while there are slight differences in protein-binding capacity that are related to age (decreased capacity in neonates and infants until 6 months of age), these are generally of little clinical significance with the exception of a few drugs (e.g. phenytoin and sulphonamides) during the neonatal period and, consequently, are not an issue for the NP in primary (Rylance 1988, Niederhausen 1997, Walson 1997).

Drug elimination (metabolism and excretion)

Differences in drug metabolism (which occurs primarily in the liver) are most acute in the immediate neonatal period (particularly in premature infants) and are related to the decreased ability of the liver and its microsomal enzyme systems. Likewise, in the kidney (the primary site of drug excretion), glomerular filtration and tubular function are less efficient in early infancy, although this is usually no longer an issue by 5 months of age. Clinical implications of decreased renal function are most pronounced in pre-term infants and, therefore, dosage adjustments should be made for drugs dependent on renal excretion for the termination of their activity: penicillins, aminoglycosides, digoxin and thiazide diuretics (Rylance 1988, Niederhausen 1997, Walson 1997).

Choice of drug, dosage/frequency, administration route, formulation, patient adherence and education

While many paediatric illnesses are self-limiting, if the NP determines that medication is required for a child's treatment, it is important that drug selection is based upon the pathophysiology of the illness and the most likely match between the causative agent/process and pharmacological activity of the drug (e.g. penicillin V for treatment of streptococcal pharyngitis). In addition, the pharmacokinetics discussed previously need to be considered along with the issues of medication cost, safety of use in paediatrics and effectiveness.

The appropriate dosage for a particular medication is largely dependent on a child's weight (this is especially true for children < 20 kg and for those medications with a narrow therapeutic range). However, certain limitations (e.g. drug concentration of an available preparation) impact the clinician's ability to request a specific milligrams per kilogram (mg/kg) dosage (keeping in mind the maximum daily dosage). The commonly accepted method of paediatric dosing among infants and young children is to calculate the optimal for each dose of medication and, subsequently, adjust it slightly to adapt it to the available preparations (cognisant of the maximum daily dose).

This is unlikely to be a problem in dosing older children and adolescents, for whom standard formulations typically apply without adjustment. Regarding dosage frequency, there should likewise be a match between drug concentration and effect that considers the number of times a day a child will need medication. For example, once-daily steroid dosing is associated with less toxicity (and likely improves adherence) while thrice (or twice) daily administration of an antibiotic is preferable to an antibiotic that needs to be administered four times a day, assuming there is no decrease in drug effectiveness (Rylance 1988).

The most common administration route for routine paediatric medications is oral; topical applications are largely reserved for dermatological conditions. Occasionally, and especially in acute situations, there is the option of rectal or parenteral administration. This route should be avoided if possible, as it is likely to be more traumatic for the child.

Drug formulation can significantly impact upon a child and family's adherence. If a child is able to manage solid preparations (and the formulation is in an acceptable dosage) there is greater accuracy of administration and usually easier storage (e.g. no need for refrigeration) as compared with liquid preparations. However, if a child cannot manage tablets, then oral medication is often a better choice than 'crushing pills' (although with unpalatable liquids, crushed medication may be more easily disguised). Care should be exercised with sustained-release preparations, because it is important that the medication is not chewed or crushed. Occasionally, a medication may come in two different strengths, thereby allowing the clinician to maintain a certain dosage while decreasing the volume of medication to be administered. This is especially helpful with uncooperative toddlers or pre-schoolers. In addition, many medications (especially liquid preparations) contain dyes, colouring agents and sucrose, to which children may be more sensitive, although the number who react is probably small (Rylance 1988). Inhaler devices are a good example of the mismatch that can result when an adult delivery system is used with children. It is crucial in paediatric asthma management that the child, device and formulation are matched.

Adherence to a medication regimen is often the most challenging aspect of medication issues in paediatrics. Difficulties arise from uncooperative children, inaccurate measurement techniques, omission of doses and conflicts such as day-care programmes or school attendance. As outlined above, a medication that is palatable, with the fewest number of doses, no special storage requirements and available in an appropriate strength that is cheap, safe and effective is ideal. Parent and child education around medications must focus on the issues that contribute to successful administration and adherence. Both groups should understand: (1) why a certain medication has been recommended; (2) what the medication should do (and what it should not do); (3) how long it should be administered for; and (4) the importance of continuing the medication for the recommended length of time (even though symptoms may subside). In addition, parents may need advice on administration techniques and aids for accurate measurement (a teaspoon is not a teaspoon is not a teaspoon).

Oral medication administration to young infants is reliant on proper positioning (head slightly elevated); accurate measurement (usually assisted with a syringe or dropper that is dispensed with the drug); and correct placement (towards the back of mouth on either side of the tongue). A gentle breath onto the baby's face often elicits a swallowing reflex, which completes the process. Warn parents that if the infant starts to choke or cough, stop giving the medicine, sit him/her up and resume administration when the infant has settled. Use of positive reinforcement (stickers, praise, etc.) is important for older children, as is a certain degree of autonomy (letting a child 'squirt' the medicine into their mouth or 'help' to measure). The child should always be approached firmly, with clear instructions on what is to be expected. If the medication is unpleasant tasting, using a straw while holding the nose is often helpful. Parents should be discouraged from putting medication into juices or bottles, as there is no way to be assured that the complete dose has been administered.

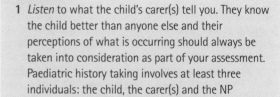

Top Tips ✓

1 *Listen* to what the child's carer(s) tell you. They know the child better than anyone else and their perceptions of what is occurring should always be taken into consideration as part of your assessment. Paediatric history taking involves at least three individuals: the child, the carer(s) and the NP

2 Flexibility is the key to a successful physical examination. Head-to-toe sequence in a cooperative adolescent or adult is frequently an unattainable goal when examining an infant, toddler or young child

3 A careful physical examination of the child presenting with an episodic illness (minimum assessment of the head to abdomen) is essential

4 Adolescent patients may be adult in their appearance but do not assume that their knowledge base is as comprehensive as that of an adult

5 The offering of a private consultation with the adolescent patient should always be an option. Hidden agendas are not uncommon

6 Always observe the child's interaction with people and the environment when considering degree of illness or level of toxicity

7 Remember signs and symptoms are developmentally related, e.g. young infants are often hypothermic when septic rather than pyrexic

8 The pyrexic child may have more than one condition which is causing the febrile episode. Observations of a localised finding does not rule out a coexisting more serious infection

9 Patient education should always include information on the expected course of illness, what would warrant further follow-up (either by phone or a visit), reassurance and praise

10 When in doubt or dealing with children at risk, always consult with a medical colleague

11 Physical findings that are not consistent with the history as provided require more careful exploration and consideration of non-accidental injury

Glossary

Aseptic meningitis Aseptic meningitis or benign viral meningitis is a term that encompasses a group of disorders in which there is some meningeal irritation but no pyogenic organism can be detected in the cerebrospinal fluid. Meningeal irritation often follows infection with the mumps virus or with one of the enteroviruses. Symptoms may include headache and signs characteristic of meningeal irritation, photophobia and pain when the eyes are moved from side to side. Most symptoms are mild and the disease is self-limiting

Bacteraemia   The presence of bacteria in the blood

Cytokines   These are proteins or glycoproteins secreted by cells participating in the immune response. They act as messengers, enabling communication among macrophages and lymphocytes

Cytomegalovirus   Any of a group of highly host-specific herpesviruses that may infect man, monkeys or rodents. They produce unique large cells with inclusion bodies. Cytomegalic inclusion disease, found in man, has been associated with a syndrome that resembles Epstein–Barr virus (EBV)

Enterovirus   A subgroup of picornaviruses infecting the gastrointestinal tract and discharged in the excreta. They include the Coxsackie virus, the poliovirus and the echovirus.

Exanthem   Any cutaneous eruptive disease or fever

Fever   Core temperature (e.g. rectal) of at least 38°C which is a symptom of an underlying process or condition that involves inflammation

Fever of unknown origin (FUO)   A prolonged fever of more than 7 days in which the source of the fever cannot be detected by history or physical examination

Fever without localising source (FWLS)   Presentation of an acute onset of fever for less than 7 days in which no source for the fever can be found from the history and physical examination

Herpangina   An infectious febrile disease found in children that is caused by Coxsackie viruses. It is marked by vesicular or ulcerated lesions on the fauces or soft palate

Occult bacteraemia (OB)   The presence of bacteria in the blood (bacteraemia) with a benign clinical appearance and no apparent source of serious infections

Periorbital oedema   Swelling around the periosteum of the bones forming the orbit or eye socket

Prodrome   A symptom indicating the beginning of a disease

Pyrexia of unknown origin (PUO)   See fever of unknown origin

Pyrogen   An agent that causes fever

Septicaemia   The presence of microorganisms in the blood with localised or systemic disease in an ill-appearing patient

Serious bacterial illness (SBI)   Potentially life-threatening diseases if allowed to progress, they include such illnesses as, meningitis, UTI, osteomyelitis, septic arthritis, pneumonia, bacterial gastroenteritis, bacteraemia and serious skin and soft tissue infections (e.g. cellulitis)

Thrombocytopenia   A decrease in the number of platelets in the blood

References

American Academy of Pediatrics 1999 Practice parameter: the diagnosis, treatment and evaluation of the initial urinary tract infection in febrile infants and young children. Pediatrics 103(4):843–852.

Baraff L J, Bass J W, Fleisher G D et al 1993 Practice guidelines for the management of infants and children 0 to 36 months of age with fever without source. Pediatrics 92(1):1–12.

Boynton R E, Dunn, E S, Bond G R 1998 Manual of ambulatory pediatrics, 4th edn. J B Lippincott, Philadelphia.

Browne G J, Ryan, J M, McIntyre P 1997 Evaluation of a protocol for selective empiric treatment of fever without localising signs. Archives of Disease in Childhood 76(2):129–133.

Feigin R D, Perlman E 1998 Bacterial meningitis beyond the neonatal period. In: Feigin R D, Cherry J D (eds) Textbook

of pediatric infectious diseases, 4th edn. W B Saunders, Philadelphia.

Goodman M H, Brady M A 1996 Infectious diseases. In: Burns C E, Barber N, Brady M A, Dunn A M (eds) Pediatric primary care: a handbook for nurse practitioners. W B Saunders, Philadelphia, 445–490.

Grover G 1996 Fever and bacteremia In: Berkowitz C D (ed) Pediatrics: a primary care approach. W B Saunders, Philadelphia, 127–132.

McCance K L, Huether S E 1994 Pathophysiology: the biologic basis for disease in adults and children, 2nd edn. St. Louis, Mosby.

McCarthy P L 1993 Identification of a sick child. In: Dershewitz R (ed) Ambulatory pediatric care, 2nd edn. J B Lippincott, Philadelphia, 664–667.

McCarthy P L 1998 Fever. Pediatrics in Review 19(12):401–407.

Millonig V L (ed). 1994 Pediatric nurse practitioner: certification review guide, 2nd edn. Health Leadership, Potomac, Maryland.

Niederhausen V P 1997 Prescribing for children: issues in pediatric pharmacology. The Nurse Practitioner 22(3):16–30.

Paller A 1993 Viral exanthems. In: Dershewitz R (ed) Ambulatory pediatric care, 2nd edn. J B Lippincott, Philadelphia, 263–268.

Rylance C W 1988 Prescribing for infants and children. British Medical Journal 296:984–986.

Uphold C R, Graham M V 1994 Clinical guidelines in family practice, 2nd edn. Barmarrae Books, Gainsville, Florida.

Vessey J A 1995 Developmental approaches to examining young children. Pediatric Nursing 21(1):53–56.

Walson P D 1997 Paediatric clinical pharmacology and therapeutics. In: Speight T M, Holford M, Nicholas H G (eds) Avery's drug treatment, 4th edn. Blackwell, London. 127–165.

Weller B F (ed) 1989 Baillière's encyclopaedic dictionary of nursing and health care. W B Saunders, London.

Willoughby R, Polack F S 1998 Meningitis: what's new in diagnosis and management. Contemporary Pediatrics 15(9):49–70.

Wilson D 1995 Assessing and managing the febrile child. Nurse Practitioner 20(11):59–74.

Wong D M, Hockenberry-Eaton M, Winkelstein, M L, Wilson, D Ahmann, E 1999 Health promotion of the adolescent and family. In: Whaley and Wong's nursing care of infants and children, 6th edn. Mosby, St. Louis, 888–925.

Zaoutis T, Klein J D 1998 Enterovirus infections. Pediatrics in Review 19(6):183–191.

Further Reading

Algranati P S 1992 The pediatric patient: an approach to history and physical examination. Williams & Wilkins, Baltimore.

Algranati P S 1998 Effect of development status on the approach to physical examination. Pediatric Clinics of North America 45(1):1–23.

Fenstermacher K, Hudson B T 1997 Practice guidelines for family nurse practitioners W B Saunders, Philadelphia.

Hopcroft K, Forte V 1999 Symptom sorter. Radcliffe Medical Press, Abingdon, Oxon.

Johnson G, Hill-Smith I, Ellis C 1997 The minor illness manual. Radcliffe Medical Press, Abingdon, Oxon.

Lommel L L, Jackson P L 1997 Assessing & managing common signs & symptoms: a decision making approach for health care providers. UCSF Nursing Press, San Francisco, California.

18

CARE OF THE OLDER ADULT

Soline Jerram and Sylvia Newson

Key Issues

- Illness is not a sequela to old age
- Symptomology in older people is often multicausal
- Quality of life is more important than quantity of years
- The aim of health promotion in the elderly is to maximise opportunities for good health
- The older person's right to self-determination should be considered within the context of his immediate environment
- Activities of daily living should form the basis of the assessment for the older person
- Older people's health status is dependent on a wide range of personal and social issues
- Older people's health involves a multi-professional, multi-agency approach
- Assessment of older people requires consideration of sensory and cognitive function
- Older people should have equal access to health information

Introduction

As with the care of children, assessment diagnosis and care planning for older adults requires a myriad of skills and knowledge.

As it is estimated that by the year 2021, one in five of the population will be over 65, understanding the needs of the older adult will become increasingly pertinent for health care practitioners. The role of the nurse practitioner (NP) and the skills and knowledge she/he brings to health care will almost certainly identify the NP as a provider to this age group.

The changes that the natural ageing process has on a person, on individual disease and the treatments used in modern medicine need to be clearly understood by the NP. It is assumed within this chapter that the NP has gained a basic understanding regarding the pathophysiology of ageing.

Older adults can suffer the same illnesses and diseases as all other age groups; however, changes in the presentation of illness or disease are often seen, and the existence of multi-pathology presents the practitioner with a jigsaw of symptoms to be unravelled.

Care of older adults is not always about cure but about improving quality of life; however, this may involve a more proactive and aggressive approach, rather than just conservative treatment. This will require the NP to develop a collaborative relationship in the care planning process to identify the individual patient's expectations and desires. This may entail working with older adults in an imaginative way to help them achieve their individual potentials.

Older adults often have to adapt to loss: loss of spouse, loss of independence, loss of their home and general loss of ability. The sensitivity and help given to an individual by the NP can aid or hinder their ability to cope.

This chapter will explore the common symptoms for which older people may present to the NP. It will consider how knowledge of the ageing process must inform the NP when developing care plans for individuals.

The holistic assessment of an older adult

An assessment involving an older person should always include sensory, social and environmental factors, all of which can impinge on good health and treatment compliance.

The NP's role in comprehensive assessment of the elderly is an area of great potential, especially within primary care. Accurately assessing the elderly, who often present with vague symptomology complicated by the effects of ageing and chronic disease, is time consuming, frequently frustrating, but ultimately extremely rewarding. A complete and comprehensive assessment will often take more than one consultation to complete, and information may be gained from a variety of sources. Through careful and systematic assessment of older people, the NP can not only identify underlying pathology but also, through the processes of education, health promotion and multi-disciplinary working, it is possible to prevent further deterioration in health status. The range of diseases found in older people are too numerous to cover in one chapter and therefore the focus will be to concentrate on a few specific areas. Some common indicators of illness in old age are (Coni & Webster 1998):

- incontinence
- immobility
- instability
- iatrogenic disease
- intellectual failure.

The patients seen by the NP will often present with some or all of the above indicators of ill health.

Any assessment process commences when the patient enters the consulting room. This period is especially important with the elderly, as it will guide you in making decisions about further assessment. The structure of your assessment will be dependent on the general condition of your patient. It may soon become clear that because of the complexity of the presenting problems you will need to focus on one aspect at a time, building up a picture over a period. Don't feel pressured into making decisions about management until you are sure you have all the information you require. Deal with any urgent or life-threatening issues and then arrange to see the patient again, either in the surgery or in their home environment, whichever seems most appropriate. When seeing an elderly patient for the first time, you start to pick up clues for further examination and/or questioning that will aid your diagnosis.

In this initial presentation stage, therefore, the key areas for elderly assessment are:

- appearance
- communication
- mobility
- mental status.

Appearance

The presenting appearance of an older person may lead you to question whether this is normal for this individual or if it is a significant change requiring further investigation. Careful questioning will be required, as a previously independent individual may not wish to admit that he is not coping. It is also important to remember that our standards for presentation and hygiene may be quite different from our patients and the fact that they are elderly may have no bearing. Apart from the risk of offending individuals, we must also remember that they may be concerned that admission to institutionalised care will ensue if they admit to problems, possibly resulting in a loss of independence.

Subjective assessment

1. Pallor, cyanosis and dyspnoea can be indicative of underlying pathology and will require further investigation.
2. Mood: anxiety, restlessness, confusion and depression. ❶ Sudden onset confused states warrants

urgent referral for investigation. Conditions leading to coma may begin with acute confusional state.

3. Facial expression: an expressionless face could be an indicator of Parkinson's disease or secondary parkinsonism, which is most commonly induced by drugs such as the phenothiazines, or may be due to trauma, infection, neoplasm or atherosclerosis.
4. Facial palsy can be indicative of upper motor neurone lesions, lower motor neurone lesions or brainstem lesions.
5. Angular stomatitis can be indicative of ill-fitting dentures which, in turn, can lead to problems with diet and nutritional status. It is also a frequent sign of anaemia.
6. Nails are a useful indicator of health status and possible neglect. Fungal infections are common in older people. Thickened misshapen toenails can be either the processes of ageing or chronic peripheral vascular disease.
7. Urine-stained clothing and/or smell of urine or faeces could be indicative of urinary tract infection and/or incontinence caused by underlying pathology. This area will be discussed in depth later in the chapter. ❶ Sudden onset urinary incontinence should be actively investigated; particularly in the elderly, it can be an indicator of physical disease. ❶ Always consider polypharmacy as a predisposing cause of symptomology in the older adult.

Communication

The initial greeting between nurse and patient can yield much information to guide the consultation process. The manner and tone of voice used in the initial greeting can be assessed for its quality, pace and articulation. Clues may be elicited which indicate underlying depression or confusion, which may require further exploration. These conditions will be discussed in more depth later in the chapter.

The normal ageing process can affect an individual's ability to communicate effectively with others. It is therefore essential for the NP to establish as early as possible in the consultation what the difficult areas may be and adapt the approach and environment to the situation accordingly.

Deafness

Up to 60% of people over the age of 70 suffer from impaired hearing. This is known as presbycusis and patients have a high tone hearing loss. You will therefore need to adapt your consultation accordingly. This may mean positioning your chair and speaking slowly and clearly so that the patient can read your lips. You may also find it helpful to write things down.

Subjective assessment

- Difficulty hearing whispered words

- Difficulty with consonants in conversational speech
- Responds to questioning in a rather loud voice
- Asks you to repeat some or all of your questions
- Seems to give slightly inappropriate responses.

Objective assessment

Testing for hearing acuity may include:
- voice test
- Weber's test
- Rinne test
- visual inspection external auditory meatus.
  Otoscopic examination of:
- external canal
- tympanic membrane.

Check the ears for the presence of any wax that may be occluding the tympanic membrane. Wax in the elderly becomes more viscous and the presence of a hearing aid prevents the normal migration of wax from the external auditory canal, causing a conductive hearing loss.

Therapeutic intervention

- If wax is found, consider whether removal is required.
- If no wax is found, but hearing is impaired, refer for audiometry.
- Often patients have been supplied with hearing aids but they forget to switch them on, turn them up or even wear them in the first place. Check the earpiece is correctly inserted into the ear and that the patient is aware of how to clean, maintain, access and replace the batteries.

Deafness can lead to social isolation, which in turn can lead to deterioration in the health of the individual: hence, the importance of correct diagnosis and management of the condition.

Eyesight

The visual acuity of the older patient usually declines gradually over a period of months or even years, causing increasing problems for the individual.

Common causes of visual impairment in the elderly are:
- cataracts
- acute glaucoma
- macular degeneration.

The loss of or reducing visual acuity can impact greatly on the older person's ability to function in his home environment and the wider community. The person with impaired vision is at greater risk of accidents, especially in the home, from falls and scalds. Social isolation arising from no longer being able to drive can lead to poor nutritional status caused by the associated problems with shopping and food preparation.

Subjective assessment

Questioning is aimed at establishing the nature and extent of any visual disturbances. All older adults should be encouraged to have regular eye inspections via the optician. This will ensure management of failing visual acuity and the identification of more severe eye disease and underlying pathology see Chapter 5 (Referral to an ophthalmologist will be in line with recommendations in Chapter 5.)

1. Decreasing acuity
2. Blurred vision
3. Diplopia
4. Strabismus
5. Pain
6. Discharge
7. Irritation
8. Watering.

Objective assessment

1. How often their eyes are tested/date of last test
2. Previous history of glaucoma/cataracts/surgery/infection
3. Use of glasses/other visual aids.

Physical examination will be dictated by patient response to questioning, but will include some or all of the following:
- visual acuity
- visual fields
- extraocular muscle function
- visual inspection of eyebrows, eyelids, eyelashes, eyeballs, conjunctiva and sclera, cornea and lens and iris and pupils
- pupillary light reflex
- accommodation
- fundoscopy to inspect optic disc, general background, retinal vessels and macula.

Plan

Once a diagnosis has been established, management of the older patient with visual/hearing problems should include:
- effect on health/lifestyle
- potential benefits versus risks of interventions
- safety
- use of aids/appliances/adaptations
- social support networks
- patient choice
- patient compliance.

Mobility

Impaired mobility is defined as (Mosby 1995):

> *a state in which an individual experiences a limitation of ability for independent physical movement*

The NP should not underestimate the effect a change in mobility can have on an individual's health status. The gradual ageing process is slow and insidious in nature, therefore allowing individuals time to adapt to the effects. They often don't present for assessment until they can no longer adapt and cope and they have developed problems with lifestyle and activities of daily living.

Loss of mobility in the elderly can be due to a range of physical, psychological, environmental and social factors or it can be caused by an acute illness episode. As individuals age there are changes to the physiology of all the systems of the body, predisposing them to certain diseases such as arthritic conditions, osteoporosis, polymyalgia rheumatica, etc. Ageing can also lead to changes in the signs and symptoms of other diseases; for example, infection in older adults may present with confusion, falling and reduced mobility without clear indication of a site of infection.

The purpose of assessment is to identify the cause and establish the effect on the individual's lifestyle and activities of daily living. There will, of course, be some problems identified in the assessment that are not easily amenable to intervention or improvement but there will also be others where simple measures can be very effective.

The main causes of mobility problems in the elderly are:
- pain
- weakness
- stiffness
- sensory loss
- imbalance
- psychological.

Subjective assessment

Pain

- Do you ever suffer problems with pain?
- Is it present all the time?
- If not, when does it occur?
- Where exactly is the pain?
- Do you get it anywhere else?
- How long have you had it?
- Does anything make it better/worse?
- Does it wake you at night?
- Can you describe the pain to me?
- Have you tried or are you taking any medication for the pain?
- How much does it help?
- Are you taking any other tablets or medicines?
- Does the affected area swell when you have the pain?
- Does the affected area ever look reddened or feel hot to the touch?

Weakness/stiffness

- How would you describe your appetite/diet?
- Have you lost/gained weight recently?
- Do you wear dentures/attend a dentist?
- Do you experience any difficulty with bathing, toileting, dressing, grooming, eating, shopping, etc?
- Do you have any aids or appliances to help you with walking/bathing/cooking, etc?

Sensory loss

- Have you noticed any change in your eyesight/hearing recently?

- Do you have glasses/hearing aid?
- Do you wear them?
- If not, why not?
- When did you last have your sight/hearing tested?
- Do you drive?

Imbalance

- Have you had any falls recently?
- Do you ever suffer from dizzy spells or feel unsteady?
- Have you noticed a change in the distance you are able to walk?
- Do you have any problems negotiating stairs or steps?
- Are you able to get out of the house when you want to?
- If not, why not?
- Do you suffer with foot pain or discomfort?
- Do you have problems getting suitable footwear?
- Do you attend a chiropodist?

Psychological

- Have you become isolated?
- Do you live alone?
- Do you have family/friends nearby?
- Can you describe your sleep pattern for me?
- What are your hobbies/interests?

Objective assessment

Physical examination of the older adult with mobility problems will depend on presenting symptoms, general observations and responses to questioning. It may include some or all of the following:
- baseline observations, including temperature, pulse, blood pressure, routine urinalysis, weight and height
- musculoskeletal assessment (see Chapter 12)
- neurological assessment (see Chapter 11)
- respiratory assessment (see Chapter 7)
- cardiovascular assessment (see Chapter 8)
- psychological assessment (see Chapter 16).

Assessment of the above systems will require the NP to utilise basic examination skills pertinent to the system of the body, along with knowledge of the pathophysiology of ageing.

Mental status

The mental health status of an individual does not necessarily change as they age; however, there are natural physiological changes such as reduction in blood flow to the brain, changes in the neurotransmitter levels and sensory deficit that can effect mental functioning.

The older adult is more prone to memory impairment, which can range from minor forgetfulness to total inability to retain information; reduced ability to process new information; and depression.

Mental health status should always form part of the holistic assessment of an older person because:

- a change in mental health status can be the first indication of underlying physical illness
- a change in mental health status can render the individual unable to maintain a safe environment for themselves
- treatment regimes have to be developed, taught, managed and monitored with any deficit in mental functioning in mind.

Confusion, dementia syndromes and depression are frequent mental health conditions that the older adult present with. For more in-depth information on the assessment process refer to the section on confusion and dementia in this chapter and Chapter 16 on mental health.

Iatrogenic disease

Any NP involved in the assessment of older people should always be aware of the possibility of iatrogenic disease. Polypharmacy is often found to be present. The changes in the rate of drug absorption, distribution, metabolism and elimination coupled with changes in physical and mental ability, and an understanding of drug interactions, dosage and timing can have a major impact on health status. Common signs and symptoms seen in the elderly, such as dizziness, confusion, constipation, urinary problems and frequent falls, can all be indicative of adverse drug reactions or incorrect dosage and administration. It is therefore essential that any assessment of older people incorporates a careful review of all medication. This must be sure to include any over-the-counter (OTC) medication and/or alternative therapies, which are both being increasingly used by all age groups. The next three sections on falls, incontinence and confusion will discuss issues regarding polypharmacy and iatrogentic disease and their implication in these symptoms.

A patient presenting following a fall

Older adults are at an increased risk of falling for a variety of reasons, added to which they are at greater risk of sustaining injury from that fall. As people grow older a fall can have a serious effect on both their physical and psychological well-being and independence.

No fall in the elderly should be considered a minor incident, without thorough consideration of the circumstances and the results.

Objective assessment

Questions should be asked which identify:
1. Any loss of consciousness. The patient may not be totally sure if, or how long they lost consciousness and, where possible, a witness view should be obtained.
2. If the fall was preceded by a particular action or movement; for example, while walking or rising from a sitting or laying position, or a twisting movement.

3. Any environmental cause. People's homes have many hazards such as frayed carpets, pets, etc., which are not noticed until the accident, or become an adjunct to failing eyesight or a shuffling gait. *Note*: Falls which occur outside or on another's property may become a legal matter and the notes of the NP may be required as evidence.
4. The person's general state of health prior to the incident: specifically, whether they had suffered symptoms such as
   - dizziness
   - chest pains and or palpitations
   - shortness of breath
   - problems with their vision.
5. Drug history, including prescribed and OTC drugs, and alcohol intake – particularly with the older adult, investigation around how and when medication is taken can identify possible links to the fall.
   ❶ Beware of the patient who tells you: 'I must have tripped'; this can indicate that they have no idea of what happened.
   ❶ Examination of an older person directly following a fall should be aimed at identifying any acute injury.
1. Examine for bony injury: shortening or rotation, dislocation, pain, poor coordination of movement. ❶ It is not unheard of for an elderly person to walk on a fractured leg!
2. Muscular injury: pain, limited movement and weakness. Remember to consider any pre-existing disease and or disability such as arthritis, previous cerebrovascular accident.
3. Neurological examination should be completed, to identify a head injury.
4. Skin for lacerations and or underlying damage. An older person is predisposed to pressure injury and care should be taken to identify areas which could have received sufficient pressure or friction to compromise the blood supply to the skin surface and its underlying structures. ❶ Such damage may be obvious at presentation; however, the damage sustained may only become evident 24–48 hours following the fall. Knowledge of the length of time the person spent on the floor will give some indication of risk.

Following assessment and treatment for any injuries sustained in the fall, a more indepth investigation should be commenced to identify any causative factors. This may not occur immediately following the fall, but should be within a few days.

The history surrounding the fall may lead you to suspect the cause; however, the signs and symptoms of illness or disease often become less obvious in older adults. Instability and or reduction in mobility leading to a fall, may be the first indication that something is wrong. Often there is no one cause but a combination of one or more of the following could be the basis for the problem. Physiological, psychological, functional and environmental reasons should all be considered.

General appearance. Look for signs of nervousness about walking and, the use of furniture as support while moving from place to place. The lack of concentration or attention to the task may indicate a psychological problem.

Vital signs. These are
- Temperature – infection in older adults can be a cause, but remember there is often a reduction in the body's responses. The mean temperature for an older person is 36.2°C (97.2°F).
- Blood pressure – this should be completed in the lying, sitting and standing position. Older adults can be susceptible to a sudden drop in blood pressure when raising from a lower position, orthostatic hypotension.
- Pulse – older adults are more likely to experience cardiac arrhythmias and conduction disturbances. Common arrhythmias that may precipitate a syncope attack are sick sinus syndrome, Stokes–Adams attacks or atrial fibrillation. Although atrial fibrillation may be tolerated by an older person the majority of the time, if ventricular response rate exceeds 60 to 90 beats per minute, serious cardiovascular compromise can result. This arrhythmia is also implicated in the formation of thrombi.

Cardiovascular assessment. This should include cardiac auscultation for further possible identification of arrhythmia, peripheral circulation, peripheral pulses, perfusion, oedema, ulceration.

Central nervous system assessment. Assess for
- Any weakness that may indicate a cerebrovascular accident.
- Peripheral neuropathy, including proprioception joint-position, and vibration sense should be performed.
- Extrapyramidal symptoms of Parkinson's disease are commonly seen, but care to distinguish these symptoms from drug-induced side effects is vital.
- Balance, including a Romberg test: an individual should be able to stand still with their eyes closed and feet together; if they sway or fall, they have a positive Romberg's sign, which is not normal at any age, and further investigation is required.
- Dizziness is a common complaint and has many causes, but attempts must be made to eliminate the more serious causes of such a symptom.
- History of the fall from a witness is often needed to rule out epilepsy as a cause.

Disorders of balance and disruption of gait can have either a neurological or musculoskeletal cause; thorough history taking and examination is needed to establish the cause.
1. Musculoskeletal:
   - Examine for joint deformity and pain often found in older adults, caused by osteoarthritis and rheumatoid arthritis. Diabetes or syphilis can also cause severely deformed joints but is often painless.
   - Muscle wasting may also be a cause of falling in the elderly and, in turn, can indicate disease processes such as thyrotoxicosis, osteomalacia, malignant disease or electrolyte abnormalities.
   - Problems with basic foot care can easily develop in older adults due to reduced flexibility. This in turn can lead to painful and debilitating conditions of the feet and nails.
2. Psychological:
   - Screen for depression and or anxiety; these conditions can particularly affect concentration levels.
   - Screen for poor memory and cognitive ability. Dementia also predisposes individuals to falling due to its effect on perception.
3. Review of all medication:
   - consider drugs that can cause postural hypotension, or those which effect the level of consciousness
   - consider nutritional and/or fluid intake.

Plan

1. Following assessment, decide on possible cause(s) of the fall
2. Investigate for any underlying pathology
3. Refer to other professionals where appropriate
4. Consider safety with the patient.

Investigations

Investigations that may be required include full blood count (FBC), erythrocyte sedimentation rate (ESR), random or fasting blood glucose level, thyroid function, liver function, urea & electrolytes (U&E), and midstream specimen of urine (MSU) for culture and sensitivity to exclude underlying pathology or presence of infection.

An electrocardiogram (ECG), a 24-hour ambulatory ECG, is often more appropriate due to the intermittent nature of arrhythmias.

Calcium blood levels should be taken, as hypercalcaemia can induce episodes of confusion and may also indicate underlying malignant disease.

Vitamin B_{12} level should be checked if FBC reveals abnormalities, and vitamin B_1 level and serology for syphilis.

Drug toxicity screening should be carried out as appropriate.

Therapeutic interventions

This will be dependent on the findings of your assessment and the level of functional ability of the individual you are assessing.
- Treatment of underlying pathology is the first priority.
- A home visit should be considered. This can give the NP an opportunity to discuss practical problems with the patient in his own environment. It can highlight potential hazards and give insight into how the individual is coping in general.

Patient education

Actions required to prevent further falls depend considerably on the identified cause. Where found, physical causes can be treated; however, standard advice can be given to all older adults to reduce risk of falls and should include:

1. Regular eye test.
2. Use of appropriate aids for confident movement, e.g. a stick or frame, rails in the house.
3. Proper footwear and regular podiatry.
4. Advice about environmental hazards, e.g. poor lighting, cluttered living space and special care when pets are running around the home.
5. Regular exercise to improve and maintain muscle strength and balance.
6. Teaching a person how to react after a fall and how to get up from the floor can give an individual a sense of control and, therefore, confidence. The involvement of carers in this education can also prevent further complications. The first response by carers is often to rush in and get the person up following a fall, thus risking further damage to the fallen person and injury to the carer.
7. Information on call systems that can summon help if required can also be supplied.

The fear of falling again can increase a persons risk and or reduce their independence. Measures to help individuals gain confidence is an important step to reducing reoccurrence.

Referral

Other professionals to which referral may be appropriate include:

■ specialists appropriate to the identified underlying cause, or a specialist in geriatric medicine where a complicated picture or repeated falling occurs
■ an occupational therapist, who can advise on adaptation and equipment around the home to aid safe independent living
■ a physiotherapist, to advise on exercise to improve and maintain posture and balance
■ a community psychiatric nurse may be required to assess the degree of mental impairment
■ social services may have a role in the provision of home help support or the provision of aids for people with sensory impairment.

A combination of the above may be needed.

Complications

■ Fear of losing independence or 'being put in a home' can lead to an older person being reluctant to reveal to the true extent of a problem.
■ Difficulty in adapting to different ways of completing activities of daily living.
■ Reluctance to accept help from others, be they statutory or volunteer services.

Falls in the older adult, whether they result in injury or not, warrant some investigation. Appropriate information and support following a fall can help maintain an individual's independence and reduce the fear of falling in the future.

Urinary incontinence

Incontinence remains a taboo subject for many. For some older adults it continues to be considered a part of growing older and is often not reported. Using questions to encourage the reporting of urinary symptoms should form part of any consultation with older adults.

Incontinence is not a normal part of ageing. There may be predisposing functional and pathological factors, which contribute to loss of bladder control within the ageing body, but often these can be treated or at least managed to lessen the impact on the person's lifestyle. For men, urinary symptoms ranging from hesitancy, frequency, urgency, poor flow and loss of continence can be the result of an enlarging prostate gland. This can either be benign or malignant, and the priority is to identify the cause and treat or refer appropriately. Women can experience loss of continence that results from changes in oestrogen levels, loss of muscle tone around the vaginal area or poor vascular profusion. Women may also have sustained damage to the pelvic floor muscles through child-bearing, which is often left untreated and exacerbates with the age-related changes.

Age-related changes, that can contribute to urinary incontinence include decreased elasticity and compliance of the bladder wall, resulting in reduced bladder capacity. Detrusor muscle stability, which is required for effective urinary storage, can be reduced due to normal age-related changes in the cerebral cortex and the spinal reflex arc.

Loss of continence in the older adult is often a symptom of underlying illness or disease. It is not a disease in itself. Common causes of incontinence include:

■ infection
■ diabetes
■ dementia
■ depression
■ cerebrovascular disease
■ neurological problems
■ drug therapy, such as sedatives, phenothiazines and diuretics
■ any disease process causing either mental confusion, or loss of functional ability, mobility, dexterity of finger movement and pain.

The most common forms of incontinence found in the elderly are now considered.

Stress incontinence. This is identified as an unintentional loss of urine during episodes of increased intra-abdominal pressure, such as coughing or laughing, or during physical exertion. For an older person this may occur when getting up from a chair or walking upstairs.

Urge incontinence. Also known as detrusor instability, urge incontinence is identified by the strong and uncontrollable urge to pass urine. If this cannot be immediately fulfilled, urinary leakage will occur. Detrusor overactivity, poor bladder storage and uncontrolled bladder contraction are responsible.

Mixed urinary incontinence. This is a combination of the symptoms of both stress incontinence and urge incontinence.

Overflow incontinence. Urine leaks from the bladder without the patient having the desire to void. This results from a distended bladder. A range of causes can result in impaired contractility of the bladder or outlet obstruction. Drugs, constipation, diabetic neuropathy, spinal cord injury or prostatic hyperplasia are just a few causes to consider.

Functional incontinence. This is urinary leakage due to external factors. Environmental barriers, drugs which effect functioning, immobility or poor dexterity can all contribute to this form of incontinence.

The treatment varies with the type of incontinence, and an holistic assessment and thorough examination is required to be able to develop a care plan tailored for the individual's ability and lifestyle.

Subjective assessment

1. Staining on clothes may be noticed when the patient attends the surgery for other reasons.
2. Noticeable odour of urine or faeces on clothing or in the house, if on a home visit.
3. Giving up outside activities or making excuses for having a home visit rather than coming to the surgery.

Objective assessment

A full assessment of an individual presenting with incontinence will not and should not be completed in one visit but, over time, all the below should be completed:

1. General assessment should include mobility, noting any difficulty in movement, difficulty with undressing, tremor or weakness in the hand movements.
2. The patient should be asked to keep a record over a period of 7 days of the following:
   - how much they drink
   - what they drink
   - when they drink
   - when they go to the toilet
   - when they are incontinent.
   A carer should be encouraged to complete this record if the patient is unable.
3. Full past medical history, including obstetric and gynaecological history.
4. Current medical problems.

5. Drug therapy – with particular consideration of diuretics, phenothiazines or sedative use.
6. Functional assessment – use of an 'activities of daily living' rating scale is often useful; reduced ability in one or more of these activities can potentiate incontinence problems.
7. Abdominal assessment, identifying any palpable bladder, kidney tenderness, general abdominal distension or areas of tenderness.
8. Neurological assessment, particularly of the lower extremities, noting any deficit in reflexes or sensation.
9. Rectal examination to identify any constipation. *For men*, the size, shape and contours of the prostate gland should be assessed when performing a rectal examination. Benign prostatic hyperplasia increases in prevalence in men from 55 years of age (Hunter et al 1994). A normal prostate will be felt on rectal examination as a rounded heart-shaped structure with two lobes either side of the sulcus. The presence of benign prostatic hyperplasia will produce findings of a symmetrically enlarged gland, smooth, slightly elastic, but the sulcus may be lost. A gland that displays an area of hardness, irregularity or extension beyond the gland is indicative of possible malignancy. There are other causes of a hard prostate such as calculi – also a negative examination, but where urinary symptoms are present can indicate lesion on the anterior surface – which cannot be felt.
   There are various scoring systems that can be used to assess the severity of urinary symptoms, e.g. the American Urological Association (AUA) symptom index for benign prostatic hyperplasia (Barry et al 1992).
10. *For women*, pelvic examination, noting any prolapse of the rectum, uterus or bladder, general health of the skin and muscles of the vagina and surrounding area. Assessment of the muscle tone and strength can be performed; see Further reading for the specific techniques. Use of the Oxford grading system can be used for monitoring change (Laycock 1991).
11. Psychological assessment – this should include assessment of memory and cognitive function as well as the psychological effect that having urinary problems is having on the individual. Social life, sexual relationships and individual self-esteem can all be affected.

Plan

- Identification of any underlying pathological or psychological cause
- Decide with the patient the review periods that will best support him as an individual
- Devise with the patient a personalised treatment plan
- Discuss with the patient the immediate practical issues suffered by him with continence problems

- Provide practical advice concerning special clothing or contact with a professional who can.

Investigations

Listed here are a range of investigations that may be appropriate. Which ones are undertaken and in what order will be based on the symptoms and history of the patient. The first two however, should be automatic.

1. Routine urinalysis to exclude urinary tract infection (UTI), which is often asymptomatic in the older adult. It is essential to test for nitrites and leucocytes. A positive result for both or either in an asymptomatic patient should be followed up with an MSU to isolate the organism and guide appropriate antibiotic therapy.
2. Random or fasting blood glucose, U&E and thyroid function, and prostate-specific antigen (PSA) for men.
3. Urinary stress test (observation of the urethra for urinary leakage as the patient coughs).
4. Post-void residual urine measurement.
5. An ultrasound scan may be useful for pre- and post-micturition assessment of the bladder.
6. Further investigations that may be required will be completed after referral to a specialist and include:
   - urodynamic assessment (test to measure the pressure and urine flow)
   - cystoscopy
   - prostatic biopsy.

Therapeutic interventions

Treatment will be decided on the findings of the assessment and on the individual's mental and physical health status. There are a range of interventions that can be utilised, including

- bladder retraining
- muscle strengthening
- medication
- surgery
- use of equipment and special clothing to reduce the impact of the problem.

Patient education

1. Discuss with the patient the time period it takes to benefit from some of the interventions, particularly bladder retraining and pelvic floor exercises. These can take weeks and months of work and dedication by the patient before results are seen. False expectations can lead to poor treatment compliance.
2. The need to drink 1–2 litres of fluid per day; older adults often reduce their intake in the belief that this will reduce their need to go to the toilet. This often potentiates the problem and increases the incidence of infection.
3. Avoid alcohol, tea and coffee, all which stimulate the bladder: in particular, prior to going to bed.
4. Avoid constipation by eating a healthy diet high in fibre and with fresh fruit and vegetables and avoid

medication that can cause constipation, where possible.
5. Advice on weight reduction if appropriate.
6. Give help and advice to aid the patient to stop smoking. Coughing places a strain on the pelvic floor muscles.
7. Information and instruction on pelvic floor exercises can reduce the incidence of incontinence and should be encouraged to be part of every woman's fitness regime.

Referral

Incontinence can often be successfully managed in general practice using the skills of the primary health care team members. The intervention selected has as much to do with the attainment of quality of life in the elderly as the diagnosis of the cause of the incontinence. According to the decided treatment plan some patients will require the services of one or more of the following. There may also be continence clinics run by any one of the below, from which a comprehensive service is available:

- Every patient should have regular follow-up appointments with a professional who has knowledge in the treatment of incontinence
- Urologist – for the assessment of surgical intervention and which is paramount for men where malignancy is suspected
- Continence advisor – an excellent source of information and support with difficult or complicated problems
- Physiotherapist – for pelvic floor strengthening, using weights or stimulation
- District nurse – for the provision of incontinence pads, or assessment equipment for such as commodes or raised toilet seats
- Social services – for help in the home with social care needs.

Complications

- Psychological barriers to continuing normal activities: some individuals find it difficult living with the problem
- Physical disability: this can increase the patient's dependence and reliance on others to maintain their continence
- Social isolation
- Skin problems
- Depression.

Confusion and dementia

Introduction

Confusion in older adults is the most common psychiatric presentation. It is, however, not common for the patients themselves to present complaining of confusion as a symptom. Confusion or forgetfulness will either be reported by a second person, or it will become apparent during a consultation on another problem.

What is confusion?

A medical dictionary definition of confusion (Churchill Livingstone 1990) is:

A mental state, which is out of touch with reality and associated with a clouding of consciousness

First, it is important to distinguish if the person is suffering an acute confusional state, or whether this is part of an ongoing mental deterioration: in other words, a dementia syndrome.

Subjective assessment

The aim is to look and listen for information, which will give an idea of the duration of the presenting problem. Some of these questions may require to be put to a person who knows the patient, or a consultation at the patient's house may be required to gain a full picture of the situation. At all times the issue of patient confidentiality must be respected.

- Is the patient able to give a history?
- Is there evidence of longer-term poor hygiene e.g. dry scaly skin with ground-in dirt?
- Are clothes poorly maintained and are they appropriate for the weather conditions?
- Is there staining from urine or faeces on the clothes?
- Is the house tidy and warm?
- Is there evidence of poor compliance with medication e.g. half-used bottles of the same medication?
- Is there alcohol use in evidence?
- Does the patient look unwell?
- What was the patient like yesterday, a week ago, and 2 months ago?
- Does the patient look as if they have lost weight recently? Is there evidence of food in the house?

Once it has been established or highly suspected to be a new episode of acute confusion, the following actions will need to be considered. These actions should also be considered where an older person who is known to have a dementia illness suddenly deteriorates or shows extreme changes in their behaviour.

Acute confusion

There are many causes of acute confusional state, and conditions which can lead to coma may begin with a confusional state. Some of the more common causes, all of which the elderly are particularly at risk from, include:

- infection within the central nervous system (a priority to exclude)
- infection within any other system
- trauma to the head
- stroke
- metabolic disorders, i.e. diabetes, thyrotoxicosis, electrolyte imbalance
- drug effects.

Objective assessment

1. General examination: complete an all-over assessment of the patient, particularly looking for pain or bruising, indicating the patient may have fallen. Examine the head for external signs of possible head injury.
2. Vital signs: the patient's temperature may range from low, below 35°C, (hypothermia in the elderly is a significant risk to health) to high, 38°C plus. Remember, however, an older person's immune system may be less effective and the patient's normal temperature may be lower than 37°C. The mean temperature for older adults is 36.2°C. This leads to less of a temperature rise even in the presence of infection. ❶ Temperature control in older adults may not be a reliable indicator of disease, i.e. hypothermia, infection.
3. Examine the respiratory system to identify infection or the effects of heart failure.
4. Complete a neurological assessment, taking care to examine the patient for signs of infection of the central nervous system. Meningitis is not only an illness of the young.
5. Abdominal assessment should be completed, assessing for abdominal masses, constipation and tenderness around the bladder or kidneys.

Confusion may cause the patient to be hostile and or frightened. The patient may not be compliant with one or any of the above. It is then up to the NP to use all her observational skills to the full.

Plan

- To gain as much knowledge about the individual as possible to aid diagnosis
- To ensure the safety of the patient while they are under your care
- To work with relevant others to ensure reoccurrence of crises situations is minimised
- To give support to the patient and carer.

Investigations

- BM stick to test blood glucose level and dipstick urine for blood, protein, nitrites and leucocyte esterase may be the first and easiest investigations to obtain.
- Essential tests are FBC, ESR, random or fasting blood glucose level, thyroid function, liver function, U&E and calcium. MSU for culture and sensitivity to exclude underlying pathology or presence of infection may be carried out, although this may not be easy to obtain.
- According to medication, drug toxicity screening may be applicable.
- A skull X-ray if there is suspicion of a head injury.

Therapeutic interventions

- Give a slow and clear explanation to the patient of each step you take. It is not always clear as to how much the patient understands. Never assume.

- Relatives and friends will need as much support and explanation in this situation as the patient.
- Treatment should be appropriate to the identified underlying cause.

Referral

To whom a referral is made will depend on the suspected diagnosis and the risk of the situation:

- A new episode of acute confusion, with no obvious cause should be referred to hospital as a medical emergency.
- If the underlying cause of the confusion is diagnosed as an obvious infection it may be relevant to treat at home. This, however, will be depend on the severity of the patient's condition, whether he lives alone and on any other coexisting pathology.
- District nurses can provide advice and support to the family and carers regarding nursing care. Rapid response teams may also be able to provide intensive home nursing for a 24–48 hour period.
- Social services will provide home care support or placement in residential care.

Patient and or carer education

- A change in a person's mental condition is a frightening experience for both the patient and the carer. Support and advice on the condition is imperative.
- Maintenance of hydration is important: reluctance to drink is often associated with older adults and, during illness, this is often a key issue.

Complications

- The safety of the patient is the clear aim. It is sometimes the case that treatment is refused or is difficult to administer with the confused patient. The use of other members of the primary health care team should be considered.
- In some situations, sections of the Mental Health Act may need to be used, and the appropriate members of the medical team approached.

Dementia

Dementia is a progressive, degenerative disease that has a profound effect on the individual's memory and cognitive and intellectual functioning. This disease increases in prevalence with age: figures released by the Alzheimer's Society in 1997 set the prevalence in the UK at 1 in 20 for the 70–80 year old and 1 in 5 for those over 80 years of age. It has been recognised that with the growing number of older people living into their eighth and ninth decade, the numbers of people suffering from dementia and needing support is set to increase further.

There are many causes of dementia syndromes, but this chapter will only touch on the two most common seen in the older adult: Alzheimer's disease and multi-infarct dementia.

Subjective assessment

1. As mentioned before in this section, general appearance may give clues to how the patient is coping with activities of daily living, e.g. clothing, hygiene, etc.
2. Is there evidence of weight loss, i.e. clothes not fitting properly.
3. Has the patient presented with health problems that could be due to poor compliance with medication?
4. Is the patient vague about the reasons he has visited you?
5. Often a relative may come with the patient and answer questions for the patient, or correct the information the patient has given. Relatives can often compensate for the patient's failing mental ability, without realising to what extent they are doing so.
6. Ask the patient how he feels about his memory.
7. How does he cope with shopping, etc?
8. Does he go out with friends or to clubs or socialise in any way?

Objective assessment

1. Assessment of memory and cognitive function: there are various assessment tools that can be used by the NP during a consultation. The most common and widely used by professionals as a brief mental status test is the mini-mental state examination (Folstein et al 1975). However, care has to be taken and scores adapted in those patients with sensory impairment (Reischies & Geiselmann 1997).
2. Assessment of activities of daily living can also inform the NP of the level of disability. Use of an assessment tool such as the Bristol activities of daily living scale (BADLS: Bucks et al 1996) can aid in diagnosis, monitoring of change and care planning. It should be considered, however, that individuals may possibly be unrealistic about what they can do and confirmation by a family member or close friend is ideal.
3. General physical assessment: vital signs and weight. As well as looking for any underlying pathology, which could be affecting the individual, it is appropriate to obtain good baseline information. As this disease progresses, changes in health need to be based on this information, as patients may become unable to give information about themselves.
4. Multi-infarct dementia is more noticeable by its stepped deterioration. An individual often displays upper motor neurone signs, and following each small stroke there is deterioration in mental and physical functioning. These patients often have a history of
   - high blood pressure
   - angina
   - heart attacks
   - peripheral vascular disease.
5. A home visit may also clarify a situation and the true level of ability. People can continue to live independently with fairly severe mental impairment undetected by outsiders for some time.

Plan

- With the patient and his carer, discuss the issues surrounding his immediate and long-term care
- Give information about support services available
- Ensure planned review and evaluation of care takes place
- Ensure honesty but sensitivity and appropriate timing when giving information.

Investigations

Blood screening, as suggested above, could be relevant according to symptoms; in addition, a serology test for syphilis.

Therapeutic interventions

1. Treatment and monitoring of blood pressure. The progress of multi-infarct dementia can be greatly influenced by good management of blood pressure.
2. Encourage and provide help with smoking cessation.
3. Use of aspirin as antithrombotic therapy is used with multi-infarct dementia; however, there is still limited evidence of its effectiveness.
4. A clear plan of action and support should be established that involves the community psychiatric services, the primary health care team and social services.
5. It is important that a key contact for the carer is established from the multidisciplinary team: a person who gets to know the patient and the family and who the family can access when they need advice.
6. A plan of regular review should be established, so that additional or different help can be instituted and new problems dealt with appropriately and quickly.
7. Management of regular time off and respite should be planned with the carer and patient.

Patient and carer education

1. Ensure that the patient and their carer are aware of their rights and entitlements and how to access information about those rights.
2. Education about the symptoms and how to deal with them can be given to empower and support the patient. However, as the disease progresses, the carer will possibly need information on a range of topics and their management:
   - dealing with incontinence
   - nutrition
   - use of medication
   - moving and handling
   - dealing with aggressive behaviour
   - coping with stress
   - legal issues.
3. Identification of appropriate support groups.

Referral

- Consultant psychiatrist
- Community mental health team
- District nursing service
- Social services
- Voluntary organisations.

Often, all of the above have a role to play in the care and support of an individual with dementia and his family. It is important that that care is coordinated. If all of these agencies work individually, it can cause confusion and frustration for the sufferer and his family and result in ineffective care. This, more than any other health problem, requires collaborative working.

Complications

The very nature of dementia will render the individual to require supervision and support on a continuum from the moment that they are diagnosed to their eventual death. The physical and mental symptoms that patients suffer, and to what degree, during that process can vary. More and more people suffering from dementia are living at home, supported by family carers in the main. Caring for a loved one 24 hours a day can be a great strain: providing intimate care for a relative who is suffering an illness that often destroys the personality. The dependent may not recognise their husband, son, daughter, for who they are, becoming frightened of them and accusing them of being a stranger in their own home. The person may be incontinent, may wander at night and at times become aggressive.

For the family there is often a total change of family life. Individual carers may have to give up work. They may find it hard to maintain a social life because (1) mum or dad cannot be left alone or (2) friends stop visiting because of the embarrassment of not knowing what to say to the older person, particularly when inappropriate antisocial behaviour is demonstrated. Where a person is living in a family unit, the effect that the situation has on the children must also be considered.

Elder abuse

Introduction

Abuse of older adults is a subject that health care professionals still find hard to address. Child abuse has become high on the list of considerations for those caring for children, with the development of well-defined actions to be taken when abuse is suspected. The recognition and action to be followed when elder abuse is suspected has yet to reach this organised state. Nurse practitioners are in a position in which older people often tell them intimate details of their lives. The way NPs consult, giving time for the patient to talk, can present the individual with an opportunity to express his feelings and fears unlike any other arena. The opportunity to get to know individuals and their families is one of the privileges that those working in primary care settings are given. With that privilege can come unique responsibilities because of the innermost secrets and fears people divulge, and these may indicate that relationships are under significant stress, which has or could lead to an abusive situation.

There have been several definitions of elder abuse. The Social Services Inspectorate of the Department of Health (1993) adopted the following:

> *Abuse may be described as physical, sexual, psychological or financial. It may be intentional or unintentional or the result of neglect. It causes harm to the older person, either temporarily or over a period of time.*

There is little research into the exact prevalence of elder abuse, due to the complexity of the subject. Ogg & Bennett (1992) identified a prevalence level of 5% for verbal abuse and 2% for physical abuse. However, this is still considered to be an underestimation, owing to the research method.

❶ Professionals who come in to contact with older adults should always be open to the possibility of elder abuse.

This section will not give answers to all the complex issues surrounding the topic but aims only to give some information on which to base further thought around the issue. It intends also to highlight the need for health professionals to be knowledgeable about or to develop policies and procedures within their working areas to deal with cases where abuse is suspected.

Elder abuse can occur wherever older adults are cared for:

- their own home
- a family home
- residential or nursing homes
- hospitals.

Most at risk of being abused are older adults who are physically or mentally dependent on another person.

The types of abuse for which older adults can be subject come under four headings:

- Physical abuse – including physical restraint, the infliction of pain or injury, the treatment of an individual without dignity or privacy and sexual assault.
- Psychological abuse – including verbal abuse, the infliction of emotional distress, intimidation and social isolation.
- Financial abuse – misappropriation of an elder's property or funds and theft.
- Environmental – withdrawal of aids, or activities and inadequate supervision. No provision of choice in daily living, the enforcement of rules and restrictions or lack of adequate supervision (Royal College of Nursing 1996).

Subjective assessment

Features which may alert the professional to suspect abuse (West Sussex County Council 1997):

- sudden or significant changes in the vulnerable person's emotional or physical state
- clear indications of neglect
- unexplained injuries
- failure to maintain adequate care standards
- changes in the carer's emotional or physical state

- any specific allegations of cruelty or abuse
- frequent presentation for medical advice on varied non-specific matters.

It is difficult to cover all factors that may predispose a caring situation to turn abusive, but some key features that have been recognised are:

1. Previous poor or abusive relationships between dependent and care provider.
2. Unstable history of the care provider, including drug or alcohol abuse, or past or present psychiatric disorder.
3. The care provider having to make major changes to their lives to maintain the caring role, which may have necessitated giving up their job and social contacts which, in turn, gives rise to feelings of resentment.
4. Poor living conditions and financial hardship.
5. Poor support from both within the family or from outside agencies.
6. The level of dependency of the older adult: individuals with diseases or disabilities, that affect them from moment to moment, such as dementia or Parkinson's disease, can be misconstrued as 'playing up'; also, individuals whose behaviour is problematic, e.g. incontinence or difficulty with or reluctance to eat.

Plan

Our society has increasingly, over the last few years, moved back to a belief that older adults have a right to be cared for at home. This can, however, lead relatives to feel under an obligation to provide appropriate support.

It must be recognised that not all people have the physical or mental resources to provide care, and being forced into a situation of care provision can severely affect family relationships. The NP must be aware of those patients who consult with her who are in the position of caring for a dependent person or those who are reliant on another for such support. The role of health care professionals should be aimed at preventing abusive situations arising. The following should be provided for any carer:

- Ongoing support and reassessment should be planned to monitor changes in the carer's health, increasing needs of the patient and changes in personal circumstances, all of which can add to the pressure of the situation.
- Patients and carers should be given the opportunity to work with health and social care providers to set clear goals through open and honest discussion about the implications of caring for a dependent person.
- Use of a tool such as the cost of care index (Kosberg & Cairl 1986) can identify potential conflict and allow appropriate care planning, without guilt on behalf of the care provider or inappropriate expectations from care agencies.

Therapeutic interventions

For situations, which have the potential for abuse to occur, the following should be provided:
- give carers time when they need to talk
- give those who are dependent on others for care the same opportunity as anyone else to have a private consultation
- provide information.

When the NP identifies a situation that leads her to believe that abuse has occurred, then she should have a clear understanding of the protocol within the workplace for the reporting of abuse and the action to take.

Patient and or carer education

As indicated in the definition, abuse can be intentional or unintentional. Unintentional abuse is often due to lack of knowledge and understanding of what caring is and what care needs the individual has. This is where input from the NP is essential in ensuring that the care provider has the knowledge and resources to do the job, with the aim that a situation will not become so stressful that abuse occurs.
1. Provide information about the illness and the effect.
2. Provide information about voluntary support groups and self-help organisations.
3. Provide access to information and or teaching on subjects such as
   - nutrition
   - use of medication
   - moving and handling
   - dealing with aggressive behaviour
   - coping with stress.

Referral

- Patients and carers and GPs, according to the situation.
- Social services are often the lead agency when abuse is suspected. The NP should ensure she is fully aware of the protocols in her area. However, in situations where there is a dependent person being cared for, it should be routine that social services are involved.
- Police: who and when they are called is dependent on the situation and local policy.
- District nursing service.
- Community psychiatric team.

Conclusion

The main focus of care by the NP should be to recognise situations that could become abusive. She should be able to plan interventions, support and practical help with the patient, carer and other agencies to protect both the patient and carer from that possibility.

This section is meant only to highlight the issue of abuse. It aims to get NPs to think about the people they care for and the difficulties they face in day to day life. Consider the strain that dependency on others for the

| **Top Tips** | |

1. Accurate assessment of the older adult will often require more than one consultation

2. Do not feel pressured into making decisions about management until you are sure you have all the information you require

3. It is important to remember that our standards for presentation and hygiene maybe quite different from our patients and the fact that they are elderly may have no bearing

4. Up to 60% of people over the age of 70 years suffer from impaired hearing; you will therefore need to adapt your consultation style accordingly

5. The nurse practitioner (NP) should not underestimate the effect that a change in mobility can have on an individual's health and social status

6. Mental health status should always form part of the holistic assessment of an older person

7. Assessment of carers, needs should form part of your treatment plan

8. Any NP involved in the assessment of the older adult should always be aware of the possibility of iatrogenic disease

9. Falls which occur outside or on another's property may become a legal matter and the notes of the NP may be required as evidence

10. Elderly care is often more successfully managed using the skills of the multidisciplinary team

basic things in life can place on individuals and families when involved in care planning.

When abuse is suspected, it becomes a minefield of ethical and legal dilemmas and no one person can deal with the situation. Safety of the patient involved is the priority but what do you do when they do not want action taken? No one person can have the answers. Discuss in your workplace what you would do if the situation arises.

References

Barry M, Fowler F, O'Leary M 1992 The American Urological Association symptom index for benign prostatic hyperplasia. Journal of Urology 148:1549–1557.

Bucks R, Ashworth D, Wilcock G, Siegfried K 1996 Assessment of activities of daily living in dementia: development of the Bristol activities of daily living scale. Age and Ageing 25:113–120.

Churchill Livingstone 1990 In: Roper N (ed), Pocket medical dictionary. Churchill Livingstone, London.

Coni N, Webster S 1998 Lecture notes on geriatrics, 5th edn. Blackwell Science, Oxford.

Folstein M, Folstein S, McHugh P 1975 Mini-mental state: a practical method for grading the cognitive status of patients for the clinician. Journal of Psychiatric Research 12:189–198.

Hunter D, McKee C, Black N, Sanders C 1994 Urinary symptoms: prevalence and severity in British men aged 55 and over. Epidemol and Community Health 48:569–575.

Kosberg J, Cairl R 1986 Cost of care index: a case management tool for screening informal care providers. The Gerontologist 26(3):273–278.

Laycock J 1991 Pelvic floor re-education for the promotion of continence. In: Roe B (ed) Clinical nursing practice: the promotion of continence. Prentice Hall, London, chapter 5.

Mosby 1995 Mosby Year Book medical encyclopedia for health professionals (available on CD rom). Mosby, St Louis.

Ogg J, Bennett G 1992 Screening for elderly abuse in the community: stress in relatives leading to elder abuse. Geriatric Medicine 22(2):63–64, 66–67.

Reischies F, Geiselmann B 1997 Age-related cognitive decline and vision impairment affecting the detection of dementia syndrome in old age. British Journal of Psychiatry 171:449–451.

Royal College of Nursing 1996 Combating abuse and neglect of older people. RCN guidelines for nurses. Royal College of Nursing, London.

Social Services Inspectorate of the Department of Health 1993 No longer afraid: the safeguard of older people in domestic settings. HMSO, London.

West Sussex County Council 1997 Adults at risk: a multi-agency approach policy, practice guidelines and procedures. West Sussex County Council Social Services, Chichester.

Further reading

Assessment

Jarvis C 1996 Pocket companion for physical examination and health assessment, 2nd edn. W B Saunders, Philadelphia.

Mosby 1995 Mosby's year book medical encyclopedia for health professionals (available on CD rom). Mosby, St Louis.

Woodward P 1998 Physiological ageing: 1. Professional Nurse 8(13):526–532.

Woodward P 1998 Physiological ageing: 2. Professional Nurse 9(13):611–614.

Iatrogenic disease

DeMaagd G 1995 High-risk drugs in the elderly population. Geriatric Nursing September/October:198–206.

Hudson S, Boyter A C 1997 Pharmaceutical care of the elderly. Pharmaceutical Journal October 25(259): 686–690.

Shepherd M. 1998 The risks of polypharmacy. Nursing Times 32(94):60–63.

Incontinence

Button D, Roe B, Webb C, Frith T, Colin-Thome D, Gardner L 1998 Consensus guidelines: continence promotion and management by the primary health care team. Whurr, London.

NHS Centre for Reviews and Dissemination 1995 Effective health care: benign prostatic hyperplasia. University of York and Nuffield Institute for Health, University of Leeds Dec 2(2).

Penn K, Lekan-Rutledge D, Marner Joers A, Stolly J, Vickrey Amhof N 1996 Assessment of urinary incontinence. Journal of Gerontological Nursing January 8:19.

Roe B (ed) 1991 Clinical nursing practice: the promotion of continence. Prentice Hall, London.

Elder abuse

Homer A, Kingston P 1992 Screening by nurse practitioners could prevent elder abuse. Care of the Elderly May:220–222.

Kosberg J, Cairl R, Keller D 1990 Components of burden: interventive implications. The Gerontologist 30(2):236–242.

United Kingdom Central Council (1999) Practitioner – client relationships and the prevention of abuse. UKCC, London.

Falls

South East Institute of Public Health 1998 Guidelines for the prevention of falls in older people. Commissioned by the Health Promotion Division of the Department of Health, London.

Confusion and dementia

Burns A, Lawor B, Craig S 1998 Assessment scales in old age psychiatry. Martin Dunitz, London.

US Department of Health and Human Services 1997 Quick reference guide for clinicians: early identification of Alzheimer's disease and related dementias. Journal of the American Academy of Nurse Practitioners 9(2):85–96.

General to elderly care

Crigger N, Forbes W 1997 Assessing neurological function in older patients: guidelines to help you distinguish effect of ageing from disease. American Journal of Nursing 97(3):37–40.

Department of Health 1999 Caring about carers: a national strategy for carers. HMSO, London.

Weightman G 1999 A real break: Guidelines for the provision of short-term breaks. HMSO, London.

INDEX

Note: References to figures and tables are in bold.

α-adrenergic agonists, 84
α-blockers, 132, 239
α-thalassaemia, 25
Abdominal massage, 144, 145
Abducens nerve, 180–182
Absence seizure, 190
Abuse, elderly, 329–331
Acarbose, 162, 165
Acarus hunt, 40
Accommodation, 69
ACE inhibitors, 55, 130, 132, 133, 162
Acheson report, 6
Achilles reflex, 177
Aciclovir, 310, 311
Acne, 54–55
Acoustic nerve, 183–185
Acquired immune deficiency syndrome *see* AIDS
Acute bronchitis, 104
Acute cholecystitis, 149–150
Acute confusion, 327–328
Acute gastrointestinal haemorrhage, 151
Acute headache, 188, 189
Acute heart failure, 134
Acute labyrinthitis, 87
Acute lymphoblastic leukaemia (ALL), 19
Acute myeloid leukaemia (AML), 19
Acute myocardial infarction, 130–131
Acute otitis media, 85–86
Acute red eye, 70–73
Acute uveitis, 72
Adolescents, 298, 301–302, **303**
AIDS, 223–224
Alcohol, 77, 153, 257
Allergens, 77
Allergic conjunctivitis, 72–73
Allergic contact dermatitis, 43–44
Allergic rhinitis, 89–90
Allopurinol, 208
Alopecia, 38
Alzheimer's disease, 197–198
Amantadine, 106, 193
Aminoglycosides, 85, 86, 315
Aminosalicylates, 152
Amitriptyline, 135
Amoxicillin, 86, 89, 311
Ampicillin, 311
Anaemia, 16–29
Anaesthetic creams, 49
Analgesics, 46, 49, 84, 85, 86, 89, 104, 107, 189, 196, 197, 213, 218, 225, 231, 237
Anatomy, paediatric patients, 299–302
Androgen, 16
Angina, 128–130

Angiography, 127
Angiotensin II antagonists, 132, 133
Ankles, 203, 209–210
Antacids, 129, 153, 155
Anterior chamber, 68
Anterior rhinoplasty, 81, **82**
Anthralin, 46
Antibiotics, 27, 31, 41, 43, 44, 47, 50, 51, 52, 54, 56, 71, 73, 77, 85, 87, 88, 104, 107, 141, 206, 225, 227, 230, 236, 237
Anticholinergics, 84, 90, 102, 103, 193
Anticholinesterase, 198
Anticoagulants, 112, 130, 194, 208
Anticonvulsants, 189, 196
Antidepressants, 49, 58, 163, 189, 234, 236
Antidiarrhoeal agents, 142, 147, 313
Antidiuretic hormones, 234
Antiemetics, 189
Antifibrinolytics, 277
Antifungal agents, 52, 57, 85, 226
Antihistamines, 42, 51, 53, 55–56, 58, 84, 89–90, 310
Antihypertensives, 132
Antimuscarinic drugs, 236
Antiplatelet agents, 194
Antipyretics, 309, 310
Antiseptic/oxidiser soaks, 41, 44
Antispasmodic therapy, 147
Antithrombotic therapy, 329
Antithyroid agents, 167
Antiviral agents, 41, 48, 49, 106, 193, 224, 231, 311
Antiyeast preparations, 53, 56, 57
Anxiolytics, 189
Aplastic anaemia, 28–29
Apomorphine, 193
Appearance, older adults, 319
Appendicitis, 148–149
Aqueous humour, 66
Arthritis, 45, 135, 205, 211–213, 214–216
Ascites, 169
Aspartate aminotransferase (AST), 125
Aspirin, 129, 130, 134, 309, 310, 329
Asthma, 99–101
Atenolol, 162
Atopic eczema, 41–42
Atrial fibrillation, 126
Atrial flutter, 126
Atrophic vaginitis, 224–225
Audiograms, 184
Aural toilet, 85
Auscultation, 98–99, 121–123, 138
Autoimmune thyroiditis, 169
Autonomy, 12
Azathioprine, 215–216
Azoles, 53

β-agonists, 100, 102, 103
β-blockers, 99, 129, 130, 132, 133, 162, 163, 189
β-thalassaemia, 25, 26–27
Bacterial conjunctivitis, 72
Bacterial infections, 38, 73, 84, 88
Bacterial vaginosis, 277–278
Barrier contraceptives, 249–251
Bartholinitis, 225
Basal cell carcinoma, **60**
Basophilic leucocytosis, 29
Bath oil, 41, 44, 46
Beau's lines, 37
Beclometasone, 90
Behavioural change, 10–11
Bell's palsy, 196–197
Bendroflumethiazide (Bendrofluazide), 163
Benign postural vertigo, 185
Benign prostatic hyperplasia (BPH), 238–239, 325
Benzhexol, 193
Betamethasone, 85
Biceps reflex, 177
Bilateral nuclear lesions, 186
Bilateral supranuclear palsy, 186
Biopsies, dermatology, 39–40
Biphasic contraceptives, 245
Bisphosphonates, 218
Blepharitis, 73
Blepharospasm, 183
Blood
    disorders, 16–31
    flow of, 117
    glucose levels, 130, 160, 162, 164, 165
    pressure, 130, 131–132, 162, 323
    tests, 39, 102–103, 125
Blood gas analysis, 103
Body maps, 35
Bouchard's nodes, 211
Bowman's membrane, 70–71
Brachial pulse, 120
Brachial reflex, 177
Breast examinations, 263–265
Breathlessness, 96, 102, 103
Bromocriptine, 193
Bronchiectasis, 108–109
Bronchiolitis, 105
Bronchodilator reversibility, 100, 102
Bronchodilators, 103
Bullae, 38
Bursitis, 205–206

Calamine, 310
Calcium, 218, 262, 323
Calcium antagonists, 132, 189
Calendar method, 255
Campylobacter, 140, 142
Cancer, **60**, 239–240, 274–275
Candida albicans, 37, 56, 223, 225

Candidiasis, 225–226
Captopril, 162
Carbamazepine, 190, 196
Carbimazole, 167
Carbon monoxide gas, 114
Cardiac auscultation, 122–123
Cardiac enzymes, 125
Cardiac murmurs, 123–125
Cardiovascular system, 116–136, 323
Carotid artery TIA, 194
Carotid pulse, 120
Carpal tunnel syndrome, 210–211
Cataract, 75
Catechol-O-methyltransferase
    (COMT), 193
Central nervous system, 223, 323
Central vertigo, 184, 185
Cerebellar ataxia, 174
Cervical cancer, 274–275
Cervical mucus method, 255
Cervical smear test, 270
Cervix, inspections, 270–271
Chemosis, 72
Chemotherapy, 228, 239
Chest examinations, 96–99
Chest pain, 96, 128, 134
Chest X-rays, 102
Chicken pox, 309–310
Chlamydia trachomatis, 225, 226–227,
    231
Chloramphenicol, 71
Chlorphenamine (Chlorpheniramine),
    84, 310
Cholecystitis, 149–150
Choroid, 66
Chronic actinic dermatitis (CAD), **60**
Chronic cholecystitis, 150
Chronic gastrointestinal bleeding,
    151–152
Chronic heart failure, 132–133
Chronic lymphatic leukaemia, 19
Chronic obstructive pulmonary disease
    (COPD), 94–95, 101–104
Chronic pelvic pain, 275
Chronic uveitis, 72
Churg-Strauss syndrome, 110
Ciliary body, 66
Cinnarizine, 87
Clioquinol, 85
Clostridium difficile, 140, 142
Clotrimazole, 85
Clubbing, 99, 119
Cluster headaches, 188, 189
Co-ordination, 174–175
Co-phenotrope, 142
Co-proxamol, 135
Cochlea, 79
Code of Professional Conduct, 282
Codeine phosphate, 142
Colchicine, 207, 208
Colds, 83–84
Collateral ligament injuries, 208–209
Colofac, 147
Colour vision, 179
Combined oral contraceptives,
    244–247, 276, 281
Commodity, health as a, 5

Common cold, 83–84
Communication, older adults, 319
Community profiling, 9
Community-acquired pneumonia, 106
Comparative needs, 6
Compression (RICE), 209
Computed tomography (CT), 103
Condoms, 249–250
Conduction system, 117, 118
Condylomata acuminata, 228–229
Confusion, older adults, 326–328
Congenital hypothyroidism, 169
Conjunctiva, 66, 68
Conjunctivitis, 72–73
Constipation, 142–146
Contact dermatitis, 43–44
Contraception, 243–257
Contraceptive history, 269
Contraceptive products, 54
Cooley's anaemia, 26–27
Cornea, 66, 68, 69, 70–72, 182
Corneal arcus, 119
Coronary artery spasm, 128, 129
Coronary heart disease, 11, 12, 130,
    162
Corticosteroid reversibility, 100, 102
Corticosteroids, 49, 51, 56, 57, 103, 110,
    152, 189, 218, 219
Costochondritis, 134
Coughs, 95–96
Cover test, 69, 181
Coxsackie viruses, 311, 312
Crackles, inspiratory, 98
'Cradle cap', 57
Cranberry juice, 236
Cranial nerves, 177–187
Creatinine kinase (CK), 125
Crepitations, 98
Cromolyns, 90
Croup, 104–105
Cryotherapy, 59
Cryptosporidium, 223
Culture, male health, 12
Cyanosis, 99, 119–120
Cyclo-oxygenase inhibitors, 213
Cyclopentolate, 179
Cystitis, 236–237

Danazol, 277, 281
De Quervain's tenosynovitis, 207
Deafness, 184, 319–320
Decongestants, 84, 89, 90
Dehydration, 140, 142
Delusions, 286–287
Dementia, 197, 198, 328–329
Deoxyribonucleic acid (DNA), 22
Depigmentation, 36
Depo Provera, 248
Dermatitis, 43–44, 56–57, **60**
Dermatoheliosis, **60**
Dermatology, 33–62
Dermatology life quality index (DLQI),
    45, **46**
Dermatomes, 175
Dermographism, 40
Descemet's membrane, 71
Desferrioxamine IV, 27

Desogestrel, 245
DEXA scan, 217
Dextrose, 165
Diabetes mellitus, 120, 130, 159–164
Diabetic retinopathy, 180
Diamorphine, 134
Dianette, 245
Diaphragm (contraceptive), 250
Diarrhoea, 142, 223
Diascopy, 40
Diastolic blood pressure (DBP), 131
Diclofenac, 276, 277
Diet, 20, 22, 153, 162, 257, 262–263
Diffuse parenchymal disease, 109–110
Digestive processes, infancy, 300
Digoxin, 133, 315
Discrimination, neurological
    examinations, 177
Disease modifying antirheumatic drugs
    (DMARDS), 215–216
Disease prevention, 11–12
Distance vision, 179
Diuretics, 133, 207, 280
Dopamine agonists, 193
Drugs
    haemolytic anaemia, 24–25
    older adults, 322, 323
    paediatric patients, 314–316
    preconceptual care, 257
    urticaria, 55
Dry eyes, 74
Dry mouth, 83
Dry powder inhalers, 101
Dydrogesterone, 277
Dysentery, 142
Dysfunctional uterine bleeding,
    276–277
Dyspareunia, 275–276
Dyspnoea, 119

Ear, 78–79, 82, 84–87
Echocardiography, 127–128
Echoviruses, 311, 312
Eczema, 41–43
Efamast, 280
Ejection click, 123
Elderly *see* Older adults
Electrocardiograms, 125–128, 323
Electrocautery, 228
Electrolytes, 125
Electromagnetic spectrum, 65
Elliptical biopsy, 40
Emergency contraception, 251–253
Emollients, 42, 43, 44, 46, 47, 48, 51, 54,
    58
Emphysema, 102, 103
Empowerment, 3, 77, 161
Empyema, 113
Endocardium, 116
Endocrine disorders, 158–170, 217
Endometrial cancer, 274
Endometriosis, 276
Endoscopy, 140
Endothelium, 71
Enemas, 144
Enterovirus infections, 311–313
Enuresis, 233–234

Environment, dermatology assessments, 33
Eosinophilic leucocytosis, 29
Ephedrine, 89
Epicardium, 116
Epididymitis, 237
Epilepsy, 190
Epithelium, 70
Epstein-Barr virus, 30, 310–311
Erectile dysfunction, 163–164, 238
Ergotamines, 189
Erythrocyte sedimentation rate (ERS), 40
Erythrocytes, 16
Erythromycin, 85, 86, 89, 311
Erythropoietin, 16
Escherichia coli, 140, 142, 306
Ethambutol, 108
Ethamyslate, 277
Ethical issues, 12
Evening primrose oil, 280
Exanthem, 311, 313–314
Exercise tests, 100, 127
Expert Patients programme, 11
Expiratory lip pursing, 99
Expressed needs, 5
Extraocular movements, 180–181
Extrinsic allergic alveolitis, 110
Eyelids, 66, 68, 73
Eyes, 65–76, 178–183
Eyesight, older adults, 320

Face, 68, 119
Facial nerve, 183
Facial sensation, 182
Falls, older adults, 322–324
Fasciculation, 183
Fatigue, 159
Felt needs, 5
Female contraception, 250–251, 256
Fevers, 96, 304–309
Fibre, 144, 145, 147
Fibromyomata (fibroids), 272–273
Finger clubbing, 99, 119
Floaters, 74–75
5-flourouracil, 228
Flucloxacillin, 85
Flumethasone, 85
Fluticasone, 90
Folate deficiency, 23
Folic acid, 22, 23, 257
Folliculitis, 227–228
Foreign bodies, corneal, 69, 70–72
Fractures, 216–217
Framycetin, 85
Fronto-temporal dementia, 198
Functional incontinence, 325
Fundoscopy, 179
Fundus, 68
Fungal infections, 51–52, 84
Furosemide (Frusemide), 134
Furunculosis, 85
Fusidic acid, 135

G6PD deficiency, 23–24
Gag reflex, 81, 185
Gait, 174

Gall bladder disease, 149
Gardnerella, 277
Gas transfer studies, 102
Gastroenteritis, 140–142
Gastrointestinal bleeding, 150–152
Gastrointestinal system, 137–156, 223
Genetic defects, haemoglobin, 25–28
Genital warts, 228–229
Genito urinary conditions, 222–240, 278
Gentamicin, 85
Gestodene, 245
Giant cell arteritis, 218–220
Giardia lamblia, 223
Gingiva, 79, 83
Glandular fever, 30, 90, 310–311
Glaucoma, 75, 180
Glibenclamide, 162, 164
Gliclazide, 162
Glossopharyngeal nerve, 185
Glucagon, 165
Glucose-6-phosphate dehydrogenase see G6PD
Glue ear, 86–87
Glyceryl trinitrate, 129, 134
Goitre, 169
Gonadorelin analogues, 277
Gonadotrophin-releasing hormone, 267, 281
Gonorrhoea, 229–230
Gout, 207–208
Gram-negative bacteria, 107
Granulocytes, 29
Grave's disease, 168
Gynaecological system, 267–281
Gynefix, 254

H$_2$ receptor antagonists, 154
Haemoglobin, 16, 20, 300
Haemoglobinopathies, 25–28
Haemolysis, 24
Haemolytic anaemias, 23–25
Haemophilus influenzae, 85, 106, 306
Hair, 38, 49
Halitosis, 83
Hallucinations, 286–287
Hands, cardiac disease, 119
Hayfever, 89–90
Head lice, 49, 50
Head and neck, 77–92
Headache, 187–189
Health models, 4–5
Health of the Nation, The, 6
Health professionals, 10, 330
Health promotion, 3–13, 77
Health protection, 11
Health Skills programme, 11
Healthy Citizens programme, 11
Hearing tests, 184
Heart
    failure, 132–134, 169
    in infants, 300
    as a pump, 116–117
Heberden's nodes, 211
Helicobacter pylori, 152–153, 154
Helping People Change, 9–10
Hemifacial spasm, 183

Heparin, 112
Hepatomegaly, 311
Hereditary haemolytic anaemia, 23–24
Herpes genitalis, 230–231
Herpes simplex, 39, 47–48, 230
Herpes zoster, 39, 48–49
Hirsutism, 38
HIV, 223
Hoarseness, 96
Homozygous disease, 27
Hormonal contraceptives, 244–249, 251–252
Hormone replacement therapy (HRT), 218, 219, 225, 236, 261–262
Hospital-acquired pneumonia, 107
Human immunodeficiency virus see HIV
Human papillomaviruses (HPV), 58, 228
Humerus, 203–204
Hydrochloride, 142
Hydrocortisone, 85
Hydroxocobalamin, 22
Hyperlipidaemia, 162–163
Hyperpigmentation, 52
Hypertension, 12, 131–132, 162
Hypertensive retinopathy, 180
Hyperthyroidism, 166–168
Hypertrophic osteoarthritis, 135
Hypoglossal nerve, 186–187
Hypoglycaemia, 164–166
Hypoglycaemics, 162
Hypostop, 165
Hypothyroidism, 168–170
Hysterectomy, 281

Iatrogenic disease, older adults, 322
Ibuprofen, 206, 277, 309, 313, 314
Imidazole, 57
Immune system, 300
Immunisation, 12, 91
Immunoglobin E (IgE), 40
Immunosuppressive agents, 90, 110, 192
Imodium, 142, 147
Impetigo, 47
Implanon, 249
Implants (contraceptive), 249
Incontinence, urinary, 235–236, 324–326
Indomethicin, 208
Infants, 296–297, 299–300
Infections
    enterovirus, 311–313
    eyelids, 73
    head and neck, 83, 84, 88
    joints, 206
    respiratory tract, 85, 86, 87, 104–113
    sexually transmitted, 223–233
    skin disorders, 38, 39, 47, 48, 51–52, 58
    urinary tract, 236–237, 307–308
Infectious mononucleosis, 30, 90, 310–311
Infertility, 278–279
Inflammation
    eye and eyelids, 72–73
    pelvis, 226–227

Influenza, 90–91, 105–106
Inhaler devices, 101
Injectable contraception, 248–249
Insecticides, 50
Insulin, 162, 164
Insulin-dependent diabetes mellitus (IDDM), 159
Intrauterine contraception, 253–254, 277
Ipratropium, 84, 90
Iris, 66
Iron, 16, 20–21, 27, 273
Irritable bowel syndrome (IBS), 146–148
Isomorphic phenomenon, 38
Isoniazid, 108, 314
Itraconazole, 85
IUD, 253–254
IUS, 254

Jaw, 182
Jendrassik manoeuvre, 177
Joints, 201–202
Jugular veins, 82
Jugular venous pressure, 120–121

Kaolin, 142
Kidneys, 139
King's Fund, 8, 9
Klebsiella, 107
Knees, 202–203, 208–209
Koebner phenomenon, 38

Labyrinthine, 87
Lacrimal apparatus, 66–67
Lactate dehydrogenase (LDH), 125
Lactic acid, 59
Lamotrigine, 190–191
Laryngitis, 87
Laxatives, 144, 145
Lens (eye), 66
Lesions, 35, 36–37, 59–61, 83
Leucocytes, 29–30
Leucocytosis, 29
Leukotriene antagonists, 100
Levodopa, 193
Levonelle-2, 251, 252
Levonorgestrel, 245, 247, 249, 254, 277
Lewy bodies, dementia with, 198
Lice, 49, 50
Life expectancy, males, 11
Lifestyle, 9–10, 12
Light, 65, 181
Light reflex, corneal, 69
Lipoproteins, 162
Lips, 79, 99
Listening, 285–287
Listeria monocytogenes, 306
Lithium, 189
Liver, 139
Lomotil, 142, 147
Loperamide, 142
Lower respiratory tract infections, 104–113
Lungs, 94–95, 111–114
Lymphadenopathy, 311
Lymphatic system, 82, **83**, 99

Lymphocytes, 30
Lymphocytosis, 30
Lymphoid cells, 30
Lymphomas, malignant, 19

M-mode, 128
McBurney's point, 148
Macrocytic anaemia, 22–23
Males
    contraception, 249–250, 256
    genito-urinary conditions, 237–240
    health promotion, 11–12
Malignant lymphomas, 19
Malignant melanomas, **60**
Maslow, hierarchy of needs, 5
Maturity-onset diabetes of youth (MODY), 159
MDI inhalers, 101
Medical histories, preconceptual care, 257
Medication, preconceptual care, 257
Medroxyprogesterone acetate, 248, 277
Mees' lines, 37
Mefenamic acid, 277
Megaloblastic anaemia, 22–23
Melanomas, malignant, **60**
Meningitis, 307
Menopause, 258–265
Menstrual cycle, 267–268
Mental fitness, health as, 4–5
Mental health, 282–293, 321–322
Mental state examinations, 286–287
Mental strength, health as, 5
Mesalazine, 152
Metformin, 162
Methotrexate, 215
Metronidazole, 277
Middle ear, 79
Migraine, 188, 189
Mini mental state examination, 198
'Mini pill', 247–248
Mirena, 277
Mites, 40, 50
Mitral valve, opening snap, 123
Mixed urinary incontinence, 325
Mobility, older adults, 320–321
Monophasic contraceptives, 245
Morbidity, 11
Mortality, 11
Mouth, 77, 79–81, 83
Movement, joints, 201–202
Multiple sclerosis, 191–192
Muscles, pain and weakness, 96
Musculoskeletal disorders, 134, 200–221, 323
MUSE, 164
Mycobacterium tuberculosis, 107, 223
Mycology, 39
Mycoplasma genitalium, 231
Mycoplasma pneumoniae, 106
Mydriatics, 179
Myocardium, 116
Myocrisin, 215, 216
Myokymia, 183
Myotome, 175

Nails, 37
Napkin dermatitis, 56

Naproxen, 208, 277
Narcotics, 189
Nasal flaring, 99
Natural contraception, 254–256
Near vision, 178
Neck, 82
Nedocromil, 90, 100
Needs assessment, 5–9
Neisseria gonorrhoea, 229
Neisseria meningitidis, 306
Neomycin, 85
Nervous system, 173–199
Neuralgia, 185, 196
Neuraminidase inhibitors, 106
Neuroleptics, 198
Neurological symptoms, 96
Neurosurgery, 195
Neutropenia, 30
Neutrophilic leucocytosis, 29, **30**
NHANES study, 42
Nikolsky sign, 38
Non-insulin-dependent diabetes mellitus (NIDDM), 159, 160
Nongonococcal urethritis, 231–232
Nonsteroidal anti-inflammatory drugs (NSAIDs), 55, 85, 99, 100, 107, 189, 206, 207, 208, 210, 213, 218, 277
Norethisterone, 245, 247, 248, 277
Norgestimate, 245
Noristerat, 248
Normative needs, 5
Normoblasts, 16
Norplant, 249
Nose, 81–82, 82–83, 178
Numbness, 192
Nystatin, 56

Observation, 285–287
Obstetric history, 269
Occult bacteraemia, 304, 306–307
Ocular motility, 69–70
Oculomotor nerve, 180–182
Oedema, 120
Oesophageal pain, 129
Oesophagitis, 223
Oestrogen, 224, 281
Older adults, 8–9, 318–331
Olfactory nerve, 178
Onycholysis, 37
Open-angle glaucoma, 75
Ophthalmic artery, 66
Optic atrophy, 179
Optic nerve, 178–180
Orofacial dyskinesia, 183
Orphenadrine, 193
Osteoarthritis, 135, 211–213
Osteoporosis, 216–218
Otitis, 84–87
Our Healthier Nation, 5, 11, 12
Outer ear, 78
Ovarian cancer, 275
Ovasite sellotape test, 40
Overflow incontinence, 325
Oxygen, 100, 103, 130, 134
Oxymetazoline, 84

Paediatric patients, 123–125, 295–317

Pain
  in muscles, 96
  neurological examinations, 176
  see also Chest pain; Oesophageal
    pain; Pelvic pain
Pallor, 119
Palpation, 37, 97, 121, 139, 201,
  264–265, 270–271
Palpitation, 119
Papaverine, 164
Papilloedema, 179–180
Paracetamol, 86, 213, 218, 309, 310,
  313, 314
Parasite sellotape test, 40
Parenchymal disease, 109–110
Parenteral iron, 21
Parkinson's disease, 192–193
Paronychia, 37
Pars flaccida, 79
Patch testing, 40
Patellar reflex, 177
Pediculosis, 49–50
Pelvic examination, 270
Pelvic inflammatory disease, 226–227
Pelvic pain, 275
Penicillin, 31, 88, 90, 225, 311, 314, 315
Penile prosthetics, 164
People-centred health promotion, 3–4
Peppermint oil, 147
Peptic ulcer disease (PUD), 152–155
Percussion, 97–98, 138–139
Perforations, eardrum, 86
Perfusion abnormalities, 94–95
Pericarditis, 134
Perimenopausal state, 258
Periorbital oedema, 311
Peripheral pulses, 120
Peripheral vertigo, 184
PERLA, 181
Personal aspects, health, 5
Personal contraceptive system, 255–256
Personal hygiene, 47, 73
Pessaries, 278
Pharyngitis, 87, 311
Pharynx, 79–81
Phenothiazines, 183, 187
Phenytoin, 190, 315
Physical fitness, 4–5
Physical growth, 300
Physical maturity, 300–301
Physiology, paediatric patients, 299–302
Phyto-oestrogens, 262–263
Pigmentation, 27, 36
Pigmented lesions, 59–61
Pill (contraceptive), 244–248
Pilocarpine, 179
Pityriasis rosea, 53–54
Pityriasis versicolor, 52–53
Pityrosporum ovale, 52
Plantar reflex, 177
Plasma, 16
Plasma glucose, 160
Pleural effusion, 114, 169
Pleural rub, 98
Pneumococcal infections, 27, 85, 106, 107
Pneumocystis infections, 223
Pneumonia, 106–107, 223

Pneumothorax, 113
Podophyllin paint, 228
Podophyllotoxin, 228
Point-to-point test, 174
Polioviruses, 311–312
Polycystic ovary syndrome, 273–274
Polymyalgia rheumatica, 218–220
Polymyxins, 85
Popliteal pulse, 120
Positional testing, 79
Post-myocardial infarction, 130–131
Postmenopausal state, 258
Potassium, 125
Potassium citrate, 236
Potassium hydroxide, 40
Pre-school children, 297, 300–301
Preconceptual care, 256–257
Prednisolone, 85, 189, 219
Premenstrual syndrome, 279–281
Prescribing, 77
Primary care
  mental health, 282–293
  older adults, 318–331
  paediatric patients, 295–317
Prochlorperazine, 87, 187
Progesterone, 281
Progestogen-only pill, 247–248
Progestogens, 245, 254, 277, 281
Prolapse, genitourinary, 278
Proprioception, 176–177
Propylthiouracil, 167
Prostaglandin E, 164
Proteus, 107
Pruritis, generalised, 57–58
Pseudogout, 207–208
Pseudomonas, 84, 107
Psoas sign, 148
Psoriasis, 44–46
Psoriasis area and severity index
  (PASI), 45
Psychological disorders, 96, 323
Pterygoid muscles, 182
Puberty, 267, 302
Pulmonary embolus (PE), 112–113
Pulse, older adults, 323
Pulses, arterial, 120
Punch biopsy, 40
Pupils, 66, 68, 181–182
Pyelonephritis, 236–237
Pyrazinamide, 108
Pyrexia, 304, 305
Pyridoxine, 280

Radial pulse, 120
Radio waves, 65
Radioallergosorbent test (RAST), 40
Radiotherapy, 239
Rashes, 35, 36–37
Reality, mental health, 284
Rectovaginal examinations, 271
Recurrent laryngeal palsy, 186
Red blood cells *see* Erythrocytes
Reflexes, neurological examinations, 177
Rehydration, 141
Respiratory system, 77, 94–115, 223, 300
Retina, 66, 179–180
Retinoid therapies, 46

Reversibility testing, 100, 102
Rheumatic disease, 211–220
Rheumatoid arthritis, 214–216
Rhinitis, 89–90
Rhinosinusitis, 88–89
Rhonchi, 98, 102
Riboflavin, 16
RICE (rest, ice, compression and
  elevation), 209
Rifampicin, 108
Rinne's test, 79, 184
Romberg test, 174
Ropinirole, 193
Roseola, 313–314
Rovsing's sign, 148
Rubella status, 257

St Vincent Declaration Action
  Programme, 162
Salicylic acid, 59
Saline drops, 84
Saline soaks, 48
Salivary glands, 80
Salmonella, 140, 142, 223, 306
Sarcoidosis, 110
Sarcoptes scabiei, 50
Saving Lives: Our Healthier Nation, 11
Scabicides, 51
Scabies, 50–51
Scalp, 38, 49
Schering PC4, 252
School-age children, 297–298, 300–301
Sclera, 65–66
Sclerotome, 175
Scotoma, 179
Screening, 12, 28, 162
Seasonal factors, 77
Seborrhoeic dermatitis, 56–57
Secretory otitis media, 86–87
Seizure disorders, 190–191
Selective serotonin reuptake inhibitors
  (SSRIs), 189, 198, 281
Selegiline, 193
Self-awareness, 284
Self-care, 77
Self-control, 284
Self-worth, 284
Semicircular canals, 183–184
Sensory neurological examinations,
  175–177
Septic arthritis, 205
Sexual history, 243–244, 269
Sexuality
  contraception, 243–257
  menopause, 258–265
Sexually transmitted infections, 223–233
Shampoo, 46, 53, 57
Sheffield risk tables, 162
Shigella, 140, 142, 223
Shingles, 39, 135
Shoulders, 203–204
Sickle cell anaemia, 27–28
Sildenafil, 164
Silent alpha thalassaemia, 25
Sinus rhythm, 125
Sinuses, paranasal, 81
Sinusitis, 88–89

Skin prick testing, 82, 100
Skin swabs, 38–39
Smoking, 10, 77, 100, 102, 114, 153, 257
Soap substitute, 41, 43, 44, 46, 47, 56, 58
Social model, health, 4
Socioeconomic factors
    male health, 12
    respiratory disease, 77
Sodium aurothiomalate, 215, 216
Sodium bicarbonate, 236
Sodium cromoglicate, 100
Sodium valproate, 190
Solar keratosis, **60**
Solar lentigo, **60**
Sore throat, 87–88
Spacer devices, 101
Speech, mental health, 286
Spinal accessory nerve, 186
Spirometry, 102
Spleen, 27, 139
Splenomegaly, 311
Splinter haemorrhages, 119
Sponging, 309
Sputum, 96, 103
Squamous cell carcinoma, **60**
Standard Medical Advisory Committee
    (SMAC), 162
Staphylococcal infections, 38, 47, 73,
    84, 107, 206, 306
Statins, 162
Steam inhalation, 84
Stein-Leventhal syndrome, 273–274
Sterilisation, 256
Sternomastoid, 82, 186
Steroids, 42, 43, 44, 46, 51, 54, 56, 85,
    89, 90, 100, 110, 189, 192, 197, 210,
    213, 219
Stethoscopes, 121–122
Strabismus, 181
Streptococcal infections, 47, 85, 87, 306
Streptokinase, 130
Stress, 38, 155
Stress incontinence, 324–325
Stridor, 98
Stroke, 11, 12, 194–196
Stroma, 71
Subconjunctival haemorrhage, 74
Sulfasalazine, 152, 215, 216
Sulphonamides, 227, 315
Sulphonylureas, 162, 164
Sun damage, 59–61
Superior vena caval obstruction
    (SVCO), 99
Supervision, mental health, 291–293
Supraspinatus tendonitis, 207
Supraventricular dysrythmias, 125–126
Supraventricular tachycardia, 126–127
Surgery, 103, 194, 195, 196, 197, 228
Swelling, joints, 201
Swimmers ear, 84
Sympto-thermal method, 255
Systolic blood pressure (SBP), 131

Tactile vocal fremitus, 97
Tar, 46, 57
Tear film supplements, 74
Tears *see* Lacrimal apparatus

Teeth, 77, 83
Telangiectasia, 37
Temperature
    neurological assessments, 176
    older adults, 323
Temperature method, 255
Temporal arteritis, 189
Tendonitis, 206–207
Tenosynovitis, 206–207
Tension headaches, 188, 189
Testicular cancer, 239–240
Thalassaemias, 25–27
Theophyllines, 100, 103
Thiazide, 315
Throat, **81**, 83, 87–88
Thrombolysis, 112, 125, 130
Thyroid function test, 125
Thyroid gland, 82
Thyroxine, 170
Tibia, 203
Tics, 183
Tinea, 37, 51–52
Tinnitus, 185
Tissue plasminogen activator (t-PA), 130
Toddlers, 297, 299–300
Tongue, 79–80
Tonic clonic seizures, 190
Tonsils, 80, 87
Toxoplasmosis, 257
Trachea, 82, 97
Tranexamic acid, 277
Tranquillisers, 189
Transient ischaemic attack (TIA),
    193–194
Transillumination, 82
Trapezius, 186
Trauma, eye and eyelids, 70–71, 73
Triceps reflex, 177
Trichomonas vaginalis, 231, 232–233
Tricyclic agents, 49, 163, 234, 236
Trigeminal nerve, 182–183
Trigeminal neuralgia, 196
Trimethoprim, 227
Triphasic contraceptives, 245
Trochlear nerve, 180–182
Troponin, 125
Tsetse's syndrome, 135
Tuberculosis, 107–108, 223
Tuning fork tests, 79, **80**
Two-dimensional echocardiography,
    128
Tympanic membrane, 78–79
Tympanometry, 79

Ulcer radiation therapy, 153
Ultrasound, 139–140
Unilateral nuclear lesions, 186
Upper respiratory tract infection
    (URTI), 85, 86, 87
Urea, 66
Ureaplasma urealyticum, 231
Urge incontinence, 325
Urinalysis, 160
Urinary conditions, 233–237, 307–308,
    324–326
Urticaria, 55–56
User involvement, health promotion, 9

Uterus, 271
UV light therapy, 54
Uveitis, 72

Vaccinations, 106
Vacuum tumescence devices, 163–164
Vagina, inspections, 270–271
Vagus nerve, 78, 185–186
Valaciclovir, 135
Variant angina, 129
Varicella, 309–310
Varicella-zoster virus, 48, 309
Varicose eczema, 42–43
Vascular dementia, 198
Vascular system, 117–118
Vasculitis, 110
Vasoactive agents, 164
Vasoconstrictors, 89
Vegan diets, 22
Ventilation abnormalities, 94
Ventricular dysrythmias, 127
Ventricular fibrillation, 127
Vertebrobasilar TIA, 194
Vertigo, 87, 184, 185, 187
Viagra, 164
Vibration, neurological examinations,
    177
Viral infections, 39, 88
Viral warts, 58–59
Visual acuity, 178–179
Visual analogue scale, **212**
Visual fields, 70, 178, 179
Visual pathway disorders, 179–180
Vitamin A, 54
Vitamin B_6, 280
Vitamin B_{12}, 22, 192, 323
Vitamin C, 16, 20–21, 84
Vitamin D, 46, 218, 262
Vitamin E, 16, 262
Vitreous humour, 66
Vomiting, 142
Vulva, inspections, 270–271

Waldeyer's ring, 80
Warfarin, 112
Warts, 58–59, 228–229
Weber's test, 184
Wegener's granulomatosis, 110
Weight loss, 96
White blood cells *see* Leucocytes
Wood's light examination, 39
Working for Patients, 6
World Health Organization (WHO), 4,
    251

X-rays, 102, 139
Xanthelasma, 119
Xanthoma, 119
Xylometazoline, 89, 90

γ-rays, 65
Yeast infections, 51
Young persons, 6–8
    see also Paediatric patients
Yuzpe method, 251, 252

Zanamivir, 106